The ESTES/AAST Emergency Surgery Course Handbook

A Practical Reference in Expecting the Unexpected

The ESTES/AAST Emergency Surgery Course Handbook

A Practical Reference in Expecting the Unexpected

www.estesonline.org
ESTES
EUROPEAN SOCIETY FOR TRAUMA AND EMERGENCY SURGERY

ESTES / AAST
EMERGENCY SURGERY COURSE
DEDICATED TO FURTHER KNOWLEDGE ON EMERGENCY GENERAL SURGERY

THE AMERICAN ASSOCIATION FOR THE SURGERY OF TRAUMA

Wolters Kluwer

Philadelphia • Baltimore • New York • London
Buenos Aires • Hong Kong • Sydney • Tokyo

Senior Acquisitions Editor: Keith Donnellan
Senior Development Editor: Ashley Fischer
Editorial Coordinator: Sunmerrilika Baskar
Marketing Manager: Kirsten Watrud
Production Project Manager: Justin Wright
Manager, Graphic Arts & Design: Stephen Druding
Manufacturing Coordinator: Beth Welsh
Prepress Vendor: Straive

1st edition

9 8 7 6 5 4 3 2 1

Printed in Mexico

Cataloging in Publication data available on request from publisher

ISBN: 978-1-9751-9065-1

shop.lww.com

QUADM1022

Dedication

This handbook is dedicated to all health care providers who selflessly care for patients in the face of mental and physical risk to themselves.

Emergency Surgery Course Steering Committee

Dr. Gary Alan Bass, Ireland/United States

Dr. Raul Coimbra, United States

Dr. Jose J. Diaz Jr, United States

Dr. David V. Feliciano, United States

Dr. Abe Fingerhut, France

Dr. Hayato Kurihara, Italy

Dr. Ari Leppaniemi, Finland

Dr. Isidro Martinez Casas, Spain

Dr. Shahin Mohseni, Sweden

Dr. Nancy Parks, United States

Dr. Andrew B. Peitzman, United States

Dr. Stephanie Savage, United States

Dr. David Spain, United States

Dr. Nicole A. Stassen, United States

Dr. Jonathan Tilsed, United Kingdom

Dr. Eric Voiglio, Monaco

Contributors

Ananya Anand, MD, MSc
Department of Surgery
Stanford Health Care
Stanford, California

Eva Barbosa, MD, MSc, FACS
Head of the Complex Abdominal Wall Unit
Department: General Surgery
Centro Hospitalar Universitário de São João
Porto, Portugal

Gary Alan Bass, MD, MBA, PhD, FEBS (EmSurg)
Assistant Professor of Surgery
Division of Traumatology, Surgical Critical Care and Emergency Surgery
Perelman School of Medicine at the University of Pennsylvania
Philadelphia, Pennsylvania

Matthew Benns, MD
Program Director, General Surgery
Associate Professor
Department of Surgery
University of Louisville School of Medicine
Louisville, Kentucky

Alan Biloslavo, MD, FACS
General Surgery Department
Cattinara University Hospital, ASUGI
Trieste, Italy

Scott C. Brakenridge, MD, FACS
Associate Professor of Surgery
Department of Surgery
University of Washington School of Medicine
UW Harborview Medical Center
Seattle, Washington

Karen Brasel, MD, MPH
Professor and Vice Chair
Assistant Dean
Department of Surgery
Oregon Health & Science University
Portland, Oregon

Alexandra Briggs, MD, FACS
Assistant Professor of Surgery
Division of Trauma and Acute Care Surgery
Department of Surgery
The Geisel School of Medicine at Dartmouth
Dartmouth Hitchcock Medical Center
Lebanon, New Hampshire

Miloš Buhavac, MD
Assistant Professor
Trauma Medical Director, John A. Griswold Trauma Center
Medical Director of the Trauma/Surgical ICU
Surgical Critical Care Fellowship Program Director
Departments of Surgery, Trauma, Critical Care, and Acute Care Surgery
Texas Tech University Health Sciences Center
Lubbock, Texas

Clay Cothren Burlew, MD, FACS
Program Director, SCC & TACS Fellowships
Division of GI, Trauma, and Endocrine Surgery
Department of Surgery
University of Colorado School of Medicine
Aurora, Colorado

Martina Ceolin, MD
Surgeon
Department of Surgery, Emergency Surgery and Trauma Section
IRCCS Humanitas Research Hospital
Rozzano, Milano, Italy

Osvaldo Chiara, MD
Professor of Surgery
Head of Emergency Surgery and Trauma
Department: Surgical Pathophysiology and Transplantation
University of Milan—ASST Niguarda
Milan, Italy

Stefania Cimbanassi, MD
Assistant Professor of Surgery
Deputy Director of Emergency Surgery and Trauma
Department: Surgical Pathophysiology and Transplantation
University of Milan—ASST Niguarda
Milan, Italy

Jamie J. Coleman, MD, FACS
Associate Professor of Surgery
Department of Surgery
University of Louisville School of Medicine
Louisville, Kentucky

Mackenzie R. Cook, MD
Assistant Professor of Trauma, Critical Care and Acute Care Surgery
Department of Surgery
Oregon Health & Science University
Portland, Oregon

Andrea Costanzi, MD
Director General and Minimally Invasive Surgery Unit
San Leopoldo Mandic Hospital, Merate
ASST Lecco
Lecco, Italy

Marie Crandall, MD, MPH, FACS
Professor of Surgery
Division Chief, Acute Care Surgery
Associate Chair for Research
Department of Surgery
Program Director, General Surgery Residency
University of Florida College of Medicine Jacksonville
Jacksonville, Florida

Jennifer Knight Davis, MD, FACS
Trauma Director, Jon Michael Moore Trauma Center
Department of Surgery
West Virginia University School of Medicine
Morgantown, West Virginia

Kimberly A. Davis, MD, MBA, FACS, FCCM
Professor of Surgery
Chief of the Division of General Surgery, Trauma, and Surgical Critical Care
Department of Surgery
Yale School of Medicine
New Haven, Connecticut

Bogdan Diaconescu, MD, PhD
General Surgery Consultant
Clinical Emergency Hospital
Associate Professor at Anatomy Department
"Carol Davila" University of Medicine and Pharmacy
Bucharest, Romania

Jose J. Diaz Jr, MD, CPE, CNS, FACS, FCCM
Professor of Surgery, Epidemiology, and Public Health
Surgery Quality Officer
University of Maryland Medical Center
Chief
Division Acute Care Surgery & Program Director Acute Care Surgery Fellowship
Program in Trauma
University of Maryland School of Medicine
Baltimore, Maryland

Linda Ding, MD
Trauma and Acute Care Surgeon
Providence Regional Medical Center
Everett, Washington

David T. Efron, MD
Medical Director and Chief of Trauma
Professor of Sugery
Department of Surgery
University of Maryland School of Medicine
RA Cowley Shock Trauma Center
University of Maryland Medical Center
Baltimore, Maryland

Tanya Egodage, MD, FACS
Assistant Professor of Surgery
Department of Surgery
Cooper Medical School of Rowan University
Cooper University Health Care
Camden, New Jersey

Fernando Ferreira, MD
Associate Professor of Surgery
Director of Upper GI Surgery and Complex Abdominal Wall Unit
Department of General and Emergency Surgery
Pedro Hispano Hospital
Local Health Unit of Matosinhos (ULSM)
The Faculty of Medicine of the University of Porto
Matosinhos, Portugal

Douglas Fraser, MD, FACS
Associate Professor of Surgery
Division Chief, Trauma Surgery, Surgical Critical Care & Emergency General Surgery
Program Director, ACS Fellowship Trauma Medical Director, UMC Trauma
Chair, ACS Nevada Committee on Trauma
Kirk Kerkorian School of Medicine at UNLV
Las Vegas, Nevada

Joseph Galante, MD, MBA, FACS
Professor of Surgery
Department of Surgery
University of California Davis School of Medicine
Associate Chief Medical Officer, Procedural Areas
Medical Director, Perioperative Services
Trauma Medical Director
UC Davis Health
Sacramento, California

Laura N. Godat, MD, FACS
Associate Professor of Clinical Surgery
Division of Trauma, Surgical Critical Care, Burns and Acute Care Surgery
Department of Surgery
University of California San Diego School of Medicine
San Diego, California

Nicole Goulet, MD, FACS
Surgical ICU Medical Director
Division of Trauma, Acute Care Surgery, Surgical Critical Care
Department of Surgery
NYU Grossman School of Medicine
NYU Langone Health
Brooklyn, New York

Emanuel Guerreiro, MD
Chief General Surgery
Department of Surgery
Institution Pedro Hispano Hospital
Oporto, Portugal

Chrissy Guidry, DO, MSc, FACS
Assistant Professor of Surgery, Trauma & Critical Care
Department of Surgery
Tulane Medical School
New Orleans, Louisiana

Oscar D. Guillamondegui, MD, MPH, FACS, RCS (glasgow)
Professor of Surgery
Carol Ann Gavin Directorship
Chief, Division of Acute Care Surgery
Department of Surgery
Vanderbilt School of Medicine
Vanderbilt University Medical Center
Nashville, Tennessee

Tobias Haltmeier, MD, FACS
Department of Visceral Surgery and Medicine
Inselspital, Bern University Hospital
Bern, Switzerland

Jennifer L. Hartwell, MD, FACS, CNSC
Section Chief, Emergency General Surgery
Division of Acute Care Surgery
Department of Surgery
University of Kansas Medical Center
Kansas City, Kansas

Paul P. Healy, FRCS, MCh, MBChB
Specialist Registrar in General Surgery
Royal College of Surgeons in Ireland
Dublin, Ireland

Sharon Henry, MD, FACS
Anne Scalea Professor of Trauma Surgery
University of Maryland School of Medicine
Director of Wound Healing and Metabolism in the Program in Trauma
University of Maryland School of Medicine
R A Cowley Shock Trauma Center
University of Maryland Medical Center
Baltimore, Maryland

Vanessa P. Ho, MPH, MPH, FACS
Associate Professor of Surgery and Population and Quantitative Health Sciences
Department of Surgery
Case Western Reserve University School of Medicine
Metro Health Medical Center
Cleveland, Ohio

Mark H. Hoofnagle, MD, PhD
Assistant Professor
Section of Acute and Critical Care Surgery
Department of General Surgery
Washington University School of Medicine
St. Louis, Missouri

Jonathan Imran, MD
Fellow
Department of Surgery
Perelman School of Medicine at the University of Pennsylvania
Philadelphia, Pennsylvania

Angela M. Ingraham, MD, MS
Assistant Professor of Surgery
Division of Acute Care and Regional General Surgery
University of Wisconsin–Madison
Madison, Wisconsin

Lillian S. Kao, MD, MS, FACS
Professor and Chief, Division of Acute Care Surgery
Vice Chair of Quality
McGovern Medical School at UTHealth Houston
Houston, Texas

Dennis Y. Kim, MD, MMEd, FRCSC, FACS
Trauma Medical Director
Island Health Trauma Services
Victoria, British Columbia, Canada

Lisa Marie Knowlton, MD, MPH, FACS, FRCSC
Assistant Professor of Surgery
Section of Trauma, Acute Care Surgery, and Surgical Critical Care
Department of Surgery
Stanford University School of Medicine
Stanford, California

Ara Ko, MD, MPH
Assistant Professor
Department of Surgery
Stanford University School of Medicine
Stanford, California

Lucy Zumwinkle Kornblith, MD, FACS
Assistant Professor of Surgery
Department of Surgery
University of California San Francisco School of Medicine
Zuckerberg San Francisco General Hospital
San Francisco, California

Rosemary A. Kozar, MD, PhD
Professor of Surgery
Co-director of the Shock Trauma Anesthesia Research Center
University of Maryland School of Medicine
Baltimore, Maryland

Hayato Kurihara, MD, FACS, FEBS (EmSurg)
Director, Emergency Surgery Unit
Adjunct Professor, General Surgery Residency Program
State University of Milan
Fondazione IRCCS Ca' Granda Ospedale Maggiore Policlinico
Milan, Italy

Joël L. Lavanchy, MD
Attending Surgeon
Department of Visceral Surgery and Medicine
Inselspital, Bern University Hospital and University of Bern
Bern, Switzerland

David H. Livingston, MD, FACS
Wesley J. Howe Professor of Surgery
Chief, Division of Trauma and Surgical Critical Care
Department of Surgery
Rutgers–New Jersey Medical School
Newark, New Jersey

Tudor Marinescu, MD, PhD
Chief of Surgery Department
"Dr. Victor Babes" Foundation–General Hospital
Assistant Professor at Anatomy Department
"Carol Davila" University of Medicine and Pharmacy
Bucharest, Romania

Enrico Marrano, MD
General Surgeon
Emergency Surgery Unit
Hospital Parc Taulí
Sabadell
Barcelona, Spain

April E. Mendoza, MD, MPH, FACS
Assistant Professor of Surgery
Director of MGH Nutrition Support Team
Division of Trauma, Emergency Surgery, and Surgical Critical Care
Department of Surgery
Massachusetts General Hospital
Harvard Medical School
Boston, Massachusetts

Shahin Mohseni, MD, PhD
Associate Professor of Surgery
Department of Surgery
Orebro University Hospital
Faculty of School of Medical Sciences
Orebro University
Orebro, Sweden

Sean F. Monaghan, MD, FACS
Assistant Professor of Surgery
Division of Trauma, Critical Care, and Acute Care Surgery and Division of Surgical Research
Department of Surgery
Warren Alpert Medical School of Brown University
Rhode Island Hospital
Providence, Rhode Island

Michela Monteleone, MD, OU
General Surgery
San Leopoldo Mandic Hospital
ASST Lecco
Lecco, Italy

Sarah A. Moore, MD, FACS
Assistant Professor
Department of Surgery
University of New Mexico School of Medicine
Albuquerque, New Mexico

Nathan T. Mowery, MD, FACS
Professor of Surgery
Program Director, Surgical Critical Care Fellowship
Program Director, Acute Care Surgery Fellowship
Director, Clinical Research, Acute Care Surgery
Wake Forest School of Medicine
Wake Forest Medical Center
Winston-Salem, North Carolina

Matthew D. Neal, MD, FACS
Roberta G. Simmons Associate Professor of Surgery
Director, Trauma and Transfusion Medicine Research Center
Department of Surgery
University of Pittsburgh School of Medicine
Pittsburgh, Pennsylvania

Ram Nirula, MD, MPH, FACS
D. Rees and Eleanor T. Jensen Presidential Chair in Surgery
Department of Surgery
Chief, Division of General Surgery
University of Utah
Salt Lake City, Utah

Nancy A. Parks, MD, FACS
Associate Clinical Professor
Department of Surgery
UCSF Fresno School of Medicine
Fresno, California

Bruno M. Pereira, MD, MSc, PhD, FACS, FCCM
Full Professor of Surgery
Vassouras University
General Surgery Residency Program Director
Campinas Holly House
Director, Acute Care General Surgery Program
Brazilian College of Surgeons
Academic Director, Terzius Institute
CEO, Surgical Group
São Paulo, Brazil

Dorin Popa, MD, PhD, FEBS MIS
Senior Consultant
Department of Surgery
University Hospital Linköping
Linköping, Sweden

Rafael G. Ramos-Jimenez, MD
Department of Surgery
UPMC Presbyterian Shadyside
Pittsburgh, Pennsylvania

Samuel Wade Ross, MD, MPH, FACS
Assistant Professor of Surgery
Division of Acute Care Surgery
Department of Surgery
Wake Forest School of Medicine
Pediatric Trauma Medical Director
Atrium Health Carolinas Medical Center
Charlotte, North Carolina

Nathália Sampaio, MD
General Surgery Residency Program
Campinas Holly House
São Paulo, Brazil

Stephanie A. Savage, MD, MS, FACS
Medical Director, Emergency General Surgery
Professor, Acute Care and Regional General Surgery
University of Wisconsin School of Medicine and Public Health
Madison, Wisconsin

Morgan Schellenberg, MD, MPH, FRCSC, FACS
Assistant Professor of Surgery
Division of Acute Care Surgery
Keck School of Medicine of USC
LAC+USC Medical Center
Los Angeles, California

Beat Schnüriger, MD
Head Acute Care Surgery Team
Department of Visceral Surgery and Medicine
Inselspital, Bern University Hospital
University of Bern
Bern, Switzerland

David Silver, MD, MPH
Department of Surgery
University of Pittsburgh Medical Center
Pittsburgh, Pennsylvania

David A. Spain, MD, FACS
David L. Gregg, MD Professor
Chief of Acute Care Surgery
Trauma Medical Director, Stanford Healthcare
General Surgery Program Director
Department of Surgery
Stanford University School of Medicine
Stanford, California

Andrea Spota, MD
General Surgery Consultant
Tissue Bank and Therapy/Trauma Team
ASST Grande Ospedale Metropolitano Niguarda
Milan, Italy

Nicole A. Stassen, MD, FACS, FCCM
Professor of Surgery
University of Rochester School of Medicine and Dentistry
Director, Kessler Family Burn Trauma Intensive Care Unit
Director, Surgical Critical Care Fellowship
Rochester, New York

Michael Sugrue, MB BCh, BAO, MD, FRCSI, FRACS
Surgeon
Department of Surgery
Letterkenny University Hospital
Donegal Clinical Research Academy
Donegal, Ireland

Dzhendov Todor, MD
University Hospital Linköping
Linköping, Sweden

Marina Troian, MD
Attending Surgeon
Department of General Surgery
ASUGI San Giovanni di Dio Hospital
Gorizia, Italy

Sonlee West, MD, FACS
Trauma Medical Director
Chief, Division of Acute Care Surgery
Associate Professor
Department of Surgery
University of New Mexico School of Medicine
Albuquerque, New Mexico

Noel G. Williams, MD, FRCSI, FRCS(Gen), FASMBS
Rhoads-Harrington Professor in Surgery
Director, Metabolic and Bariatric Surgery
Department of Surgery
Perelman School of Medicine at the University of Pennsylvania
Philadelphia, Pennsylvania

Salina M. Wydo, MD, FACS
Program Director, Surgical Critical Care
Associate Director, Trauma/Surgical ICU
Department of Surgery
Cooper Medical School of Rowan University
Cooper University Hospital
Camden, New Jersey

Brian S. Zuckerbraun, MD, MBA, FACS
Henry T Bahnson Professor of Surgery
Chief, Division of General and Trauma Surgery
University of Pittsburgh School of Medicine
VA Pittsburgh Healthcare System
Pittsburgh, Pennsylvania

Preface

The optimal management of the patient requiring emergency surgical treatment is a global challenge. The magnitude of the surgical burden is increasing as the population ages and thus requires operations more often. Multiple studies have documented the mortality of 10%-20% for emergency general surgery (EGS) admissions, with high interhospital variability in mortality (as high as a 10-fold difference).

With the high morbidity and mortality in this high-risk population, the inconsistent quality and timeliness of patient care must be addressed. An educational initiative to promulgate unified treatment guidelines is essential in this quest. *The ESTES/AAST Emergency Surgery Course Handbook: A Practical Reference in Expecting the Unexpected* has been developed as a joint effort of the *European Society for Trauma and Emergency Surgery* and the *American Association for the Surgery of Trauma*. The goal of the Emergency Surgery Course and this handbook is to provide easily accessible knowledge for the surgeon on EGS call.

Contents

CHAPTER

1 "Why an Emergency General Surgery Course?"

Ara Ko, Ananya Anand, and David A. Spain

In 2012, the American Association of Trauma Surgery (AAST) set out to define what constitutes emergency general surgery (EGS). A dedicated committee on Patient Assessment and Outcomes defined the EGS patient as "any patient (inpatient or emergency department) requiring an emergency surgical evaluation (operative or nonoperative) for diseases within the realm of general surgery…." EGS was outlined to encompass clinical conditions including gastrointestinal and biliary disease, hernias, skin and soft tissue infections, colorectal, vascular, cardiothoracic, and those requiring acute resuscitation. The optimal treatment and management of the EGS population pose a global health challenge.

Based on 10-year National Inpatient Sample (NIS) data in the United States, over 3 million patients were found to suffer from one or more of these conditions annually, with >50% requiring emergency admission and more than a quarter undergoing surgery during their hospitalization. This accounts for 7%-8% of total nationwide hospital admissions and an estimated $28-$38 billion in health care expenditures due to EGS-related diagnoses per year. Over time, the nationwide cost estimate is projected to increase 45% by 2060, primarily due to an aging population. In terms of incidence per population, the burden of disease from EGS supersedes other public health problems, including injury, new diagnoses of diabetes or cancer, and hospitalizations due to heart disease or incidence of stroke.

Commissioned by The Royal College of Surgeons of England in 2016, the Nuffield Trust conducted analyses on data from 154 National Health Service (NHS) hospitals, revealing that 22% of high-risk emergency patients underwent a major general surgical procedure. In those who had surgery, 30-day in-hospital mortality was >10%, with high interhospital variability. A recent 1-year study of EGS diagnosis–related admissions in Scotland reported that up to 25% of all EGS admissions required an operation, with high all-cause mortality of up to 20% in patients older than 75 years. Furthermore, data compiled from the World Health Organization and other surveys in low- and middle-income countries estimate the disease burden from EGS to be 1%-3% of all deaths and all disability-adjusted life years.

EGS patients represent a complex population, half of which comprises those over age 60 and the majority presenting with comorbidities. Consequently, up to half of those undergoing emergent or urgent surgery experience at least one postoperative complication. It is also acknowledged that compared to patients undergoing elective surgery, EGS patients cannot undergo medical optimization before surgical procedures, further contributing to higher rates of medically related complications. In line with more significant postoperative morbidity, up to 6% 30-day readmission rates have been observed, with 17% requiring another operation during readmission. Additionally, the EGS population may be more vulnerable to fragmentation of care, with up to 17% of EGS patients readmitted to hospitals different from the index admission and subsequently enduring worse outcomes.

With a population subject to such high morbidity and mortality rates, it is essential to address variations in EGS care and attempt to eliminate discrepancies in management. Variance in practice and, subsequently, outcomes can be seen globally. Data from the United Kingdom in 2012 demonstrated that for patients undergoing emergency laparotomy in different NHS hospitals, mortality ranged from 3.6% to 41.7%. The 2015 National Emergency Laparotomy Audit also found significant variations in practice and compliance with essential standards in managing EGS patients. According to the United States' 2010 NIS data, significant outcome variations exist across hospitals around the country, even after risk adjustment. Namely, differences in death rates are widely variable in high- vs low-mortality hospitals and may be attributed to institutional variances in quality of care and processes for EGS. Variations in outcomes may reflect inconsistencies in practice patterns, suggesting a need to develop and disseminate a unified treatment guideline among surgeons who manage the EGS patient worldwide.

Despite the seemingly vast breadth of EGS conditions, there are seven common operations that allow the general surgeon to manage up to 85% of all EGS cases. This includes colon resection, small bowel resection, procedures for peptic ulcer disease, exploratory laparotomy, cholecystectomy, appendectomy, and lysis of adhesions. Accurate diagnosis and timely intervention of EGS conditions are critical and lifesaving. These subsequent chapters were written for surgeons practicing non-trauma emergency surgery to give broad exposure to common problems in EGS. We hope to provide the knowledge to help hone the decision-making skills needed for the surgeon taking EGS call.

SUGGESTED READINGS

Gale SC, Shafi S, Dombrovskiy VY, Arumugam D, Crystal JS. The public health burden of emergency general surgery in the United States: a 10-year analysis of the Nationwide Inpatient Sample—2001 to 2010. *J Trauma Acute Care Surg*. 2014;77(2):202-208. doi:10.1097/TA.0000000000000362

Havens JM, Olufajo OA, Cooper ZR, Haider AH, Shah AA, Salim A. Defining rates and risk factors for readmissions following emergency general surgery. *JAMA Surg*. 2016;151(4):330-336. doi:10.1001/jamasurg.2015.4056

McCord C, Ozgediz D, Beard JH, et al. General surgical emergencies. In: Debas HT, Donkor P, Gawande A, et al., eds. *Essential Surgery: Disease Control Priorities*. 3rd ed. Volume 1. The International Bank for Reconstruction and Development/The World Bank; 2015. Chapter 4.

McCoy CC, Englum BR, Keenan JE, Vaslef SN, Shapiro ML, Scarborough JE. Impact of specific postoperative complications on the outcomes of emergency general surgery patients. *J Trauma Acute Care Surg*. 2015;78(5):912-918; discussion 918-919. doi:10.1097/TA.0000000000000611

McCrum ML, Cannon AR, Allen CM, Presson AP, Huang LC, Brooke BS. Contributors to increased mortality associated with care fragmentation after emergency general surgery. *JAMA Surg*. 2020;155(9):841-848. doi:10.1001/jamasurg.2020.2348

Ogola GO, Crandall ML, Shafi S. Variations in outcomes of emergency general surgery patients across hospitals: a call to establish emergency general surgery quality improvement program. *J Trauma Acute Care Surg*. 2018;84(2):280-286. doi:10.1097/TA.0000000000001755

Ogola GO, Gale SC, Haider A, Shafi S. The financial burden of emergency general surgery: National estimates 2010 to 2060. *J Trauma Acute Care Surg*. 2015;79(3):444-448. doi:10.1097/TA.0000000000000787

Saunders DI, Murray D, Pichel AC, Varley S, Peden CJ; UK Emergency Laparotomy Network. Variations in mortality after emergency laparotomy: the first report of the UK Emergency Laparotomy Network. *Br J Anaesth*. 2012;109(3):368-375. doi:10.1093/bja/aes165

Shafi S, Aboutanos MB, Agarwal S Jr, et al.; AAST Committee on Severity Assessment and Patient Outcomes. Emergency general surgery: definition and estimated burden of disease. *J Trauma Acute Care Surg*. 2013;74(4):1092-1097. doi:10.1097/TA.0b013e31827e1bc7

Shafi S, Aboutanos MB, Brown CV, et al.; American Association for the Surgery of Trauma Committee on Patient Assessment and Outcomes. Measuring anatomic severity of disease in emergency general surgery. *J Trauma Acute Care Surg*. 2014;76(3):884-887. doi:10.1097/TA.0b013e3182aafdba

Spain DA, Miller FB. Education and training of the future trauma surgeon in acute care surgery: trauma, critical care, and emergency surgery. *Am J Surg*. 2005;190(2):212-217. doi:10.1016/j.amjsurg.2005.05.014

Watson R, Crump H, Imison C, Currie C, Gaskins M. Emergency general surgery: challenges and opportunities. 2016. Research Report. Nuffield Trust.

Wohlgemut JM, Ramsay G, Jansen JO. The changing face of emergency general surgery. *Ann Surg*. 2020;271(3):581-589. doi:10.1097/SLA.0000000000003066

CHAPTER

2

Initial Assessment and Resuscitation of the Emergency Surgery Patient

Beat Schnüriger, Joël L. Lavanchy, and Tobias Haltmeier

CASE PRESENTATION

A 76-year-old woman is admitted by ambulance to the emergency department (ED). Her complaints are diffuse abdominal pain and vomiting lasting 8 hours.

The patient is awake, alert, and oriented. Physical examination reveals a midline laparotomy scar; the abdomen is distended with signs of local peritonitis in the left lower quadrant. The qSOFA score is 2 (systolic blood pressure 95 mm Hg and a respiratory rate of 28 breaths/min, with an O_2 saturation of 86%). Arterial lactate level is 3.4 mmol/L. Nasal high-flow oxygen (10 L/min) is started and 1500 mL of crystalloid solution is administered, which improved the patients' systolic blood pressure to 110 mm Hg. The patient's past medical history includes a left-sided colectomy for cancer 20 years ago and an open appendectomy almost 60 years ago. She has no known allergies. Adhesive small bowel obstruction is suspected; in the ED, a nasogastric tube is inserted and 700 mL of gastric fluid are rapidly evacuated. Blood cultures are obtained, and intravenous antibiotic therapy is started.

Secondary survey reveals a moderately obese patient with a body mass index of 32 kg/m^2. She is taking a β-blocker for chronic hypertension and metformin for type 2 diabetes. A contrast-enhanced computed tomography (CT) of the chest and abdomen reveals distended small bowel loops up to 4 cm and intraperitoneal free fluid. Moreover, there is a segment of small bowel with wall thickening, fat stranding, and the suspicion of pneumatosis intestinalis just proximal to a transition zone.

Question: *What diagnosis do you suspect?*

Answer: *Strangulated small bowel obstruction.*

The patient is consented for an exploratory laparotomy and taken to the operating room 4.5 hours post-ED admission. Laparotomy revealed an adhesive small bowel obstruction with a necrotic segment of small bowel requiring resection.

INTRODUCTION

Expeditious and systematic initial assessment and resuscitation of the emergency surgery patient, in particular those requiring emergency laparotomy, is critical. Appropriate early evaluation of these patients will determine the course of treatment early in their care, with a direct impact on overall outcome. The history and careful physical examination are the cornerstones of the initial assessment, as these clinical findings are major determinants with the surgical decision-making. In contrast to elective surgery, emergency cases limit the time for resuscitation and prehabilitation in preparation for laparotomy. Initial care requires timely diagnosis with simultaneous resuscitation. Furthermore, a sense of urgency for intervention is key for improving postoperative outcomes. This is even more important in the fastest growing group of emergency surgical patients, the elderly, with limited physiological reserves. They are often frail and burdened by multiple comorbidities. The elderly also often present late in their disease course, enduring major physiological stress with limited ability to compensate.

INITIAL ASSESSMENT

The emergency surgery patient population may present with a wide range of acute diseases. The focus of this chapter will be on the initial assessment of the acute abdomen (see also Chapter 3: Evaluation of the Acute Abdomen). However, the principles described here can be translated to other organ systems where similar pathophysiological interactions and treatment pathways may apply, such as the management of sepsis and surgical source control in a thoracic empyema or soft tissue infections. As a principle, these acutely ill patients need a systematic initial assessment with simultaneous prompt interventions or treatments and efforts to diagnose the underlying cause of the acute illness. The initial management is often treat

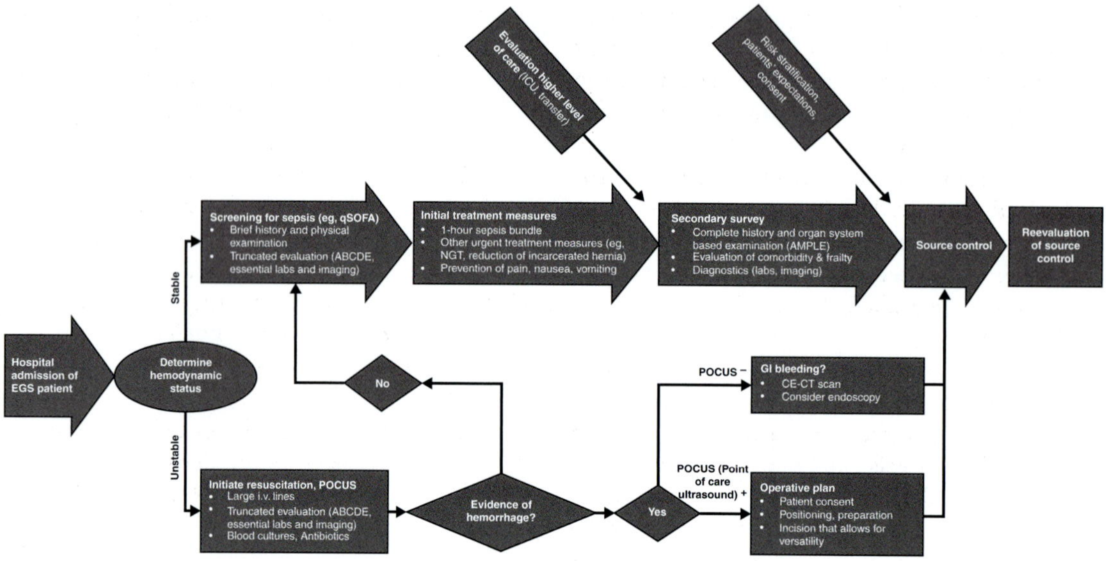

Figure 2.1 Principles of initial assessment and management of the emergency surgery patient.

and then diagnose. For example, this includes the synchronized assessment of the specific diseased organ and its systemic sequelae, followed by a tailored treatment and reassessment (**Figure 2.1**). In practice, this includes the following:

1. Determination of hemodynamic status with screening for hemorrhage
2. Initiation of resuscitation and a rapid primary survey including screening for sepsis
3. Initiation of urgent treatment measures
4. A secondary survey including a comprehensive organ system–based assessment of the patient
5. Source control
6. Reevaluation of source control

PRIMARY SURVEY INCLUDING SCREENING FOR SEPSIS

Similar to ATLS, the goal of the primary survey in the emergency surgery patient is to identify and treat immediate threats to life, often treating empirically without a specific diagnosis. After securing the airway, the next priority is to identify and control hemorrhage as the etiology of the patient's hypotension. Exsanguination is the major threat to life in an undifferentiated emergency surgery patient. After doing so, or excluding bleeding as the pathology, determine the systemic effects of the underlying disease and assess the urgency of initial treatment measures. The primary survey includes a focused medical history and brief physical examination. This will allow the formulation of a working diagnosis and the simultaneous initiation of primary treatment measures. The presence of bleeding or sepsis should be considered in all emergency surgical patients. Other less common causes of shock in this setting include tension pneumothorax, pulmonary embolism, and cardiogenic shock. Sepsis and septic shock comprise up to 20% of cases admitted to emergency surgical services with high morbidity and mortality, particularly in the elderly. Screening for sepsis using a validated score is mandatory during the primary survey.

Brief History

The art in medical history taking is to balance the patients' urge to report their complaints comprehensively and the doctor's need to acquire the relevant information in a short time. Therefore, using a scheme is helpful and timesaving:

- Main complaint
- OPQRST history (**O**nset, **P**rovocation/ **P**alliation, **Q**uality, **R**egion/ **R**adiation, **S**everity, **T**ime)
- Existing diagnoses
- Previous interventions

Brief Physical Examination

Physical examination may provide information in regard to the underlying pathology as well as direct initial management and interventions based on the findings. The initial physical examination should be performed in a structured and organ-based manner:

- Airway
  The risk of aspiration is assessed, especially in patients with suspected small bowel obstruction. In patients presenting with nausea and

vomiting, nasogastric tube (NGT) insertion to decompress the stomach and drain its contents is mandatory. A patient with hematemesis and massive UGI bleeding should also be intubated preemptively.

Hemodynamically unstable and neurologically impaired patients may require intubation. The need to protect the airway and to perform rapid sequence induction of anesthesia should be evaluated early.

- **B**reathing
  The respiratory rate and breathing excursions are assessed. The typical Kussmaul breathing (deep and labored breathing) may indicate metabolic acidosis. Diabetic ketoacidosis, lactic acidosis due to sepsis, and kidney failure are common reasons for metabolic acidosis. Breathing can be impaired due to a distended abdomen or abdominal compartment syndrome. Suspicion of aspiration pneumonia mandates early antibiotic treatment. Pulmonary embolism should always be considered when respiratory symptoms are nonspecific.
- **C**irculation
  Assessment of the heart rate and arterial blood pressure is crucial in the primary assessment of the emergency surgery patient. Tachycardia, although nonspecific, may reflect hypovolemia, pain, or atrial fibrillation. A systolic arterial blood pressure <100 mm Hg or mean arterial pressure <65 mm Hg requires fluid resuscitation. If hemorrhage is suspected, hypotensive patients should be resuscitated with packed red blood cells, fresh frozen plasma and platelets in a balanced transfusion ratio, or whole blood if available. If accessible, thromboelastography (TEG) as a point-of-care assessment of coagulation may guide blood product transfusion. A narrowed pulse pressure (systolic − diastolic blood pressure) may indicate hypovolemic shock due to insufficient preload and reduced cardiac output. In hypovolemic patients, monitoring of the urine output and a measure of global perfusion such as lactate levels or base deficit is recommended.
- **D**isability
  The level of consciousness is assessed using the Glasgow Coma Scale (GCS) score. Three categories of response (motor, verbal, and eye opening) are assessed. The GCS score ranges from 3 to 15 points. Coma is defined as GCS score of 3.
- **E**xamination
  Clinical examination during initial assessment is focused on the organ system associated with the primary complaint. Abdominal examination consists of inspection and manual palpation of the abdomen. The presence and location of scars suggest the surgical history of the patient. Assess scars and predilection sites for abdominal wall hernias (epigastric, umbilical, inguinal). Caput medusae is periumbilical portosystemic shunts seen in portal hypertension. Periumbilical (Cullen sign) or bilateral discolorations in the flanks (Grey-Turner sign) are suspicious for severe acute pancreatitis or a ruptured retroperitoneal vessel (ruptured abdominal aortic aneurysm). Assess local or diffuse peritonitis by palpation of the abdomen. The value of abdominal auscultation in the diagnosis of ileus is questionable. Therefore, routine auscultation of the abdomen is not recommended.

Sequential Organ Failure Assessment Score

In 2016, the third international consensus definitions for sepsis and septic shock (Sepsis-3) were published, in which sepsis was defined "as a life-threatening organ dysfunction caused by a dysregulated host response to infection." For clinical practice, the Sequential Organ Failure Assessment (SOFA) score was suggested as a measure to define sepsis. The previous definition of sepsis was based on the systemic inflammatory response syndrome (SIRS) criteria. However, according to the updated Sepsis-3 guidelines, SIRS criteria, often present in many hospitalized patients including those without infection, does not necessarily represent a dysregulated host response, which is part of the current definition of sepsis. Furthermore, the discrimination for in-hospital mortality using the SOFA score is superior compared to the SIRS criteria.

The SOFA score is based on six individual criteria including following organ systems: respiratory, cardiovascular, hepatic, coagulation, renal, and neurological system. The individual organ scores are summed to generate the SOFA score (**Table 2.1**).

While sepsis is defined as life-threatening organ dysfunction caused by dysregulated host response to infection, organ dysfunction is defined as an increase in two points or more in the SOFA score. The definition of septic shock includes vasopressor requirements to maintain a mean arterial blood pressure of 65 mm Hg and serum lactate level >2 mmol/L (18 mg/dL) (see also Chapter 5: Abdominal Sepsis).

TABLE 2.1 ■ Sequential Organ Failure Assessment (SOFA) Score

	Score				
System	**0**	**1**	**2**	**3**	**4**
Respiration					
PaO_2/FiO_2, mm Hg (kPa)	≥400 (53.3)	<400 (53.3)	<300 (40)	<200 (26.7) with respiratory support	<100 (13.3) with respiratory support
Coagulation					
Platelets, $\times 10^3/\mu L$	150	<150	<100	<50	<20
Liver					
Bilirubin, mg/dL (μmol/L)	<1.2 (20)	1.2-1.9 (20-32)	2.0-5.9 (33-101)	6.0-11.9 (102-204)	>12.0 (204)
Cardiovascular					
Mean arterial blood pressure	≥70 mm Hg	<70 mm Hg	Dopamine <5 μg/kg/min or dobutamine (any dose)	Dopamine 5.1-15 or epinephrine ≤0.1 or norepinephrine ≤0.1 μg/kg/min	Dopamine >15 or epinephrine >0.1 or norepinephrine >0.1 μg/kg/min
Central nervous					
Glasgow Coma Scale score	15	13-14	10-12	6-9	<6
Renal					
Creatinine, mg/dL (μmol/L)	<1.2 (110)	1.2-1.9 (110-170)	2.0-3.4 (171-299)	3.5-4.9 (300-440)	>5.0 (440)

PaO_2, partial arterial pressure of oxygen; FiO_2, fraction of inspired oxygen.
Adapted from Springer: Springer. Vincent et al. The SOFA (Sepsis-related Organ Failure Assessment) score to describe organ dysfunction/failure. On behalf of the Working Group on Sepsis-Related Problems of the European Society of Intensive Care Medicine. *Intensive Care Med*. 1996;22:707-710 and From Singer M, Deutschman CS, Seymour CW, et al. The third international consensus definitions for sepsis and septic shock (Sepsis-3). *JAMA*. 2016;315(8):801-810.

The criteria of the SOFA score such as the PaO_2/FiO_2 ratio or mean arterial pressure are not always available in the initial management of the septic patient. For patients in the prehospital setting, ED, or surgical ward, the quick SOFA (qSOFA) score has been developed. This score includes only three criteria: altered mentation, systolic blood pressure ≤100 mm Hg, and a respiratory rate of ≥22 breaths/min. Patients with suspected infection are likely to have poor outcomes if two or more criteria of the qSOFA score are present. A qSOFA score of 2 or greater prompts further investigation for organ dysfunction, escalation of therapy, and evaluation for intensive care unit (ICU) admission.

In clinical research, the SOFA score is increasingly used as an outcome measure in response to treatment.

INITIAL TREATMENT MEASURES

The concept of sepsis as a medical emergency is of paramount importance for the clinical management in patients with suspected sepsis (see also Chapter 5: Abdominal Sepsis). These critically ill patients need urgent initial assessment and treatment, including fluid resuscitation while pursuing source control, obtaining further laboratory studies, and attaining more precise measurements of hemodynamic status. Early identification and appropriate immediate management improve outcomes.

The 1-Hour Sepsis Bundle

In 2018, the Surviving Sepsis Campaign updated their recommendations and the 1-hour sepsis bundle. The elements of the 2018 bundle, intended to be initiated within the first hour, are listed in

TABLE 2.2 ■ Bundle Elements With Strength of Recommendations and Underpinning Quality of Evidence

Bundle Element	Grade of Recommendation and Level of Evidence
Measure lactate level. Remeasure if initial lactate is >2 mmol/L	Weak recommendation, low quality of evidence
Obtain blood cultures prior to administration of antibiotics	Best practice statement
Administer broad-spectrum antibiotics	Strong recommendation, moderate quality of evidence
Rapidly administer 30 mL/kg crystalloid for hypotension or lactate ≥4 mmol/L	Strong recommendation, low quality of evidence
Apply vasopressors if patient is hypotensive during or after fluid resuscitation to maintain an MAP ≥ 65 mm Hg	Strong recommendation, moderate quality of evidence

Adapted from Levy MM, Evans LE, Rhodes A. The surviving sepsis campaign bundle: 2018 update. *Crit Care Med*. 2018;46(6):997-1000.

Table 2.2. More than 1 hour may be required for resuscitation to be completed, but initiation of resuscitation and treatment, including blood samples for lactate measurements and blood cultures, administration of fluids and antibiotics, and, in the case of severe hypotension, initiation of vasopressor therapy, are all started immediately. With the delivery of high-flow oxygen (15 L/min) and commencement of an accurate measurement of urine output, these measures comprise the "Sepsis Six" standards, which have been endorsed by multiple professional organizations.

It is important to note that these interventions and especially the time dependency of early sepsis treatment bundles are highly debated. The evidence of these recommendations is of moderate quality, and a direct time dependency of treatment bundles on mortality could not been established in recent studies. Moreover, there is even potential harm, for example, when administrating unnecessary IV fluids. Therefore, all interventions in this group of critically ill patients need careful and repeated evaluation as well as close monitoring.

Other Urgent Preoperative Treatment Measures

Preoperative optimization of patients with abdominal sepsis not only includes the "1-hour sepsis bundle" but also treatment maneuvers such as the reduction of incarcerated hernias or the insertion of an NGT in patients with ileus to prevent aspiration pneumonia. The insertion of an NGT in the alert patient is the safest way to empty the stomach in a patient with a mechanical bowel obstruction. These rather simple interventions should not delay definitive surgical treatment but can be lifesaving. Of note, aspiration pneumonia in hospitalized surgical patients has been reported to be associated with a mortality rate of ~30%.

In addition, acute pharmacological treatments should be considered and initiated as early as possible. Sufficient analgesia and prevention of nausea and vomiting will improve patient outcomes. Many of the emergency surgery patient population are elderly, and comorbidities are common. In this group of frail patients, pharmacological anticoagulation is common, and its reversal needs to be considered preoperatively. On the other hand, in patients with acute mesenteric ischemia, early anticoagulation with heparin should be initiated with planned prompt revascularization, if possible, and resection of infarcted bowel (see Chapter 12: Mesenteric Ischemia).

EVALUATION FOR ICU ADMISSION AND TRANSFER TO HIGHER LEVEL OF CARE

At an early stage in the evaluation of emergency surgery patients, consider the potential need for a higher level of care. Advanced age, high body mass index, and the presence of comorbidities are risk factors for unplanned ICU admissions in emergency surgery patients. Ideally, critically ill patients scheduled for emergency general surgery are evaluated by an interdisciplinary team including surgeons, anesthesiologists, and intensivist. The surgical procedure including the possibility of damage control procedures with planned relaparotomy, anticipated postoperative treatment measures such as mechanical ventilation, renal replacement therapy, and the need for prolonged critical care treatment should be discussed preoperatively with the patients and the patient's relatives whenever possible.

SECONDARY SURVEY

The aim of the secondary survey is to set the acute illness of the emergency surgery patient—after primary assessment and simultaneous initiation of the initial treatment—in context to the medical history and existing diagnoses. Furthermore, the clinical examination is completed, and supplementary diagnostics (blood tests and imaging) are ordered. The impact of comorbidities and frailty on the treatment plan and individual risks need to be assessed carefully.

History and Complete, Organ System–Based Examination

For a comprehensive completion of the history taken during primary assessment, the mnemonic AMPLE is helpful:

Allergies to drugs, food, contrast agents, and latex
Medications, with special attention to immunosuppressive or anticoagulant drugs
Past medical history
Last oral intake
Events surrounding the begin of the complaints

Comorbidities and Fitness for Surgery

As societies in the Western world are aging, the average age of the emergency general surgery population is increasing, as well. With older age, the likelihood of concomitant comorbidities also increases. There are multiple scores for the evaluation of comorbidities. Of these, the American Society of Anesthesiologists (ASA) score is the most popular in clinical and scientific use. First published in 1941, and adopted in the actual form in 1963, the ASA score aims to stratify the perioperative risks of patients based on a classification of their comorbidities. It has five classes ranging from 1 (healthy person) to 5 (a moribund patient who is not expected to survive without operation). Another commonly utilized score that describes the impact of comorbidities on mortality is the Charlson Comorbidity Index (CCI). In 1987, the CCI was first described by Mary E. Charlson compiling comorbidities of 10 organ systems for a composite score. Based on this score, a 1-year mortality rate of 26%, 52%, and 85% is predicted by CCI scores of 1-2, 3-4, and ≥5, respectively. However, the CCI is not validated for emergency surgery patients, and its applicability in patients with occult comorbidities is limited.

Frailty

Frailty can be defined as an age-related decline of the general state of the patient, characterized by an increased vulnerability to adverse outcomes and a reduced resilience. As the concept of frailty encompasses both physical and psychological aspects, frailty is difficult to assess. Accordingly, multiple competing assessment tools have been proposed. In 2012, Morley and colleagues compiled the following frailty questionnaire (**Table 2.3**).

Risk Stratification

For every surgical intervention, the potential benefit and the risk to the patient must be weighed against each other. The quantification of the potential benefit of an operation is based on the experience and the knowledge of the treating

TABLE 2.3 ■ Frailty Questionnaire

	Question	1 Point	0 Points
Fatigue	How much of the time during the past 4 weeks did you feel tired?	Most of the time	Fewer
Resistance	By yourself and not using aids, do you have any difficulty walking up 10 steps without resting	Yes	No
Ambulation	By yourself and not using aids, do you have any difficulty walking several hundred yards?	Yes	No
Illnesses	Did your doctor ever tell you that you have hypertension, diabetes, cancer, chronic lung disease, heart attack, congestive heart failure, angina, arthritis, stroke, or kidney disease?	≥5 illnesses	≤4 illnesses
Loss of weight	How much do you weight with your clothes compared to 1 year ago?	>5% weight loss	<5% weight loss

Frailty scale scores range from 0 = best to 5 = worst and represent frail (3-5 points) and prefrail (1-2 points) and robust health (0 points) patients.
Adapted from Morley JE, Malmstrom TK, Miller DK. A simple frailty questionnaire (FRAIL predicts outcomes in middle aged African Americans. *J Nutr Health Aging*. 2012;16(7):601-608.

interdisciplinary team. The risk for complications and mortality in an individual patient can be assessed using risk calculators. One of the most comprehensive risk calculators is the American College of Surgeons National Surgical Quality Improvement Program risk calculator using 21 patient variables validated with data from over 4.3 million operations.

Patient Expectations and Goals of Care

Even if there is a clear indication for surgery from a medical point of view, patients need to understand the indications and provide their informed consent. The decision of a competent patient not to undergo surgery should be respected. In patients who lack the capacity to give informed consent, surgeons should act in the patient's best interest and where possible involve the patient's relatives in this decision.

Blood Tests

Laboratory tests can help to confirm a diagnosis (eg, elevated lipase levels in patients with acute pancreatitis) or indicate the severity of disease (eg, white blood count in patients with intra-abdominal infection). However, broad laboratory testing may also result in incidental findings that may confound the clinical picture of the acute disease.

Basic laboratory testing in emergency surgery patients should include a complete blood count, metabolic panel with glucose, electrolytes, liver function tests, creatinine, and blood urea nitrogen, as well as serum lipase or amylase, coagulation parameters, blood type and cross match, blood gas analysis, and urine analysis. Further laboratory analyses, such as blood cultures, stool cultures, endocrine laboratory tests, and measures of the nutritional status, are ordered for specific diagnostic questions.

Diagnostic Imaging

The importance of early and liberal imaging in the elderly population with undifferentiated abdominal pain cannot be overstated and is strongly emphasized in the emergency medicine literature. However, radiological investigations should not delay lifesaving interventions and should be carried out simultaneously with initial resuscitation.

At primary survey, abdominal evaluation with point of care ultrasound (POCUS) provides excellent imaging of free abdominal fluid (eg, blood, ascites). Furthermore, in experienced hands, systemic fluid status can be assessed by ultrasound based on the diameter of the inferior vena cava and the pulmonary edema. Moreover, in the nontrauma situation, fluid collections (eg, intraabdominal abscess), the hepatobiliary system (intra- and extrahepatic biliary dilatation, wall thickening of the gallbladder, sonographic Murphy sign), bowel motility, or volume of stomach can be visualized. In patients with cholecystitis or appendicitis, abdominal sonography may yield definitive diagnosis. Of note, sonography highly depends on the experience of the sonographer and patient characteristics (eg, obesity, subcutaneous air).

At the secondary survey, further imaging modality is guided by the clinical condition and suspected diagnosis. However, in the critically ill patients, computed tomography with intravenous contrast (regardless of the kidney function) is recommended.

Contrast-associated acute kidney injury (CA-AKI) may occur after the administration of iodinated contrast agents. Usually a mild increase in serum creatinine is observed 24-48 hours after contrast exposure. Most patients with CA-AKI are not oliguric, although oliguria can develop in patients with preexisting kidney disease. CA-AKI is usually transient, and most patients return to their baseline kidney function. In critically ill patients with acute surgical emergencies, intravenous contrast should not be omitted for imaging, as the benefits of an accurate imaging-based diagnosis outweigh the risk for CA-AKI.

URGENCY OF SOURCE CONTROL

Nontraumatic hemorrhagic shock caused by a ruptured aortic/splenic artery aneurysm, spontaneous splenic rupture, etc., is an indication for immediate laparotomy. For this group of patients, concepts similar to trauma care are applied. In acute septic abdominal emergencies, however, the management is different. In contrast to the traumatic acute abdomen with peritonitis—which is an indication for immediate operative exploration—the patient with nontraumatic acute abdomen will benefit from a brief period of fluid resuscitation and antibiotics. Nevertheless, following initial resuscitation, the infectious focus suspected to cause septic shock should be controlled expeditiously. According to the third international consensus (Sepsis-3) guidelines, source control not later than 6-12 hours after diagnosis appears to be sufficient for most cases. However, patients

TABLE 2.4 ■ Delay to Surgical Source Control

Time to Surgical Source Control	Indication
Immediate	Hemorrhagic shock (eg, ruptured aortic aneurysm, spontaneous splenic rupture, etc.)
≤6 h	Severe abdominal sepsis/septic shock (eg, hollow viscus perforation, ileus with signs of strangulated bowel, incarcerated hernia, abdominal compartment syndrome, toxic megacolon, etc.)
6-12 h	Severe intra-abdominal infection with peritonitis *without* sepsis/septic shock (eg, early hollow viscus perforation, postoperative anastomotic leakage, complicated appendicitis/cholecystitis)
12-24 h	Ileus *without* suspected bowel strangulation, abdominal infection *without* signs of peritonitis/sepsis (eg, uncomplicated appendicitis/cholecystitis, swallowed foreign bodies)

with mesenteric ischemia for any reason (incarcerated hernia, adhesive small bowel obstruction with possible strangulated bowel segments, mesenteric arterial occlusion, etc.) should be operated on earlier as "time is bowel" (**Table 2.4**). Moreover, there is growing evidence, that systemic sepsis–related pathophysiological changes become irreversible as time without adequate source control passes.

SUMMARY

The emergency surgery patient population may present with a wide range of acute diseases. Therefore, expeditious and systematic initial assessment and resuscitation is critical. In practice, this includes the following:

1. Determination of hemodynamic status with screening for hemorrhage
2. Initiation of resuscitation and a primary survey including screening for sepsis
3. Initiation of urgent treatment measures
4. A secondary survey including a comprehensive organ system–based assessment of the patient
5. Source control
6. Reevaluation of source control

A sense of urgency for intervention is key for improving postoperative outcomes; diagnostic and treating maneuvers may be applied simultaneously. This is even more important in the fastest growing group of emergency surgical patients, the elderly, with limited physiological reserves.

SUGGESTED READINGS

Becher RD, DeWane MP, Sukumar N, et al. Hospital volume and operative mortality for general surgery operations performed emergently in adults. *Ann Surg.* 2020;272(2):288-303.

Bilimoria KY, Liu Y, Paruch JL, et al. Development and evaluation of the universal ACS NSQIP surgical risk calculator: a decision aid and informed consent tool for patients and surgeons. *J Am Coll Surg.* 2013;217(5):833-842.e831-e833.

Debas HT, Gawande A, Jamison DT, Kruk ME, Mock CN. Essential surgery: disease control priorities. In: Debas HT, Donkor P, Gawande A, et al., eds. *Essential Surgery: Disease Control Priorities*. 3rd ed. Volume 1. The World Bank; 2015.

Dellinger RP, Levy MM, Rhodes A, et al. Surviving sepsis campaign: international guidelines for management of severe sepsis and septic shock: 2012. *Crit Care Med.* 2013;41(2):580-637.

Diaconescu B, Uranues S, Fingerhut A, et al. The Bucharest ESTES consensus statement on peritonitis. *Eur J Trauma Emerg Surg.* 2020;46:1005-1023.

Freund Y, Lemachatti N, Krastinova E, et al. Prognostic accuracy of sepsis-3 criteria for in-hospital mortality among patients with suspected infection presenting to the emergency department. *JAMA.* 2017;317(3):301-308.

Lavanchy JL, Holzgang MM, Haltmeier T, et al. Outcomes of emergency abdominal surgery in octogenarians: a single-center analysis. *Am J Surg.* 2019;218(2):248-254.

Levy MM, Evans LE, Rhodes A. The surviving sepsis campaign bundle: 2018 update. *Crit Care Med.* 2018;46(6):997-1000.

Morley JE, Malmstrom TK, Miller DK. A simple frailty questionnaire (FRAIL) predicts outcomes in middle aged African Americans. *J Nutr Health Aging.* 2012;16(7):601-608.

Onwochei DN, Fabes J, Walker D, et al. Critical care after major surgery: a systematic review of risk factors for unplanned admission. *Anaesthesia.* 2020;75(Suppl 1):e62-e74.

Roger C, Morel J, Leone M. Low level of evidence in Surviving Sepsis Campaign guidelines: should we throw the baby out with the bathwater? *Anaesth Crit Care Pain Med.* 2020;39(4):491-492.

Sartelli M, Catena F, Abu-Zidan FM, et al. Management of intra-abdominal infections: recommendations by the WSES 2016 consensus conference. *World J Emerg Surg*. 2017;12:22.

Sartelli M, Chichom-Mefire A, Labricciosa FM, et al. The management of intra-abdominal infections from a global perspective: 2017 WSES guidelines for management of intra-abdominal infections. *World J Emerg Surg*. 2017;12:29.

Sartelli M, Guirao X, Hardcastle TC, et al. 2018 WSES/SIS-E consensus conference: recommendations for the management of skin and soft-tissue infections. *World J Emerg Surg*. 2018;13:58.

Seymour CW, Gesten F, Prescott HC, et al. Time to treatment and mortality during mandated emergency care for sepsis. *N Engl J Med*. 2017;376(23):2235-2244.

Singer M, Deutschman CS, Seymour CW, et al. The third international consensus definitions for sepsis and septic shock (Sepsis-3). *JAMA*. 2016;315(8):801-810.

Tolonen M, Coccolini F, Ansaloni L, et al. Getting the invite list right: a discussion of sepsis severity scoring systems in severe complicated intra-abdominal sepsis and randomized trial inclusion criteria. *World J Emerg Surg*. 2018;13:17.

van de Groep K, Verhoeff TL, Verboom DM, et al. Epidemiology and outcomes of source control procedures in critically ill patients with intra-abdominal infection. *J Crit Care*. 2019;52:258-264.

CHAPTER

3 Evaluation of the Acute Abdomen

April E. Mendoza, Douglas Fraser, and Nancy A. Parks

CASE PRESENTATION

A 68-year-old man presents to the emergency department with severe abdominal pain. He reports that the pain started suddenly, 8 hours prior to arrival, and was centered over the epigastrium. However, the pain rapidly became more severe and spread across his abdomen. He is currently unable to identify a point of maximal tenderness and reports that the pain is everywhere. He had one episode of bilious emesis and complete loss of appetite. The patient states that he does not have any known medical conditions, although he does not regularly see a physician. He is a long time smoker. In the emergency department, the patient is tachycardic with a heart rate in the 130bpm and his blood pressure is 95/72 mm Hg. His respiratory rate is 22/min and temperature 37.1 °C. On examination, the patient appears pale and has mildly increased work of breathing. Other than his respiratory effort, he is laying completely still and motionless on the bed with his knees bent. His abdomen is flat with no visible scars. On auscultation, bowel sounds are notably hypoactive. Abdomen is somewhat tympanic to percussion and diffusely tender to even light palpation. His abdominal wall is rigid with involuntary guarding. Rectal exam is normal with soft, brown stool and no palpable masses. However, the difficulty that the patient experiences while turning to his side for the rectal examination is noteworthy. Initial laboratory studies are significant for a leukocytosis of 17 000/mm^3 with 31% bands, hemoglobin of 17 g/dL, and platelets of 196 000 mm^3. His electrolytes are normal except for hypokalemia of 3.1 mmol/L. Renal function is notable for a BUN of 41 mg/dL and a creatinine of 2.4 mg/dL. Lactic acid is elevated at 4.4 mmol/L.

Question: *What is the patient's diagnosis? And what are the immediate priorities in management for this patient?*

Answer: *This patient is in septic shock with the likely source being intra-abdominal. In the emergency department, he is hypotensive and tachycardic and has increased work of breathing, acute kidney injury, and a lactic acidosis. His abdominal examination is consistent with peritonitis. The priorities of management for this patient are rapid initiation of intravenous (IV) fluid resuscitation and planning for urgent surgical intervention. While it is important to avoid delay to operation, the patient needs adequate intravascular volume to prevent acute decompensation, and even potential cardiac arrest, during the induction of anesthesia. While IV fluids are rapidly being administered, a nasogastric tube and urinary catheter are placed. Broad-spectrum IV antibiotics are initiated. An upright chest x-ray done in the emergency department shows free air under the bilateral diaphragms. The patient's blood pressure improves with 3 L of IV fluids and he is taken to the OR for laparotomy.*

INTRODUCTION

Emergency general surgery accounts for 11% of all hospital admissions in the United States—and approximately half of all surgical mortality. Emergency laparotomy has a particularly high mortality rate, estimated between 14% and 20% overall. Patients presenting with acute intra-abdominal pathology therefore require rapid and nuanced evaluation by an experienced surgeon. This evaluation should begin with a detailed history and physical examination—these clinical findings are the cornerstone of evaluation. Useful adjuncts to the history and physical examination include laboratory studies and imaging. Taken together, the history, physical examination, laboratory values, and imaging allow the rapid identification of patients requiring urgent operative intervention for stabilization and those patients that can be safely managed nonoperatively.

PRINCIPLES OF MANAGEMENT

History

A detailed patient history will provide the experienced surgeon with significant information in a short period of time—and it is the basis upon which the remainder of the evaluation will build. The history begins with a thorough history of present illness (HPI), which is then followed by a detailed past medical and surgical history. When eliciting the history, remember that a wide variety of intra-abdominal, thoracic, and medical diseases can cause abdominal pain (**Tables 3.1 and 3.2**).

TABLE 3.1 ■ Acute Abdominal Pain—Abdominal Causes Vary by Location

Right upper quadrant	Biliary pathology: symptomatic cholelithiasis
	  Acute cholecystitis
	  Choledocholithiasis
	  Cholangitis
	  Gallstone pancreatitis
	Hepatitis
	Right lower lobe pneumonia

Epigastric	Pancreatitis Peptic ulcer disease Biliary pathology Gastritis Myocardial ischemia
Left upper quadrant	Peptic ulcer disease Gastritis Splenic pathology: infarction, rupture
Periumbilical	Small bowel pathology Early appendicitis Proximal colonic pathology

Right lower quadrant	Appendicitis
	Inflammatory bowel disease
	Diverticulitis
	Gynecologic pathology: ectopic pregnancy
	  Ovarian torsion or cyst
	  Pelvic inflammatory disease
	  Tubo-ovarian abscess
	Nephrolithiasis (radiating to ipsilateral groin)

Hypogastric	Colonic obstruction Bladder obstruction Uterine pathology

Left lower quadrant	Diverticulitis
	Gynecologic pathology: ectopic pregnancy
	  Ovarian torsion or cyst
	  Pelvic inflammatory disease
	  Tubo-ovarian abscess
	Nephrolithiasis (radiating to ipsilateral groin)

History of Present Illness

In evaluating a new patient, the surgeon begins with open-ended questions focused on the patient's abdominal pain. It is important to start by letting the patient describe the pain in his or her own words, before asking more direct and focused questions. This balance between open-ended questions and closed-ended questions allows the surgeon to take a history efficiently, while keeping the initial differential diagnosis wide and avoiding leading questions.

Onset

Ask the patient to describe how the abdominal pain began. Determining the timing and progression of abdominal pain provides a good deal of information about the acuity of the underlying process. For example, an abrupt onset of severe pain is suggestive of a process that may require urgent intervention such as perforation of a peptic ulcer, rupture of an abdominal aortic aneurysm, or rupture of an ectopic pregnancy. Causes of pain with more gradual onset tend to be due to progression of an inflammatory or infectious process such as acute cholecystitis, diverticulitis, or worsening intestinal obstruction.

Location and Radiation

The location of the pain and how it radiates or migrates over time provide key insights into the potential underlying etiology. Classic examples of localized pain include biliary pathology presenting as right upper quadrant pain and acute diverticulitis presenting as left lower quadrant pain. Pain that radiates can also be highly suggestive of the pathology: Biliary pain commonly radiates to the right scapular region, pain from pancreatitis radiates to the back, and pain from a ureteral stone classically

TABLE 3.2 ■ Extra-abdominal Causes of Abdominal Pain

Cardiac	Myocardial infarction
Pulmonary	Lower lobe pneumonia or infarct
Vascular	Dissecting thoracic aneurysm
Endocrine	Diabetic ketoacidosis
Hematologic	Sickle cell disease
	Henoch-Schonlein purpura
Immunologic	Polyarteritis nodosa
	Systemic lupus

radiates from the flank to the groin. Migration is also important to note. The most classic example is acute appendicitis beginning as periumbilical pain that subsequently radiates to the right lower quadrant. This is because in early appendicitis only the appendix itself is inflamed and this inflammation is perceived as referred visceral pain to the periumbilical area. However, as the inflammation spreads from the appendix to the surrounding parietal peritoneum, the pain becomes localized as right lower quadrant pain.

Character

Pain may fall into two broad categories: visceral and somatic. Visceral pain is caused by distention of the underlying viscera (intestine, biliary tree, or liver) and causes a nonspecific pain that can be difficult to localize but is vaguely midline in the upper abdomen (from the upper abdominal structures), the periumbilical region (from the small intestine, appendix, and proximal colon), or the hypogastrium (from the colon, uterus, or bladder). This pain may be intermittent in nature, or colicky, as the distended organ contracts against a distal obstruction such as a bowel obstruction or a stone in the biliary tree. Other classic descriptions of visceral pain include the burning pain of a perforated peptic ulcer and the tearing pain of a dissecting aortic aneurysm. Visceral pain may also be constant and progressive, leading to peritonitis. Somatic pain is caused by inflammation of the parietal peritoneum and can present as localized or diffuse peritonitis. Patients with diffuse peritonitis report that the entire abdomen hurts and are unable to localize a single area of maximal pain.

Associated Symptoms

It is important to ask the patient about any symptoms that are associated with the pain. Common examples include fever, anorexia, nausea, vomiting, diarrhea, constipation, change in bowel habits, scleral icterus, jaundice, acholic stools, melena, and bright red blood per rectum. Each of these symptoms helps narrow the differential diagnosis. For example, when discussing emesis, it is important to ask about the nature (bilious or bloody) and the timing of emesis. Emesis that began after the onset of abdominal pain is more likely to be caused by surgical pathology, while patients who present with vomiting as the initial symptom are more likely to have a gastroenteritis. The timing of emesis is also important. Emesis that starts soon after the pain may be due to an attack of biliary colic or an intestinal obstruction that is in the proximal small bowel. In contrast, with a large bowel obstruction, vomiting may not occur until days after the onset of pain.

Alleviating and Aggravating Factors

The description of how eating or activity affects the abdominal pain aids in the diagnosis. Pain that is ameliorated by food is typically due to peptic ulcer disease. On the contrary, biliary colic, pancreatitis, or bowel obstructions will worsen with any oral intake. The patient who prefers to lie still and describes that any bump of the bed causes significant pain likely has peritonitis. Patients with pancreatitis may be less uncomfortable in an upright position leaning forward.

Past Medical History

Once completing the HPI, it is imperative that a full history be taken. The past medical history provides important information to aid in narrowing the current differential diagnosis and to assess the patient's overall physical reserve. For example, a patient with known vascular disease or paroxysmal atrial fibrillation is at risk for mesenteric ischemia. Patients with medical conditions such as chronic obstructive pulmonary disease, congestive heart failure, or pulmonary hypertension will require careful perioperative management of their underlying disease process. It is important to include an obstetric and gynecologic history in female patients—and pregnancy should always be excluded in women of childbearing age.

Take a detailed ***past surgical history***. Previous surgery may place the patient at risk for a specific complication—such as marginal ulceration or internal hernias after laparoscopic Roux-en-Y gastric bypass. Previous abdominal surgery places the patient at risk for an adhesive small bowel obstruction.

Ask about all current ***medications*** the patient is taking. Many of these can affect incidence as well as management of the underlying pathology. Chronic NSAID use places individuals at risk for peptic ulcer disease, while anticoagulation may predispose patients to hemorrhage—and also may need to be corrected prior to urgent surgical intervention. Patients on beta blockade may not exhibit tachycardia despite intra-abdominal pathology and impending sepsis. Patients on chronic steroids can exhibit wound healing difficulties or hypotension from acute adrenal insufficiency requiring stress dose steroids, particularly in the setting of concomitant septic shock.

Family history provides information regarding potential pathologies the patient may be at increased risk of developing. Family history of cancer, particularly in first-degree relatives or individuals with diagnosis at a young age, is particularly important. Problems with coagulation and anesthesia in close family members can also be relevant to any surgical intervention. A full ***social history*** focusing on tobacco, alcohol, and illicit drug may alert the surgeon to monitor for alcohol withdrawal or associated conditions such as cardiomyopathy or heart failure in patients with significant methamphetamine use. A detailed ***sexual history*** may also reveal risk factors for sexually transmitted infections or pelvic inflammatory disease.

In the setting of emergency general surgery, time may not allow further evaluation or optimization of a patient's underlying comorbidities prior to intervention. However, it is still crucial to perform a full ***review of systems***. Knowledge of an individual's baseline exercise tolerance, ambulatory status, exertional angina, or dyspnea provides necessary information for the anesthesia and surgery teams to provide individualized and judicious perioperative care. It is also important as it enables surgeons to counsel patients and their families with realistic expectations regarding potential surgical outcomes.

PHYSICAL EXAMINATION

After completing the history, the surgeon already has an idea of the potential cause of the patient's abdominal pain (**Figure 3.1**). The physical examination should further solidify this differential diagnosis (**Table 3.3**). Perform a full physical examination beginning with careful observation of the patient's overall appearance noting any overt distress, pallor, or diaphoresis, which may indicate an impending crisis. A full set of current vital signs, as well as any changes in vital signs since arrival in the emergency department or in response to IV fluid administration, is critical information in assessing the overall acuity of the patient. If a nasogastric tube or urinary catheter has been placed, monitor the volume and character of the output. Altered mental status and lethargy are both grave signs of sepsis, particularly in the elderly. Auscultation of the lungs may demonstrate evidence of decreased respiratory expansion due to abdominal pain or distant breath sounds due to an effusion, atelectasis, or consolidation. The heart rate and rhythm may reveal a new-onset arrhythmia placing the patient at risk for mesenteric emboli

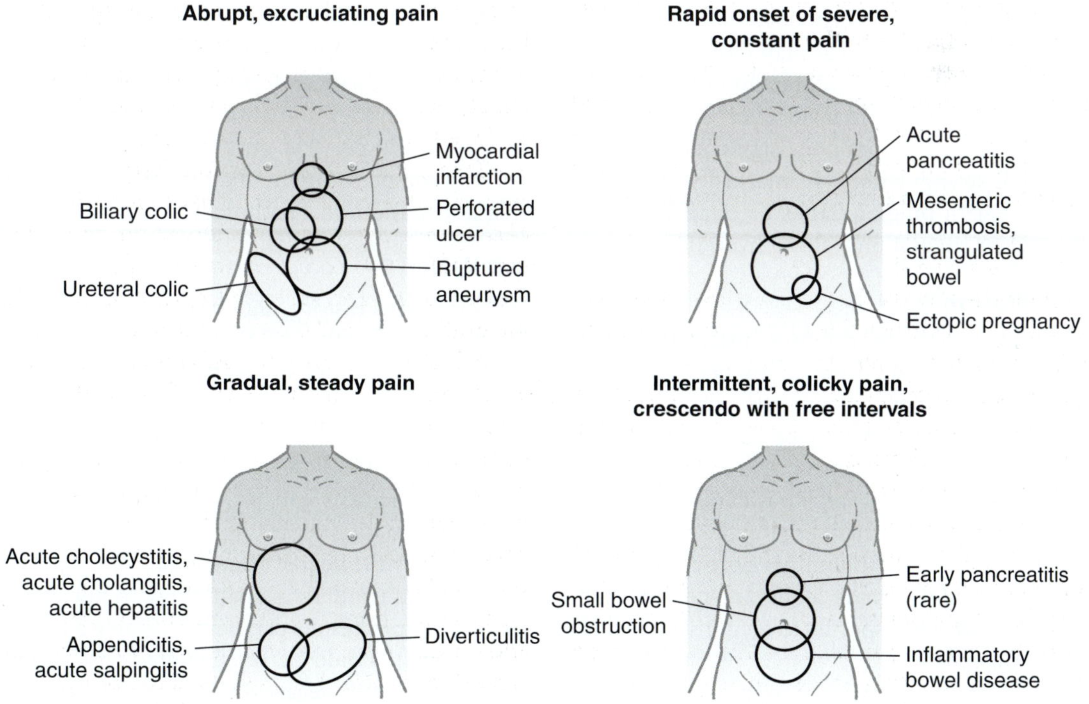

Figure 3.1 Location and character of pain are helpful in the differential diagnosis of the acute abdomen. (From Peitzman AB, Yealy DM, Fabian TC, C. W Schwab CW, Guyette FX, Seamon MJ, Zuckerbraun BS. *The Trauma Manual*. 5th ed. Wolters Kluwer; 2020. Figure 52.1.)

TABLE 3.3 ■ Classic Findings on Physical Examination

Sign	Physical Examination Findings	Associated Diagnosis
Murphy sign	Pause in inspiration with deep palpation of the right upper quadrant	Acute cholecystitis
Iliopsoas sign	Pain with passive hyperextension of the right hip	Acute appendicitis (retrocecal appendix)
Rovsing sign	Palpation of the left lower quadrant causes pain in the right lower quadrant	Acute appendicitis
Obturator sign	Pain with internal rotation of the flexed right hip	Acute appendicitis (pelvic appendix)

or sinus tachycardia from a systemic inflammatory response.

The focus of the examination should be on the abdomen and is comprised of four basic steps to be performed in the following order: inspection, auscultation, percussion, and palpation.

Inspection

To begin, uncover and carefully inspect the abdomen, bilateral flanks, and groins. Attention to the patient's respiratory pattern and movement of the abdominal wall with breathing may reveal a rigid abdominal wall that barely moves during respiration due to underlying peritonitis. Take note of external changes to the skin such as scars from prior operations, ecchymoses or flank hematomas consistent with retroperitoneal hemorrhage, or superficial cellulitis, which may indicate underlying deep pathology. A protuberant bulge, particularly in the groin, may indicate a hernia—overlying skin changes are an ominous sign concerning for intestinal strangulation. A markedly distended abdomen with bulging flanks or dilated periumbilical veins suggest underlying liver disease.

Auscultation

The next step is to carefully listen for bowel sounds. This is done prior to any percussion and palpation as they may alter the frequency of bowel sounds. Bowel sounds may be absent or hypoactive with an ileus and hyperactive or high pitched in the case of a partial small bowel obstruction. A bruit may also be heard overlying the epigastrium in patients with an abdominal aortic aneurysm. Note that bowel sounds alone are neither sufficiently sensitive nor specific to definitively exclude a given diagnosis.

Percussion

Gentle percussion may reveal a dull fluid-filled abdomen, a dull mass, or a tympanic abdomen with significant gaseous distention of the bowels or pneumoperitoneum. Patients with peritonitis will experience diffuse tenderness to even light percussion.

Palpation

It is best to start with gentle palpation remote from the site of maximal pain. If the patient tolerates this, proceed to deep palpation. Palpation will determine whether the abdomen is tense, rigid, and the amount of tenderness. Involuntary guarding and a rigid abdominal wall are both classic findings in peritonitis.

Perform a digital rectal examination to assess for fecal impaction, masses, blood in the stool, or potential pelvic abscesses or carcinomatous implants. If the patient has a stoma, it should also be digitalized to ensure that it is patent and not stenotic. Females with abdominal pain should have a thorough pelvic examination to determine if there is significant cervical motion tenderness concerning for pelvic inflammatory disease, adnexal masses, or additional pathology.

ADJUNCTS

Although the history and physical examination form the basis of the initial evaluation of the acute abdomen, laboratory studies and imaging findings are useful adjuncts.

Laboratory Studies

Laboratory studies can provide significant additional information regarding a suspected diagnosis and quantify the degree of metabolic derangement caused by the underlying pathology. While abnormal laboratory results can help reinforce a clinical diagnosis, it should be remembered that normal labs alone do not negate other clinical findings. A clinical diagnosis of peritonitis in a patient with sudden onset of severe abdominal pain warrants surgical exploration—even if the white blood cell

(WBC) count or other labs are normal. In such cases, normal labs should not be considered reassuring or delay operative intervention. Such a delay could have a devastating outcome for the patient.

When evaluating a patient with acute abdominal pain, a complete blood count (CBC) can be quite useful. The WBC count is a generalized sign of infection and can reinforce a surgeon's list of differential diagnoses. In a patient with an acute abdomen, fever, and tachycardia, a leukocytosis of 20 000 mm^3 strengthens a diagnosis of perforated diverticulitis, perforated appendicitis, gangrenous cholecystitis, or possibly a perforated ulcer. If the WBC was markedly elevated at 50 000 mm^3 in a patient with acute abdominal pain and diarrhea, this would suggest a diagnosis of clostridium difficile with toxic megacolon. The hemoglobin is also important to follow in patients with evidence of ongoing intra-abdominal or gastrointestinal bleeding. In other cases, the hemoglobin may be falsely elevated due to hemoconcentration and significant dehydration from a complete bowel obstruction. Platelet levels may be elevated as an acute phase reactant in patients with ongoing inflammation or decreased in patients with chronic liver disease.

Electrolytes and renal function values should be obtained in patients with acute intra-abdominal pathology. Gastrointestinal losses may lead to hypokalemia, dehydration, and acute kidney injury. Markedly elevated glucose levels suggest previously undiagnosed diabetes. During an evaluation of a patient with history and physical examination findings suggesting biliary or pancreatic pathology, obtain a liver function panel and lipase. A classic example would be a patient who presents with a prior history of gallstones, severe epigastric tenderness, fever, an elevated WBC count, and lipase all pointing to a diagnosis of gallstone pancreatitis. (See Chapter 14.)

Additionally, laboratory studies can be a surrogate for adequacy of resuscitation and perfusion. For example, a patient who presents with a remote history of myocardial infarction, severe abdominal pain out of proportion to findings on examination, and an elevated lactic acid level is a classic example of mesenteric ischemia and the operating room should be prepped and at the ready. As the patient undergoes surgical intervention and resuscitation for the ischemic bowel, lactic acid levels should trend back to normal. It is important to remember, however, that normal lactic acid levels should not be reassuring if the remainder of the clinical picture is consistent with ischemic bowel. (See Chapter 12.)

Urine should also be collected for a urinalysis and toxicology screen in patients presenting with acute abdominal pain. Finally, all women of childbearing age require a pregnancy test at the time of initial evaluation.

The skilled clinician uses a variety of diagnostic tools to arrive at the appropriate diagnosis, and laboratory values should be considered as one tool to use in context with the overall patient presentation.

Imaging

Advanced imaging techniques have evolved rapidly over the past decades. Current imaging provides significant information and has improved diagnostic accuracy in many arenas. (See Chapter 6.) For example, increasing use of preoperative computed tomography (CT) has lowered negative appendectomy rates over the last several decades. In spite of these advances, it is important that imaging still be considered as an adjunct to a detailed history and physical examination. The most common imaging techniques in use today are plain radiographs, ultrasound, CT scanning, and magnetic resonance imaging (MRI).

Plain Radiographs

While plain radiographs do still play a role in imaging of the acute abdomen, with the advent of more widely available advanced imaging techniques, the role of plain x-rays has become limited. Plain films are useful in patients with peritonitis on examination and suspected pneumoperitoneum. In most settings, x-rays can be performed more quickly than a CT scan and therefore can expedite surgical intervention. Additionally, portable x-rays can be performed at the bedside for patients who are not stable for transport and have suspected intra-abdominal pathology. x-rays are also useful in patients with significant abdominal distention and may show evidence of a small bowel obstruction, colonic ileus, or volvulus.

Ultrasound

The great advantages of ultrasound are that it is portable, does not expose the patient to radiation, and can be repeated. It is the imaging study of choice for biliary pathology, early detection of a leaking abdominal aortic aneurysm, hemoperitoneum, or for appendicitis in children and pregnant women. Despite these benefits, ultrasound remains operator dependent.

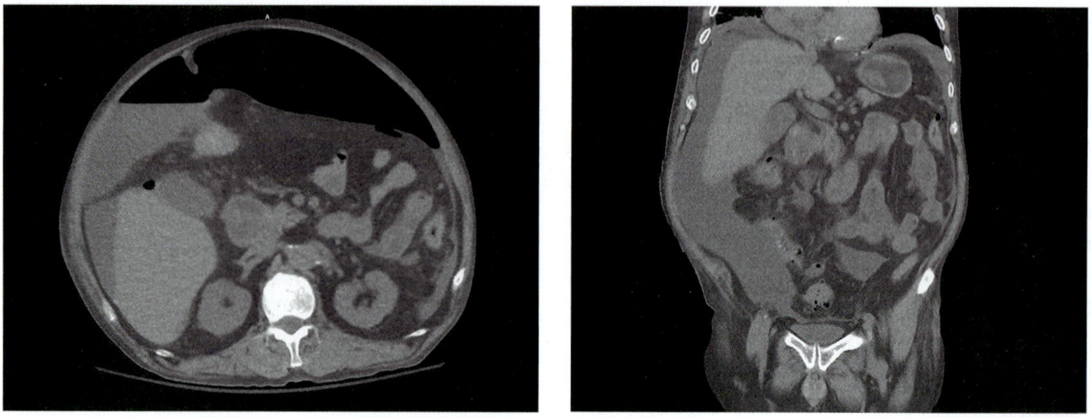

A B

Figure 3.2 CT scan showing pneumoperitoneum **(A)** and free fluid tracking down the right paracolic gutter **(B)** in a patient with a perforated duodenal ulcer.

Computed Tomography

In recent decades, CT technology has become widely available and increasingly fast and has very high resolution leading to excellent diagnostic detail (**Figure 3.2 A and B**). This has led to CT becoming the initial imaging study for most patients with significant intra-abdominal pathology (**Figure 3.3**). Disadvantages of CT include that patients must be stable for transport to the scanner, exposure to radiation, and contrast-enhanced scans inducing acute kidney injury and contrast-induced nephropathy.

Magnetic Resonance Imaging

MRI has a limited role in the initial evaluation of the acute abdomen. MRI is not universally available and takes time to perform, and some patients are not candidates for MRI (either due to implanted medical devices or anxiety/claustrophobia). However, there are certain instances where MRI may be appropriate in the evaluation of stable patients with abdominal pain. Pregnant women with suspected appendicitis, with a non-diagnostic ultrasound, may undergo MRI to avoid both the ionizing radiation of a CT scan and also the risks of a negative appendectomy. Magnetic resonance cholangiopancreatography (MRCP) can also be useful in patients with potential concern for a common duct stone that do not have a clear indication for endoscopic retrograde cholangiopancreatography (ERCP).

SPECIAL CONSIDERATIONS

Certain patient populations warrant additional consideration when evaluating the acute abdomen.

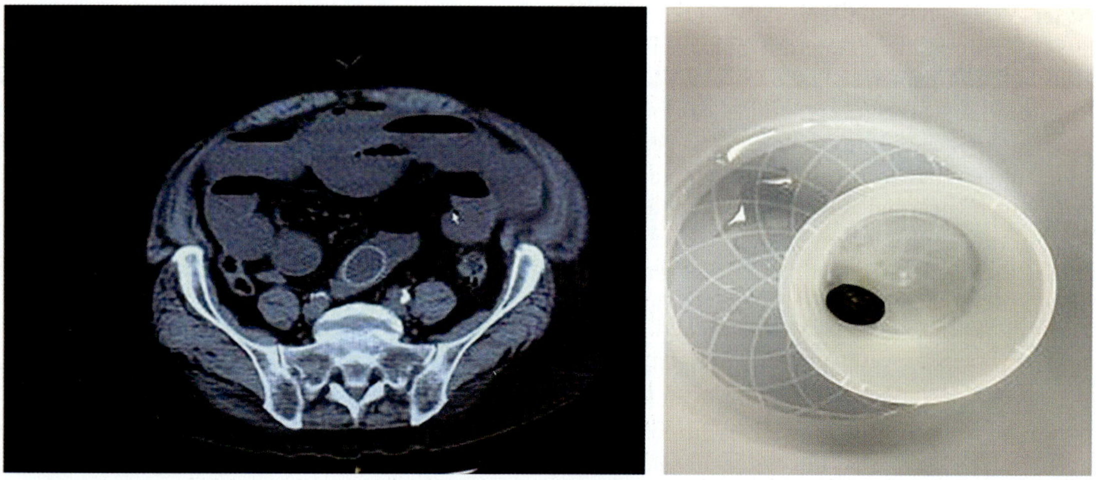

Figure 3.3 CT scan showing a gallstone ileus (*left*); gallstone after removal (*right*).

Pregnant Patients

Nonobstetrical surgical procedures are performed on ~ 2% of all pregnancies, with acute appendicitis being the most common surgical emergency during pregnancy. (See Chapter 24.) The diagnosis of acute appendicitis is complicated by the gravid uterus and physiologic changes of pregnancy. However, it is important to confirm the diagnosis efficiently and accurately, since fetal loss may occur in as many as 36% of patients with appendiceal perforation. Additionally, a negative appendectomy in a pregnant patient is associated with potential fetal loss. Therefore, ultrasound is the initial imaging study of choice. If nondiagnostic, MRI can be used with high sensitivity and specificity. If MRI is unavailable, a CT of the abdomen and pelvis is within the acceptable limits of fetal radiation exposure established by the American College of Obstetricians and Gynecologists. Laparoscopic appendectomy can be performed safely during pregnancy. The second most common cause of emergency general surgery during pregnancy is biliary disease. Recurrent attacks of biliary symptoms are common during pregnancy and laparoscopic cholecystectomy is safe. Therefore, proceeding with cholecystectomy during pregnancy is considered safe. Pregnant patients should be managed in conjunction with their obstetrician and utilize fetal monitoring in viable pregnancies of 24 weeks or more gestation.

Elderly Patients

As the population is aging, elderly patients with acute abdominal pathology present a particular challenge. Many elderly patients present with significant comorbidities or a poor baseline functional status placing them at high risk for significant morbidity and mortality. Scoring systems such as the American College of Surgeons Risk Calculator and the frailty index aid in risk stratification. However, the urgent nature of emergency general surgery results in limited time for in depth preoperative discussion surrounding goals of care. Formal palliative care consultation is rarely available prior to deciding on surgical intervention. Therefore, surgeons should discuss the possible options for intensity of care, as well at the likelihood of functional recovery with patients and their families before surgery and throughout their hospital course. Increasing access to palliative care in this patient group may improve patient-centered care and reduce futile or unwanted care.

SUMMARY

The evaluation of the acute abdomen is built upon the foundation of a thorough, but focused, history and physical examination. Useful adjuncts to the evaluation include laboratory and imaging studies as described. Patients who are acutely ill require ongoing resuscitation with IV fluids and antibiotics during the initial evaluation. Synthesizing all the information obtained will provide the emergency general surgeon with a good assessment as to the patient's diagnosis and need for potential operative intervention.

SUGGESTED READINGS

ACOG Committee Opinion Number 775: Nonobstetric Surgery During Pregnancy. *Obstetr Gynecol.* 2019;133(4):e285-e286.

Arkenbosch JHC, van Ruler O, de Vries AC. Non-obstetric surgery in pregnancy (including bowel surgery and gallbladder surgery). *Best Pract Res Clin Gastroenterol.* 2020;44-45:1-7.

Baimas-George M, Yelverton S, Ross SW, Rozario N, Matthews BD, Reinke CE. Palliative care in emergency general surgery patients: reduced inpatient mortality and increased discharge to hospice. *Am Surg.* 2021;87(7):1087-1092.

Bickley LS, Szilagyi PG, Hoffman RM, Soriano RP. *Bates' Guide to Physical Examination and History Taking.* 13th ed. Lippincott Williams & Wilkins; 2021. Print.

Diegelmann L. Nonobstetric abdominal pain and surgical emergencies in pregnancy. *Emerg Med Clin N Am.* 2012;30(4):885-901.

DuBose JJ, Lissauer M, Maung AA, et al. Pneumatosis Intestinalis Predictive Evaluation Study (PIPES): a multicenter epidemiologic study of the Eastern Association for the Surgery of Trauma. *J Trauma Acute Care Surg.* 2013;75(1):15-23.

Gans SL, Pols MA, Stoker J, Boermeester MA. Guideline for the diagnostic pathway in patients with acute abdominal pain. *Dig Surg.* 2015;32:23-31.

Havens JM, Neiman PU, Campbell BL, Croce MA, Spain DA, Napolitano LM. The future of emergency general surgery. *Ann Surg.* 2019;270(2):221-222.

Joseph B, Zangbar B, Pandit V, et al. Emergency general surgery in the elderly: too old or too frail? *J Am Coll Surg.* 2016;222:805-813.

Lameris W, van Randen A, van Es HW, et al. Imaging strategies for detection of urgent conditions in patients with acute abdominal pain: diagnostic accuracy study. *BMJ.* 2009;339:b2431.

Moore LR, Todd SR. *Common Problems in Acute Care Surgery.* 2nd ed. Springer International Publishing; 2017. Web.

Nateson S, Lee J, Volkamer H, Thoureen T. Evidence-based medicine approach to abdominal pain. *Emerg Med Clin N Am.* 2016;34:165-190.

Panebianco NL, Jahnes K, Mills AM. Imaging and laboratory testing in acute abdominal pain. *Emerg Med Clin N Am.* 2011;29:175-193.

Pearl JP, Price RP, Tonkin AE, Richardson WS, Stefanidis D. SAGES guidelines for the use of laparoscopy during pregnancy. *Surg Endosc.* 2017;31:3767-3782.

Pisano M, Allievi N, Gurusamy K, et al. 2020 World Society of Emergency Surgery updated guidelines for the diagnosis and treatment of acute calculus cholecystitis. *World J Emerg Surg.* 2020;15:61.

Silen W, Cope Z. *Cope's Early Diagnosis of the Acute Abdomen.* 21st ed./revised by William Silen. Oxford University Press; 2005. Print.

To KB, Kamdar NS, Patil P, et al. Acute care surgery model and outcomes in emergency general surgery. *J Am Coll Surg.* 2019;228:21-28.

Wagner M, Tubre DJ, Asensio JA. Evolution and current trends in the management of acute appendicitis. *Surg Clin N Am.* 2018;98:1005-1023.

CHAPTER

4 General Surgery Issues in the MICU and CTICU

Lisa Marie Knowlton, Jennifer Knight Davis, and Clay Cothren Burlew

CASE PRESENTATION

A 67-year-old male is 8 days post aortic arch repair. His clinical course has been complicated by an ST-elevation myocardial infarction (STEMI) and cardiac arrest requiring placement of a balloon pump. The ICU team contacts you regarding concern for increasing abdominal distension over the past 24 hours, as well as a rising WBC to 28k and elevated lactate of 7.0 g/dL. CTA of the abdomen and pelvis does not reveal any obvious intravascular thrombosis and his mesenteric vessels appear patent; however, there are patches of bowel wall hypoenhancement near the terminal ileum concerning for ischemia.

Question: *What is the diagnosis and optimal approach?*

Answer: *Intestinal ischemia requiring operative exploration and likely resection.*

INTRODUCTION

Intra-abdominal diseases requiring operative intervention occur in 4% of ICU patients, with the general surgeon consulted in up to 20%. The diagnosis of an acute abdominal process in the Medical Intensive Care Unit (MICU) or CTICU is difficult due to intubation, sedation, dementia, comorbidity, and distracting diseases or operations. The most common etiologies are intestinal ischemia, bowel perforation or obstruction, cholecystitis, or complications of a procedure such as a feeding tube, angioembolization, or a therapeutic endoscopy/colonoscopy. Postoperative mortality is 40% or greater, with mesenteric ischemia and colonic ischemia as the most common causes of death. These are also the most common abdominal processes that are delayed or missed in diagnosis and therapy. The highest mortality occurs in patients who require decompression for abdominal compartment syndrome (ACS) or operation for a feeding tube complication.

INTESTINAL ISCHEMIA

Intestinal ischemia can affect the small or large intestine and can be caused by any process that reduces intestinal blood flow, such as arterial occlusion, venous occlusion, or arterial vasospasm. (See also Chapter 12.) Patients experiencing acute symptoms require prompt evaluation, as the clinical consequences can include sepsis, septic shock, bowel infarction, perforation, and death. Ischemia affecting the small intestine is referred to as *mesenteric ischemia*, whereas ischemia affecting the large intestine is referred to as *colonic ischemia or ischemic colitis*.

The main blood supply to the bowel is the superior mesenteric artery (SMA) and inferior mesenteric artery (IMA). The SMA supplies the small bowel, except for the proximal duodenum. The SMA and IMA share blood supply to the colon. Venous drainage occurs through the superior mesenteric vein (SMV) and the inferior mesenteric vein (IMV), draining into the portal circulation. The intestines also receive collateral blood flow from branches of the celiac axis. "Watershed" areas prone to ischemia include the splenic flexure (Griffiths point is the arterial supply between the ascending left colic artery and the marginal artery of Drummond), as well as the rectosigmoid junction (Sudeck point is the arterial supply where the last sigmoid arterial branch from the IMA meets the branch from the superior rectal artery).

Acute mesenteric ischemia refers to the sudden onset of small intestinal hypoperfusion, which can be due to occlusive or nonocclusive obstruction of the arterial blood supply or obstruction of venous outflow. Occlusive arterial obstruction is due to an acute embolism or thrombosis and most commonly affects the SMA or its branches. Venous thrombosis is due to obstruction of the intestinal outflow tract, including the superior and IMVs and the splenic and portal veins. Nonocclusive mesenteric ischemia (NOMI) is a result of a low-flow state and is most commonly due to vasoconstriction from low cardiac output or the use of vasopressors. Additionally, twisting of the bowel (ie, volvulus) around a fixed attachment (ie, adhesion, mesenteric defect) or incarceration and strangulation of intestinal contents within a hernia can lead to intestinal ischemia involving both arterial and venous occlusion.

Ischemic injury to the intestine develops when there is insufficient delivery of oxygen and nutrients required for cellular metabolism. Intestinal injury can be caused both by tissue hypoxia and reperfusion. Reperfusion injury occurs following restoration of blood flow after a period of ischemia, releasing free oxygen radicals and toxic by-products of ischemic injury, which can lead to multisystem organ failure. Chronic mesenteric ischemia usually develops in patients with mesenteric atherosclerosis and will not be discussed here. Certain risk factors predispose to intestinal ischemia (**Table 4.1**).

In patients presenting with intestinal ischemia, abdominal pain is the most common symptom. This may be described as "pain out of proportion" to the physical examination. Acute colonic ischemia may be accompanied by rectal bleeding or bloody diarrhea. As bowel ischemia progresses and transmural bowel infarction develops, the abdomen becomes grossly distended and peritoneal signs may develop. Patients may develop a marked leukocytosis and a metabolic acidosis with elevated serum lactate. It is important to note that neither a normal lactate nor lack of guaiac-positive or bloody stools rule out bowel ischemia. For patients with a suspicion for intestinal ischemia, computed tomography angiography (CTA) of the abdomen is the test of choice (**Figure 4.1**). Imaging can help identify mesenteric ischemia as a possible cause of worsening sepsis and metabolic acidosis in a critically ill patient. For those patients who present with peritonitis or obvious bowel perforation (eg, free air on abdominal imaging), emergent exploration should be performed. In questionable cases, colonoscopy or sigmoidoscopy can establish the diagnosis of ischemic colitis.

TABLE 4.1 ■ Predisposing Factors for Intestinal Ischemia

Cardiac disease
Aortic surgery
Peripheral arterial disease
Hemodialysis
Vasoconstrictive medications
Thrombotic conditions (acquired, hereditary)
Hypovolemia
Inflammation/infection
Segmental ischemia from bowel strangulation

The initial management of intestinal ischemia includes fluid resuscitation, hemodynamic monitoring and support, correction of electrolyte abnormalities, pain control, systemic anticoagulation under most circumstances, and initiation of broad-spectrum antibiotics. Gastrointestinal decompression can be performed with a nasogastric tube (NGT). For patients with acute intestinal ischemia due to mesenteric arterial or venous occlusion, or NOMI, initiate systemic anticoagulation to prevent thrombus formation and propagation, unless patients are actively bleeding. For patients requiring abdominal exploration, anticoagulation is typically started perioperatively and continued during and after surgery to prevent new thrombus formation. Start broad-spectrum antibiotic therapy immediately.

Preoperative CTA of the abdomen can help to evaluate areas of potential ischemia as well as the presence of thrombus or emboli in mesenteric vessels. In these situations, revascularization via endovascular or open approaches should be discussed with a vascular surgeon. Patients for whom there is a high index of clinical suspicion for intestinal ischemia should undergo prompt operative evaluation. The goal is to restore intestinal blood flow as rapidly as possible by treating the underlying cause. For example, acute mesenteric arterial embolism requires surgical

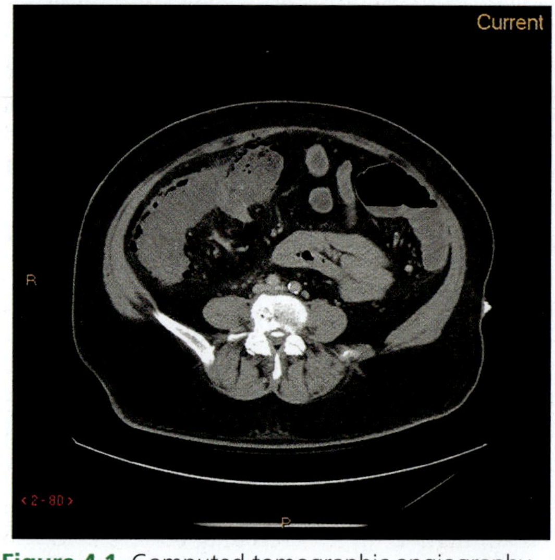

Figure 4.1 Computed tomographic angiography (CTA) of the abdomen may demonstrate thickened, hypoperfused bowel or pneumatosis.

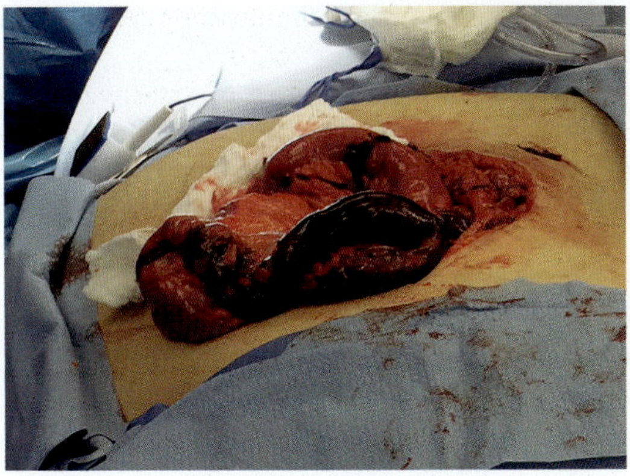

Figure 4.2 At abdominal exploration, areas of frank bowel ischemia should be resected; areas that are questionable may be left for repeat evaluation at second-look laparotomy.

laparotomy with embolectomy. For patients with a volvulus or mechanical obstruction leading to ischemia of surrounding intestine, the bowel should be detorsed, adhesions lysed, or ischemic areas resected. Areas of frank ischemia should be resected to viable margins (**Figure 4.2**). Surgery should not be delayed in patients suspected to have intestinal infarction or perforation.

In critically ill patients with intestinal ischemia, leave the bowel in discontinuity and the abdomen open with a vacuum-assisted closure (VAC) dressing with return to the operating room 24-48 hours later for further inspection of the bowel. This "second-look" laparotomy is intended to rule out additional areas of ischemia and necrosis. In addition to clinical judgment, adjuncts such as laser fluorescence angiography (eg, Spy Elite) can help determine bowel wall perfusion. A fluorescent dye (eg, indocyanine green, 0.2-0.5 mg/kg) is injected in a bolus dose into the patient intravenously, and after a delay of time, the dye fluoresces using NIR laser light allowing analysis of the tissue of interest. This approach allows a waiting period of revascularization that may render salvageable bowel that on first look was deemed borderline ischemic. Additionally, this damage-control approach facilitates a more rapid return to the ICU for continued resuscitation in patients who are tenuous and not able to tolerate prolonged operations much less a bowel anastomosis. Regardless of etiology, mortality rates for acute ischemic intestinal events remain high, at times exceeding 60%. The key to a more favorable prognosis is maintaining a high index of suspicion and intervening early.

SEVERE ACUTE OR NECROTIZING PANCREATITIS

The most common etiology of severe acute or necrotizing pancreatitis in the critically ill patient is obstructive biliary tract disease, representing ~40% of cases. (See also Chapter 14.) Other common etiologies include alcohol abuse, procedural manipulation (endoscopic retrograde cholangiopancreatography [ERCP]), abdominal trauma, anatomic abnormalities (eg, pancreas divisum), hypertriglyceridemia, or idiopathic reasons. Acute pancreatitis can be classified as (1) mild acute pancreatitis, which denotes the absence of organ failure or local and systemic complications; (2) moderately severe pancreatitis, which is characterized by transient organ failure and/or local or systemic complications that resolve within 48 hours; and (3) severe acute pancreatitis, which is characterized by persistent organ failure affecting one or multiple organs.

Classic symptoms of epigastric abdominal pain radiating to the back may not always be evident in ICU patients. Therefore, in a patient who is tachycardic, hypotensive, or has suspicion for intra-abdominal pathology, the clinician's differential diagnosis should include pancreatitis; liver function tests including a serum lipase and cross-sectional imaging of the abdomen should be obtained.

Several scoring systems have been developed to classify the severity of acute pancreatitis. The severity of pancreatitis and associated risk of mortality is classically estimated using the Ranson criteria (**Table 4.2**). Severe pancreatitis is defined by the presence of three or more Ranson criteria or if the patient has evidence of shock. In general, however, the severity of pancreatitis is most readily characterized by the presence of persistent organ(s) failure (>48 hours). Although the Ranson criteria continue to be used, a recent meta-analysis found this score to be a poor predictor of severity. Many other scoring systems exist including the Acute Physiology and Chronic Health Examination (APACHE) II score, the CT severity index (Balthazar score), and the Systemic Inflammatory Response Syndrome (SIRS) score. Many favor the SIRS score as it can be readily calculated at the bedside, and the presence of SIRS is associated with increased mortality (**Table 4.3**). In one validation study, mortality rates were 25%, 8%, and 0% in those with persistent SIRS from admission, SIRS at admission but not persistent, and no SIRS, respectively.

TABLE 4.2 ■ Ranson Criteria

Present on Admission	Detected After 48 Hours
Age >55 years	Calcium <8.0 mg/dL
WBC > 16 000	Hematocrit decreased >10%
Blood glucose >200 g/dL	Hypoxemia (PaO_2 < 60 mm Hg)
AST > 250 IU/L	BUN increased by >5 mg/dL
LDH > 350 IU/L	Base deficit >4 mEq/L
Ranson score of:	Sequestration of fluids >6 L
1-2 = 1% mortality	
3-4 = 15% mortality	
5-6 = 40% mortality	

Clinical severity is guided by clinical examination to assess for early fluid losses, organ failure, and SIRS score elements. Routine abdominal computed tomography (CT) is useful in evaluating patients with abdominal pain that is not resolving, biochemical markers that are not improving, or patients who are showing systemic clinical deterioration. Imaging of these more severe cases enables the clinician to identify any peripancreatic edema, presence of fluid collections, and areas of necrosis (**Figure 4.3**).

While most patients with mild pancreatitis recover with conservative management, it is important to note that severe pancreatitis is associated with mortality rates >15%. Admission to a monitored or intensive care unit is indicated for patients demonstrating signs of shock or organ failure. Initial management of the patient with severe pancreatitis includes continuous monitoring, fluid resuscitation, and pain control. As with all critically ill patients, monitoring of vital signs including oxygenation is important. Patients may be fed enterally via nasogastric or nasojejunal tube.

TABLE 4.3 ■ SIRS Score

Two or more of the following conditions:
Temperature >38.3 °C or <36.0 °C
Heart rate of >90 beats/min
Respiratory rate of >20 breaths/min or $PaCO_2$ of <32 mm Hg
WBC count of >12 000 cells/mm³, <4000 cells/mm³, or >10% immature (band) forms

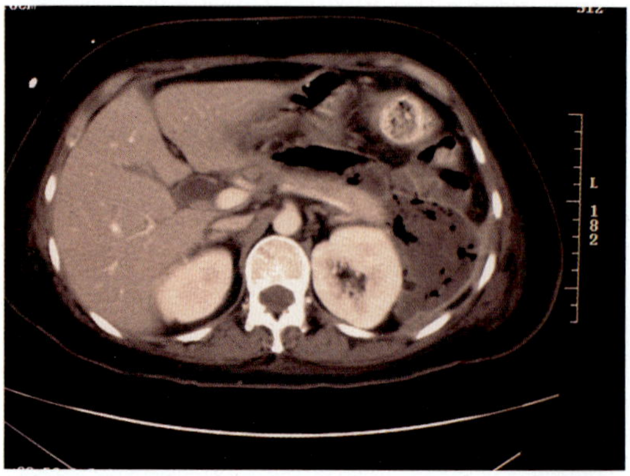

Figure 4.3 Computed tomographic (CT) imaging of the abdomen can demonstrate sequelae of acute pancreatitis such as infected fluid collections.

If the patient does not tolerate enteral feeds or the target rate is not achieved, supplemental parenteral nutrition should be provided within 7 days.

Pancreatitis can elicit a dramatic SIRS syndrome. Non-necrotizing pancreatitis should be treated with supportive care and nonoperative management. In the absence of documented infection, antibiotic therapy is not warranted. Fluid collections should not be drained in the acute phase unless there is evidence of abscess and infection. Both acute necrotic collections and walled-off necrosis (WON) are initially sterile but may become infected if intervened upon. Infection should be suspected in patients with pancreatic or extrapancreatic necrosis who deteriorate or fail to improve after 7-10 days of hospitalization. In patients with suspected infected necrosis, empiric antibiotics are preferred over CT-guided fine needle aspiration (high false negative rate).

In patients who develop necrosis, allowing time for necrotic regions of the pancreas to demarcate will minimize the resection of potentially viable pancreas. The step-up approach of starting with minimally invasive strategies is associated with lower mortality rate. Nearly one-third of patients can be treated with percutaneous drainage of infected collections. Every attempt should be made to delay intervention until 4 weeks after initial presentation to allow the infected necrosis to become walled off. If additional debridement is required, endoscopic debridement can be performed by accessing necrotic collections via the stomach. Minimally invasive surgical options, such as videoscopic-assisted retroperitoneal debridement (VARD) or laparoscopic surgical debridement, are alternatives if the collection is not readily accessible from the stomach or

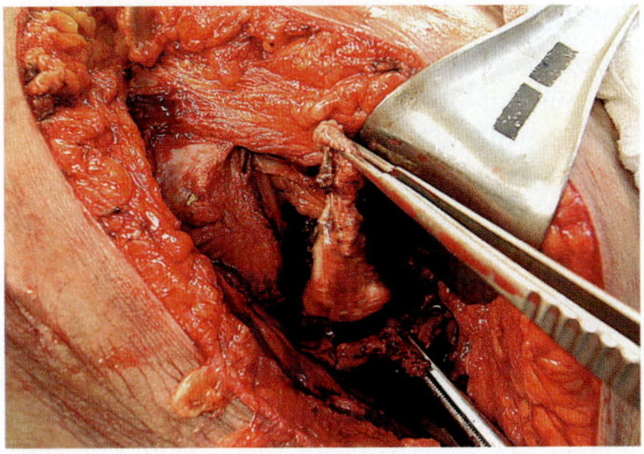

Figure 4.4 Open necrosectomy can be performed through an anterior approach via the lesser sac or via a retroperitoneal 12th rib left lateral approach as seen here.

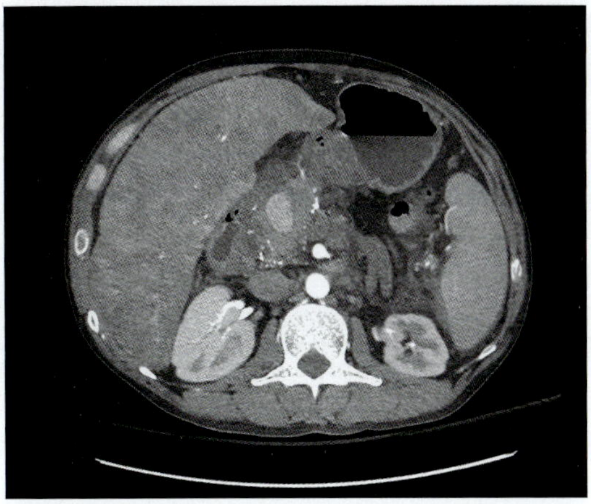

Figure 4.5 Sequelae of severe pancreatitis include pseudoaneurysms that may rupture and bleed; endovascular control of hemorrhage is advocated.

if additional debridement of necrotic tissue is required. Open pancreatic necrosectomy may be considered in patients who are refractory to less invasive options, though morbidity and mortality are high (**Figure 4.4**).

Patients undergoing massive resuscitation for pancreatitis are at risk of developing ACS. This may be signaled by abdominal distention, decreased urine output, elevated bladder pressures, and difficulty ventilating/high airway pressures. Prompt surgical depression is the treatment of choice; if there is a significant intra-abdominal fluid component on bedside ultrasound, percutaneous drain may be placed. If drainage of abdominal resuscitation-associated ascites does not lower the intra-abdominal pressure significantly and reverse end-organ derangements, perform decompressive laparotomy. In patients undergoing operative debridement of their pancreas, complications such as intra-abdominal and retroperitoneal hemorrhage, as well as superimposed infections, can occur. Longer term pseudocysts and fistulae can form, as well as vascular complications such as splanchnic venous thrombosis and pseudoaneurysm (**Figure 4.5**). Follow-up imaging is required to identify and manage these sequelae. Ultimately, those with severe pancreatitis are at risk for endocrine and exocrine dysfunction.

ACALCULOUS CHOLECYSTITIS

Acalculous cholecystitis is typically seen in patients who are hospitalized and critically ill, particularly those who have undergone major trauma, cardiac or vascular intervention, or who are immunosuppressed from bone marrow transplantation. Rarely patients with acalculous cholecystitis can present in the outpatient setting. (See also Chapter 15.) Acalculous cholecystitis results from gallbladder stasis and ischemia, which then cause a local inflammatory response in the gallbladder wall. While primary infections such as acquired immunodeficiency syndrome (AIDS) may predispose to acalculous cholecystitis, it typically occurs secondary to some other major physiologic insult. Gallbladder stasis and distention can result, leading to ischemia and eventually necrosis. Associated infection with enteric pathogens, such as *Escherichia coli*, *Enterococcus faecalis*, *Pseudomonas*, *Klebsiella* spp, *Proteus* spp, and *Bacteroides fragilis*, is common. In rare cases, gangrene and perforation of the gallbladder wall may be seen.

In critically ill patients, the appearance of unexplained sepsis may be the first indicator of underlying acalculous cholecystitis. Typical signs and symptoms include fever, abdominal pain, leukocytosis, and/or elevated liver function tests. The physical examination may reveal right upper quadrant tenderness, a palpable right upper quadrant mass, or rarely jaundice. In advanced cases, the distended gallbladder or a phlegmon can cause extrinsic compression of the common bile duct resulting in a Mirizzi-type syndrome with hyperbilirubinemia. The history and presentation are similar to that seen in calculous cholecystitis, with fever, severe right upper quadrant pain with tenderness to palpation, and a positive Murphy sign (pain elicited during inspiration while palpating the right upper quadrant). Laboratory tests are usually nonspecific. Abdominal ultrasound should be ordered, and if the diagnosis is still uncertain, a contrast-enhanced abdominal CT scan can be

TABLE 4.4 ■ Radiographic Features of Acalculous Cholecystitis

Ultrasound or CT Abdomen Pelvis
Gallbladder wall thickening (>3 mm)
Sonographic Murphy sign
Pericholecystic fluid/subserosal edema
Lack of gallstones
Distended gallbladder
Mucosal sloughing
Intramural gas
Hyperdense bile (sludge)
Gallbladder distention (>5 cm)

obtained (**Table 4.4**). For stable patients in whom the diagnosis is unclear after ultrasonography and abdominal CT scan, a hepatic iminodiacetic acid scan can be used as an adjunct.

The initial treatment of acalculous cholecystitis is fluid resuscitation and broad-spectrum antibiotics. Typical antibiotic regimens should offer Gram-positive, Gram-negative, and anaerobic coverage. Patients may require percutaneous gallbladder drainage procedure under radiologic guidance if they have an overall worsening clinical status. Decompressing the gallbladder with a percutaneous cholecystostomy allows both local inflammation and systemic illness to subside. Cholecystostomy tubes usually have low failure rates, but complications can include bleeding, sepsis, bile peritonitis, pneumothorax, intestinal perforation, secondary infection of the gallbladder, and catheter dislodgement.

Cholecystostomy tube is effective and is less invasive than cholecystectomy and is often the preferred approach in critically ill patients who may not be able to tolerate an operation. Their overall risk of recurrent cholecystitis is low. Once the episode of acalculous cholecystitis has resolved, cholecystectomy is typically not required in the absence of concurrent gallstones or sludge. If patients' symptoms are severe (eg, gangrenous, emphysematous, or perforated gallbladders) and they do not clinically improve within 48 hours of percutaneous drainage, a small percentage may require emergency cholecystectomy. Overall, perforation occurs in <10% of patients with acalculous cholecystitis, which may result in a cholecystoenteric fistula, abscess formation, or free perforation with generalized peritonitis. If treatment is delayed, mortality rates from acalculous cholecystitis range up to 75%.

Clostridium difficile Infection

Clostridium difficile infections (CDI) are the leading cause of hospital-associated infectious diarrhea. (See also Chapter 18.) CDI primarily affects the colon where exotoxins disrupt the cytoskeleton of the enterocyte, opening the tight junctions with fluid release into the intestinal lumen and eventual cell death. These toxins, produced by the spore-forming Gram-positive bacteria, also cause an intense inflammatory response resulting in neutrophilic infiltration of the colonic wall. CDI can progress to fulminant pancolitis, systemic inflammation, sepsis, and death.

Clostridium difficile infections are increasing in both incidence and severity. Predisposing factors include antibiotic use, commonly fluoroquinolones, cephalosporins, and clindamycin, which are implicated in more than 90% of hospital cases of CDI. Conversely, the majority of antibiotic-associated diarrhea is not caused by CDI. Other predisposing factors include older age, immunosuppression, gastrointestinal surgery, inflammatory bowel disease, and hospitalization. Gastric acid suppressants such as proton pump inhibitors (PPI) and H_2 blockers also may be associated with increased risk of CDI. The diagnosis of CDI should be considered in any patient with greater than three bowel movements per day, blood or mucus in the stool, and/or abdominal pain. About 30% of patients have fever and ~50% of patients have a leukocytosis. Diarrhea may be absent with toxic megacolon.

Diagnosis of a CDI is based on a combination of clinical findings and laboratory testing positive for the *C difficile* antigen and toxin. Although the clinical presentation can vary, up to 10% of cases are considered severe or "fulminant." Original stratification proposed by Dallal et al. describes fulminant disease with heart rate >120 beats/min, >30% bands, mechanical ventilation, severe oliguria, and vasopressor requirements; in this subset of patients, mortality is over 50%. In patients who undergo sigmoidoscopy, pseudomembranes may only be present in 50% of patients with CDI colitis. The historical cornerstones of treatment for CDI include antimicrobial therapy, discontinuing any inciting antibiotics, and organ support. Antibiotic treatment options for hospitalized patients with CDI include intravenous metronidazole, oral vancomycin, and vancomycin enemas in patients with a marked ileus. Newer therapies have focused on fecal transplantation in highly selected patients with refractory CDI. Suggested indications for

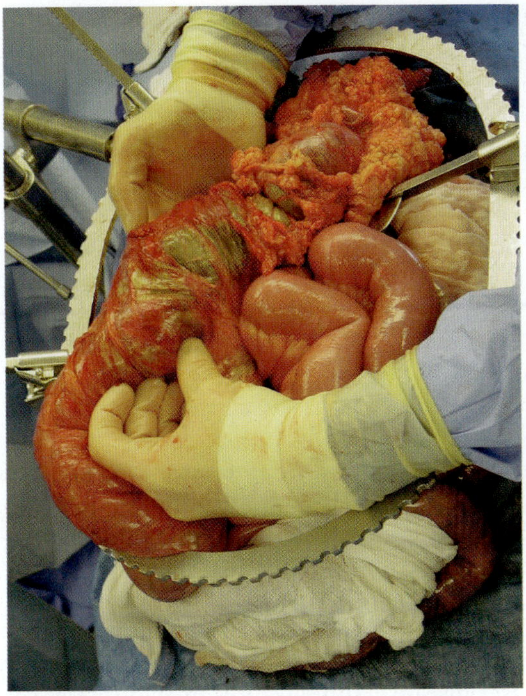

Figure 4.6 Patients with fulminant *C difficile* colitis may require total colectomy for ischemia, perforation, or unremitting organ failure.

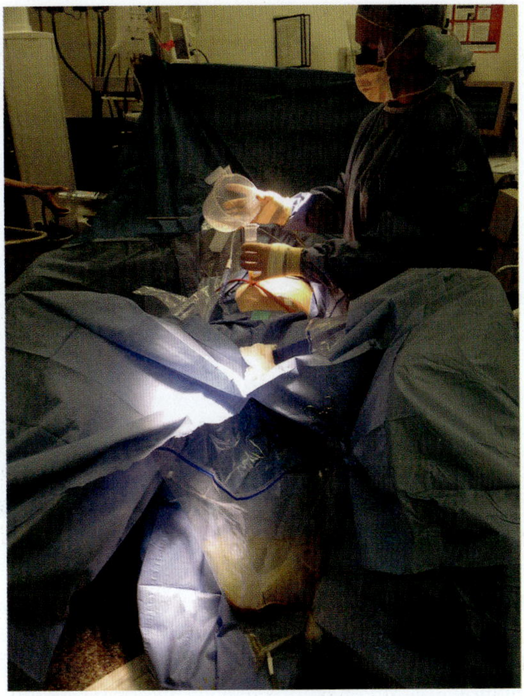

Figure 4.7 Following diverting loop ileostomy, antegrade lavage is performed with 8 L of GoLytely in patients with *C difficile* colitis.

fecal transplantation include patients who are refractory to medical therapy, those with two documented recurrences after completing adequate antimicrobial treatment, or potentially those who have not had symptomatic relief after 1 week of adequate therapy.

Surgical management of CDI is reserved for patients with marked clinical deterioration, peritonitis, or shock. Colectomy with end ileostomy is the definitive surgical option and is required in patients with perforation, ischemia, or ACS (**Figure 4.6**). For patients who are identified early, prior to complete organ failure, colon-sparing surgery using a laparoscopic diverting loop ileostomy and intraoperative, high-volume colonic lavage should be considered. Intraoperative antegrade lavage via the newly created loop ileostomy with 8 L of GoLytely is directed at eradication of the toxin from the mucosal surface (**Figure 4.7**). Postoperatively, patients are treated with antegrade vancomycin colon enemas for 10 days. Series to date demonstrate mortality rates of 35%-80% for patients undergoing total colectomy for fulminant colitis, and survivors often require permanent ileostomy. Reported mortality rates for patients undergoing diverting loop ileostomy and colon lavage average 20% in this select patient population.

PEPTIC ULCER DISEASE/UPPER GASTROINTESTINAL BLEEDING

Acute upper gastrointestinal hemorrhage (UGIB) is the most common complication of peptic ulcer disease. Other complications include perforation, penetration, and gastric outlet obstruction. (See also Chapters 13 and 16.) With the introduction of PPI and the identification of *Helicobacter pylori* and its treatment, peptic ulcer disease has become largely a medically managed disease. For acute UGIB, restrictive transfusion strategies should attempt to maintain a hemoglobin of 7-9 g/dL depending on whether the patient has a cardiovascular history. High-dose PPI therapy IV for 3 days should be given to patients with bleeding ulcers with high-risk stigmata and then oral PPI therapy twice a day for 14 days before decreasing to once daily treatment. For esophageal or gastric varices from cirrhosis, antibiotics and vasoactive drugs are recommended. Investigating for the presence of *H pylori* and treating when detected are recommended as is documentation of its eradication.

For acute UGIB, endoscopy should occur within 24 hours and thermocoagulation and sclerosant injection are recommended; clips suggested

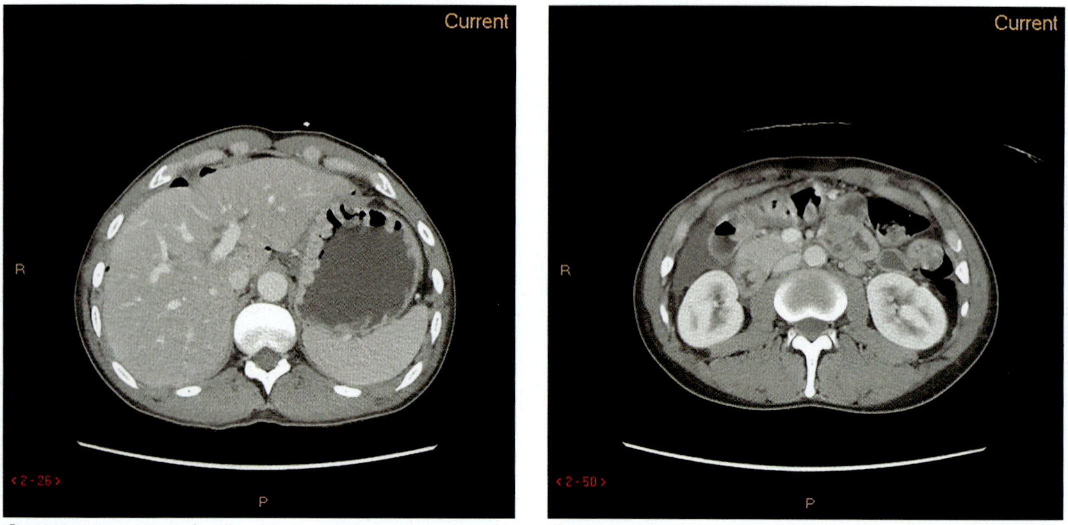

A B

Figure 4.8 CT imaging in perforated peptic ulcer disease may demonstrate free air **(A)** or free fluid **(B)**.

for endoscopic therapy in patients with high-risk stigmata. Other endoscopic interventions could include ligation of esophageal varices or tissue glue for gastric varices. Very early (<12 hours) upper GI endoscopy should be considered in high-risk clinical features of hemodynamic instability that persists despite goal-directed resuscitation, bloody emesis or NG output, or if anticoagulation cannot be stopped. Repeat attempt at endoscopic control of bleeding is only recommended if previous success was achieved. CT angiography is a valuable tool to aide in identifying the bleeding source especially in the event of an obscure UGIB and is equivalent to angiography. If endoscopic attempts at hemorrhage control are unsuccessful, transcatheter angiographic embolization should be considered.

Historically, surgical management was the mainstay of treatment for symptomatic peptic ulcer disease. With advances in acid suppressive medications, surgical intervention is reserved for acute and chronic complications. Acute perforation presents with acute onset of severe abdominal pain, tachycardia, and peritonitis and carries a mortality rate as high as 30%. Patients typically have fever and leukocytosis, and free intra-abdominal air may be present on plain abdominal radiograph or CT imaging (**Figure 4.8**). Treatment with an omental patch is recommended (**Figure 4.9**). Giant ulcers often require resection and reconstruction such as antrectomy and either Billroth I or II; vagotomy is often added to this procedure. Conservative management for perforated PUD should only be considered in extremely

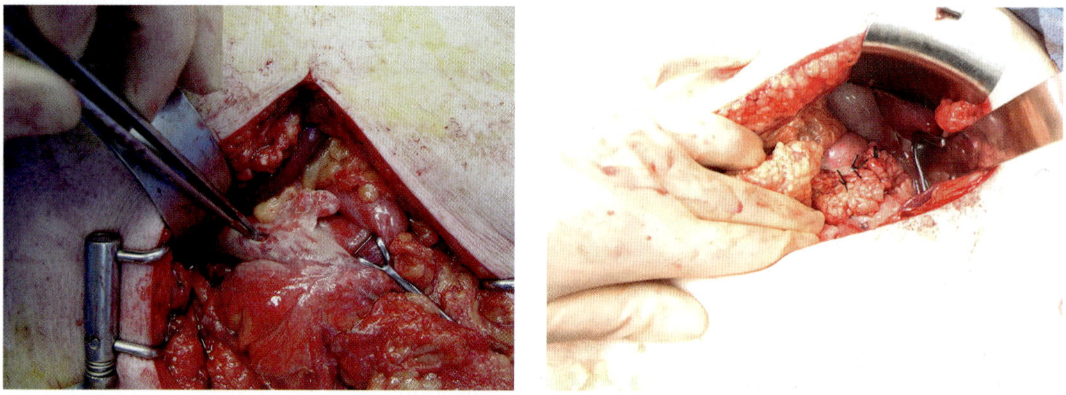

A B

Figure 4.9 At exploration, identification of a small punctate ulcer **(A)** can be repaired with an omental patch, typically called a Graham patch **(B)**.

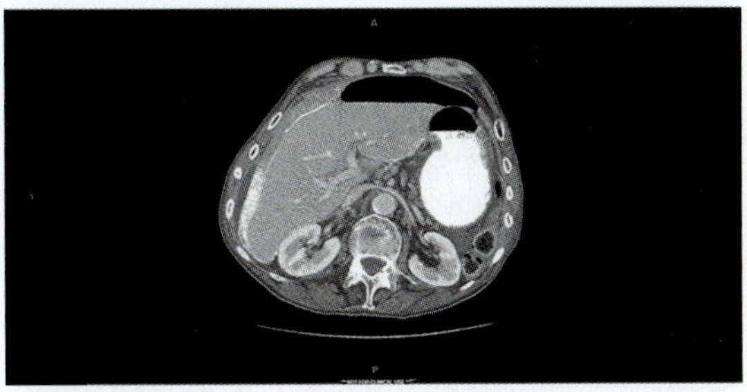

Figure 4.10 On CT imaging, free contrast extravasation from perforated PUD is a contraindication to nonoperative management.

high-risk patients who do not have free contrast extravasation into the peritoneum (**Figure 4.10**); perform additional imaging with fluoroscopic upper gastrointestinal contrast imaging to ensure a contained leak prior to the institution of treatment with nasogastric decompression, *nil-per-os*, and total parenteral nutrition.

Gastric outlet obstruction, as a chronic complication of PUD, is most commonly associated with a duodenal or pyloric ulcer. Gastric cancer must always be excluded in this setting. Patients will present with bloating, nausea and vomiting, early satiety, anorexia, and weight loss. There is potential to reverse this condition with aggressive medical management; however, when this fails despite 1-2 weeks of intensive treatment, endoscopic dilation can be considered. Surgical indications include inability to stop NSAID use, inability to tolerate a medical regimen, or recurrence/persistence of disease while on PPI therapy. Surgical management includes truncal vagotomy with pyloroplasty, truncal vagotomy with antrectomy, or truncal vagotomy with subtotal gastrectomy. Reconstruction options include Billroth I, Billroth II, and Roux-en-Y.

ABDOMINAL COMPARTMENT SYNDROME

Abdominal compartment syndrome and intra-abdominal hypertension (IAH) result from increased intra-abdominal pressures within the confines of the abdominal cavity. (See also Chapter 10.) This elevation in pressure leads to impairment of the cardiac, pulmonary, renal, gastrointestinal, hepatic, and central nervous system function. While there is some elasticity to this compartment, should the volume of any of the contents of this space increase, the pressure within the space will increase as well. The resting pressure within the abdomen is 5-7 mm Hg in hospitalized patients and is affected by body mass index. The World Society of Abdominal Compartment Syndrome has defined IAH as a graded disease process; Grade I: IAP 12-15 mm Hg, Grade II: 16-20 mm Hg, Grade III: 21-25 mm Hg, Grade IV: IAP > 25 mm Hg. The ACS is the combination of IAH causing end-organ dysfunction. Typically, intra-abdominal pressures >20 mm Hg are seen in ACS, but end-organ derangements may occur at lower abdominal pressures.

As a potential complication in critically ill patients, ACS can be caused by either a surgical or nonsurgical cause and can occur as an acute or chronic problem. ACS can also be classified by primary abdominal pathologies or secondary to nonabdominal causes. Acute causes of ACS are intra-abdominal or retroperitoneal hemorrhage, peritonitis or intra-abdominal abscess, pancreatitis, bowel distention from ileus, obstruction or pseudo-obstruction, tight fascial closure after abdominal surgery, repair or reduction of a larger hernia, and burns. Chronic causes of ACS include intra-abdominal or retroperitoneal tumor, ascites from liver failure or malignancy, pregnancy, and obesity. Secondary causes of ACS are respiratory ventilator support with high positive end expiratory pressure, massive fluid resuscitation, prone positioning, and peritoneal dialysis.

End-organ dysfunction that results from IAH can affect many organ systems. The cardiovascular effects are (1) decreased preload to the heart due to venal caval compression and (2) increased afterload due to increased systemic vascular resistance from compression of the abdominal aorta. The respiratory impact of IAH occurs when increased abdominal pressure is transmitted across the diaphragm to the chest; respiratory failure worsens as tidal volumes decrease and intrathoracic pressures increase. Renal perfusion is compromised resulting in decreased urine output. Gastrointestinal absorption and motility are impaired. Liver function is decreased and direct hepatocellular damage can occur.

The diagnosis of ACS is not always straightforward. The combination of elevated intra-abdominal pressures and the direct consequence on organ function makes the diagnosis. Signs and symptoms may be missed in critically ill patients as the organ failure may be mistaken for other etiologies, that is, sepsis, cardiac dysfunction, acute kidney injury, or acute respiratory distress syndrome. Physical examination findings that suggest elevated intra-abdominal pressures include abdominal distention or guarding. However, the physical examination is unreliable in up to 40% of patients. Other signs include increased need for ventilator support either by the need for increased pressure or volume needed depending on the mode of ventilation being used. Poor urine output or feeding intolerance may also be a sign of organ dysfunction.

No imaging study reliably diagnoses ACS. Plain radiographs may show distended bowel loops. Ultrasonography may show the presence or an increase of abdominal free fluid. CT imaging can show abdominal pathologies that may lead to or be a result of increased abdominal pressure, such as bowel edema or ischemia, pancreatitis, intra-abdominal hemorrhage, or flattening of the venal cava. While none of these findings diagnose ACS, they add to the information needed to make the diagnosis in a critically ill patient. Measurement of intra-abdominal pressures remains the most accurate means to diagnose IAH. IAP measurements from the foley after instillation of saline into the bladder and clamping are most commonly used. However, nasogastric or direct measurement through an intraperitoneal catheter is an alternative if the foley cannot be used (ie, bladder rupture).

Preventative efforts are the first-line options for treatment of IAH before it progresses to the ACS. Fluid overload in the setting of intra-abdominal sepsis, bowel obstruction, and hemorrhage control are the lead causes of elevated intra-abdominal pressures. Effective diuresis of this excess fluid can be difficult; avoid the fluid overload preemptively. Early detection of elevated pressures with mitigation of inciting events and treatment can prevent progression to end-organ dysfunction. It is recommended that patients with ACS (ie, IAH and signs of organ dysfunction) should undergo decompressive laparotomy (**Figure 4.11**). For patients with a significant intra-abdominal fluid component, percutaneous drain placement at the bedside may reduce the IAP significantly and laparotomy may be avoided. Following decompression, there is often an immediate resolution of cardiopulmonary effects and an increase in urine output. A summary of the 2013 World Society of the Abdominal Compartment Syndrome's management recommendations for noninvasive and minimally invasive treatment is listed in **Table 4.5**.

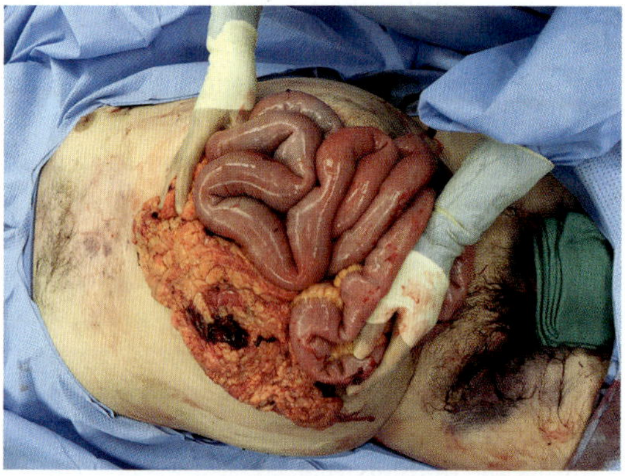

Figure 4.11 Decompressive laparotomy allows egress of edematous bowel and intra-abdominal fluid with resultant improvement in the patient's physiology.

LONG-TERM ENTERAL ACCESS IN MICU PATIENTS

Early total enteral nutrition (TEN) is important in the critically ill population, particularly in reducing septic complications. (See also Chapter 7.) The specific type of enteral feedings, stomach vs duodenum vs small bowel, appears to be less important; tolerance of enteral nutrition through each of these routes appears to be equivalent unless there is upper gastrointestinal pathology. Enteral access for nutrition can be obtained via multiple options. NGTs, most commonly placed for gastric decompression, can be used for enteral feeding once gastric motility is assured and NGT output decreases. Dobhoff tubes or longer nasoenteric tubes provide postpyloric access and can be particularly advantageous in patients with a gastric ileus. Obtain radiographs confirming placement prior to use to prevent inadvertent placement in the lung or pleural space (**Figure 4.12**). Longer term access, typically quantified by a need for access >4-6 weeks, is best obtained with gastrostomy or jejunostomy tubes. Gastrostomy tubes can be either percutaneously placed at the bedside in the ICU or operatively placed.

For intubated patients, a first attempt at placement should be performed at the bedside unless the patient has prior abdominal surgical history that would preclude safe placement. Upper endoscopy is performed with transillumination of the abdominal wall to confirm apposition of the stomach (**Figure 4.13**). Standard technique results in percutaneous endoscopic gastrostomy (PEG) placement in the left upper quadrant. Repeat endoscopy should confirm the flange is pulled snug within the stomach with the exterior bolster/fastener adjusted. The position of the external fastener should be noted (ie, PEG bolster at 3 cm) and documented daily. If the height of the bolster changes, concern for accidental tube manipulation should be pursued. If the height is shorter, for example reading at 1-2 cm rather than 3 cm, the

TABLE 4.5 ■ Management Recommendations for IAH and ACS

Treatment	Recommended (Yes or No or Suggest)	Comments
Sedation and analgesia	Suggest	Suggest that optimal pain and anxiety relief be achieved.
Neuromuscular blockade	Suggest	Brief trials as a temporizing measure.
Body positioning	Suggest	Some body positions may elevate IAP.
Nasogastric/colonic decompression	Suggest	Liberal use when the stomach or colon is dilated in the presence of IAH/ACS.
Promotility agents	Suggest	Neostigmine be used for the treatment of established colonic ileus not responsive to simple measures.
Negative or neutral fluid balance	Suggest	A protocol to avoid positive accumulative fluid balance.
Diuretics	No recommendation	There is lack of evidence to support this intervention.
Renal replacement therapies	No recommendation	There is lack of evidence to support this intervention.
Albumin	No recommendation	There is lack of evidence to support this intervention.
Damage control resuscitation	Suggest	Use of enhanced ration of plasma/packed red blood cells for massive hemorrhage.
Paracentesis	Suggest	May be useful when obvious intraperitoneal fluid is present in preventing the decompressive laparotomy.

tube may be dislodged with the flange (and tube feeds) in the subcutaneous tissue. If the height is longer, then the tube may need to be pulled snug to prevent leakage from the stomach. PEG tubes are often placed to gravity for 12 hours after initial insertion. Patients may have evidence of free air

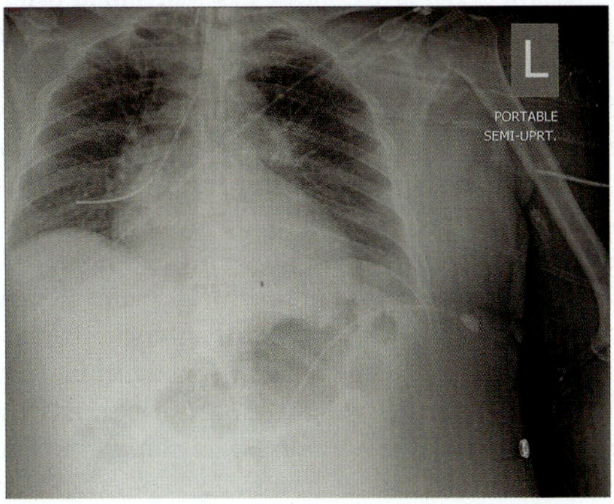

Figure 4.12 Following Dobhoff tubes placement, plain radiographs should be obtained to confirm there has not been inadvertent placement in the lung.

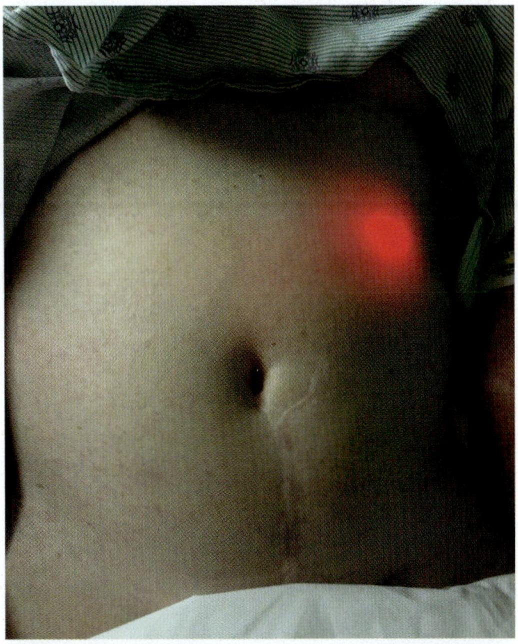

Figure 4.13 Transillumination of the abdominal wall confirms apposition of the stomach prior to percutaneous endoscopic gastrostomy (PEG) placement.

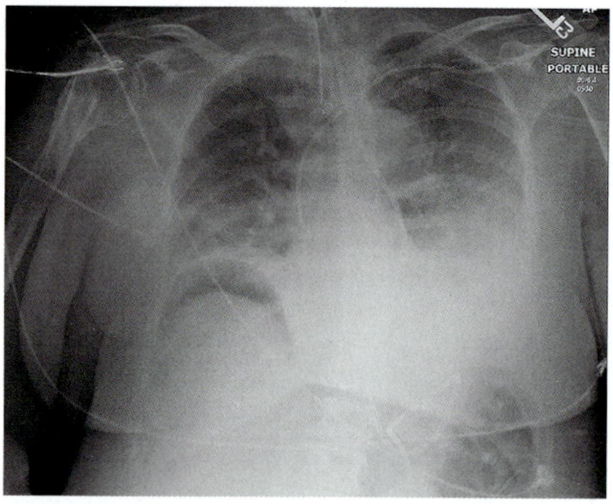

Figure 4.14 Patients may have an incidental finding of free air on abdominal plain radiographs immediately following PEG placement.

on abdominal plain radiographs immediately following PEG placement and should not in isolation cause alarm (**Figure 4.14**). Jejunal feeding tubes are typically placed in the operating room and provide long-term distal feeding access.

Complications following enteral access can include tube dislodgement and clogging (**Figure 4.15**). For patients with maturation of the tract, complete dislodgement can be temporized by placing a foley catheter down the tract. Confirmatory contrast study with bedside plain radiograph as well as aspiration of gastric contents should be performed. Rarely PEG tubes may inadvertently be placed through the transverse colon into the stomach. CT imaging is confirmatory with operation warranted. Jejunostomy tubes can result in bowel obstruction if kinked or twisted, so careful monitoring of examination and awareness of bowel function are important.

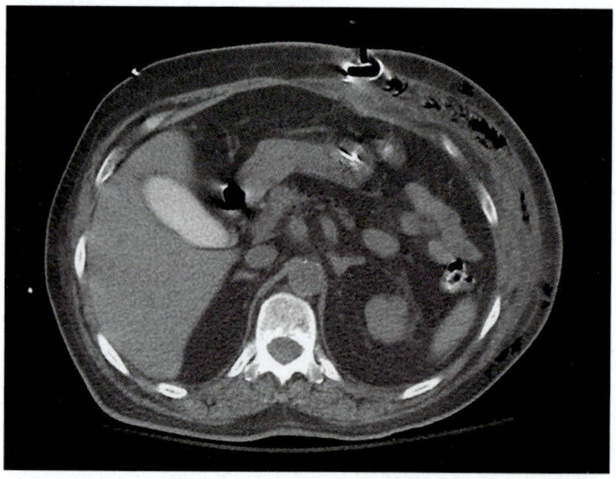

Figure 4.15 Following PEG placement, the tube may become dislodged with the flange (and tube feeds) in the subcutaneous tissue.

Routine wound care and examination should alert the team to the development of cellulitis or abscess formation.

POSTOPERATIVE PATIENT ON THE MICU SERVICE

At times, patients who have undergone surgery are managed by the MICU physicians, either for associated comorbidities or for the underlying medical diagnosis that resulted in an operative intervention. While there can be a wide variety of etiologies leading to primary management of a postoperative patient by the MICU service, the postoperative course of a patient should be relatively straightforward. The MICU intensivist should be aware of specifics of acute postoperative resuscitation, routine postoperative care, as well as potential postoperative complications.

On arrival to the MICU, patient assessment includes several critical components: (1) determination of current physiologic status; (2) delineation of operative course including vasopressor agents, resuscitation, and estimated blood loss (EBL); (3) pending imaging or diagnostics; and (4) past medical history. For patients who arrive in the MICU physiologically *in extremis*, resuscitation should optimize tissue perfusion, ensure normothermia, and correct coagulopathy. Initial volume loading with crystalloid or blood products as indicated should be the first measure followed by the use of vasopressors once adequate preload in ensured. Typically, resuscitation endpoints include normalization of arterial base deficit or serum lactate. During the acute resuscitation, low urine output is most likely related to hypovolemia, and diuretics should not be administered. Viscoelastic assays (TEG or ROTEM) facilitate blood product transfusion and limit immunologically active component therapy to only necessary agents. In turn, the risk of transfusion-associated lung injury and multiple organ failure should be lower. The intraoperative blood product transfusion requirements as well as the EBL can help the intensivist anticipate events in the postoperative period.

Despite operative intervention, patients may still require imaging or other diagnostic maneuvers following the OR. These may include CT imaging, endoscopy, angiography, or even repeat operation. Routine postadmission studies include laboratory studies and chest radiograph. The chest radiograph is important to determine central line catheter, endotracheal tube, NGT, or tube thoracostomy positions, as any of these could become dislodged with transport. Critical elements of a patient's past medical history include any conditions that impact the current care and resuscitation. These can include a history of cardiopulmonary disease, specifically any past myocardial infarctions, use of steroids or β-blockers, chronic hepatic failure, and chronic renal insufficiency or failure.

The operating surgeon must effectively communicate to the intensivist the critical intraoperative findings and procedures, including any tenuous operative repairs and location of drains. Anticipated problems or complications, including the potential for bleeding or potential for abscess development or even septic shock should be discussed. Although uncommon in MICU patients, there may be a need for open abdomen management or expected repeat operative exploration. Bleeding is the most common complication in the postoperative period; this is often heralded by a drop in hemoglobin or bloody output from drains placed during laparotomy. Substantial hemorrhage may cause hemodynamic instability and a persistent metabolic acidosis. Infectious complications typically occur 3-7 days following initial operative management and may include surgical site infection or deep space infection. An anastomotic leak with sepsis due to intra-abdominal contamination often results in fevers, generalized pain, and a leukocytosis; at times, respiratory distress with tachypnea may be the first sign of a postoperative enteric complication. CT imaging is diagnostic and operative intervention may be necessary. (See also Chapter 27.)

Following operative intervention, some general postoperative considerations should be discussed with the intensivists. For gastrointestinal conditions requiring a bowel anastomosis, one should ensure some return of bowel function prior to aggressive feeding. If an ileostomy or colostomy was created, this should be examined daily to evaluate for output and to ensure it is neither retracted nor ischemic in appearance. The laparotomy incision may be closed at the skin or may be managed with local wound care. Wounds should be examined daily to ensure there is no evidence of cellulitis or developing abscess. Drains are most commonly placed for abscess cavities or pancreatic procedures, less commonly for bowel resections. Intra-abdominal drains are most commonly closed suction drains such as Blake or Jackson-Pratt drains. The drain locations should be clearly communicated, and these are often left on bulb suction. The amount and character of drain output (blood, succus, bile, pus, etc.) should be recorded daily. Drain removal should be discussed with the surgeon. Finally need for antibiotics and duration of therapy will be dictated by the infectious condition and overall source control combined with the physiologic status of the patient. (See also Chapter 5.)

SURGICAL FUTILITY

There may be situations where operative management in a critically ill patient can be performed, but if it should be done is another challenging question. Taking time to discuss the risk and benefit of proceeding with an operation in a critically ill patient should be carefully considered with the patient and their family. There is, however, no clear definition of medical futility.

Emergency laparotomy is associated with a 14% mortality rate. However, patients with age >90, ASA class V, septic shock, dependent functional status, and abnormal WBC have <10% probability of survival according to a 5-year look at the NSQIP database. There are also certain patient populations that carry higher risk for emergency laparotomy procedures performed on patients in a cardiac or medical ICU, associated with a 71.4% and 70% mortality, respectively.

Early implementation of end-of-life decisions in the ICU setting can decrease the need for surgical intervention in the setting of death is certain, medical futility with minimal response to maximal care, and the presence of underlying malignancy. These discussions should include best-case and worst-case scenarios. Consideration of the patient's frailty and quality of life prior to the operation is vital. Criteria suggested for getting palliative care consultation when considering surgery in the ICU setting include family request, multisystem organ failure of >3 systems in a patient > 60 years old, when tracheostomy or PEG tube is needed in traumatic brain injury, carcinomatosis or unresectable malignancy, and >2 surgical ICU admissions during the same hospital stay. In the patient who is marginal, physician and family agreement to operative management on a time-limited postoperative course based on physiologic response may be a reasonable approach.

SUMMARY

With the increasing clinical complexity of patients admitted to intensive care units, the intensivist must have a low threshold to suspect and diagnose general surgical emergencies. General surgeons are consulted in up to 20% of ICU patients and perform operative interventions in 4%-5% of patients. A larger percentage of patients undergo interventional procedures including angioembolization, percutaneous drainage, and placement of feeding tubes. Postoperative mortality remains high if a surgical disease process is not recognized early. This chapter reviews the most common etiologies and suggests management approaches ranging from damage control resuscitation to definitive operative management. Equally important is the ability to recognize and discuss surgical futility with patients and families in a select subset of patients whose perioperative mortality is prohibitively high. A continued multidisciplinary approach to these complex patients is warranted.

SUGGESTED READINGS

Al-Temimi MH, Griffee M, Enniss TM, et al. When is death inevitable after emergency laparotomy? Analysis of the American College of Surgeons National Surgical Quality Improvement Program Database. *J Am Coll Surg*. 2012;215(4):503-511.

Anderson JE, Chang DC, Talamini MA. A nationwide examination of outcomes of percutaneous cholecystostomy compared with cholecystectomy for acute cholecystitis, 1998–2010. *Surg Endosc*. 2013;27:3406.

Barie PS, Eachempati SR. Acute acalculous cholecystitis. *Gastroenterol Clin North Am*. 2010;39:343.

Barkun AN, Almadi M, Kuipers EJ, et al. Management of nonvariceal upper gastrointestinal bleeding: guideline recommendations from the international consensus group. *Ann Intern Med*. 2019;171(11):805-822.

Bradley CT, Brasel KJ. Developing guidelines that identify patients who would benefit from palliative care services in the surgical intensive care unit. *Crit Care Med*. 2009;37(3):946-950.

Briggs A, Handzel RM, Kutcher ME, et al. Predisposed to failure? The challenge of rescue in the medical intensive care unit. *J Trauma Acute Care Surg*. 2019;87:774-781.

Briggs A, Rosengart MR. Acute abdomen in ICU patients. In: Peitzman AB, Yealy DM, Fabian TC, et al., eds. *The Trauma Manual*. Wolters Kluwer; 2020:651-660.

Callaway DW, Shapiro NI, Donnino MW, Baker C, Rosen CL. Serum lactate and base deficit as predictors of mortality in normotensive elderly blunt trauma patients. *J Trauma*. 2009;66(4):1040-1044.

Cudnik MT, Darbha S, Jones J, et al. The diagnosis of acute mesenteric ischemia: a systematic review and meta-analysis. *Acad Emerg Med*. 2013;20:1087.

Dellinger EP, Tellado JM, Soto NE, et al. Early antibiotic treatment for severe acute necrotizing pancreatitis: a randomized, double blind, placebo controlled study. *Ann Surg*. 2007;245:674-683.

Expert Panels on Vascular Imaging and Gastrointestinal Imaging; Singh-Bhinder N, Kim DH, Holly BP, et al. ACR appropriateness criteria® nonvariceal upper gastrointestinal bleeding. *J Am Coll Radiol*. 2017;14(5S):S177-S188.

Ferrada P, Callcut R, Zielinski MD, et al.; EAST Multi-Institutional Trials Committee. Loop ileostomy versus total colectomy as surgical treatment for *Clostridium difficile*-associated disease: an Eastern Association for the Surgery of Trauma multicenter trial. *J Trauma Acute Care Surg*. 2017;83(1):36-40.

Gonzalez E, Moore EE, Moore HB, Chapman MP, Silliman CC, Banerjee A. Trauma-induced coagulopathy: an institution's 35 year perspective on practice and research. *Scand J Surg*. 2014;103(2):89-103.

Gralnek IM, Dumonceau JM, Kuipers EJ, et al. Diagnosis and management of nonvariceal upper gastrointestinal hemorrhage: European Society of Gastrointestinal Endoscopy Guidelines. *Endoscopy*. 2015;47(10):a1-a46.

Grant SB, Modi PK, Singer EA. Futility and the care of surgical patients: ethical dilemmas. *World J Surg*. 2014;38(7):1631-1637.

Hasenboehler E, Williams A, Leinhase I, et al. Metabolic changes after polytrauma: an imperative for early nutritional support. *World J Emerg Surg*. 2006;1:29.

Kavitt RT, Lipowska AM, Anyane-Yeboa A, Gralnek IM. Diagnosis and treatment of peptic ulcer disease. *Am J Med*. 2019;132(4):447-456.

Kirkpatrick A, Roberts D, Waele J, et al. Intra-abdominal hypertension and the abdominal compartment syndrome: updated consensus definitions and clinical practice guidelines from the World Society of the Abdominal Compartment Syndrome. *Intensive Care Med*. 2013;39:1190-1206.

Kougias P, Lau D, El Sayed HF, et al. Determinants of mortality and treatment outcome following surgical interventions for acute mesenteric ischemia. *J Vasc Surg*. 2007;46:467.

Lee YL, Ong YY, Thong SY, et al. A retrospective study of end-of-life care decisions in the critically ill in a surgical intensive care unit. *Indian J Palliat Care*. 2018;24(1):17-24.

Martin ND, Sagar P, Chreiman K, et al. Emergency laparotomy in the critically ill: futile at the bedside. *Crit Care Res Pract*. 2018;2018:6398917.

Mofidi R, Duff MD, Wigmore SJ, Madhavan KK, Garden OJ, Parks RW. Association between early systemic inflammatory response, severity of multiorgan dysfunction and death in acute pancreatitis. *Br J Surg*. 2006;93(6):738.

Moore FA, McKinley BA, Moore EE, et al. Inflammation and the Host Response to Injury, a large-scale collaborative project: patient-oriented research core—standard operating procedures for clinical care. III. Guidelines for shock resuscitation. *J Trauma.* 2006;61:82-89.

Moore FA, Moore EE, Haenel JB. Clinical benefits of early post-injury enteral feeding. *Clin Intensive Care.* 1995;6:21-27.

Mounzer R, Langmead CJ, Wu BU, et al. Comparison of existing clinical scoring systems to predict persistent organ failure in patients with acute pancreatitis. *Gastroenterology.* 2012;142:1476.

Neal MD, Alverdy JC, Hall DE, Simmons RL, Zuckerbraun BS. Diverting loop ileostomy and colonic lavage: an alternative to total abdominal colectomy for the treatment of severe, complicated *Clostridium difficile* associated disease. *Ann Surg.* 2011;254(3):423-427.

Ouellet JF, Roberts DJ, Tiruta C, et al. Admission base deficit and lactate levels in Canadian patients with blunt trauma: are they useful markers of mortality? *J Trauma Acute Care Surg.* 2012;72(6):1532-1535.

Sanchez NC, Tenofsky PL, Dort JM, et al. What is normal intra-abdominal pressure? *Am Surg.* 2001;67:243.

Santvoort HC, Besselink MG, Bakker OJ, et al. A step-up approach or open necrosectomy for necrotizing pancreatitis. *N Engl J Med.* 2010;362:1491-1502.

Solomkin JS, Mazuski JE, Bradley JS, et al. Diagnosis and management of complicated intra-abdominal infection in adults and children: guidelines by the Surgical Infection Society and the Infectious Diseases Society of America. *Clin Infect Dis.* 2010;50:133.

Spira RM, Nissan A, Zamir O, et al. Percutaneous transhepatic cholecystostomy and delayed laparoscopic cholecystectomy in critically ill patients with acute calculus cholecystitis. *Am J Surg.* 2002;183:62.

Stanley AJ, Laine L. Management of acute upper gastrointestinal bleeding. *BMJ.* 2019;364:l536.

Wang A, Yerxa J, Agarwal S, et al. Surgical management of peptic ulcer disease. *Curr Probl Surg.* 2020;57(2):100728.

Zhao Y, Yin H, Yao C, et al. Management of acute mesenteric ischemia: a critical review and treatment algorithm. *Vasc Endovascular Surg.* 2016;50:183.

CHAPTER

5 Abdominal Sepsis

Scott C. Brakenridge, Mackenzie R. Cook, and David H. Livingston

CASE PRESENTATION

The patient is a 52-year-old male with no past medical history diagnosed with a tubular polyp in the sigmoid colon and a mass in his appendix. The polyp was not amenable to endoscopic removal, and he underwent a laparoscopy-assisted appendectomy and sigmoid colectomy. The final pathology returned noninvasive adenocarcinoma of the colon and a mucinous neoplasm of the appendix. On the night of postoperative day 2, the patient had an episode of atrial fibrillation with rapid ventricular response that was successfully treated. The cardiac evaluation was negative. Chest x-ray revealed bibasilar atelectasis, a large gastric bubble, and air in the splenic flexure of the colon. He was afebrile with a normal white blood cell count. He had passed no flatus or bowel movement, and abdominal examination revealed diffuse pain and distension without overt peritoneal signs. Surgical incision sites were dry and nonerythematous. Over the next 2 days, he was able to tolerate limited oral intake. On the night of postoperative day 4, the patient had a sudden increase in abdominal pain, tachycardia, and hypotension (systolic blood pressure of 80 mm Hg). He remained afebrile, but his repeat white blood cell count returned 3200/mm^3 with 35% bands. A chest radiograph demonstrated free air (**Figure 5.1**). He underwent an abdominal CT scan (**Figure 5.2**), which further delineated the free air (star). During an open laparotomy, a perforation of the left colon proximal to the anastomosis was identified. There was a large amount of inflammation throughout the left upper quadrant but no discrete abscess. During the operation, the patient required pressor support with vasopressin to maintain his blood pressure. The perforated section was resected, and a colostomy was created. The abdomen and skin were closed.

Over the next 48 hours, the patient was weaned from the vasopressors. Five days from the re-exploration, the ostomy was functional and oral intake was started. On reoperative day 6, he spiked a temperature to 101.8 °F (38.8 °C), and murky drainage was noted from the midline wound. The physical examination disclosed diffuse tenderness. The white blood cell count was 19 400/mm^3. An abdominal CT demonstrated fluid throughout the abdomen and within loops of the bowel (**Figures 5.3 and 5.4**). He returned to the operating room and at re-exploration, the abdominal closure was necrotic with evidence of fasciitis. The dissection was difficult, multiple intra-loop abscesses were identified, and murky fluid in the right and left gutters (arrows) was found. All collections grew multiple multidrug-resistant gram-negative organisms. Due to visceral edema and the need for debridement of the abdominal wall, the abdomen could not be closed and was left open. The viscera were covered with a hydrophilic sponge, and a negative pressure dressing was applied. On postoperative day 18 from the original re-exploration, succus was noted from the midline wound. The presence of a fistula without any further drainable fluid collection was confirmed on a CT scan (**Figures 5.5 and 5.6**).

Question: *What is the optimal diagnostic approach to initial and subsequent post-operative abdominal infection?*

Answer: *CT scanning, with appropriately timed contrast administration, remains the mainstay of radiologic diagnosis. In post-operative patients, the most important mindset is to have a high index of suspicion in any patient that is not progressing appropriately following a laparotomy. Lastly, there remains a group of patients who have signs and features of abdominal infection but whose CT scan is "not positive" where abdominal exploration is the diagnostic modality of choice.*

Question: *What is the optimal approach to source control?*

Answer: *The goal of source control is to fully and completely evacuate infected fluid, debride or remove infected or dead tissue, remove infected devices or foreign bodies, and control enteric spillage. The optimal approach is guided by the patient's physiology and the findings on radiologic imaging or at* *laparotomy. In some patients, one percutaneous drain will suffice where others may require multiple open interventions over several days.*

Question: *What is the optimal timing of re-exploration/intervention?*

Answer: *The optimal timing of re-exploration is often as soon as the infection is diagnosed or suspected. Ideally, this should be prior to any end-organ dysfunction is apparent.*

Question: *What is the role of damage control in patients with abdominal sepsis?*

Answer: *The use of damage control laparotomy in patients with abdominal sepsis remains controversial. In almost all cases it is better to close the peritoneal cavity and treat any subsequent infection as needed. However there does remain a small subset of patients whose deranged physiology and/or visceral edema preclude closing the abdomen. In these patients, damage control techniques may be lifesaving. The goal in these patient should be to achieve abdominal closure as soon as possible*

Question: *How best to manage the fistula?*

Answer: *The management of fistulae include control of effluent and delivery of adequate nutritional (preferably enteral) support and fluid and management.*

INTRODUCTION

The diagnosis and treatment of abdominal infection are some of the defining features of emergency general surgery. The breadth and scope of potential abdominal infections that challenge the emergency general surgeon are large and varied. The goal of this chapter is to provide a general understanding of the optimal diagnostic and treatment strategies for intraabdominal infection that challenge acute care surgeons.

DEFINITIONS AND TYPES OF INTRA-ABDOMINAL INFECTIONS

Intra-abdominal infections have been defined and characterized using several schemas. The simplest and most straightforward is dividing them into uncomplicated or complicated infections. *Uncomplicated intra-abdominal infections* are confined to the pathologic organ (eg, acute appendicitis or cholecystitis). While not part of this definition, physiologic perturbations are generally uncommon. The diagnostic and therapeutic approaches to organ-specific abdominal infectious processes are covered in depth in other chapters. *Complicated infections*, by comparison, involve tissues and organs beyond the initial site of infection into the peritoneal cavity. Complicated intra-abdominal infections most commonly are accompanied by more significant physiologic abnormalities and patients typically present with a degree of peritonitis. Although simple, this dichotomy does little to aid the surgeon in determining the optimal diagnostic and treatment for an individual patient.

Peritonitis can be defined as primary, secondary, or tertiary (persistent). Primary peritonitis is bacterial contamination of the normally sterile peritoneal fluid without an obvious break in the

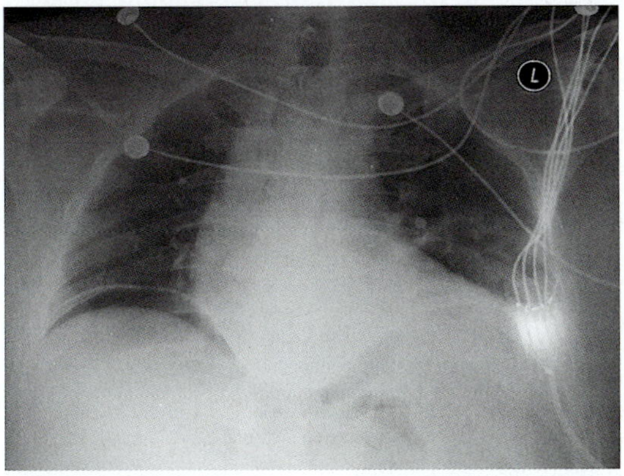

Figure 5.1 Upright chest x-ray demonstrating a large amount of free air between the liver and the right hemidiaphragm.

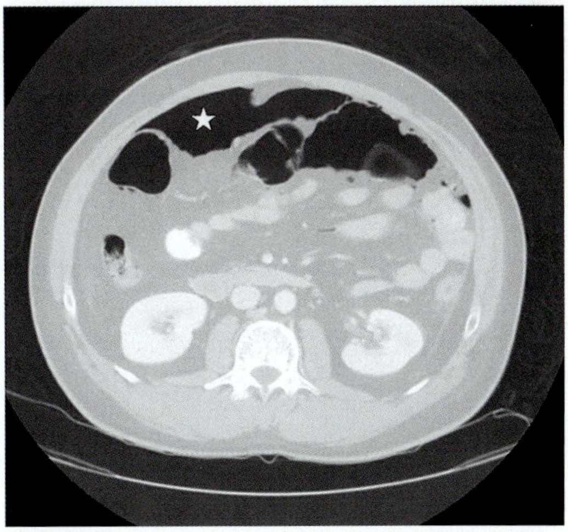

Figure 5.2 CT scan further demonstrating extensive free air (*star*) distinct from the air within the intestinal lumen.

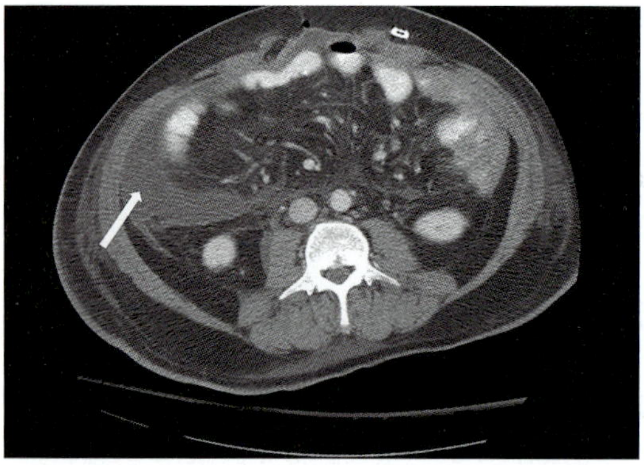

Figure 5.3 CT scan demonstrating an extensive amount of fluid in the right gutter (*arrow*) and inflammation within the mesentery.

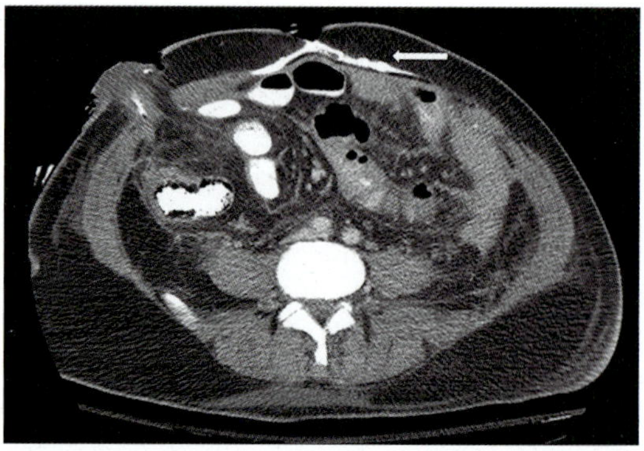

Figure 5.5 CT scan demonstrating extravasation of contrast from the midline wound (*arrow*) confirming the presence of a leak and fistula. There are no drainable collections noted.

integrity of the bowel or abdominal walls. Most commonly encountered as spontaneous bacterial peritonitis in patients with advanced liver disease, the management usually includes antibiotics and ascites mitigation. There is a rare need for a source control procedure. Historically, pathologic organisms include gram-negative bacteria with an increasing incidence of gram-positive, quinolone resistant, and multidrug resistant bacteria. Spontaneous bacterial peritonitis in this group is associated with poor long-term survival and a 60% mortality at 1 year following the first episode.

Secondary peritonitis most commonly occurs due to a breach in the gastrointestinal tract wall or occasionally through significant external contamination secondary to traumatic abdominal wall injury. Secondary peritonitis accounts for about 1% of urgent or emergent hospital admissions worldwide and is the second most common cause of sepsis in the intensive care unit (ICU) setting (pulmonary sepsis is most common). Up to 20% of patients with secondary peritonitis will develop organ failure with an overall mortality of 6%. Pathologic organisms typically include aerobic and anaerobic bacteria usually with relatively benign antibiotic resistance patterns.

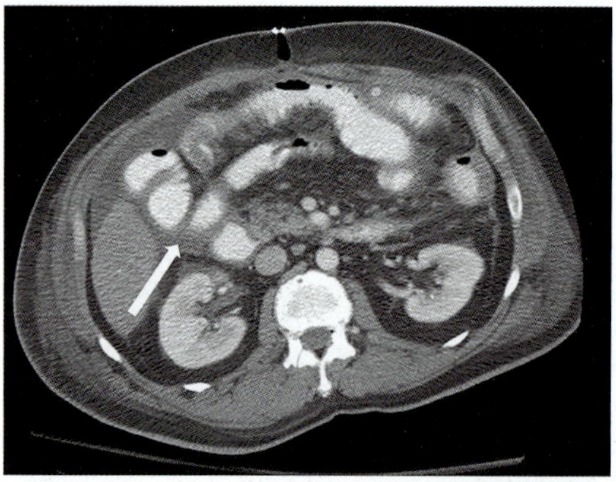

Figure 5.4 Another image from the same CT scan as **Figure 5.3** demonstrating fluid is also present within loops of bowel (*arrow*).

Tertiary peritonitis (persistent peritonitis) is a pathologic entity on a spectrum from secondary peritonitis. It is defined as the persistence or recurrence of an intra-abdominal infection following presumed adequate treatment (ie, appropriate antibiotics and source control) of primary or secondary peritonitis. As opposed to secondary peritonitis, pathologic organisms in tertiary peritonitis often reflect the patient's hospital course. They typically include resistant gram-negative bacilli as well as resistant *Enterococcus*, *Staphylococcus*, and fungal species. As with secondary peritonitis, tertiary peritonitis frequently requires source control procedures and, in surgical patients, the need for complex fistula and wound management are not uncommon. The case presented demonstrates many of these aspects of secondary and tertiary peritonitis.

In addition to the anatomic and pathologic components, the patient's physiologic status is

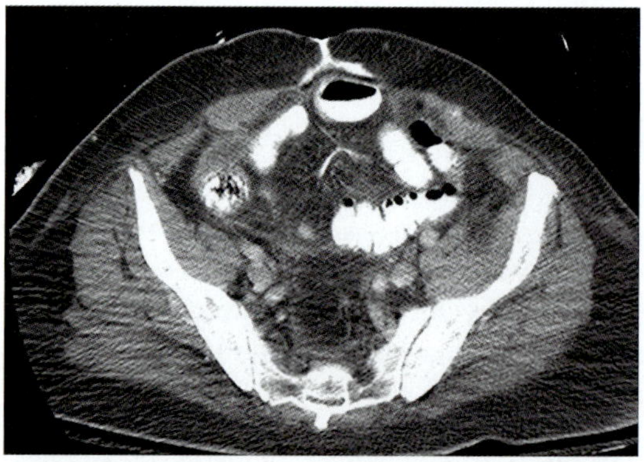

Figure 5.6 Another image from the same CT scan as **Figure 5.5** demonstrating the fistula and the leak.

essential when categorizing and describing intra-abdominal infections. The degree of physiologic compromise associated with the intra-abdominal infection not only drives the urgency of source control but the range of diagnostic and therapeutic options. Sepsis is a heterogeneous clinical syndrome, and the clinical priority is recognizing patients at risk for deterioration. The Third International Consensus Definitions for Sepsis and Septic Shock (Sepsis-3) was published in 2016 (**Table 5.1**). The recommendations and updated definitions replaced the previous definitions that were detailed in the Surviving Sepsis Campaign guidelines. Within the structure of Sepsis-3, sepsis is a life-threatening organ dysfunction caused by a dysregulated host immune system. This is clinically recognized as an increase in the Sequential Organ Failure Assessment (SOFA) score by 2 or more points. Septic shock is defined as a state of profound physiologic perturbation with severe circulatory, cellular, and metabolic abnormalities. It is recognized clinically by the need for vasopressors to maintain a mean arterial pressure (MAP) ≥65 mm Hg and a serum lactate >2 mmol/L.

The SOFA score, while helpful from a research perspective, is difficult to quickly calculate, as it requires information on six physiologic systems: respiratory, coagulation, liver, cardiovascular, central nervous system, and renal, all scored across a 0-4 range. Far more useful at the bedside is the quick SOFA (qSOFA). This score helps identify patients who are at risk for poor outcomes. A high-risk patient is recognized if presenting with ≥2 of the following: respiratory rate ≥22/minute, altered mental status (eg, Glasgow coma score <15), or systolic blood pressure of <100 mm Hg. The qSOFA is used to prompt additional investigations and not replace the complete SOFA score as physiologic data become available. Importantly, the astute clinician should not defer further workup of a potentially infected patient if the SOFA/qSOFA threshold is not met, as neither score was intended to be a stand-alone definition of sepsis.

TABLE 5.1 ■ Sepsis-3 Consensus Criteria

- Sepsis is defined as life-threatening organ dysfunction caused by a dysregulated host response to infection.
- Organ dysfunction can be identified as an acute change in total SOFA score ≥2 points consequent to the infection.
- Septic shock is a subset of sepsis in which underlying circulatory and cellular/metabolic abnormalities are profound enough to substantially increase mortality.
- Patients with septic shock are those with persisting hypotension requiring vasopressors to maintain MAP ≥65 mm Hg and serum lactate level >2 mmol/L (18 mg/dL) despite adequate volume resuscitation.

DIAGNOSTIC APPROACH TO ABDOMINAL INFECTIOUS PROCESSES

Clinical Examination

The diagnostic approach to a patient with a suspected intra-abdominal infection begins with a careful history and physical examination. In patients presenting with obvious peritonitis and septic shock—little else is required to proceed to the operating room. History is invaluable as it provides critical clinical information about the duration and severity of the symptoms, the type of any recent or remote surgery, and the patient's prehospital nutritional and functional status.

While the approach to patients presenting to the emergency department with abdominal pathology may be straightforward, the identification of abdominal infection in patients following recent abdominal surgery is more nuanced and complicated. The aim in this group is to identify those at risk for physiologic decline and intervene before peritonitis and physiologic collapse occur, that is, *surgical rescue.* (See Chapter 27: Surgical Complications and Surgical Rescue.) This hinges on repeated and detailed history and physical examinations throughout the hospital course and prompt recognition of subtle changes that may portent future complications. Often these patients "fall off" of the expected trajectory of recovery. In the case presented, the early physiologic derangements followed by a slow return of bowel function were subtle signs of the subsequent peritonitis from the colonic perforation. At any point in time along this trajectory, the patient may "look okay"; however, the astute clinician will notice the warning signs. When the entire course is considered, it becomes clear that the recovery has stalled, or the patient is deteriorating. In patients with tertiary peritonitis, these signs can even be more difficult to determine when the start of therapy and the aid of further diagnostic studies are often necessary.

The physical examination of a patient with an abdominal infectious process remains critically important and influenced by an understanding of the dual innervation of the abdomen. The parietal peritoneum is innervated by somatic and visceral afferent nerves and receives sensory branches from the lower intercostal and upper lumbar nerves. The visceral peritoneum is not innervated *per se*, but the subperitoneal tissue is innervated through the sympathetic and parasympathetic fibers. The visceral peritoneum is driven by distension and chemical irritation, interpreted as deep, poorly localized or periumbilical pain and pressure. This is often paroxysmal and described as "colicky." The most common example is observed in patients with early appendicitis. In the case presented here, the ongoing abdominal discomfort in the early postoperative period was related to the colonic ischemia that preceded the frank perforation. However, the parietal peritoneum is sensitive to laceration, temperature, and pressure, experienced as a sharp, constant, and localized pain with rigidity of local muscle groups. Inflammation that progresses and involves the parietal peritoneum results in reflexive muscle rigidity and physical examination maneuvers, causing the parietal peritoneum to contact intra-abdominal pathology, resulting in localized pain and tenderness. Again, this is classically observed later in appendicitis when the inflammation progress and the pain becomes localized in the right lower quadrant. In contrast to palpation, auscultation in the physical examination of acute abdominal pain has little role.

The validity and reliability of the physical examination in abdominal infectious processes do not appear to be limited by early prescription of opioids, and analgesia should not be delayed for a patient in acute pain. A reliable physical examination will be valid even with prior dosing of narcotics. However, the reliability of the physical examination may be degraded in patients with morbid obesity or significant immunosuppression. Within this population, sinus tachycardia may be the only physical examination finding suggestive of a progressive intra-abdominal catastrophe. Great care should be taken when examining these patients with concern for intra-abdominal infection.

Laboratory Testing

The results from most laboratory studies are nonspecific and often inappropriately weighted in clinical decision-making. Except for serum lipase in the diagnosis of acute pancreatitis, most laboratory values provide greater insight into the patient's physiologic status than the presence or etiology of the intra-abdominal infection. While it is beyond the scope of this chapter to describe the utility of every laboratory test in the evaluation of an abdominal infectious process, a few specific tests warrant mention:

- Procalcitonin: In a noninflamed status, procalcitonin is selectively synthesized in the thyroid, although in the setting of bacterially induced inflammation, procalcitonin synthesis is induced in many tissues. This has led to its use in nonsurgical populations to help distinguish between bacterial and nonbacterial infections. The nonspecific nature of procalcitonin and its potential elevation due to trauma or surgery limit its routine use in the diagnosis and management of secondary and tertiary peritonitis.
- Lactate: An elevated lactate has been associated with mortality in septic surgical patients and is a reliable, nonspecific marker of compromised physiology. There are two types of lactic acidosis. Type A acidosis represents an increase in serum lactate due to anaerobic metabolism driven by impaired perfusion resulting from hypovolemia, cardiac failure, distributive shock, or cardiac arrest. Type B lactic acidosis is **NOT** driven by tissue hypoperfusion but by a variety of other biochemical mechanisms. Most pertinently in the acutely ill, β-adrenergic stimulation occurs with endogenous or exogenous epinephrine. While not proven, the proposed mechanism is that high-level β-adrenergic stimulation increases glycolysis in skeletal muscles, resulting in pyruvate conversion to lactate while decreasing hepatic uptake of serum lactate. Thus, in Type B, lactate concentrations are unrelated to tissue perfusion status. It may be that the lactic acidosis seen early in sepsis is a Type B lactic acidosis, or at least mixed type A and B, driven by high levels of endogenous β-adrenergic stimulation.
- Base deficit: The base deficit is a calculated and derived measurement expressed on arterial blood gas analysis and reflects the amount of base that must be added to a sample to return to a normal pH. More useful than the pH in assessing the degree of metabolic acidosis, the base deficit is not subject to the compensatory mechanisms designed to moderate changes in pH. As with lactate, the base deficit has utility in stratifying patients along a spectrum of physiologic derangement. In contrast to its use in patients with hemorrhagic shock, the base deficit is too nonspecific to aid in the diagnosis of a specific intra-abdominal problem.

Imaging

The search for a potential abdominal source of infection usually involves imaging to confirm a clinically suspected diagnosis and guide management options. It is important and needs to be continually emphasized that preoperative imaging is

NOT required in a patient with sepsis and clinically suspected intra-abdominal infection.

While most often nonspecific and nondiagnostic, plain upright and lateral decubitus x-rays are easy to obtain. As with the case presented, these studies are useful if positive (see **Figure 5.1**). The presence of free air is diagnostic of intestinal perforation; these patients require no further investigation, and the initial CT scan (see **Figure 5.2**) in our case was unnecessary. These radiographs in optimal circumstances can demonstrate as little as 1 mL of extra-luminal air. However, the sensitivity of the plain radiograph for free air can be variable, ranging from 30% to 89%, likely reflecting variations in technique, exposure, and interpretation.

In most patients, the diagnostic modality of choice is a high-quality computed tomography (CT) scan of the abdomen. A complete study should include the lower chest and the entire pelvis. Advanced imaging has an increasingly important role in patients with alterations in consciousness, significant obesity, or underlying immunosuppression as the diagnostic utility of the history and physical examination in these patients is degraded. There is no doubt that CT imaging revolutionized and radically changed the diagnostic and treatment options of intraabdominal infections. CT allows grading of infections such as in perforated diverticulitis and can easily differentiate patients with localized and contained perforations, which can be managed with antibiotics and percutaneous drains from those with more advanced disease requiring an emergent sigmoid colectomy.

One important caveat concerning advanced imaging is the physiologic state of the patient. The decision to transport a critically ill patient out of their current care site (ie, the ICU) should not be taken lightly. Careful consideration must be given as to the information gained by the study versus the risk of moving the patient for the study. In critically ill patients, particularly those with complicated tertiary peritonitis or profound septic shock, the rate of adverse events and clinical misadventures during intrahospital transportation is high. In patients with high suspicion for abdominal pathology and profound instability, presumptive laparotomy in the ICU may be the best diagnostic and therapeutic option.

While all the details of CT scan interpretation are beyond the scope of this chapter, the use of oral and intravenous (IV) contrast in patients with suspected abdominal infection warrants additional discussion. Noncontrast CT scans should be used sparingly, if at all, because their diagnostic yield in this population is minimal. Thus, they may pose a significant risk without benefit. Oral contrast requires a period between administration and imaging, which may delay intervention. Its use may not be advisable in the emergent setting. In addition, for most patients, oral contrast does not add to the diagnostic value of the study. Oral contrast is useful for patients with possible bowel obstruction or suspected contained anastomotic leaks and to help delineate the nature, course, and features of enterocutaneous and enteroatmospheric fistulae (see **Figure 5.6**). In contrast, IV contrast significantly improves the diagnostic accuracy of a CT scan of the abdomen and pelvis. Fears of renal toxicity have historically limited the use of IV contrast in patients with acute and chronic renal dysfunction. This concern has been debunked with the use of modern contrast agents. Renal failure attributed to the use of contrast is far more likely due to untreated sepsis, even in the setting of preexisting acute kidney injury.

The surgeon should always review the CT scans and correlate them to their understanding of the patient's anatomy and condition. Consultation with a skilled radiologist is invaluable, and direct communication between the surgeon and the radiologist is strongly encouraged as this combination often leads to greater clinical insight. As a note of caution, CT imaging in the early postoperative period can be misleading. It can be exceedingly difficult to differentiate benign and pathologic free fluid and inflammation. When there is clinical suspicion for complications and/or ongoing infectious processes in the early postoperative period, the surgeon should not be assuaged by an otherwise "negative" CT scan. Readers are encouraged to think of CT scans without identified pathology in this setting as "not positive" rather than "negative."

A few specific CT findings warrant additional comments. As CT imaging technology has improved, increasing numbers of patients have small volume pneumoperitoneum despite being asymptomatic. A patient presenting with any abdominal pain and pneumoperitoneum should be considered to have a perforated viscus and treated accordingly. Asymptomatic patients with no abdominal pathology, except for a small volume pneumoperitoneum, should be observed for a short period. The etiology of the pneumoperitoneum is often unknown but benign. Similar to small volume pneumoperitoneum, emergency general surgeons are frequently asked to evaluate an increasing number of patients who have *pneumatosis intestinalis* identified on CT scanning. Gas within the wall of the bowel or the portal venous system may portend a very ominous diagnosis and be the only radiographic correlate of bowel ischemia. Pneumatosis with elevated lactate (>2.0 mmol/L) can be associated with up to an 80% mortality rate. While there are benign explanations for incidentally discovered pneumatosis (eg, chronic obstructive pulmonary disease, cystic fibrosis, immunosuppression with atrophy of Peyer patches, unknown, etc.), distinguishing between pathologic and benign causes of pneumatosis can be difficult on radiographic imaging alone. This highlights the importance of correlating history and physical examination. In a multicenter study from the American Association for the Surgery of Trauma, 62% of patients had benign disease; however, those with elevated lactate and small bowel pneumatosis and those with peritoneal signs were more likely to have full-thickness necrosis. Ultrasound evaluation in patients with a suspected intra-abdominal infection is primarily used when there is concern for biliary or renal etiology due to its ability to identify biliary tract stones, dilated ducts or collecting systems, and perihepatic or perinephric fluid collections. Bowel edema, bowel gas, and abdominal wall edema often limit additional evaluations in the acute setting.

Magnetic resonance imaging (MRI) is of limited utility in the acute evaluation of abdominal infection. While occasionally used in evaluating pregnant patients with suspected appendicitis, there is limited utility for this imaging modality in the acute setting due to the time required for image acquisition.

TREATMENT

The fundamental goals in the treatment of abdominal sepsis are the administration of broad-spectrum antibiotics and volume resuscitation followed by obtaining adequate source control (**Table 5.2**). In some patients, a transfer to the ICU for a "few hours" of initial resuscitation to restore end-organ perfusion and improve the patient's overall physiologic state takes precedence over immediate surgical source control. This is especially true of patients in septic shock. Evidence-based sepsis protocols to restore physiology have been shown to decrease the absolute risk of sepsis mortality by as much as 10%. However, what constitutes a "few hours" is similarly important, and it needs to be emphasized that restoration of "normal physiology is not the goal. It should be possible, and in fact, necessary to improve a patient's physiology over a relatively short period (<2-4 hours) of initial resuscitation as most patients will not regain normal physiology until sometime after source control is achieved. This was observed in the case presented where vasopressor support could not be weaned for 48 hours. A reasonable assessment that adequate initial resuscitation has been achieved is objective repletion of hypovolemia or achieving a steady state of vasopressor titration. It should also be recognized that some patients will never improve without source control.

TABLE 5.2 ■ Approach to Abdominal Sepsis

- Blood cultures drawn prior to antibiotics
- Antibiotics infused within 1 hour of presentation to the hospital
- Broad spectrum antibiotics, active against enteric organisms
- Fluid resuscitation and support of organ function
  - Avoid excessive fluid resuscitation
    - Add vasopressors if the patient is hypotensive after fluid resuscitation to maintain ≥MAP 65 mm Hg (first-line: norepinephrine; second-line: vasopressin)
- Expeditious source control

Following resuscitation, the next priority is to achieve adequate source control. Source control is defined as "any and all means necessary to eradicate a focus of infection, as well as modification of factors that maintain the infection, such as leaking intestinal contents." This stage aims to evacuate infected fluid, debride or remove infected or dead tissue, remove infected devices or foreign bodies, and control enteric spillage. This may be achieved by percutaneous or operative intervention depending on the size, location, and source of the infection. The appropriate choice of source control intervention may be significantly affected by the timing of the event from any index operative procedure or pathologic event. Depending on the underlying cause and the patient's ongoing condition, serial interventions may be required to achieve complete and definitive source control over several days.

Percutaneous Drainage

The introduction of image-guided percutaneous drainage in the 1980s revolutionized the management of surgical infections. In many cases, percutaneous drainage is considered first-line therapy for the management of infected abdominal fluid collections. General requirements for this approach include a fluid collection that is localized and well-defined, along with a safe anatomic window for percutaneous access. Examples of abdominal infections that are well managed by

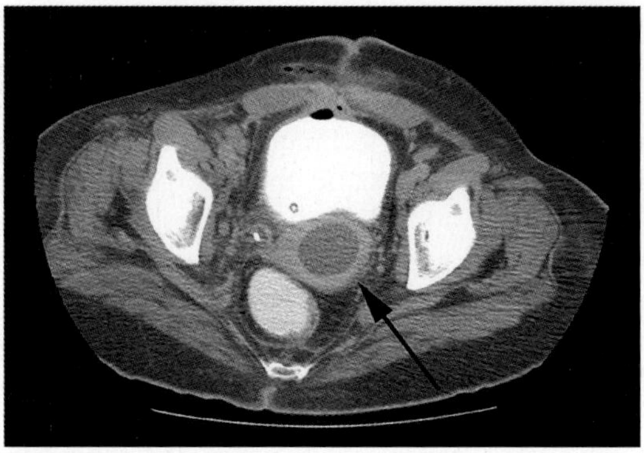

Figure 5.7 Pelvic abscess following ruptured appendicitis (*arrow*). Note the contained unilocular abscess with a thick wall. This is the ideal abscess for percutaneous drainage.

percutaneous drainage include Hinchey Ib or II diverticulitis, postsplenectomy abscess, and post-appendectomy pelvic abscess (**Figure 5.7**). Gross intestinal spillage, multiloculated fluid collections, or inter loop abscesses of the intestines (as in the case presented) are commonly not amenable to adequate source control by percutaneous drainage. These infections need to be treated by more invasive approaches (ie, laparoscopy or laparotomy). It is important to consider the underlying cause of the infected fluid collection, as percutaneous drainage alone may be inadequate when the source is due to intestinal perforation or necrotic tissue. Patients with generalized peritonitis, massive free air, or septic shock often are best served using a prompt open operative approach. However, percutaneous drainage can be the safest initial management option for ongoing intestinal spillage in patients with a hostile "frozen" abdomen or in special circumstances such as low rectal anastomotic leaks. Percutaneous drainage achieves initial source control in these situations by allowing external decompression of enteric contents until either the leak seals or a mature fistula tract develops.

Laparoscopy

Laparoscopy is now a standard skill set for general surgeons, so it is not surprising that the breadth and scope of laparoscopic approaches to intra-abdominal diagnosis and source control continue to increase. While CT imaging has become the gold-standard diagnostic modality for acute intra-abdominal processes, in the stable and resuscitated patient, laparoscopy can often provide diagnostic confirmation as well as definitive intervention. A laparoscopic approach requires a degree of hemodynamic stability, as under-resuscitated patients may not tolerate pneumoperitoneum due to decreased cardiac performance. Additionally, laparoscopic procedures may be limited by the patient's past or recent surgical history. Abdominal entry and achieving adequate surgical exposure in the setting of severe adhesive disease can be limited or impossible. Severe abdominal distension also can make laparoscopic procedures difficult due to the inability to create sufficient pneumoperitoneum. The highest yield for diagnostic laparoscopy is in the naive, acute abdomen when CT imaging does not yield a definitive diagnosis. This can be observed in some patients with perforated peptic ulcer disease, where CT findings may be vague, with findings of free air and fluid but without definitive identification of the source of perforation. Once identified, anterior duodenal perforations are particularly amenable to laparoscopic repairs, such as a modified Graham patch technique. In multiloculated or intraloop abscesses not amenable to percutaneous drainage laparoscopy may be useful, especially in those due to complex diverticular disease or late appendicitis. Laparoscopic unroofing of abscess cavities, washout, and drain placement is commonly successful and effective. However, laparoscopic intervention for some indications remains controversial. Studies evaluating the use of laparoscopic washout and drainage for perforated (Hinchey III or IV) diverticulitis have shown mixed results. (See also Chapter 18: GI Inflammatory Diseases.)

The utility of laparoscopic approaches to intra-abdominal source control in the postoperative period varies depending on the stability of the septic patient, the nature of the initial operation, and the timing of needed intervention from the index procedure. Early reoperative laparoscopy for washout and drain placement after an index laparoscopic procedure can be a safe and effective option. Examples include laparoscopic washout and drainage of an infected postcholecystectomy subhepatic biloma or source control or drain placement in an early bariatric roux-en-y gastric pouch leak. In contrast, a laparoscopic approach to multiple interloop abscesses in a patient 2 weeks after laparotomy for feculent peritonitis is unlikely to be safe or effective. A postoperative patient with diffuse peritonitis, septic shock, and suspected or confirmed abdominal source should be managed with an emergent laparotomy. Overall, laparoscopic approaches to intra-abdominal sepsis diagnosis and source control in the stable patient are reasonable but must be tailored to the individual situation.

Open Laparotomy and the Role of "Damage Control Surgery" in Sepsis

Laparotomy remains the gold standard for patients in septic shock from an intraabdominal source. Open laparotomy is also the approach of choice for ongoing gross intestinal spillage, necrotic bowel, or other tissue necrosis requiring resection or debridement. The extent of the operation performed is dictated by the patient's physiologic status and the organs involved. The primary goal of the initial operation is complete drainage of abscesses, infected fluid or succus, control of intestinal spillage, and resection of dead or devitalized tissues. After the evacuation of free peritoneal fluid or succus, the first task is identifying an inciting source of intestinal perforation. In cases of intraabdominal infection without an obvious perforation, unroofing and drainage of all abscess cavities and infected fluid collections is likely adequate. Most commonly, this will identify the likely source of the infection. The role of leaving intraperitoneal drains in these situations remains controversial and is based more on surgical dogma than evidence-based medicine. In our opinion, drains are ineffective at preventing subsequent abscess formation.

In most cases, intestinal perforation should be managed by bowel resection. It is often helpful to temporarily control intestinal spillage with a figure-of-eight stitch or Babcock clamp while completing the initial exploration. While it is tempting it is to "simply close" a small bowel or colon perforation, the inflamed and edematous bowel will break down resulting in a second leak. The perforated segment needs to be resected. The primary exception to this rule is in duodenal perforation, where a modified Graham patch or equivalent procedure is the operation of choice. Bowel resection should be the procedure of choice in *de novo* intestinal perforations at or distal to the Ligament of Treitz. In the proximal jejunum, perform resection and primary anastomosis. Management after resection of distal small bowel or colonic perforation is more nuanced. The surgeon must consider the risk-to-benefit ratio of anastomosis compared to the creation of an ostomy. Remember that the anastomosis never made will never leak! The presence of healthy, perfused, and non-inflamed bowel is an absolute necessity for creating a primary anastomosis in these settings. A primary anastomosis with diverting ileostomy may be considered in patients who are not in shock and with localized inflammatory (usually diverticular) disease for selected colonic resections. In other cases, primary colostomy should be the operation of choice. (See Chapter 18: GI Inflammatory Diseases.)

There continues to be debate and controversy over the preferred technique of stapled versus handsewn anastomosis in the emergency setting. Several observational studies suggest an equivalence between stapled and handsewn anastomosis in the emergency setting. These studies suffer from surgeon and inclusion bias. Most staplers were not designed for edematous and inflamed bowel, and most experienced surgeons choose to perform handsewn anastomoses in this setting. Additionally, the patient's hemodynamic stability and physiologic state need to be considered in determining whether to perform any intestinal reconstruction during the index procedure or in subsequent operations.

The benefit of damage control surgery (DCS) was first recognized in severely injured patients in hemorrhagic shock. This concept has been broadened to include patients with abdominal sepsis. In this setting, DCS includes obtaining control of intestinal spillage, resecting devascularized or grossly necrotic tissues, and performing a temporary abdominal closure (TAC) to prioritize physiologic resuscitation in the ICU. Definitive anatomic reconstruction is deferred to subsequent operations following the restoration of the patient's physiologic state. While DCS is life-saving for trauma patients in hemorrhagic shock, its usage and benefit in patients undergoing laparotomy for intraabdominal sepsis remain ill defined. Deferring intestinal reconstruction after initial source control until after the patient's physiologic resuscitation is restored is a reasonable extrapolation from the trauma experience.

In contrast to trauma, there may be a temptation to defer definitive management and abdominal closure of an otherwise stable patient because of perceived "gross contamination and ongoing inflammation." The peritoneal cavity and contents may appear less hospitable to the surgeon during subsequent take-back operations than the initial procedure due to fibrinous exudate from the post-sepsis inflammatory response. These patients are at higher risk of being left with an "open abdomen," as bowel edema and fascial retraction progress over subsequent days. The rate of failed abdominal fascial closure requiring management of the open abdomen is higher in patients with intra-abdominal sepsis than severe trauma. Thus, while DCS remains a key component of the surgical strategy to the surgical patient in septic shock, a diligent and aggressive approach to obtain abdominal closure as quickly as possible is safe and feasible.

The best results are achieved using a protocol-driven approach accepting residual inflammation in the absence of ongoing enteric spillage to the rapidly closure of the open abdomen. Thus, close the abdomen at the index procedure and reexplore the abdomen only when clinical changes mandate another operation—*re-laparotomy on demand*. On the other hand, indications for a planned reexploration are appropriate when: (1) source control cannot be achieved at the first operation, (2) significant visceral edema or the presence of abdominal packs prohibit abdominal closure, (3) the patient's physiology does not tolerate abdominal closure, (4) concern for viability of the bowel due to ischemic changes, or (5) planned "deferred anastomosis."

It is critical to note that the abdominal microbiome changes with the number of operations for persistent peritonitis. Although culturing the abdominal contents at the index operation for feculent peritonitis has little utility, culture of the abdominal contents at subsequent operations is necessary. Fewer gram-positive cocci and anaerobes will be found, with increasing emergence of multidrug-resistant gram-negative rods, MRSA, and fungi and the need for adjusting antibiotics based on these repeated cultures. Importantly, the repeated cultures also allow de-escalation of antibiotics. If source control is achieved, 4 days of antibiotics should suffice. In patients with evidence of ongoing infection, the approach to antibiotics must be individualized. If the patient has signs of ongoing infection after 5-7 days of approach antibiotics, search for an undrained source.

Achieving definitive source control in the septic patient due to a postoperative complication such as an anastomotic leak or iatrogenic injury can be extremely challenging. Especially if it has been several days from the index procedure and/or the entire peritoneum and bowel is severely inflamed due to prolonged exposure to intestinal spillage. Dense inflammatory intestinal adhesions and friable tissues are a setup for creating additional enterotomies during the operative exposure. Often the offending area of the bowel cannot be safely or adequately mobilized to perform an adequate resection. As outlined previously, when an intestinal anastomotic leak is the offending source, it is often tempting to close or imbricate the leak with a few simple sutures. However, this is almost always fails, and a recurrent leak is a near certainty. In cases where the initial repair attempt fails or in the postoperative "frozen abdomen" setting, it may not be possible to achieve definitive surgical source control. In these situations, the goal becomes controlling the intestinal effluent with the primary purpose of creating a controlled fistula.

Enterocutaneous and Enteroatmospheric Fistulas

While the development of a fistula is not a perfect outcome, it is preferable to ongoing peritoneal sepsis. With diligence and care, these patients will recover and may regain intestinal continuity without subsequent operation. Although a complete discussion of the pathophysiology of intestinal fistulas and their management is beyond the scope of this chapter, there are essential concepts for emergency general surgeons to understand. In most cases, the acute care surgeon will not be dealing with fistulas secondary to cancer, radiation, or inflammatory bowel disease. These fistulas are specifically difficult to manage and rarely close spontaneously. For the acute care surgeon, the need to create or manage a fistula is most commonly following drainage of an abscess or a perforation or in the setting of a frozen abdomen where resection and reconstruction are not possible. In these cases, the pressure differential between the intestinal lumen and the outside world will keep the fistula open. As long as it takes less "effort" due to a lower pressure gradient for the intestinal content to come out of the fistula tract, the fistula will remain open. The volume of fluid has no bearing on subsequent closure rates. Understanding this simple concept will help the acute care surgeon manage these challenging patients. The difference between an enterocutaneous and enteroatmospheric fistula is the presence of an intact abdominal wall. In the former, the abdominal wall acts as an important source of external pressure. Thus, these fistulas may close spontaneously. In contrast, an enteroatmospheric fistula is similar to a stoma (**Figure 5.8**). Even before epithelization around the fistula occurs, there will always be a significant pressure difference between the intestinal lumen and the outside, and these fistulas will not close without surgery. Occasionally, a small enteroatmospheric fistula at the edge of an open abdomen may close spontaneously as the wound contract and full-thickness abdominal wall covers the fistula.

The use of intraluminal rubber or latex tubes such as T-tubes or Malecot drains to create inflammation along the fistula tract is invaluable (**Figure 5.9**). The inflammation creates a higher pressure differential in the fistula tract, greater than the normal physiologic route. In an abscess cavity, adequate peritoneal drainage is necessary to ensure

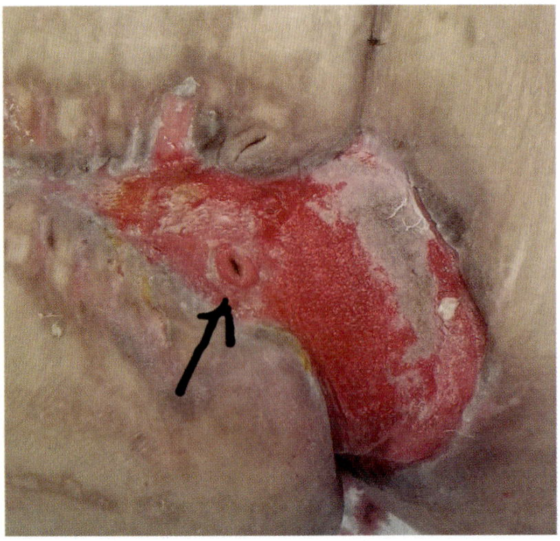

Figure 5.8 Enteroatmospheric fistula in a patient with an open abdomen secondary to loss of the abdominal wall. These fistulas appear as a small stoma. Due to the irregular contour, controlling the effluent can be challenging. The next step in management is further skin grafting to help close the wound.

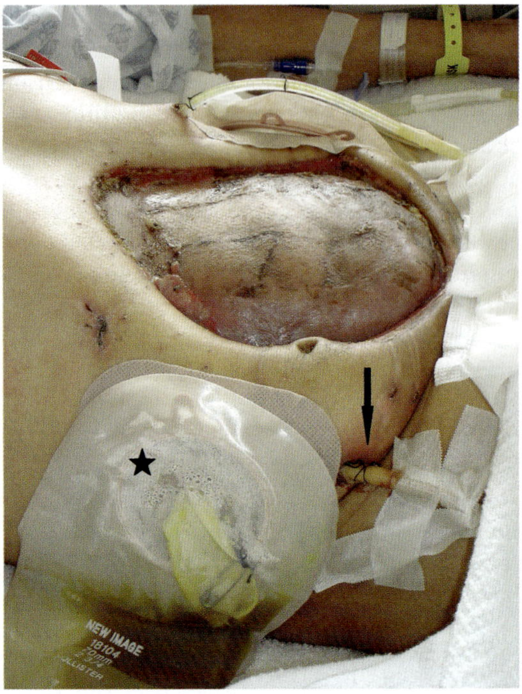

Figure 5.9 Patient with a duodenal fistula from an iatrogenic perforation following a right hemicolectomy. Control of the effluent is accomplished with a large Malecot catheter in the duodenal lumen (*arrow*) and dependent drainage using multiple Penrose drains (*star*). Note the lateral and dependent position of all drains. Following 3 months of care, all drains were removed, and the fistula closed spontaneously.

that there is no potential space for intestinal effluent to accumulate. Any space will act as a low-pressure reservoir, which will prevent the fistula from ever closing. Since the advent of suction drains, there is less concern on drain placement and the path that drains exit the peritoneal cavity. In managing these complex patients, the acute care surgeon must take gravity and patient positioning into account. As most patients are in the supine position, drains and fistula tubes should exit from the abdomen through the shortest path and as lateral and posterior as possible. This dependent placement will aid egress of intestinal contents and further prevent the pooling of intestinal contents in the peritoneal cavity.

The keys to successful fistula management are control of effluent and delivery of adequate fluid and nutrition. The systems necessary to control effluent in the setting of an enteroatmospheric fistula require ingenuity and constant vigilance. Enlisting the aid of a stomal therapist can be lifesaving. Commonly, these systems need to be changed multiple times per day, which can challenge the nursing and physician staff. In addition, what worked on a Monday may no longer work on Friday as the abdomen heals and the architecture of the wound and fistula changes. In the setting of an open abdomen, aggressive skin grafting with thin grafts will help contract the wound and ultimately provide a better surface to control the effluent. These skin grafts are often better treated open to prevent the effluent from dissolving the graft before it incorporates. Even in the setting of a high-output intestinal fistula, nutrition and fluids can usually be supplied enterally. Occasionally, the architecture of a fistula may require total parental nutrition. Other times, a combination of IV fluid and/or some parenteral nutrition is required. The goal is to achieve positive nitrogen balance that aids wound healing. Surgical closures of these complex fistulas are usually not attempted until at least 6 months after the patient recovers from the initial operation. Earlier attempts at 3-6 months are reserved for patients who have difficulty or complications related to maintaining their nutritional or fluid status.

SUMMARY

The management and treatment of patients with intraabdominal infections can challenge even the most experienced general and acute care surgeons. As this chapter outlined, while the spectrum of disease is great, the concepts remain simple and can help guide surgeons. These concepts include rapid diagnosis, adequate resuscitation and hemodynamic support, appropriate antimicrobial coverage, and source control using operative or percutaneous approaches. For the novice or early career surgeon, it is also these cases where consultation and even scrubbing with and more senior colleague can be lifesaving for the patient.

SUGGESTED READINGS

Alhaj Saleh A, Esquivel EC, Lung JT, et al. Laparoscopic omental patch for perforated peptic ulcer disease reduces length of stay and complications, compared to open surgery: a SWSC multicenter study. *Am J Surg*. 2019;218(6):1060-1064.

American College of Chest Physicians/Society of Critical Care Medicine Consensus Conference: definitions for sepsis and organ failure and guidelines for the use of innovative therapies in sepsis. *Crit Care Med*. 1992;20(6):864-874.

Anaya DA, Nathens AB. Risk factors for severe sepsis in secondary peritonitis. *Surg Infect (Larchmt)*. 2003;4:355-362.

Attard AR, Corlett MJ, Kidner NJ, Leslie AP, Fraser IA. Safety of early pain relief for acute abdominal pain. *BMJ*. 1992;305:554-556.

Azagra JS, De Simone P, Goergen M. Is there a place for laparoscopy in management of postcholecystectomy biliary injuries? *World J Surg*. 2001;25(10):1331-1334.

Bansal J, Jenaw RK, Rao J, Kankaria J, Agrawal NN. Effectiveness of plain radiography in diagnosing hollow viscus perforation: study of 1,723 patients of perforation peritonitis. *Emerg Radiol*. 2012;19:115-119.

Brundage SI, Jurkovich GJ, Hoyt DB, et al. Stapled versus sutured gastrointestinal anastomoses in the trauma patient: a multicenter trial. *J Trauma*. 2001;51(6):1054-1061.

Bruns BR, Morris DS, Zielinski M, et al. Stapled versus hand-sewn: a prospective emergency surgery study. An American Association for the Surgery of Trauma multi-institutional study. *J Trauma Acute Care Surg*. 2017;82(3):435-443.

Clec'h C, Fosse JP, Karoubi P, et al. Differential diagnostic value of procalcitonin in surgical and medical patients with septic shock. *Crit Care Med*. 2006; 34(1):102.

Connelly CR, Schreiber MA. Endpoints in resuscitation. *Curr Opin Crit Care*. 2015;21:512-519.

Cothren CC, Moore EE, Johnson JL, Moore JB, Burch JM. One hundred percent fascial approximation with sequential abdominal closure of the open abdomen. *Am J Surg*. 2006;192(2):238-242.

Dandona P, Nix D, Wilson MF, et al. Procalcitonin increase after endotoxin injection in normal subjects. *Clin Endocrinol Metab*. 1994;79(6):1605.

Dellinger RP, Levy MM, Rhodes A, et al.; Surviving Sepsis Campaign Guidelines Committee including the Pediatric Subgroup. Surviving sepsis campaign: international guidelines for management of severe sepsis and septic shock: 2012. *Crit Care Med*. 2013;41: 580-637.

Felder S, Margel D, Murrell Z, Fleshner P. Usefulness of bowel sound auscultation: a prospective evaluation. *J Surg Educ*. 2014;71:768-773.

Ferrada P, Callcut R, Bauza G, et al. AAST Multi-institutional Trials Committee Pneumatosis Intestinalis Predictive Evaluation Study: a multicenter epidemiologic study of the American Association for the Surgery of Trauma. *J Trauma Acute Care Surg*. 2017;82:451-460.

Gauzit R, Péan Y, Barth X, Mistretta F, Lalaude O; Top Study Team. Epidemiology, management, and prognosis of secondary non-postoperative peritonitis: a French prospective observational multicenter study. *Surg Infect (Larchmt)*. 2009;10:119-127.

Gilbert DN. Role of procalcitonin in the management of infected patients in the intensive care unit. *Infect Dis Clin North Am*. 2017;31(3):435.

Henny CP, Hofland J. Laparoscopic surgery: pitfalls due to anesthesia, positioning, and pneumoperitoneum. *Surg Endosc*. 2005;19(9):1163-1171.

Jang JH, Kim HC, Huh JW, et al. Anastomotic leak does not impact oncologic outcomes after preoperative chemoradiotherapy and resection for rectal cancer. *Ann Surg*. 2019;269(4):678-685.

Kohl A, Rosenberg J, Bock D, et al. Two-year results of the randomized clinical trial DILALA comparing laparoscopic lavage with resection as treatment for perforated diverticulitis. *Br J Surg*. 2018;105(9):1128-1134.

Levy MM, Fink MP, Marshall JC, et al.; International Sepsis Definitions Conference. 2001 SCCM/ESICM/ACCP/ATS/SIS International Sepsis Definitions Conference. *Intensive Care Med*. 2003;29(4):530-538.

Levy MM, Rhodes A, Phillips GS, et al. Surviving Sepsis Campaign: association between performance metrics and outcomes in a 7.5-year study. *Intensive Care Med*. 2014;40(11):1623-1633.

Loftus TJ, Efron PA, Bala TM, et al. The impact of standardized protocol implementation for surgical damage control and temporary abdominal closure after emergent laparotomy. *J Trauma Acute Care Surg*. 2019;86(4):670-678.

Loftus TJ, Jordan JR, Croft CA, et al. Temporary abdominal closure for trauma and intra-abdominal sepsis: different patients, different outcomes. *J Trauma Acute Care Surg*. 2017;82(2):345-350.

Lovell MA, Mudaliar MY, Klineberg PL. Intrahospital transport of critically ill patients: complications and difficulties. *Anaesth Intensive Care*. 2001;29(4):400-405.

Marciano S, Díaz JM, Dirchwolf M, Gadano A. Spontaneous bacterial peritonitis in patients with cirrhosis: incidence, outcomes, and treatment strategies. *Hepat Med*. 2019;11:13-22.

Matsuda M, Nishiyama M, Hanai T, Saeki S, Watanabe T. Laparoscopic omental patch repair for perforated peptic ulcer. *Ann Surg*. 1995;221(3):236-240.

Montravers P, Dufour G, Guglielminotti J, et al. Dynamic changes of microbial flora and therapeutic consequences in persistent peritonitis. *Crit Care*. 2015;19:70. doi:10.1186/s13054-015-0789-9

Moore LJ, McKinley BA, Turner KL, et al. The epidemiology of sepsis in general surgery patients. *J Trauma.* 2011;70:672-680.

Pace S, Burke TF. Intravenous morphine for early pain relief in patients with acute abdominal pain. *Acad Emerg Med.* 1996;3:1086-1092.

Pieracci FM, Barie PS. Management of severe sepsis of abdominal origin. *Scand J Surg.* 2007;96:184-196.

Rhodes A, Evans LE, Alhazzani W, et al. Surviving sepsis campaign: International Guidelines for Management of Sepsis and Septic Shock: 2016. *Crit Care Med.* 2017;45(3):486-552.

Ross JT, Mattay MA, Harris HW. Secondary peritonitis: principles of diagnosis and intervention. *BMJ.* 2018;361:k1407.

Sawyer RG, Claridge JA, Nathens AB, et al. Trial of short-course antimicrobial therapy for intraabdominal infection. *N Engl J Med.* 2015;372:1996-2005.

Schultz JK, Wallon C, Blecic L, et al. One-year results of the SCANDIV randomized clinical trial of laparoscopic lavage versus primary resection for acute perforated diverticulitis. *Br J Surg.* 2017;104(10):1382-1392.

Schultz JK, Yaqub S, Wallon C, et al. Laparoscopic lavage vs primary resection for acute perforated diverticulitis: the SCANDIV randomized clinical trial. *JAMA.* 2015;314(13):1364-1375.

Singer M, Deutschman CS, Seymour CW, et al. The Third International Consensus Definitions for Sepsis and Septic Shock (Sepsis-3). *JAMA.* 2016;315(8):801-810.

Tang A, Huddleston P, Attaluri P, Cruz A, Joseph S, Lavy D. Clinical cases of nonsurgical pneumoperitoneum: categorizing the disease and treatment options. *Am Surg.* 2015;81:E206-E208.

van Baal JO, Van de Vijver KK, Nieuwland R, et al. European Society of Intensive Care Medicine. *Intensive Care Med.* 1996;22(7):707-710.

Vincent JL, Moreno R, Takala J, et al. The SOFA (Sepsis-related Organ Failure Assessment) score to describe organ dysfunction/failure. On behalf of the Working Group on Sepsis-Related Problems of the Yurcisin BM, DeMaria EJ. Management of leak in the bariatric gastric bypass patient: reoperate, drain and feed distally. *J Gastrointest Surg.* 2009;13(9):1564-1566.

Zhang Z, Xu X. Lactate clearance is a useful biomarker for the prediction of all-cause mortality in critically ill patients: a systematic review and meta-analysis. *Crit Care Med.* 2014;42(9):2118-2125.

CHAPTER

6 Imaging in Emergency General Surgery

Sarah A. Moore and Stephanie A. Savage

CASE PRESENTATION

A 36-year-old woman, gravida 2 para 1, who is 28 weeks pregnant with an uncomplicated pregnancy, presents with pain in the midright abdomen for 24 hours. She has had nausea and vomiting associated with the pain and a low-grade elevation in her temperature. The patient has class I obesity with a BMI of 32 kg/m^2, and her past history includes only gestational diabetes. She has never had an abdominal surgery, takes prenatal vitamins and insulin, has no allergies, and does not smoke, drink, or use drugs. The initial physical examination identified a sinus tachycardia of 110 bpm, a blood pressure of 140/95 mm Hg, and tenderness to palpation in the right upper, middle, and lower abdomen. She does not have diffuse peritonitis, has no vaginal discharge, and the fetus is appropriate for gestational age in no distress. Laboratory studies include a white blood cell count of 22 × 10^3/mm^3, a hemoglobin of 10.5 g/dL, and a platelet count of 225 × 10^9/L. Basic chemistry studies are normal except for a serum glucose of 225 mmol/L. Liver function tests demonstrate an aspartate transaminase (AST) of 45 U/L, an alanine transaminase of 50 U/L, an alkaline phosphatase of 300 U/L, and a total bilirubin of 0.3 mg/dL.

Question: *What is the optimal choice for diagnostic imaging in this patient?*

Answer: *Magnetic resonance imaging*

This patient does not have a history of physical examination indicating the need for immediate operative exploration. Although CT would provide helpful information, the patient is stable and does not require emergent diagnosis, so avoiding ionizing radiation for the patient and fetus is relatively more important.

Right-sided abdominal pain in this patient may have multiple etiologies. Still, the most likely diagnoses in the differential include biliary pathology and appendicitis, as the location of pain may be atypical when the gravid uterus displaces the appendix. Although ultrasound is an excellent diagnostic modality for biliary and appendiceal pathology, the patient's obesity renders this modality less accurate. MR will allow visualization of the entire abdominal cavity, excellent evaluation of the biliary tree, and will not expose the fetus to ionizing radiation.

INTRODUCTION

Whether to Image

Evaluation of patients with emergency surgical complaints relies heavily on imaging. Four to five percent of all patients presenting to the emergency department (ED) complain of acute abdominal pain. Rapid and accurate diagnosis is important to facilitate early correction of potentially life-threatening complaints, as well as to decrease ED length of stay and maintain efficient patient flow. On the hospital wards and in the intensive care unit, hospitals with dedicated acute care surgery (ACS) services are in part defined by rapid access to imaging modalities at all hours, attending-level interpretation of imaging studies readily available, even in the middle of the night, and continuous, emergent access to interventional radiology services.

However, the ready access to imaging in nearly all centers in the current era comes at a cost. Computed tomography (CT), readily available and highly sensitive and specific, is heavily relied upon to diagnose abdominal pathology. From 1996 to 2005, the use of CT in the evaluation of acute abdominal pain increased by 141%. Not infrequently, CT imaging is obtained before or despite diagnostic physical examination findings. CT imaging may unnecessarily prolong a patient's length of stay, delay indicated therapies, and, most importantly, expose patients to ionizing radiation. Although it is difficult to isolate or quantify the exact increase in cancer risk attributable to ionizing radiation from CT,

Mathews et al. postulated that every sievert of effective dose may cause 0.125 cancers and 1 in 4000 brain scans leads to subsequent brain cancer. These alarming statistics do not even consider the monetary cost associated with the studies.

The burden is on the medical community to be responsible stewards of these diagnostic modalities. The first step in this process should always be a careful physical examination after a comprehensive patient interview. A patient with evident peritonitis, a soft tissue lesion with crepitus, fluctuance, or pain out of proportion to examination likely needs operative intervention *in lieu* of additional diagnostic tests. Imaging in all modalities should be reserved for unclear pathology or when the information provided will alter decision-making or surgical approach.

When imaging is indicated, the choice of modality should meet several criteria. (1) The modality chosen should have the ability to effectively provide the information needed. For example, although ultrasound is effective in the diagnosis of acute appendicitis in many patients, it may not be highly accurate in a morbidly obese patient. Additionally, an imaging modality such as CT may be preferred when the underlying pathology is unclear or when rapid diagnosis is imperative. (2) The modality chosen should minimize exposure to ionizing radiation. In patients with right upper quadrant pain but without concerns for choledocholithiasis, ultrasound is an excellent modality to diagnose acute cholecystitis without exposing the patient to radiation. Conversely, if there is a high likelihood that CT will be necessary for diagnosis, it is reasonable to go directly to this option and defer plain radiographs that may represent additional cost and radiation without providing additional information. (3) The modality chosen should be available when needed. Although magnetic resonance (MR) imaging is highly sensitive and specific and spares the patient's exposure to ionizing radiation, it is often unavailable during off-hours or at smaller medical centers.

For some emergency surgical diseases, proposed scoring systems may decrease or eliminate the need for imaging. Multiple scoring systems have been developed to predict the likelihood of acute appendicitis, with varying success. The Alvarado score (**Table 6.1**) has demonstrated a good association between higher scores (≥9 in males or ≥10 in females) and a positive diagnosis of acute appendicitis. Scores ≤1 in males or ≤2 in females were also predictive of negative appendicitis diagnosis. The pediatric appendicitis score has demonstrated better predictive ability in children, compared to the Alvarado score. The Fenyö-Lindberg score is not as widely used but has been proposed as helpful in predicting appendicitis in women of child-bearing years.

TABLE 6.1 ■ AS Calculation

RLQ tenderness	2 points
Rebound tenderness	1 point
Temperature >37.3 °C	1 point
Migration of pain to RLQ	1 point
Nausea or vomiting	1 point
Anorexia	1 point
WBC count >10 000	2 points
WBC left shift	1 point
Total	10 points

RLQ, right lower quadrant; WBC, white blood cell.
Based on Coleman JJ, Carr BW, Rogers T, et al. The Alvarado score should be used to reduce emergency department length of stay and radiation exposure in select patients with abdominal pain. *J Trauma Acute Care Surg*. 2018;84(6):946-950. doi:10.1097/TA.0000000000001885

The American Association for the Surgery of Trauma (AAST) has developed a comprehensive series of grading scales for most emergency general surgery (EGS) diseases. Grading may be based on one to four categories derived from clinical presentation, radiologic studies, operative findings, and pathologic results. The "clinical" category of these scales may be helpful to the clinician to determine the need for further imaging vs the need for earlier operative intervention.

Necrotizing soft tissue infections (NSTI) may also be evaluated using the LRINEC score (see also Chapter 21: Necrotizing Soft Tissue Infections). Using various laboratory markers, including white blood cell count, hemoglobin, sodium level, serum glucose, serum creatinine, and C-reactive protein, scores of ≥6 should raise concerns for NSTI. However, validation studies have indicated that the LRINEC score may not be as accurate as initially proposed. As with all disease processes and all scoring systems, a scoring system should not be used in isolation to make a diagnosis. Instead, these scoring systems may help direct subsequent diagnostic choices or may be a final piece of data confirming a management plan.

UTILITY OF PLAIN FILMS IN EMERGENCY GENERAL SURGERY—IS THERE A ROLE TODAY?

In 1895, Wilhelm Roentgen, a German physicist, developed the technology to create plain radiographs (x-rays) using an electron beam tube. This was described in the New York Medical news as a "weird and wonderful discovery destined to enrich medicine with possibly the most valuable diagnostic process, which recent years have witnessed," and earned him the first Nobel Prize in Physics in 1901. With the advances of the subsequent 125 years in medical imaging, x-rays are often dismissed as nonspecific and inadequate for diagnosis, especially in patients with complex surgical pathology. The American College of Radiology (ACR) has issued guidelines (updated in 2016) on the use of abdominal radiography, with indications including evaluation and follow-up of abdominal distention, bowel obstruction, or ileus; placement of medical devices; evaluation of possible pneumoperitoneum or toxic megacolon; and others (**Table 6.2**). In general, only 10% of abdominal radiographs will demonstrate an abnormality in patients with acute abdominal pain; additional views (upright, lateral) provide little utility in the evaluation of generalized abdominal pain. When combined with history, examination, and laboratory analysis, abdominal x-rays have a sensitivity of 56% and specificity of 81% to predict the need for urgent intervention in the first 24 hours. Given this limited utility to evaluate generalized abdominal pain, plain abdominal x-rays should be limited to the indications listed in **Table 6.2**.

Advantages of abdominal radiographs include the utility in unstable patients who may not tolerate transport for more advanced imaging studies such as CT, as well as the lower radiation dose: two abdominal radiographs imply an overall radiation dose of 1.4 mSv in comparison to a standard CT of the abdomen, which is in range of 10-20 mSv depending on technique.

Pneumoperitoneum

Standard surgical teaching suggests that in the presence of physical examination findings of acute abdominal pathology, pneumoperitoneum on abdominal radiographs should be considered an absolute indication for surgical exploration (**Figure 6.1**). However, abdominal radiographs may have a false-positive diagnosis of pneumoperitoneum. Chilaiditi sign, first described in 1910, is seen when the colon is interposed between the inferior surface of the right hemidiaphragm and the superior surface of the liver and will result in the appearance of pneumoperitoneum on x-ray (**Figure 6.2**). Abdominal radiographs have a reported specificity of between 53% and 89%, so false-positive diagnosis is of real concern. However, in a retrospective evaluation of 43 patients with pneumoperitoneum and acute surgical pathology, CT added no additional clinical information or improvement in outcomes. The authors

TABLE 6.2 ■ American College of Radiology Practice Parameter for the Performance of Abdominal Radiography Indications

- Evaluation and follow-up of abdominal distension, bowel obstruction, or nonobstructive ileus
- Constipation, especially assessment of fecal load in children
- Evaluation for necrotizing enterocolitis, particularly in the premature newborn
- Evaluation of congenital gastrointestinal abnormalities
- Follow-up of the postoperative patient, including detection of inadvertent retained surgical foreign bodies
- Evaluation and follow-up of urinary tract calculi, including assessment of lithotripsy patients
- Evaluation of ingested or other introduced foreign bodies
- A scout radiograph prior to a planned imaging examination, that is, fluoroscopy
- Evaluation of the placement of medical devices
- Evaluation for pneumoperitoneum
- Evaluation of possible toxic megacolon
- Evaluation of unstable patients after blunt trauma to the abdomen
- Evaluation of a palpable mass in an infant or child
- Localization of pancreatic duct stone prelithotripsy and endoscopic stone removal
- Evaluation for suspected retained video endoscopy capsule and determination of location of patency capsule
- Evaluation of colon transit time using the simplified radiodense marker colon transit test

American College of Radiology. ACR-SPR practice guideline for the performance of abdominal radiography. 2016.

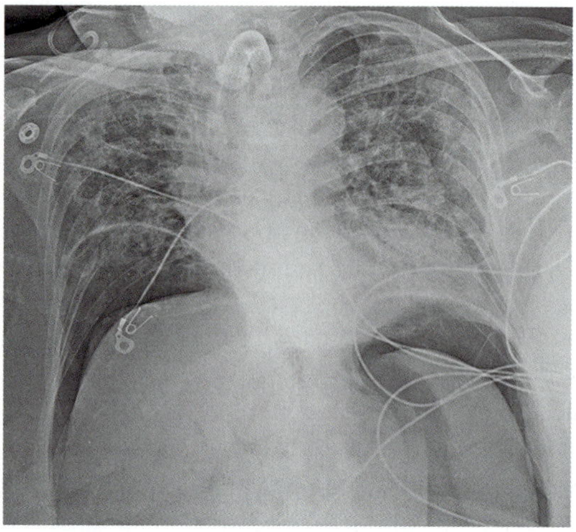

Figure 6.1 Plain radiograph of the chest shows massive pneumoperitoneum in a patient with acute respiratory distress syndrome (ARDS) from viral pneumonia.

concluded that in patients with peritonitis and pneumoperitoneum on x-ray, CT delays surgery without providing any benefit.

Clinicians should also note that there are a multitude of nonsurgical causes of pneumoperitoneum. These include retained postoperative air, peritoneal dialysis catheter placement, mechanical ventilation, cardiopulmonary resuscitation, pneumothorax, and others. Care should be taken to correlate radiographic pneumoperitoneum with clinical assessment when deciding to pursue surgical intervention.

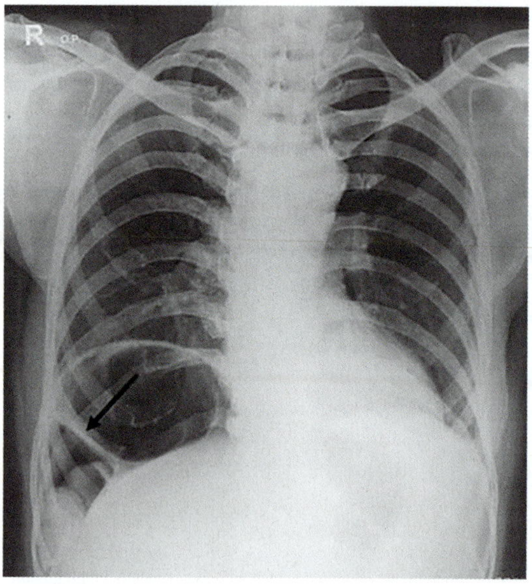

Figure 6.2 Plain radiograph of the chest shows interposition of hepatic flexure with haustral folds, between the liver and right diaphragm (Chilaiditi sign). Note the haustral fold (*arrow*). (From Indiran V, Kannan K, Ramachandra Prasad T, Maduraimuthu P. Chilaiditi sign. *Abdom Radiol (NY)*. 2017;42(8):2188-2189. doi:10.1007/s00261-017-1104-9)

Volvulus

Colonic volvulus is responsible for ~15% of large bowel obstructions in the United States (see also Chapter 11: Bowel Obstruction). The "coffee-bean" sign, an inverted U shape extending upward from the pelvis on abdominal radiographs, is a classic diagnostic finding of sigmoid volvulus (**Figure 6.3**). The dilated bowel generally arises in the left pelvis and extends to the right upper quadrant. Abdominal radiographs are diagnostic in 60%-80% of patients. Absence of rectal gas may also suggest sigmoid volvulus. A cecal volvulus has a much less classic radiographic appearance. Radiographs will definitively diagnose cecal volvulus in <20% of patients, although suspicion is high for this diagnosis in nearly half of patients.

Bowel Obstruction

Abdominal radiographs are commonly used in the initial evaluation of a patient with suspected ileus or bowel obstruction. Radiographs may distinguish large bowel obstruction from small bowel obstruction. Small bowel obstruction (80%) is far more common than large bowel obstruction (20%) (see also Chapter 11: Bowel Obstruction). Location, diameter, and the presence of haustra suggest

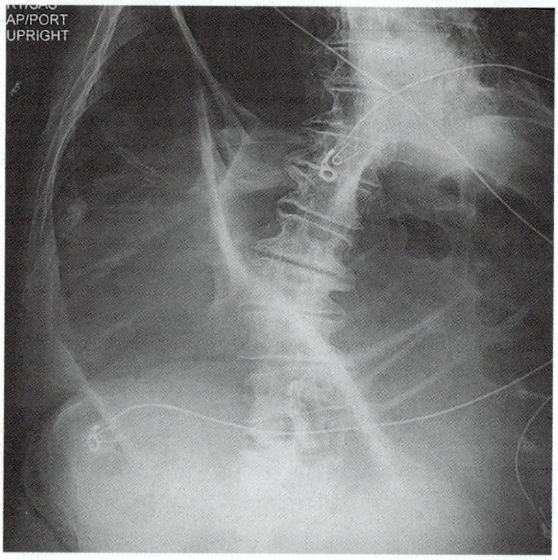

Figure 6.3 Plain radiograph of the abdomen shows sigmoid volvulus with "coffee bean sign."

colonic dilatation. The diameter of the colon, particularly the cecum, should be noted. Any suggestion of a cutoff in intraluminal air, as with an obstructing sigmoid cancer, should be sought. Radiographic signs of small bowel obstruction include distended small bowel loops (>3 cm), air-fluid levels, or visible prominence of the valvulae conniventes. These findings vary with the severity and duration of the obstruction. In one large study, the overall sensitivity of radiographs was ~70%, and specificity is 57%. Radiographs were more sensitive and specific with high-grade obstruction when compared to low-grade obstruction. In addition, there is significant variation in accuracy ranging from 59% to 93% depending on the training level of the radiologist, when comparing residents up through senior faculty. Of multiple objective findings present on abdominal imaging in small bowel obstruction, the presence of air-fluid levels of different height in the same bowel loop and the presence of a mean air-fluid level width of greater or equal to 25 mm were found to have the strongest predictive value (odds ratio of 4.5 and 7.2, respectively). When both findings are present, patients have an 86% chance of having a high-grade partial or complete small bowel obstruction.

Timed, serial abdominal radiographs with the use of oral, water-soluble contrast (Gastrografin) have arguably revolutionized the management of small bowel obstruction over the past two decades. This protocol is advocated as both a diagnostic and therapeutic tool in the management of adhesive small bowel obstruction. Passage of the Gastrografin to the colon within a defined time period is generally predictive of successful nonoperative management (**Figure 6.4**). In addition, the hyperosmotic property of this oral contrast theoretically draws edema out of the obstructed, edematous bowel wall and helps reduce the obstruction. The first randomized controlled trial was published in 1994 with 99 patients and demonstrated a reduction in need for operative management and decreased length of stay without increased complications. Since this initial trial, multiple studies have been published demonstrating the utility of this protocol in both expeditious diagnosis of patients requiring operative treatment as well as therapeutic effect in resolving obstruction. The largest multicenter prospective observational study enrolled 316 patients, 173 in the Gastrografin group and 143 patients in the non-Gastrografin group. Patients in the Gastrografin protocol group had lower rates of abdominal exploration (20.8% vs 44.1%) and shorter length of hospital stay (4 vs 5 days), with a similar rate of complications. On multivariable analysis, Gastrografin treatment was an independent predictor of successful nonoperative management. This protocol has been extrapolated in to use in other clinical scenarios of bowel obstruction, such as pediatric patients, patients with a history of abdominal or pelvic malignancy, postoperative bowel obstruction, and others, with positive results.

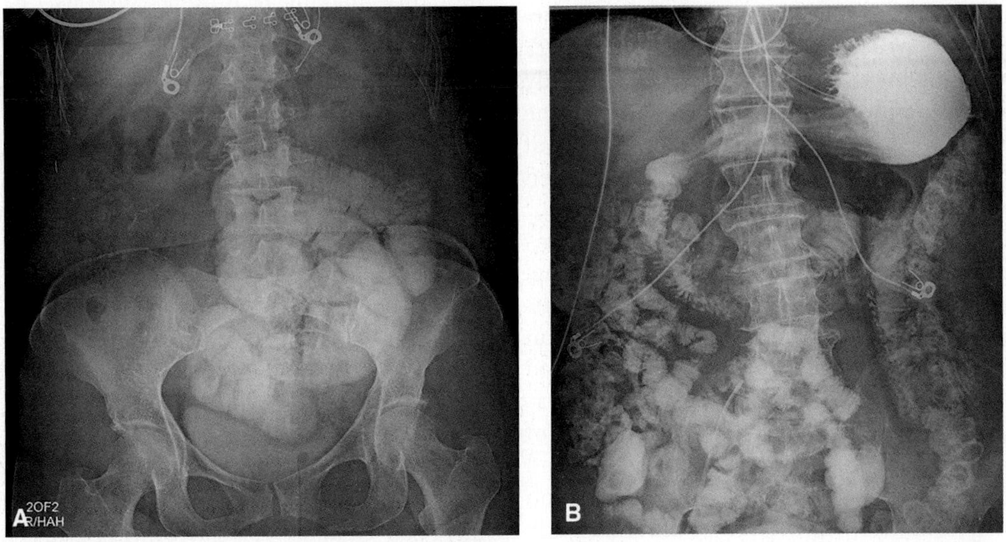

Figure 6.4 Plain radiographs of the abdomen with demonstrating small bowel obstruction evaluated with Gastrografin challenge, showing no passage of contrast in to the colon **(A)** and passage of contrast in to the colon at 4 hours **(B)**.

ADVANCED IMAGING IN EMERGENCY GENERAL SURGERY

The options for advanced imaging in patients with suspected EGS diagnoses are numerable, and it is challenging for a clinician to select the most appropriate imaging test(s). This section will focus on the options for advanced imaging, with a detailed discussion of each imaging modality and how best to image various diagnoses.

Imaging Modalities

Ultrasound

Ultrasound has a multitude of advantages in the evaluation of emergency surgical patients. Ultrasound utilizes a beam of sound waves that is sent into the tissues; the waves are then reflected back to the transducer as an echo depending on the acoustic impedance of the tissue and tissue interfaces. Ultrasound involves no ionizing radiation and can be done with portable machines, making it extremely useful for bedside diagnosis, especially in critically ill patients. Some authors have likened it to a "modern stethoscope equivalent" given its point-of-care utility in patient evaluation. Microbubble ultrasound contrast agents were approved by the FDA in 2016 for noncardiac indications, and these have allowed further improvements in the detection of perfusion and blood flow. Ultrasound limitations include that it is highly operator dependent and is affected by body habitus.

Computed Tomography

Computed tomography, or CT, utilizes a motorized x-ray source that rotates around the patient's body, propelling x-ray beams through the body and detecting them after they pass through the patient. Over the past 40 years, a multitude of technological developments have revolutionized the process of CT scanning, including helical or spiral CT, multidetector CT, multiplanar reconstructions (MPR), electrocardiographic gating, three-dimensional reconstruction, and others. These developments have made the acquisition of CT images extremely fast and have allowed high-resolution images with expanded capabilities of CT angiography. Disadvantages of CT include exposure to ionizing radiation and iodinated contrast agents, cost, and degradation of image quality with motion artifact or body habitus.

Magnetic Resonance Imaging

Magnetic resonance (MR) imaging uses powerful magnets that produce a strong magnetic field that forces protons in the body to align with that field. As a radiofrequency current is pulsed through the patient, protons are stimulated to spin, and sensors detect the energy released as protons realign with the magnetic field. The varying magnetic properties of the protons allow the detection of different tissue types. MR was first introduced in clinical medicine in the early 1980s, and as with CT, a multitude of technological advances over the past several decades have allowed MR to be utilized in a broad spectrum of diagnoses and diseases. Recent advancements in MR include contrast-enhanced MR angiography, time-of-flight MR angiography, functional MR, and others. Disadvantages of MR include its generally longer image acquisition time, cost, and relative contraindication in patients with various ferromagnetic implantable devices or other foreign bodies.

Nuclear Medicine

Nuclear medicine involves a wide variety of imaging techniques, with the critical uniting feature being the use of radiopharmaceuticals for both diagnostic and therapeutic purposes. Radiopharmaceuticals can provide information on both structure and function of numerous different organs by emitting small amounts of radiation that are detected as they accumulate in different tissues at different rates. Multimodality imaging techniques such as PET/CT, PET/MR, and others have allowed for advancements in diagnostics, particularly for oncologic evaluation. While nuclear medicine studies have a minor role in the initial diagnosis of most EGS conditions, these studies can be quite helpful if diagnoses are unclear after initial workup or if further characterization is needed based on this workup.

Disease-Specific Imaging

Upper Gastrointestinal Tract: Nonvariceal Upper Gastrointestinal Bleeding

Despite significant advances in endoscopic therapy, upper gastrointestinal bleeding (UGIB) is a significant cause of morbidity and mortality (see also Chapter 13: Gastrointestinal Hemorrhage in Emergency Surgery). Defined as bleeding proximal to the ligament of Treitz, UGIB may result from peptic ulcer disease, varices, Mallory-Weiss tears, malignancy, angiodysplasia, vascular malformations, or iatrogenic complications, among others. After resuscitation, identifying and treating the source of bleeding is paramount. The ACR has issued a consensus statement on the role of imaging in nonvariceal UGIB. Endoscopy remains the most appropriate initial imaging modality, based on its ability for both diagnosis and treatment, with early endoscopy (<24 hours from admission) having a favorable impact on hospital length of stay and requirement for blood transfusion. If endoscopy is unsuccessful in controlling overt hemorrhage in an unstable patient, angiography with embolization should be performed. Angiography can identify a bleeding source in up to 80% of patients and embolization has a primary success rate of 80%. Angioembolization has been associated with lower overall complication rates and a trend toward lower 30-day mortality rates when compared to surgical intervention but with higher rates of rebleeding.

CT angiography (CTA) has a growing role in the evaluation of UGIB. It is considered a reasonable next test if endoscopy fails to localize or control an UGIB in a stable patient. In addition, CTA is often performed prior to endoscopy due to its convenience and rapid availability. CTA can detect bleeding rates as low as 0.3 mL/min, in comparison to 0.5-1.0 mL/min for conventional angiography and 0.2 mL/min for Tc-99m–labeled RBC scintigraphy. In one large study, CTA had a sensitivity of 85.2% and specificity of 92.1% for detecting active, acute GI bleeding. CTA has the disadvantage of not offering any therapeutic role, and sensitivity depends on the presence of active bleeding at the time of imaging. Of note, CT enterography and CT without IV contrast generally have no role in the acute evaluation of UGIB. CT enterography may be useful to evaluate intermittent small bowel bleeding in occult gastrointestinal bleeding.

Tc-99m–labeled RBC scintigraphy can be used to localize an UGIB that has failed to localize with both endoscopy and CTA. It can detect bleeding rates as low as 0.05-0.1 mL/min, making it quite sensitive for slow bleeding. However, it has both high false-positive and high false-negative rates, making its role in the evaluation of UGIB controversial.

Upper Gastrointestinal Tract: Gastric Volvulus

Gastric volvulus often presents with a triad of severe epigastric pain, retching, and inability to pass a nasogastric tube (Borchardt triad). Volvulus occurs when rotation of the stomach leads to gastric outlet obstruction, which may progress to gastric ischemia or rupture if not treated. The volvulus can occur along the long axis from the gastroesophageal junction to the pylorus (mesenteroaxial volvulus) or more commonly along the axis from the lesser curvature to the greater curvature of the stomach (organoaxial volvulus) (**Figure 6.5**). Primary gastric volvulus occurs when the laxity of the anchoring ligaments of the stomach allows excessive mobility of the stomach, and secondary gastric volvulus occurs due to other causes, such as congenital or traumatic diaphragmatic hernias or paraesophageal hernias. The gold standard for diagnosis of gastric volvulus is a fluoroscopic upper gastrointestinal series, but this is often not the first test performed, as the presentation may be more insidious and vague. Most patients will undergo CT for further evaluation and characterizing gastric volvulus vs paraesophageal hernia can be difficult. In one large series of patients with surgically proven gastric volvulus, the most frequent and sensitive signs of gastric volvulus were stenosis at the hernia neck and transition point at the pylorus, with CT yielding 90% accuracy in identifying gastric volvulus. CT can suggest gastric necrosis when

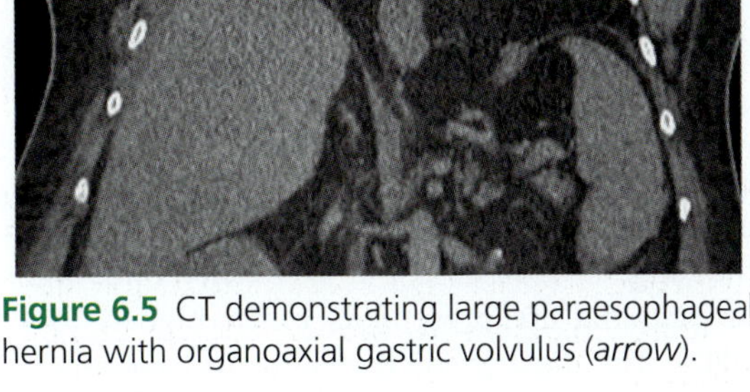

Figure 6.5 CT demonstrating large paraesophageal hernia with organoaxial gastric volvulus (*arrow*).

pneumatosis of the gastric wall, free gas and fluid outside the gastric wall within the hernia sac, or lack of contrast enhancement of the gastric wall is visualized.

Upper Gastrointestinal Tract: Gastroduodenal Perforation

Upper gastrointestinal perforation may occur from various causes, including ulcer disease, foreign body ingestion, malignancy, and iatrogenic perforation. As noted earlier, abdominal radiographs with evidence of pneumoperitoneum, combined with clinical signs of peritonitis, should prompt surgical intervention instead of further imaging. However, if abdominal radiographs are nondiagnostic, CT with IV contrast is indicated. In a recent Italian series of 166 patients with surgical findings of gastroduodenal perforation, 12% were diagnosed based on clinical examination alone without further imaging. Of the remaining 146 patients undergoing imaging evaluation, 85.5% of patients were diagnosed by abdominal radiograph, 1.8% with both radiograph and sonographic assessment, and 12.7% by CT findings.

Small Bowel: Small Bowel Obstruction

In the absence of an obvious hernia causing small bowel obstruction, imaging workup of suspected small bowel obstruction is warranted. While abdominal radiographs have a reported accuracy of 50%-67% for the diagnosis of small bowel obstruction, CT imaging with IV contrast has higher accuracy, in the range of 70%-94%. CT findings consistent with small bowel obstruction include caliber change of small bowel from dilated (>2.5 cm) proximally to decompressed distally, air-fluid levels, small bowel feces sign (**Figure 6.6**), presence of a transition point, bowel wall thickening (>0.3 cm), intraperitoneal fluid, mesenteric inflammation, and a mesenteric whirl sign.

The goal of CT imaging in small bowel obstruction is to evaluate the severity of the obstruction, identify the site and etiology of obstruction, and detect the presence of complications such as ischemia, closed-loop obstruction, or volvulus. CT sensitivity for ischemia is low, in the range of 15%-40%, but specificity, once signs of ischemia are present, is much higher, 89%-100%. The most predictive signs of ischemia on multivariate logistic regression include reduced bowel wall enhancement, reduced enhancement of mesenteric veins, and lack of engorgement of mesenteric veins. CT is also valuable to predict the need for operative intervention. In two large studies of >100 patients with small bowel obstruction, the findings of intraperitoneal free fluid, mesenteric edema, lack of small bowel feces sign, history of vomiting, and high-grade or complete obstruction were the most significant predictors of need for surgery.

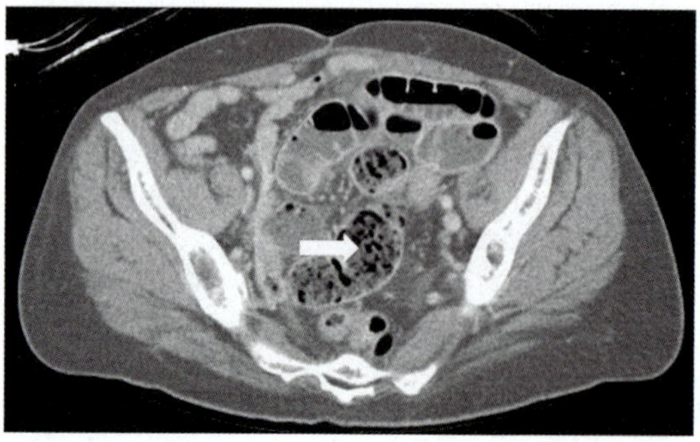

Figure 6.6 CT demonstrating multiple loops of dilated small bowel and small bowel feces sign (*arrow*) secondary to adhesive small bowel obstruction.

Small Bowel: Mesenteric Ischemia

Acute mesenteric ischemia is a group of disease processes that result in a lack of adequate blood supply to the small intestine, with resulting inflammation and ischemia (see also Chapter 12: Mesenteric Ischemia). The incidence is low, accurate diagnosis can be challenging, and mortality is high in the range of 50%-80%. As such, accurate radiographic assessment and diagnosis are paramount.

Mesenteric ischemia can be occlusive, from mesenteric arterial embolism or thrombus or mesenteric venous thrombus, or can be nonocclusive from low flow (NOMI). Timely CT angiography is the cornerstone of diagnosis. Comprehensive CTA should include precontrast scans (to detect vascular calcifications, hyperattenuated intravascular thrombus, and intramural hemorrhage), arterial and portal venous phases, and MPR to best assess the origin of the mesenteric arteries. CTA has a sensitivity and specificity between 90% and 100% to diagnose mesenteric ischemia. CT findings suggest both signs of vascular insufficiency and signs of ischemic intestinal injury. Intraluminal defects or occlusions of the mesenteric vessels (present in 12%-75% of cases) are quite specific for mesenteric

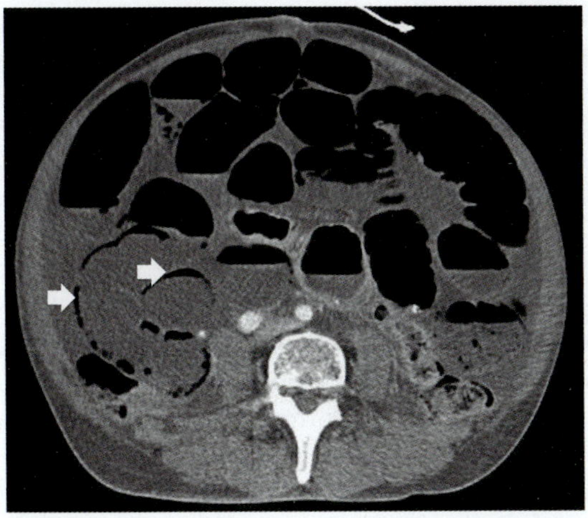

Figure 6.7 CT demonstrating severe small bowel pneumatosis (*arrows*) and small bowel dilation with multiple air-fluid levels secondary to small bowel ischemia.

ischemia. Signs of bowel ischemia include bowel wall thickening, lack of bowel wall enhancement, bowel dilation, pneumatosis intestinalis, portal venous gas, and mesenteric stranding (**Figure 6.7**). Pneumoperitoneum is indicative of necrosis with perforation. The prognostic value of pneumatosis is debatable; in several series, between 47% and 59% of patients with pneumatosis on CTA had bowel necrosis. Duplex ultrasonography plays a role in chronic mesenteric ischemia but does not have a significant role in the diagnosis of acute mesenteric ischemia.

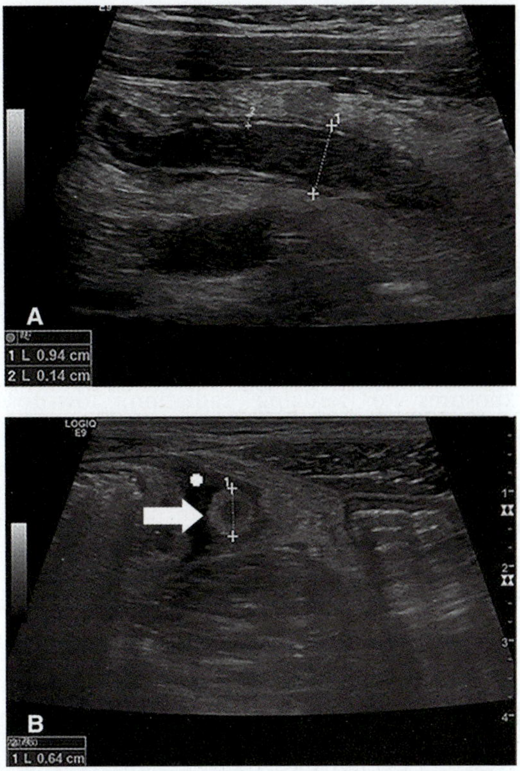

Figure 6.8 Ultrasound scan of acute appendicitis demonstrating appendiceal wall thickening, target sign (*arrow*), diameter >6 mm, and surrounding free fluid in longitudinal **(A)** and transverse **(B)** planes. (From Mostbeck G, Adam EJ, Nielsen MB, et al. How to diagnose acute appendicitis: ultrasound first. *Insights Imaging*. 2016;7(2):255-263. doi:10.1007/s13244-016-0469-6)

Colon: Appendicitis

If clinical scoring systems are inconclusive in a patient with suspected appendicitis, imaging is warranted to establish or refute the diagnosis (see also Chapter 17: Appendicitis). The most common modalities used to diagnose appendicitis are ultrasound, CT, and MR. Attempts to decrease the dependence on CT imaging have led to an increased interest in the use of ultrasound and MR, as well as the development of low-dose CT protocols.

Graded compression ultrasound involves protocolized compression of the right lower quadrant and optimizes visualization of the appendix via ultrasound. Ultrasound findings of appendicitis include noncompressibility, diameter >6 mm, wall thickness >3 mm, "target sign," presence of appendicolith, hypervascularity in early appendicitis, and hypo- to avascularity in abscess or necrosis (**Figure 6.8**). The diagnostic performance of ultrasound varies widely in the United States, with reported sensitivity of 21%-96%, specificity of 71%-98%, PPV of 41%-94%, and NPV of 49%-90%. Appendix visualization also has significant variability, with ranges of 35%-81% of nonvisualization or incomplete visualization. Visualization rates and diagnostic accuracy are higher in male patients and nonobese patients.

MR has a growing role in diagnosing appendicitis, especially in the pediatric and pregnant patient populations. Improvements in protocols have allowed rapid image acquisition in as little as 15 minutes. Techniques such as free-breathing image acquisition and diffusion-weighted imaging sequences have decreased motion artifact from peristalsis and respiration. In general, for appendicitis, MR has a sensitivity of 96%-100% and a specificity of 81%-96% with experienced radiologists. The administration of gadolinium contrast has not been demonstrated to improve diagnostic accuracy and is not recommended.

CT has several advantages in the diagnosis of appendicitis. It is highly accurate, with sensitivity and specificity of >98%. In addition, the use of CT has reduced the negative appendectomy rate from 17% to 9%. CT also offers the advantage of accurately diagnosing the presence of complicated appendicitis with phlegmon or abscess, as well as establishing the presence of alternative diagnoses if appendicitis is not present. Given the growing concern over repeated exposures to ionizing radiation, low-dose abdominal CT has been suggested to replace standard-dose CT to evaluate suspected appendicitis. A large trial of 891 patients randomized to low-dose CT vs standard-dose CT established noninferiority for negative appendectomy rates, rate of appendiceal perforation, or need for additional imaging tests.

Colon: Diverticulitis

The incidence of diverticulosis increases with age, ranging from 30% to 50% in individuals over 50 years and more than 65% in individuals over 80 years of age (see also Chapter 18: Gastrointestinal Inflammatory Diseases). Up to 25% of patients with diverticulosis will develop complicated diverticular disease in their lifetime, with abscess, phlegmon, fistula, obstruction, or perforation. When evaluating patients with suspected diverticulitis, abdominal radiographs can demonstrate pneumoperitoneum indicating free perforation. However, the majority of patients with suspected diverticulitis undergo CT scan evaluation. The traditional Hinchey classification was developed before the routine use of CT scans for diagnosis, but the grading is still applicable to CT images. Both the Western Trauma Association and the AAST have developed grading systems for diverticulitis; these are outlined in **Table 6.3**. Comparatively, the AAST

TABLE 6.3 ■ Comparison of the Hinchey, Modified Hinchey, American Association for the Surgery of Trauma (AAST), and Western Trauma Association (WTA) Grading Systems for Acute Colonic Diverticulitis

Grade	Hinchey	Modified Hinchey	AAST (Frequency)	WTA
I	Pericolic abscess or phlegmon	IA: phlegmon IB: pericolic or mesenteric abscess	Colonic inflammation (26%)	IA: phlegmon with no abscess IB: phlegmon with abscess <4 cm
II	Pelvic, intra-abdominal, or retroperitoneal abscess	Walled off pelvic abscess	Colon microperforation or pericolic phlegmon without abscess (37%)	Phlegmon with abscess >4 cm
III	Generalized purulent peritonitis	Generalized purulent peritonitis	Localized pericolic abscess (23%)	Purulent peritonitis (no hole in colon)
IV	Generalized fecal peritonitis	Generalized fecal peritonitis	Distant abscess (5%)	Feculent peritonitis (persistent hole in colon)
V			Free colonic perforation with generalized peritonitis (9%)	

Moore FA, Moore EE, Burlew CC, et al. Western Trauma Association critical decisions in trauma: management of complicated diverticulitis. *J Trauma Acute Care Surg*. 2012;73:1365-1371.
Shafi S, Priest EL, Crandall ML, et al. Multicenter validation of American Association for the Surgery of Trauma grading system for acute colonic diverticulitis and its use for emergency general surgery quality improvement program. *J Trauma Acute Care Surg*. 2016;80:405-410; discussion 410-401.
Hinchey EJ, Schaal PG, Richards GK Treatment of perforated diverticular disease of the colon. *Adv Surg*. 1978;12:85-109.
Kaiser AM, Jiang JK, Lake JP, et al. The management of complicated diverticulitis and the role of computed tomography. *Am J Gastroenterol*. 2005;100:910-917.

grades and the original Hinchey classification are based on clinical, radiologic, operative, and pathologic findings, while the WTA grading system and modified Hinchey classification are based on CT scan findings.

CT also has utility in predicting the development of complicated diverticulitis. When evaluating 528 patients with acute diverticulitis, CT findings predictive of a complicated course were the presence of a fluid collection and a longer inflamed colon segment, while pericolic extraluminal air was not predictive. CT is generally the mainstay of diagnostic imaging, although ultrasound has a limited role in evaluating suspected diverticulitis. Ultrasound can identify local bowel wall thickening, mesenteric inflammation, and paracolic abscess, and is useful in serial evaluations of diverticulitis, especially in nonobese patients.

Colon: Volvulus

Colonic volvulus is the third most common cause of large bowel obstruction and accounts for 10%-15% of all colon obstructions in the United States (see also Chapter 11: Bowel Obstruction). Sigmoid volvulus is most common, followed by cecal volvulus, and rarely transverse colon or splenic flexure volvulus. Cecal volvulus may represent a true volvulus or may be a cecal bascule, where the cecum folds on itself in an anterosuperior direction. As discussed earlier, sigmoid volvulus has a classic "coffee bean" shape on an abdominal radiograph. In contrast, cecal volvulus shows a dilated loop of distended bowel with haustral markings that extends to the left upper quadrant. X-ray is diagnostic in >60% of sigmoid volvulus cases. However, in cecal volvulus, radiographs are suggestive in less than half of patients and diagnostic in only 17%.

CT with IV contrast is useful to establish the diagnosis of both sigmoid and cecal volvulus. CT findings of sigmoid volvulus include swirling of the sigmoid colon mesentery, dilated sigmoid colon, intestinal air-fluid levels, and one sigmoid colon transition point. CT findings of cecal volvulus include whirl sign, ileocecal twisting, decompression of the distal colon, a centralized appendix, and cecal apex in the left upper quadrant. Two additional CT signs of both sigmoid and cecal volvulus are the "X marks the spot" sign, which is convergent, crossing transition points, and the "split-wall sign," where mesenteric fat is seen between two loops of bowel, giving the impression of a split in a single twisted loop of bowel.

The endoscopic and fluoroscopic evaluation may be both diagnostic and therapeutic in sigmoid volvulus, if the diagnosis remains unclear. Nonoperative detorsion and decompression are the most appropriate initial management strategies for sigmoid volvulus unless frank ischemia or perforation is suspected. In cecal volvulus, barium enema has an accuracy of up to 88%, with a classic finding of a "bird's beak," where the bowel loops taper, ending at the site of torsion in the right colon. In general, endoscopy has little role in cecal volvulus, and operative detorsion is the primary treatment modality.

Colon: Lower Gastrointestinal Bleeding

As with UGIB, lower gastrointestinal bleeding (LGIB) management follows the same principles of resuscitation and stabilization, followed by prompt localization of the bleeding source (see also Chapter 13: Gastrointestinal Hemorrhage in Emergency Surgery). Triphasic (precontrast, arterial phase, and portal venous phase) CTA of the abdomen and pelvis has become the initial diagnostic test of choice for patients with LGIB as it is widely available and convenient, with fast acquisition and high accuracy of ~89% in patient with active GI bleeding. CTA also has excellent sensitivity and specificity, 90% and 92%, respectively. CTA is also an attractive option in patients who cannot tolerate a bowel prep. However, CTA does not provide a therapeutic option. Colonoscopy as the initial procedure in evaluating LGIB can both diagnose and treat. Diagnostic yield of colonoscopy for acute LGIB ranges from 48% to 90%. The terminal ileum should also be intubated to rule out a proximal bleeding source. However, colonoscopy in the unprepped colon is difficult. Bowel preparation for appropriate visualization and safe endoscopic hemostasis is recommended, and the American College of Gastroenterology recommends against unprepped colonoscopy. A fully prepped colon in the setting of initial major LGIB is unlikely.

Noncolonoscopic interventions include tagged red blood cell scintigraphy, CT angiography, and catheter-based angiography. Tagged red blood scintigraphy localizes bleeding in only 26%-80% of LGIB but does allow repeated scans, making it useful for intermittent, occult GI bleeding. Depending on CTA findings, patients can be appropriately stratified to needing emergent surgery or angioembolization. Conventional angiography localizes a LGIB source in 25%-70% of examinations and, similar to colonoscopy, allows both diagnosis and treatment. Angioembolization is usually done in a super-selective manner to minimize the risk of ischemia, <8% in modern series. Rates of rebleeding after angioembolization are comparable to colonoscopic rebleeding rates, with 8%-33% rebleeding for angioembolization compared to 16%-22% rebleeding rates for colonoscopy.

Colon: Ischemic Colitis

As with acute mesenteric ischemia, ischemic colitis results from inadequate blood flow to meet the metabolic demands of the colon (see also Chapter 12: Mesenteric Ischemia). In comparison to mesenteric ischemia, ischemic colitis often occurs without a specific original insult. Most commonly, ischemic colitis occurs in an elderly patient with diffuse microvascular disease and multiple comorbidities, while hypoperfusion states such as heart failure, hypovolemia, sepsis, or other physiologic insults may exacerbate the underlying microvascular disease. Medications, infections, hypercoagulability, and iatrogenic causes such as aortic reconstruction also may result in ischemic colitis. Ischemic colitis most commonly affects the left colon (75%), splenic flexure, and isolated right colon in 10% of cases, with isolated right colon ischemia associated with a worse prognosis. Abdominal radiographs are abnormal in up to 21% of patients, but CT is by far the most commonly used diagnostic test, as most patients present with vague abdominal pain. CT demonstrates bowel wall thickening, thumb-printing, pericolonic stranding, and a "target sign" (**Figure 6.9**). Vascular occlusion in the inferior mesenteric artery may be seen. In addition, signs of severe ischemia include pneumatosis, portal venous gas, peritoneal fluid, and pneumoperitoneum in the setting of perforation. CT angiography is frequently obtained, but in one multicenter study reviewing 118 patients with ischemic colitis, CTA did not provide additional information that altered management or prognosis.

Colonoscopy is useful if CT findings are nonspecific. This allows evaluation of degree of ischemia as well as biopsy if diagnosis is unclear. Ultrasound has some limited utility in evaluating suspected ischemic colitis, when colon wall thickening is seen and the clinical suspicion is high. CT and CT angiography remain the most useful radiographic tests in ischemic colitis.

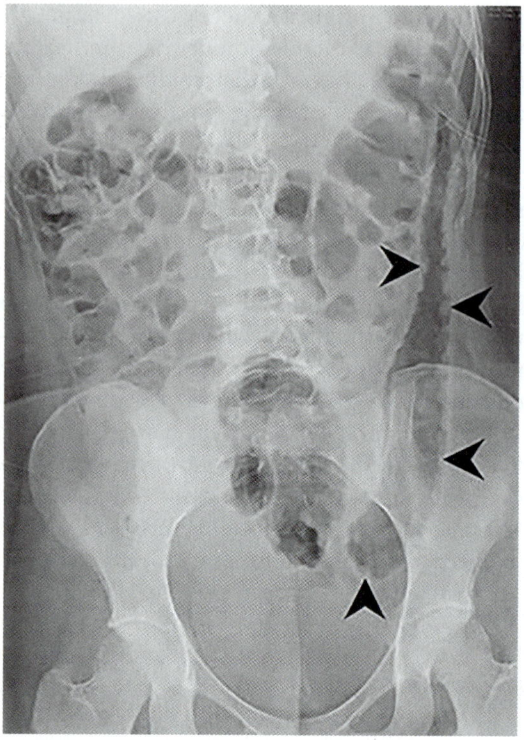

Figure 6.9 Radiograph demonstrating edematous sigmoid colon with "thumbprinting" (*black arrowheads*) from ischemic colitis. (Reprinted by permission from Springer: Chawla A, Tim WL, Lim TC. The colonic thumbprinting sign. *Abdom Imaging*. 2015;40(7):2918-20. Figure 2.)

Intraoperative Imaging

Other surgical specialty fields such as orthopedics and neurosurgery rely heavily on intraoperative imaging to guide the performance of procedures. EGS uses intraoperative imaging much less frequently, most commonly in hepatobiliary surgery.

Intraoperative cholangiography (IOC) was introduced in the 1930s by Mirizzi, and there has been great debate about the indications for cholangiography in laparoscopic cholecystectomy. Some surgeons advocate routine IOC, others advise selective IOC, and some do none. IOC is suggested to evaluate common bile duct (CBD) stones, delineate biliary anatomy, and provide an early warning for misidentification of the CBD as the cystic duct. The American Society for Gastrointestinal Endoscopy (ASGE) and the Society of American Gastrointestinal and Endoscopic Surgeons (SAGES) guidelines suggest that IOC performance depends on institutional strategy and the patient's risk of presenting a CBD stone. Multiple large trials have failed to support or refute the use of IOC to prevent retained CBD stones or major bile duct injury. IOC may be technically challenging in the acutely inflamed gallbladder. However, in a large trial of >500 patients undergoing emergency cholecystectomy, all but three were able to have IOC performed successfully, suggesting that IOC is nearly always technically feasible even in acute cholecystitis.

As an alternative to IOC, both ultrasound and fluorescent imaging have been utilized to identify CBD stones and bile duct anatomy. Laparoscopic intraoperative ultrasound (LUS) was developed in the early 1980s, after technology allowed the development of appropriate ultrasound probes for laparoscopic access. LUS has been found to have similar diagnostic accuracy to IOC in several large prospective studies. In addition, LUS has several advantages, including lack of ionizing radiation, less need for dissection of the cystic duct, risk of CBD injury during duct cannulation, and the ability for serial examinations during dissection. However, it is operator dependent and does not allow panoramic view of the entire biliary tree.

Intraoperative near-infrared fluorescence with indocyanine green (ICG) has recently become available in various surgical settings and is used for various applications. For cholangiography, ICG is administered intravenously before surgery and a specialized imaging system for near-infrared fluorescence imaging is used (**Figure 6.10**). Similar to LUS, fluorescence imaging can be performed multiple times throughout the operation and does not require cannulation of the cystic duct or use of fluoroscopy. In several smaller trials, this technique has been demonstrated to be safe, effective, and provide similar visualization rates of critical structures similar to IOC.

Fluorescence-guided imaging can also be used to identify intestinal perfusion. This is particularly relevant in cases of gastrointestinal ischemia (**Figure 6.11**). In both small bowel and colonic ischemia, ICG fluorescence angiography can help identify areas of intestinal perfusion to allow a better definition of resection margins. In one study of 52 patients undergoing surgical resection for small bowel and colon ischemia, ICG fluorescence angiography provided additional information that changed operative strategy in 11.5% of patients and resulted in clinical benefit. ICG fluorescence angiography has also been used to evaluate anastomotic perfusion in colorectal surgery, with findings of decreased anastomotic leak rate in a meta-analysis of over 1000 patients undergoing resection for colon cancer. Of note, these findings have not yet been reproduced in an EGS cohort.

Imaging Controversies

Diagnosis of Appendicitis in Pregnancy

Appendicitis and cholecystitis are the most common causes of acute abdominal pain in pregnancy. Acute appendicitis accounts for approximately one-quarter of nonobstetrical surgeries in this population. Ultrasound is a reasonable first-line approach in pregnant patients. The appendix will appear enlarged and may not compress or may be fluid filled. However, ultrasound may be limited by body habitus, and the quality of images is operator dependent. Additionally, the gravid uterus may displace the appendix, making it more challenging to identify.

MR is the optimal second choice for diagnosis to avoid ionizing radiation. Similar to ultrasound, the appendix will appear enlarged, and fluid and inflammatory stranding are evident on T2-weighted images. When gadolinium is used for contrast, clinicians should be aware that the contrast agent may cross the placenta and will be excreted by the fetus. If a study provides adequate information without gadolinium, contrast should be avoided, as definitive safety for the fetus is unknown. However, if needed to make an accurate diagnosis, gadolinium should be used as most evidence suggests that it does not significantly impact the fetus.

The approach outlined for appendicitis is appropriate for most other surgical emergencies in pregnant patients. Ultrasound vs MRI should be considered depending on the differential diagnosis and available resources. However, blunt abdominal trauma is different. In the case of suspected injury, rapid and accurate diagnosis is imperative to protect the life of both the mother and fetus. In this circumstance, CT is recommended.

Imaging the Gallbladder

Imaging of the biliary tree depends heavily on the underlying pathology. The spectrum of acute cholecystitis, symptomatic cholelithiasis, choledocholithiasis, and cholangitis are some of the most common causes of acute abdominal pain seen in

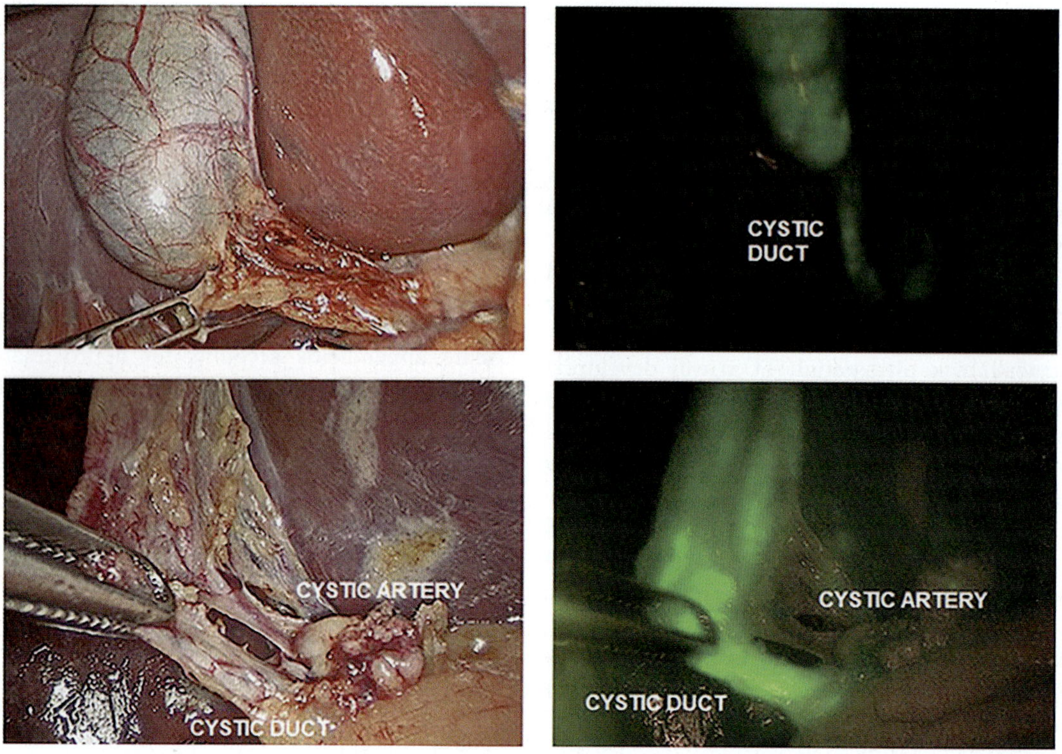

Figure 6.10 Intraoperative indocyanine green fluorescent cholangiography during dissection of cystic duct and cystic artery under white light (left) and fluorescent light (right). (Copyright © 2020 Esposito, Settimi, Del Conte, Cerulo, Coppola, Farina, Crocetto, Ricciardi, Esposito and Escolino. In: Esposito C, Settimi A, Del Conte F, et al. Image-guided pediatric surgery using Indocyanine Green (ICG) fluorescence in laparoscopic and robotic surgery. *Front Pediatr*. 2020;8:314. Figure 4. This is an open-access article distributed under the terms of the Creative Commons Attribution License (CC BY).

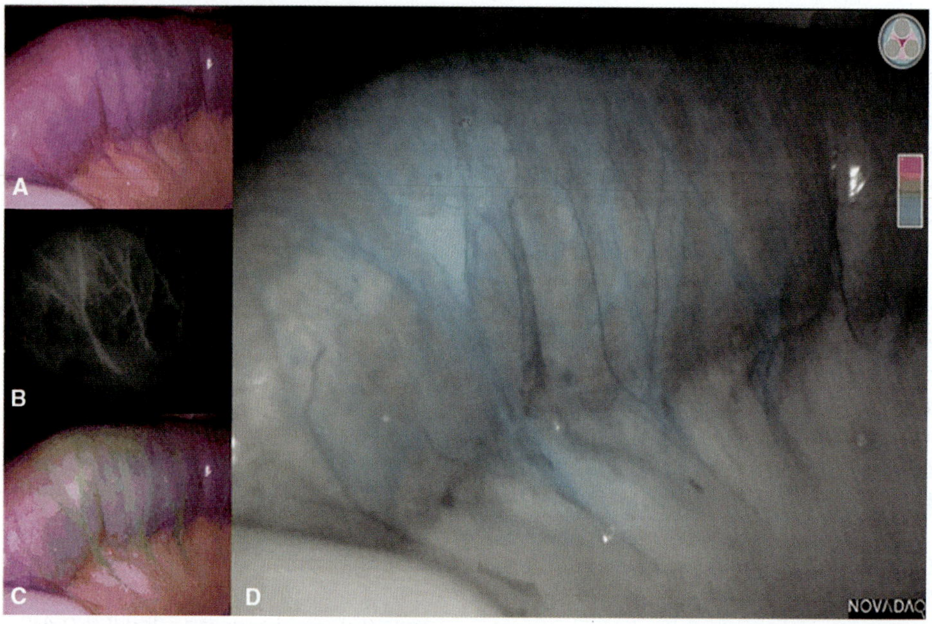

Figure 6.11 Intraoperative indocyanine green fluorescent evaluation of bowel ischemia using visual inspection (**A**), and three different fluorescent imaging devices **(B-D)**. (Reprinted by permission from Springer: Springer Nature. From Karampinis I, Keese M, Jakob J, et al. Indocyanine green tissue angiography can reduce extended bowel resections in acute mesenteric ischemia. *J Gastrointest Surg*. 2018;22(12):2117-2124. doi:10.1007/s11605-018-3855-1)

the ED. CT is often the initial imaging modality, as it is readily available and provides imaging of the entire abdomen.

However, as a first-line imaging modality, for biliary tract disease, ultrasound is superior. Multiple studies have indicated ultrasound has a sensitivity of 81%-97% and a specificity of 83%-95% for detection of biliary pathology, compared to CT with a sensitivity of 92.5%-94% and a specificity of 59%. Sonographic findings consistent with acute cholecystitis include distention of the gallbladder, wall thickening, pericholecystic fluid, Murphy sign with sonographic compression (right upper quadrant pain with compression by the ultrasound probe), hyperemia of the gallbladder wall, and the presence of gallstones. This information is available without the use of ionizing radiation, and CT is not as accurate in the detection of gallstones. When other imaging modalities are equivocal regarding the diagnosis of acute cholecystitis, cholescintigraphy is superior to all other modalities in establishing the diagnosis. Cholescintigraphy may not be available at all medical centers.

The diagnosis of choledocholithiasis may also require imaging beyond ultrasound or CT. Intrahepatic biliary dilatation and dilation of the CBD, especially in the setting of elevated direct bilirubin or amylase, is highly suspicious for obstruction of the biliary tree. In some centers, concerns for choledocholithiasis will be referred directly to gastroenterology for endoscopic retrograde cholangiopancreatography (ERCP). However, magnetic resonance cholangiopancreatography (MRCP) is an excellent noninvasive diagnostic tool with a sensitivity and specificity of 95% and 97%, respectively (**Figure 6.12**). MRCP is not limited by gallstone composition, unlike CT, which is much more accurate with calcium-dense stones. MRCP also has excellent accuracy with small stones and in differentiating benign from malignant strictures.

Overall, ultrasound is an excellent first-line imaging modality for acute biliary complaints. Cholescintigraphy should be considered when suspicion remains high but other imaging is not conclusive. MRCP is the preferred imaging modality for obstructive pathology of the biliary tree.

Imaging in the Setting of Necrotizing Soft Tissue Infections

Necrotizing soft tissue infections are a surgical emergency. Surgical residents have classically been told to call the attending with the consult from the OR, so rapidly should they be moving toward surgical debridement. One of the most significant contributors to morbidity and mortality in NSTI is delay in diagnosis. Delays occur, as the diagnosis is often difficult to make, with an NSTI and cellulitis at times difficult to differentiate.

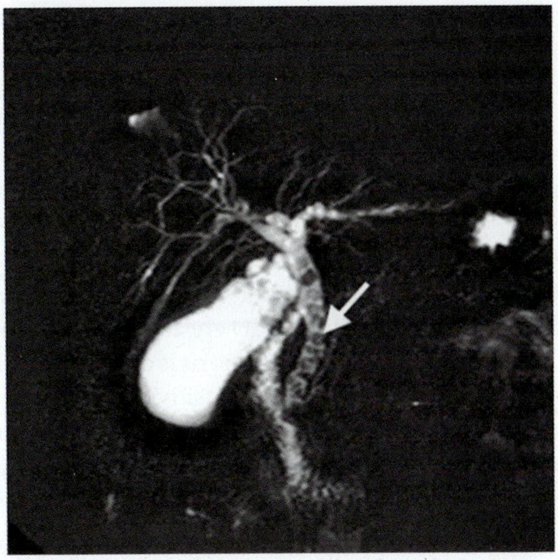

Figure 6.12 Magnetic resonance cholangiopancreatography (MRCP) of choledocholithiasis demonstrating dilated common bile duct with multiple stones (*arrow*). (From Thomas S, Jahangir K. Noninvasive imaging of the biliary system relevant to percutaneous interventions. *Semin Intervent Radiol.* 2016;33(4):277-282. doi:10.1055/s-0036-1592328. © Georg Thieme Verlag KG.)

The role of imaging in the diagnosis of NSTI remains unclear. Certainly, the gold standard for diagnosis remains incision and inspection of the tissue planes, although this exposes the patient to risks of anesthesia, wounds, and pain. Imaging has the potential to improve diagnostic accuracy before, or instead of, surgical intervention. In general, ultrasound and MR are not routinely used due to limited emergent availability, especially during off-hours. Historically, CT has not been considered accurate in the diagnosis of NSTI, although this may be changing with more modern equipment that can take finer cuts and produce more accurate images.

There is consensus that CT is superior to plain radiographs in the diagnosis of NSTI. Subcutaneous emphysema is pathognomonic for NSTI on imaging, yet not all causative organisms produce gas, and emphysema, when present, may be a late finding. In addition to subcutaneous emphysema, other CT findings that should raise suspicion include evidence of tissue inflammation and ischemia, especially in an asymmetrical distribution; signs of muscle necrosis; and fluid collections along tissue planes. As these findings are relatively nonspecific, CT imaging may ultimately be too sensitive, resulting in a lower predictive ability. Evidence supporting the role of imaging in the diagnosis of NSTI is 2C at best. Imaging should not delay operative intervention when suspicion is high.

Imaging in Pediatric Patients

The most common emergent surgical concerns for children presenting to the ED are acute appendicitis and trauma. Accurate diagnosis is essential in all cases, but the degree of time sensitivity will greatly affect the modality chosen. In circumstances such as trauma, the need for rapidly obtained, highly accurate imaging usually necessitates CT.

The risk of ionizing radiation is real, however, and has a greater impact on children. For a 1-year-old child, the lifetime risk of malignancy due to radiation is 0.18%, only decreasing slightly to 0.11% in a 15-year-old undergoing similar CT imaging. The use of protocols designed to minimize radiation is critical in protecting pediatric patients. When possible, alternative imaging modalities such as ultrasound are preferred in children. Finally, serial examinations may be another alternative that spares pediatric patients unnecessary imaging.

Contrast

The choice of contrast agents and modalities has important implications for the effectiveness of the study. In CT imaging, intravenous (IV) contrast is sensitive and specific for bowel-related pathology. IV contrast is also mandatory to assess vascular structures. In general, oral contrast is no longer utilized for initial workup of generalized acute abdominal pain, as studies have shown it does not significantly increase diagnostic accuracy, often does not even reach the site of pathology by the time of imaging and may contribute to delays in imaging and diagnosis. Enteral contrast may be indicated for specific diagnoses related to the upper gastrointestinal tract, colon, or rectum.

Intravenous iodinated contrast is often avoided in patients with reduced renal function due to the fear of worsening an acute kidney injury or causing a patient with marginal renal function to develop complete renal failure. The exact risk of contrast administration to renal function is unclear. However, in patients with a decreased glomerular filtration rate (<30 mL/min/1.73m^2, possibly 30-44 mL/min/1.73m^2), prophylactic hydration with IV solutions such as normal saline is indicated and provides some renal protection. Clinicians must weigh the risks and benefits of administering contrast and how effective the imaging will be with or without contrast to make the optimal decision for the patient.

For patients with a contrast allergy, the clinician must weigh the same risks and benefits. A careful history to determine the type and severity of allergy is important in decision-making. When IV contrast is indicated, most radiology departments have well-protocolized pretreatment algorithms to include antihistamines and steroids. Of course, these patients should be monitored closely during and after the administration of the contrast agent.

While MRI using gadolinium contrast is often considered safer than iodinated contrast for CT, reactions to gadolinium are widely reported. Anaphylaxis may occur following the administration of gadolinium. The most serious complication, nephrogenic systemic fibrosis, is characterized by fibrosis of the skin and soft tissues and occasionally leads to multiorgan failure and death. This complication occurs more frequently in patients with acute renal failure or stage 4 or 5 chronic kidney disease. However, nephrogenic systemic fibrosis remains exceedingly rare even in this population, with a rate of 0.07%. Overall, adverse reactions to MR-related contrast occur in 0.17%-0.24%. In regard to contrast, MR has a more favorable safety profile compared with CT.

SUMMARY

Current imaging modalities provide critical tools in the diagnosis and often treatment of the EGS patient. The hemodynamic status of the patient is a critical determinant of appropriate imaging in the EGS patient. The proximity of CT scanners to the ED, the rapidity of the test, and detailed information obtained has made this a vital tool in the evaluation of the EGS patient. Ultrasonography is the test of choice in the patient with suspected biliary tract disease, often appendicitis and obstetrical/gynecologic emergencies. Angiography and embolization are the usual next step if endoscopic therapy cannot control GI bleeding.

SUGGESTED READINGS

Adler DG, Leighton JA, Davila RE, et al. ASGE guideline: the role of endoscopy in acute non-variceal upper-GI hemorrhage. *Gastrointest Endosc.* 2004;60:497-504.

Ai T, Morelli JN, Hu X, et al. A historical overview of magnetic resonance imaging, focusing on technological innovations. *Invest Radiol.* 2012;47:725-741.

Aldrich JE. Basic physics of ultrasound imaging. *Crit Care Med*. 2007;35:S131-S137.

Alvarado A. A practical score for the early diagnosis of acute appendicitis. *Ann Emerg Med*. 1986;15:557-564.

Assalia A, Schein M, Kopelman D, Hirshberg A, Hashmonai M. Therapeutic effect of oral Gastrografin in adhesive, partial small-bowel obstruction: a prospective randomized trial. *Surgery*. 1994;115:433-437.

Atamanalp SS, Ozturk G. Sigmoid volvulus in the elderly: outcomes of a 43-year, 453-patient experience. *Surg Today*. 2011;41:514-519.

Bala M, Kashuk J, Moore EE, et al. Acute mesenteric ischemia: guidelines of the World Society of Emergency Surgery. *World J Emerg Surg*. 2017;12:38.

Ballantyne GH, Brandner MD, Beart Jr RW, Ilstrup DM. Volvulus of the colon. Incidence and mortality. *Ann Surg*. 1985;202:83-92.

Blanco-Colino R, Espin-Basany E. Intraoperative use of ICG fluorescence imaging to reduce the risk of anastomotic leakage in colorectal surgery: a systematic review and meta-analysis. *Tech Coloproctol*. 2018;22:15-23.

Brenner DJ, Elliston CD, Hall EJ, Berdon WE. Estimates of the cancer risks from pediatric CT radiation are not merely theoretical: comment on "point/counterpoint: in x-ray computed tomography, technique factors should be selected appropriate to patient size. against the proposition". *Med Phys*. 2001;28:2387-2388.

Chakraborty A, Ayoob A, DiSantis D. Coffee bean sign. *Abdom Imaging*. 2015;40:2904-2905.

Chang WC, Ko KH, Lin CS, et al. Features on MDCT that predict surgery in patients with adhesive-related small bowel obstruction. *PLoS One*. 2014;9:e89804.

Chaudhry AA, Baker KS, Gould ES, Gupta R. Necrotizing fasciitis and its mimics: what radiologists need to know. *AJR Am J Roentgenol*. 2015;204:128-139.

Chong WK, Papadopoulou V, Dayton PA. Imaging with ultrasound contrast agents: current status and future. *Abdom Radiol (NY)*. 2018;43:762-772.

Coleman JJ, Carr BW, Rogers T, et al. The Alvarado score should be used to reduce emergency department length of stay and radiation exposure in select patients with abdominal pain. *J Trauma Acute Care Surg*. 2018;84:946-950.

ASGE Standards of Practice Committee; Maple JT, Ben-Menachem T, Anderson MA, et al. The role of endoscopy in the evaluation of suspected choledocholithiasis. *Gastrointest Endosc*. 2010;71:1-9.

Copin P, Zins M, Nuzzo A, et al. Acute mesenteric ischemia: a critical role for the radiologist. *Diagn Interv Imaging*. 2018;99:123-134.

Dane B, Hindman N, Johnson E, Rosenkrantz AB. Utility of CT findings in the diagnosis of cecal volvulus. *AJR Am J Roentgenol*. 2017;209:762-766.

Daniel VT, Ingraham AM, Khubchandani JA, et al. Variations in the delivery of emergency general surgery care in the era of acute care surgery. *Jt Comm J Qual Patient Saf*. 2019;45:14-23.

Davenport MS, Perazella MA, Yee J, et al. Use of intravenous iodinated contrast media in patients with kidney disease: consensus statements from the American College of Radiology and the National Kidney Foundation. *Radiology*. 2020;294:660-668.

Davila RE, Rajan E, Adler DG, et al. ASGE Guideline: the role of endoscopy in the patient with lower-GI bleeding. *Gastrointest Endosc*. 2005;62:656-660.

DeBarros J, Rosas L, Cohen J, et al. The changing paradigm for the treatment of colonic hemorrhage: superselective angiographic embolization. *Dis Colon Rectum*. 2002;45:802-808.

Eisenberg RL, Heineken P, Hedgcock MW, Federle M, Goldberg HI. Evaluation of plain abdominal radiographs in the diagnosis of abdominal pain. *Ann Surg*. 1983;197:464-469.

Enochsson L, Gudbjartsson T, Hellberg A, et al. The Fenyo-Lindberg scoring system for appendicitis increases positive predictive value in fertile women—a prospective study in 455 patients randomized to either laparoscopic or open appendectomy. *Surg Endosc*. 2004;18:1509-1513.

Expert Panel on Gastrointestinal Imaging; Chang KJ, Marin D, Kim DH, et al. ACR appropriateness criteria® suspected small-bowel obstruction. *J Am Coll Radiol*. 2020;17:S305-S314.

Expert Panel on Gastrointestinal Imaging; Garcia EM, Camacho MA, Karolyi DR, et al. ACR appropriateness criteria® right lower quadrant pain-suspected appendicitis. *J Am Coll Radiol*. 2018;15:S373-S387.

Expert Panels on Vascular Imaging and Gastrointestinal Imaging; Singh-Bhinder N, Kim DH, Holly BP, et al. ACR appropriateness criteria® nonvariceal upper gastrointestinal bleeding. *J Am Coll Radiol*. 2017;14:S177-S188.

Feuerstadt P, Brandt LJ. Colon ischemia: recent insights and advances. *Curr Gastroenterol Rep*. 2010;12:383-390.

Ford JA, Soop M, Du J, Loveday BP, Rodgers M. Systematic review of intraoperative cholangiography in cholecystectomy. *Br J Surg*. 2012;99:160-167.

Garcia-Blazquez V, Vicente-Bartulos A, Olavarria-Delgado A, et al. Accuracy of CT angiography in the diagnosis of acute gastrointestinal bleeding: systematic review and meta-analysis. *Eur Radiol*. 2013;23:1181-1190.

Garcia-Bournissen F, Shrim A, Koren G. Safety of gadolinium during pregnancy. *Can Fam Physician*. 2006;52:309-310.

Garzelli L, Nuzzo A, Copin P, et al. Contrast-enhanced CT for the diagnosis of acute mesenteric ischemia. *AJR Am J Roentgenol*. 2020;215:29-38.

Gerhardt RT, Nelson BK, Keenan S, et al. Derivation of a clinical guideline for the assessment of nonspecific abdominal pain: the Guideline for Abdominal Pain in the ED Setting (GAPEDS) Phase 1 Study. *Am J Emerg Med*. 2005;23:709-717.

Gingold D, Murrell Z. Management of colonic volvulus. *Clin Colon Rectal Surg*. 2012;25:236-244.

Gorter RR, Eker HH, Gorter-Stam MA, et al. Diagnosis and management of acute appendicitis. EAES consensus development conference 2015. *Surg Endosc.* 2016;30:4668-4690.

Grassi R, Romano S, Pinto A, Romano L. Gastro-duodenal perforations: conventional plain film, US and CT findings in 166 consecutive patients. *Eur J Radiol.* 2004;50:30-36.

Hinchey EJ, Schaal PG, Richards GK. Treatment of perforated diverticular disease of the colon. *Adv Surg.* 1978;12:85-109.

Hsiao CT, Chang CP, Huang TY, Chen YC, Fann WC. Prospective validation of the laboratory risk indicator for necrotizing fasciitis (LRINEC) score for necrotizing fasciitis of the extremities. *PLoS One.* 2020;15:e0227748.

Huprich JE, Fletcher JG, Fidler JL, et al. Prospective blinded comparison of wireless capsule endoscopy and multiphase CT enterography in obscure gastrointestinal bleeding. *Radiology.* 2011;260:744-751.

Iranmanesh P, Tobler O, De Sousa S, et al. Feasibility, benefit and risk of systematic intraoperative cholangiogram in patients undergoing emergency cholecystectomy. *PLoS One.* 2018;13:e0199147.

Ittyachen AM, Eapen M, Kumar R. Chilaiditi's sign. *Eur J Intern Med.* 2016;28:e5-e6.

Jakimowicz JJ. Intraoperative ultrasonography in open and laparoscopic abdominal surgery: an overview. *Surg Endosc.* 2006;20(Suppl 2):S425-S435.

Jung JW, Kang HR, Kim MH, et al. Immediate hypersensitivity reaction to gadolinium-based MR contrast media. *Radiology.* 2012;264:414-422.

Kaiser AM, Jiang JK, Lake JP, et al. The management of complicated diverticulitis and the role of computed tomography. *Am J Gastroenterol.* 2005;100:910-917.

Karampinis I, Keese M, Jakob J, et al. Indocyanine green tissue angiography can reduce extended bowel resections in acute mesenteric ischemia. *J Gastrointest Surg.* 2018;22:2117-2124.

Kessner R, Barnes S, Halpern P, Makrin V, Blachar A. CT for acute nontraumatic abdominal pain-is oral contrast really required? *Acad Radiol.* 2017;24:840-845.

Kiewiet JJ, Leeuwenburgh MM, Bipat S, et al. A systematic review and meta-analysis of diagnostic performance of imaging in acute cholecystitis. *Radiology.* 2012;264:708-720.

Kim K, Kim YH, Kim SY, et al. Low-dose abdominal CT for evaluating suspected appendicitis. *N Engl J Med.* 2012;366:1596-1605.

Kossoff G. Basic physics and imaging characteristics of ultrasound. *World J Surg.* 2000;24:134-142.

Krajewski S, Brown J, Phang PT, Raval M, Brown CJ. Impact of computed tomography of the abdomen on clinical outcomes in patients with acute right lower quadrant pain: a meta-analysis. *Can J Surg.* 2011;54:43-53.

Lappas JC, Reyes BL, Maglinte DD. Abdominal radiography findings in small-bowel obstruction: relevance to triage for additional diagnostic imaging. *AJR Am J Roentgenol.* 2001;176:167-174.

Lee SY, Coughlin B, Wolfe JM, et al. Prospective comparison of helical CT of the abdomen and pelvis without and with oral contrast in assessing acute abdominal pain in adult Emergency Department patients. *Emerg Radiol.* 2006;12:150-157.

Leichtle SW, Tung L, Khan M, Inaba K, Demetriades D. The role of radiologic evaluation in necrotizing soft tissue infections. *J Trauma Acute Care Surg.* 2016;81:921-924.

Levin DC, Rao VM, Parker L, Frangos AJ, Sunshine JH. Ownership or leasing of CT scanners by nonradiologist physicians: a rapidly growing trend that raises concern about self-referral. *J Am Coll Radiol.* 2008;5:1206-1209.

Levsky JM, Den EI, DuBrow RA, Wolf EL, Rozenblit AM. CT findings of sigmoid volvulus. *AJR Am J Roentgenol.* 2010;194:136-143.

Machi J, Tateishi T, Oishi AJ, et al. Laparoscopic ultrasonography versus operative cholangiography during laparoscopic cholecystectomy: review of the literature and a comparison with open intraoperative ultrasonography. *J Am Coll Surg.* 1999;188:360-367.

Maglinte DD, Reyes BL, Harmon BH, et al. Reliability and role of plain film radiography and CT in the diagnosis of small-bowel obstruction. *AJR Am J Roentgenol.* 1996;167:1451-1455.

Mathews JD, Forsythe AV, Brady Z, et al. Cancer risk in 680,000 people exposed to computed tomography scans in childhood or adolescence: data linkage study of 11 million Australians. *BMJ.* 2013;346:f2360.

Mazaheri P, Ballard DH, Neal KA, et al. CT of gastric volvulus: interobserver reliability, radiologists' accuracy, and imaging findings. *AJR Am J Roentgenol.* 2019;212:103-108.

McCarthy E, Little M, Briggs J, et al. Radiology and mesenteric ischaemia. *Clin Radiol.* 2015;70:698-705.

Mervak BM, Wilson SB, Handly BD, Altun E, Burke LM. MRI of acute appendicitis. *J Magn Reson Imaging.* 2019;50:1367-1376.

Mirizzi PL. Functional disturbances of the main bile duct and operative cholangiography. *Prensa Med Argent.* 1947;34:2273-2276.

Moore FA, Moore EE, Burlew CC, et al. Western Trauma Association critical decisions in trauma: management of complicated diverticulitis. *J Trauma Acute Care Surg.* 2012;73:1365-1371.

Mostbeck G, Adam EJ, Nielsen MB, et al. How to diagnose acute appendicitis: ultrasound first. *Insights Imaging.* 2016;7:255-263.

Moszkowicz D, Mariani A, Tresallet C, Menegaux F. Ischemic colitis: the ABCs of diagnosis and surgical management. *J Visc Surg.* 2013;150:19-28.

Mularski RA, Sippel JM, Osborne ML. Pneumoperitoneum: a review of nonsurgical causes. *Crit Care Med.* 2000;28:2638-2644.

Nakashima K, Ishimaru H, Fujimoto T, et al. Diagnostic performance of CT findings for bowel ischemia and necrosis in closed-loop small-bowel obstruction. *Abdom Imaging.* 2015;40:1097-1103.

Nakatsu S, Yasuda H, Maehata T, et al. Urgent computed tomography for determining the optimal timing of colonoscopy in patients with acute lower gastrointestinal bleeding. *Intern Med.* 2015;54:553-558.

O'Grady HL, Hartley JE. Radiographic work-up and treatment of lower gastrointestinal bleeding. *Clin Colon Rectal Surg.* 2008;21:188-192.

Ohle R, O'Reilly F, O'Brien KK, Fahey T, Dimitrov BD. The Alvarado score for predicting acute appendicitis: a systematic review. *BMC Med.* 2011;9:139.

Osayi SN, Wendling MR, Drosdeck JM, et al. Near-infrared fluorescent cholangiography facilitates identification of biliary anatomy during laparoscopic cholecystectomy. *Surg Endosc.* 2015;29:368-375.

Puylaert JB. Ultrasound of colon diverticulitis. *Dig Dis.* 2012;30:56-59.

Rabinovici R, Simansky DA, Kaplan O, Mavor E, Manny J. Cecal volvulus. *Dis Colon Rectum.* 1990;33: 765-769.

Radiology ACo. ACR—SPR practice guideline for the performance of abdominal radiography. 2016.

Roentgen's discovery. *Am J Dent Sci* 1896;30:33-36. https://www.ncbi.nlm.nih.gov/pmc/articles/PMC6118566/pdf/amjdentsci81545-0040.pdf

Rosenblat JM, Rozenblit AM, Wolf EL, et al. Findings of cecal volvulus at CT. *Radiology.* 2010;256:169-175.

Rosines LA, Chow DS, Lampl BS, et al. Value of gadolinium-enhanced MRI in detection of acute appendicitis in children and adolescents. *AJR Am J Roentgenol.* 2014;203:W543-W548.

Rubin GD. Computed tomography: revolutionizing the practice of medicine for 40 years. *Radiology.* 2014;273:S45-S74.

Samuel M. Pediatric appendicitis score. *J Pediatr Surg.* 2002;37:877-881.

Sarli L, Costi R, Gobbi S, et al. Scoring system to predict asymptomatic choledocholithiasis before laparoscopic cholecystectomy. A matched case-control study. *Surg Endosc.* 2003;17:1396-1403.

Sarr MG. How useful is methylglucamine diatrizoate solution in patients with small-bowel obstruction? *Nat Clin Pract Gastroenterol Hepatol.* 2006;3:432-433.

Shafi S, Aboutanos M, Brown CV, et al. Measuring anatomic severity of disease in emergency general surgery. *J Trauma Acute Care Surg.* 2014;76:884-887.

Shafi S, Priest EL, Crandall ML, et al. Multicenter validation of American Association for the Surgery of Trauma grading system for acute colonic diverticulitis and its use for emergency general surgery quality improvement program. *J Trauma Acute Care Surg.* 2016;80:405-410; discussion 410-401.

Shah AH, Olivero JJ. Gadolinium-induced nephrogenic systemic fibrosis. *Methodist Debakey Cardiovasc J.* 2017;13:172-173.

Sherid M, Samo S, Sulaiman S, et al. Is CT angiogram of the abdominal vessels needed following the diagnosis of ischemic colitis? A multicenter community study. *ISRN Gastroenterol.* 2014;2014:756926.

Shriki J. Ultrasound physics. *Crit Care Clin.* 2014;30: 1-24, v.

Smith JE, Hall EJ. The use of plain abdominal x rays in the emergency department. *Emerg Med J.* 2009;26:160-163.

Solis CV, Chang Y, De Moya MA, Velmahos GC, Fagenholz PJ. Free air on plain film: do we need a computed tomography too? *J Emerg Trauma Shock.* 2014;7:3-8.

Stoker J, van Randen A, Lameris W, Boermeester MA. Imaging patients with acute abdominal pain. *Radiology.* 2009;253:31-46.

Strate LL, Gralnek IM. ACG clinical guideline: management of patients with acute lower gastrointestinal bleeding. *Am J Gastroenterol.* 2016;111:459-474.

Suri S, Gupta S, Sudhakar PJ, et al. Comparative evaluation of plain films, ultrasound and CT in the diagnosis of intestinal obstruction. *Acta Radiol.* 1999;40:422-428.

Tabibian JH, Wong Kee Song LM, Enders FB, Aguet JC, Tabibian N. Technetium-labeled erythrocyte scintigraphy in acute gastrointestinal bleeding. *Int J Colorectal Dis.* 2013;28:1099-1105.

Tarasconi A, Baiocchi GL, Pattonieri V, et al. Transcatheter arterial embolization versus surgery for refractory non-variceal upper gastrointestinal bleeding: a meta-analysis. *World J Emerg Surg.* 2019;14:3.

Theodoropoulou A, Koutroubakis IE. Ischemic colitis: clinical practice in diagnosis and treatment. *World J Gastroenterol.* 2008;14:7302-7308.

Thoeni RF, Cello JP. CT imaging of colitis. *Radiology.* 2006;240:623-638.

Thomas S, Jahangir K. Noninvasive imaging of the biliary system relevant to percutaneous interventions. *Semin Intervent Radiol.* 2016;33:277-282.

Thompson WM, Kilani RK, Smith BB, et al. Accuracy of abdominal radiography in acute small-bowel obstruction: does reviewer experience matter? *AJR Am J Roentgenol.* 2007;188:W233-W238.

Tominaga GT, Staudenmayer KL, Shafi S, et al. The American Association for the Surgery of Trauma grading scale for 16 emergency general surgery conditions: disease-specific criteria characterizing anatomic severity grading. *J Trauma Acute Care Surg.* 2016;81:593-602.

van Dijk ST, Daniels L, Nio CY, et al. Predictive factors on CT imaging for progression of uncomplicated into complicated acute diverticulitis. *Int J Colorectal Dis.* 2017;32:1693-1698.

Vandenberghe W, Hoste E. Contrast-associated acute kidney injury: does it really exist, and if so, what to do about it? *F1000Res.* 2019;8:F1000.

Vaz SC, Oliveira F, Herrmann K, Veit-Haibach P. Nuclear medicine and molecular imaging advances in the 21st century. *Br J Radiol.* 2020;93:20200095.

Wallace GW, Davis MA, Semelka RC, Fielding JR. Imaging the pregnant patient with abdominal pain. *Abdom Imaging.* 2012;37:849-860.

Wong CH, Khin LW, Heng KS, Tan KC, Low CO. The LRINEC (Laboratory Risk Indicator for Necrotizing

Fasciitis) score: a tool for distinguishing necrotizing fasciitis from other soft tissue infections. *Crit Care Med.* 2004;32:1535-1541.

Woolen SA, Shankar PR, Gagnier JJ, et al. Risk of nephrogenic systemic fibrosis in patients with stage 4 or 5 chronic kidney disease receiving a group II gadolinium-based contrast agent: a systematic review and meta-analysis. *JAMA Intern Med.* 2020;180:223-230.

Yi WS, Garg G, Sava JA. Localization and definitive control of lower gastrointestinal bleeding with angiography and embolization. *Am Surg.* 2013;79:375-380.

Zacharias N, Velmahos GC, Salama A, et al. Diagnosis of necrotizing soft tissue infections by computed tomography. *Arch Surg.* 2010;145:452-455.

Zielinski MD, Eiken PW, Bannon MP, et al. Small bowel obstruction—who needs an operation? A multivariate prediction model. *World J Surg.* 2010;34:910-919.

Zielinski MD, Haddad NN, Cullinane DC, et al. Multi-institutional, prospective, observational study comparing the Gastrografin challenge versus standard treatment in adhesive small bowel obstruction. *J Trauma Acute Care Surg.* 2017;83:47-54.

CHAPTER

7 Nutrition

Jennifer L. Hartwell and Rosemary A. Kozar

CASE PRESENTATION

The patient is a 64-year-old male who presents to the emergency department (ED) with a 6-hour history of severe abdominal pain. He states he awoke from his sleep with severe pain and nausea. He had one episode of emesis and one episode of blood-tinged diarrhea. His pain is crampy and has not resolved. He has a past medical history of hypertension, diabetes, coronary artery disease status post percutaneous cardiac stenting 4 years ago, atrial fibrillation (Afib), chronic kidney disease (CKD) stage 2, and chronic mesenteric ischemia complicated by a recent weight loss of 40 pounds. His medications include metoprolol, amlodipine, atorvastatin, metformin, warfarin, and sertraline, all of which he is compliant with. He has smoked ½ pack per day of cigarettes for the past 40 years and has two to three cocktails every evening.

A full assessment is completed in the ED. His heart rate (HR) is 124 beats/min, and he is noted to be in Afib, blood pressure (BP) 90/60, temperature 38.5 °C, respiratory rate 22 breaths/min, height 191 cm, and weight 67 kg (body mass index [BMI] 18.4, underweight by definition). He is awake and alert but appears to be in moderate distress. He complains of severe abdominal pain. On examination, his abdomen is soft but diffusely tender. His skin is cool, and his radial and dorsalis pedis pulses are weakly palpable. He has obvious muscle wasting at his temples and in all four extremities. Rectal examination reveals maroon-tinged stool but no masses. Pertinent laboratory values obtained include white blood cell count of 13.5 k/mm^3, platelets of 254 k/mm^3, hemoglobin 11.6 g/dL, sodium 146 mmol/L, potassium 3.4 mmol/L, creatinine 1.6 mg/dL (baseline 1.3 mg/dL), INR 2.6, total bilirubin 1.4 mg/dL, and lactate 3.1 mmol/L. Intravenous fluids resuscitation is initiated, and he undergoes a computed tomography scan with intravenous contrast revealing the following (**Figure 7.1**):

Question: *What is the diagnosis?*

Answer: *Acute on chronic mesenteric ischemia complicated by underweight and protein-calorie malnutrition.*

The patient is given prothrombin complex concentrate (PCC) to reverse his INR, 2 L of lactated Ringer's, and begun on broad-spectrum antibiotics. He is taken emergently to the operating suite where an exploratory laparotomy is performed. Intraoperative findings include ischemia of the distal 150 cm of the small intestine, the cecum, and the ascending colon. The affected bowel is resected. He remains in hypovolemic shock during the operation, requiring large volume crystalloid resuscitation, high-dose vasopressor support, and transfusion of 4 units of packed red blood cells and 4 units of fresh frozen plasma. Because of his instability, the decision is made to abbreviate the operation, leave the bowel in discontinuity, and place a temporary abdominal closure device.

He is brought to the intensive care unit (ICU) with ongoing hypotension, acute on chronic renal failure, acute respiratory failure, and coagulopathy. Due to oliguria, hyperkalemia, and refractory acidemia, he requires continuous renal replacement therapy (CRRT) and prolonged ventilatory support. He undergoes an ileostomy at the second operation and facial closure at the third. On hospital day 14, he undergoes tracheostomy and percutaneous endoscopic gastrostomy (PEG) tube placement and is weaned from the ventilator by hospital day 18. He is transferred from the ICU to the surgical ward, where his course is complicated by ongoing delirium, ileus and feeding intolerance, debility, central line–associated bloodstream infection (CLABSI), and a surgical site infection of his midline abdominal wound. Ultimately, he participates in intensive physical and occupational therapy and is discharged to a rehabilitation facility on hospital day 32.

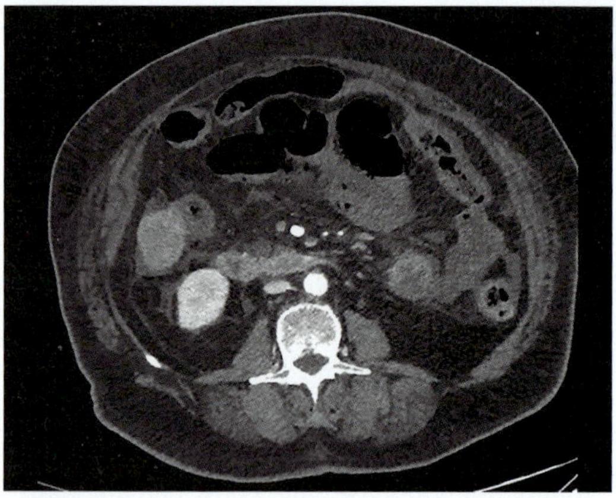

Figure 7.1 CT scan: thickened and hypoenhanced small bowel, mesenteric stranding, free fluid.

DISCUSSION OF CASE MANAGEMENT

Diagnosis

Intestinal ischemia results from progressive atherosclerotic disease, prolonged hypoperfusion of the viscera in cases of hypovolemic or hemorrhagic shock, or as in the case of this patient, a sudden embolic event precipitated by Afib. The classic presentation of acute mesenteric ischemia is pain out of proportion to physical examination findings. The patient will often describe the pain as crampy and unrelenting, associated with nausea, emesis, and occasionally bloody diarrhea. As the disease progresses, septic shock ensues. Common laboratory findings include leukocytosis, metabolic acidosis, and an elevated lactate level. The gold standard for diagnosis of mesenteric ischemia is computed tomographic angiography (CTA), which has a 96% sensitivity and 94% specificity and provides the evaluation of both the bowel and the vasculature that supplies it. CTA findings suggestive of bowel ischemia include bowel wall thickening, dilatation, hypoenhancement, mesenteric edema, pneumatosis, portal venous gas, and pneumoperitoneum. Prompt diagnosis and intervention for mesenteric ischemia are paramount as the disease has a high mortality, ranging from 30% to 90%.

Operative Considerations

The basic principles of surgical management include pre-, intra-, and postoperative resuscitation with an aim for euvolemia; correction of electrolyte disturbances and metabolic acidosis; revascularization; and resection of infarcted bowel. Overly aggressive resuscitation will result in bowel edema, anasarca, and is a known risk factor for acute renal failure. Options for revascularization include percutaneous endovascular techniques such as thrombectomy or thrombolysis, or stenting. If endovascular techniques are unavailable or the patient is too unstable to tolerate such a procedure, an arteriotomy and embolectomy should be performed at the time of surgery. All infarcted bowel should be immediately resected, and the remaining bowel examined thoroughly for areas of patchy necrosis. Frequently, the decision is made from the outset that the operation will be abbreviated to allow for a "second look" after revascularization and resuscitation. Bowel that is not overtly ischemic may be left *in situ* and reevaluated at this "second-look" operation. It is essential that no more bowel than is absolutely necessary be resected to limit the risk of short bowel syndrome, which is the presence of only 150-200 cm of the small bowel (SB). As such, the patient will be left in bowel discontinuity for 12-24 hours or until end points of resuscitation are met. The surgeon should ensure adequate placement of a nasogastric tube for bowel decompression during this period. At the "second-look" operation, the surgeon may find some bowel that previously appeared threatened now appears viable and will not require resection. Alternatively, some additional bowel may be necrotic after revascularization and will require resection. The decision to perform a bowel anastomosis or ostomy depends on the patient's age, comorbid conditions, and the intraoperative findings of the bowel. Edematous bowel is at risk for an anastomotic leak, and performing an ostomy will likely be safer. Regardless of whether an anastomosis or ostomy is created, the surgeon should consider what route will be used for nutrition in the coming days at the time of the final operation. Placing a small-bore nasojejunal (NJ) feeding tube can easily be accomplished with the assistance of the anesthesiologist. The surgeon can manually position the NJ tube in the third portion of the duodenum. If the indication is present for more durable feeding access, a device such as a gastrostomy or gastrojejunal tube can be placed before definitive abdominal closure.

Occasionally, due to ongoing abdominal distention or bowel edema, even after bowel continuity is reestablished, the abdomen cannot be closed. A temporary abdominal closure device can be utilized and subsequent attempts at fascial closure can be made over the ensuing days. If the fascia cannot be closed within 7-10 days, most surgeons will elect to perform a skin-only closure or utilize a bridging mesh to protect the bowel and limit the risk of enteroatmospheric fistula formation.

ICU Management

The initial nutritional management of a critically ill patient will depend on the rapidity with which resuscitation goals are met, including resolution of acidosis, coagulopathy, and electrolyte disturbances; normothermia; stabilization of blood pressure without the use of vasopressor agents; and normal urine output. The decision regarding the type and timing of nutrition administration in the ICU is determined by the patients' nutrition status on admission and the ability to tolerate enteral nutrition (EN). Patients with a history of chronic tobacco, alcohol, or illicit drug use are at high risk for malnutrition, as are sedentary obese patients and those who are institutionalized or dependent upon others for their care. Patients who are admitted with malnutrition (discussed below) will be candidates for early parenteral nutrition (PN) beginning within the first 24-48 hours of admission, bearing in mind that PN is not a resuscitative fluid and should not be used to replace intravascular fluid volume, which is best accomplished by crystalloid and blood product transfusion to meet resuscitation goals. Once hemodynamics are stabilized, PN should be started via a dedicated central venous access line. In patients who are not malnourished, attempts at EN should be made when bowel continuity is restored and resuscitation is complete. Evidence supports that early EN, even in critically ill surgical patients, is associated with less inflammation and portends improved overall outcomes. However, in previously healthy patients, tolerance up to 5-7 days of NPO status is acceptable, after which time, if EN is not tolerated, PN should be considered. Patients who are critically ill require higher doses of protein administration than noncritically ill patients, up to 1.2-2.0 g/kg/d, with even higher requirements (2.5 g/kg/d) for patients requiring renal replacement therapy in the ICU.

INTRODUCTION

Principles of Nutrition Management

We will review the principles of nutritional assessment, initiation, and continuation, emphasizing unique challenges in critically ill surgical patients.

Malnutrition, also referred to as undernutrition, occurs from lack of sufficient intake of calories and micronutrients with an increasing appreciation for the role of disease-associated inflammation as a major contributing factor. Although the association of preexisting malnutrition to poor surgical outcomes is well established, a uniform definition of malnutrition is lacking. New guidelines by the American Society for Parenteral and Enteral Nutrition (ASPEN) focus on the presence of fat or muscle wasting, fluid accumulation, or signs of micronutrient deficiencies on physical examination, history of weight loss and reduced nutrition intake, and alterations in serum proteins on laboratory studies to help define malnutrition. A recently convened Global Leadership in Malnutrition (GLIM) group proposed using a combination of phenotypic and etiologic criteria to define malnutrition. Phenotypic criteria include weight loss, low body mass, and low muscle mass. The etiologic criteria are reduced intake and inflammation. To meet the definition of malnutrition, at least one phenotypic and one etiologic criteria must be present. Several recent studies have validated the utility of GLIM.

There are several nutrition risk screening tools available, which include the Mini Nutritional Assessment, the Malnutrition Universal Screening Tool, the Short Nutritional Assessment Questionnaire, the Subjective Global Assessment (SGA), preoperative nutrition screening (PONS), the Nutrition Risk Screening Score (NRS-2002), and the Nutrition Risk in Critically ill (NUTRIC). A number of the tools target different patient populations. For instance, the PONS is for preoperative assessment in outpatients, while NUTRIC is for critically ill patients. The NUTRIC score incorporates age, Acute Physiology and Chronic Health Evaluation (APACHE II) score, baseline Sequential Organ Failure Assessment (SOFA) score, comorbidities, days from hospital admission to ICU admission, and serum interleukin-6 (IL-6). A more recent update deleted the requirement for IL-6, making it a more feasible score to calculate. Preoperative nutrition screening is not possible with emergency surgery, but an assessment postoperatively by a nutritionist should be completed. Identified high nutrition risk patients are at risk for surgical complications and may benefit most from aggressive postoperative nutrition supplementation. **Figure 7.2** reviews the potential benefits of perioperative nutrition screening and intervention.

Role of Enteral Nutrition

After resuscitation goals are achieved, including resolution of metabolic acidosis, stabilization of

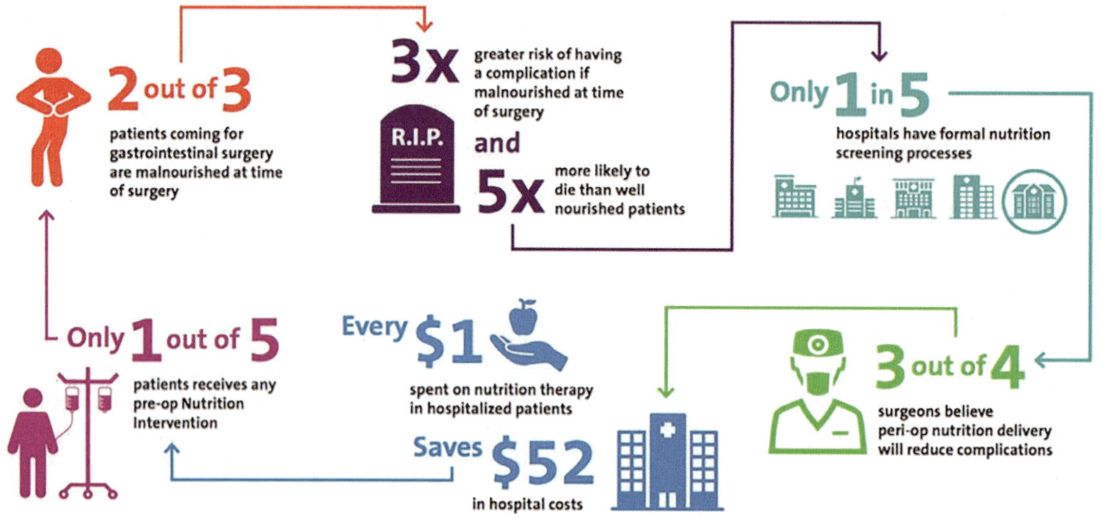

Figure 7.2 Potential benefits of perioperative nutrition screening and intervention. (Reprinted with permission from Wischmeyer PE, Carli F, Evans DC, et al. American Society for Enhanced Recovery and Perioperative Quality Initiative Joint Consensus Statement on Nutrition Screening and Therapy Within a Surgical Enhanced Recovery Pathway [published correction appears in Anesth Analg. 2018 Nov;127(5):e95]. *Anesth Analg*. 2018;126(6):1883-1895.)

blood pressure with no or only low-dose vasopressors, it is not only safe but advantageous to begin EN. Early EN (within 24-48 hours of admission) has been demonstrated to reduce infectious complications. There is no evidence to support awaiting the return of bowel function, as evidenced by flatus or bowel movement, to begin EN. It is safe to start EN even in patients with an open abdomen.

Optimal Site for Delivery of Enteral Nutrition: Gastric vs Postpyloric

The gastric route for enteral access is often the simplest and is generally well-tolerated, although no high-quality studies have addressed this issue in surgical patients. ASPEN/SCCM recommends that most critically ill patients can be safely fed into the stomach unless intolerance is demonstrated or the patient poses a high risk of aspiration. Many emergency general surgery and trauma patients are at increased risk, but in general, it is safe to initiate gastric feeding in most patients.

For patients who fail gastric feeding or are at high risk for aspiration, bedside placement of an NJ feeding tube has also proven safe and effective. It is frequently accomplished by the nurse in the critical care unit to facilitate SB feeding. Some patients tolerate SB feeding better than gastric feeding, especially patients with gastroparesis or reflux. Regardless of the location chosen for the EN feeding access, radiographic confirmation of tube placement is required before the initiation of EN.

Initiation of Enteral Nutrition

Once access has been established, a prescription for EN should be developed. EN should provide 25-35 kcal/kg/d (based on ideal body weight), and protein supplements can be added to EN to achieve the recommended 1.2-1.5 g/kg/d protein. Be mindful of additional sources of nonprotein calories and fluid that patients may receive, such as propofol or medications mixed in dextrose-containing solutions. Specific prescriptions for EN can be determined in collaboration with dietitians and clinicians trained in nutrition support. EN should be initiated and the rate advanced based on institutional protocols, typically at 20 mL/h every 4 hours to goal.

Strategies to Optimize Nutritional Delivery

To increase the likelihood of achieving protein and calorie delivery, consider utilization of a volume-based feeding protocol (**Table 7.1**). These protocols use a 24-hour volume-based goal rather than an hourly goal and empower the bedside nurse to calculate missed EN periods and adjust the hourly rate of EN delivery to accommodate for NPO periods. These protocols can be utilized with both gastric and SB access sites. A recent prospective randomized controlled trial in surgical and trauma ICU patients failed to show a benefit with this method, but there were issues with the study and enrollment. A study by Lee et al. using a multi-targeted feeding strategy to include volume-based

TABLE 7.1 ■ Strategies to Optimize Enteral Nutrition Intake

Strategy	Nutrition Goal
Early institution of EN	Begin EN within 24 hours of ICU admission
Avoidance of NPO prior to surgery[a]	Reduced fasting time and increased nutrition intake
Volume based or catch-up protocol	Recommended if reduced adequacy

[a]In patients with secured airway and not undergoing intestinal or airway procedure.
NPO, nil per OS.
Adapted from Lee JC, Williams GW, Kozar RA, et al. Multitargeted feeding strategies improve nutrition outcome and are associated with reduced pneumonia in a level 1 trauma intensive care unit. *JPEN J Parenter Enteral Nutr.* 2018;42(3):529-537.

feeding demonstrated a significant increase in nutrition adequacy and a significant reduction in pneumonia. This strategy can be considered to improve nutrition delivery if there is concern over adequacy with traditional protocols.

Enteral Intolerance

Intolerance of EN is demonstrated by the constellation of clinical findings of abdominal distention, pain, nausea, emesis, and/or radiographic findings of severe ileus or obstruction.

If a patient is intolerant of gastric feeding, a trial of SB feeding should be considered. Additionally, the early use of promotility agents such as erythromycin or metoclopramide may improve tolerance of EN. The routine assessment of gastric residual volumes (GRV) is no longer recommended as part of monitoring and treatment of intolerance. GRV measurement can lead to prolonged periods of NPO status with resulting deficits in the delivery of protein, calories, and nutrients. Additionally, studies have not revealed that higher GRV is associated with increased rates of pneumonia in the ICU. In patients who have required opioid medications for pain control, the constipating effects of these drugs can be mitigated with methylnaltrexone bromide, a μ-opioid receptor antagonist. Lastly, it is historically believed that ileus mandated NPO status while awaiting the return of bowel function. However, it is currently recommended to "feed through an ileus" as NPO status can promote instead of mitigating the ileus. As the definition of ileus can vary widely, an Intake, Feeling nauseated, Emesis, physical Exam, and Duration of symptoms (I-FEED) scoring system has been proposed as a more functional definition of postoperative gastrointestinal dysfunction that encourages intake through moderate intolerance.

Role of Parenteral Nutrition

Despite attempts to deliver adequate EN, it is not always possible or done effectively. ASPEN guidelines recommend using supplemental PN after 7-10 days for patients unable to meet at least 60% of their energy and protein requirements by the enteral route alone regardless of nutritional status or risk. However, a prospective randomized trial examining the early administration of supplemental PN in critically ill patients with acute respiratory failure suggested a benefit in functional outcomes in patients at high nutrition risk, defined in this study as low BMI. A definite trial to address at-risk populations has not been performed and represents a gap in our current knowledge.

For patients with a contraindication or complete intolerance to EN, ASPEN recommends low nutrition risk patients not receive total PN (TPN) for the first 7 days. A change from prior guidelines is that high nutrition risk or severely malnourished patients receive TPN upon ICU admission. Examples of contraindications to EN include bowel obstruction, short bowel syndrome, high-output enterocutaneous fistula, and bowel discontinuity.

For patients requiring PN, recent data support the use of omega-3 fatty acid–enriched PN. Pradelli et al. in a systematic review and meta-analysis of 49 randomized trials compared omega-3 fatty acids to standard lipid emulsions. The authors found a significant reduction in infections and reduced ICU and hospital length of stay with the use of omega-3 fatty acid–enriched PN.

The use of PN is not without complications. Overfeeding, refeeding syndrome, hyperglycemia, hypertriglyceridemia, hepatic dysfunction, and infections have all been reported. However, with stricter protocols for central line insertion and additional focus on central line care, infectious complications associated with PN have been reduced, with some studies showing no increase.

Challenges in the Critically Ill Surgical Patient

Feeding Above an Intestinal Anastomosis

Once bowel continuity has been restored, it is safe to begin EN even in the setting of SB anastomosis or fresh ostomy. It is not necessary to await the return of bowel function as evidenced by flatus or stool.

Feeding the Open Abdomen

It is common for patients to have a period before definitive fascial closure in which a temporary abdominal closure device is utilized. It is safe to begin EN in these patients once bowel continuity is restored and the end points of resuscitation have been met. Early use of EN in patients with an open abdomen is associated with reduced rates of ventilator-associated pneumonia, earlier primary fascial closure, and fewer enteroatmospheric fistula formation.

Feeding the Patient on Vasopressors

The benefits of EN extend beyond the provision of calories to the maintenance of gut integrity. Although critically ill patients requiring vasopressors are at high risk for gut dysfunction, they may, in fact, benefit most from early EN. However, this must be balanced with the potential for gut ischemia. Nonocclusive bowel necrosis resulting from EN can occur in critically ill patients on vasopressors, with higher rates in surgical patients than other patient populations. These studies, however, are older and performed when excess crystalloid resuscitation was common and may not apply to in the modern-day practice of minimization of fluids.

Based on available data, which is primarily retrospective or observational, EN can be initiated and maintained in patients on low and probably moderate dose vasopressors after initial resuscitation is complete and pressor needs have stabilized. This is primarily based on two recent studies. Ohbe et al. performed a propensity-matched study of intubated patients in shock receiving early (within 2 days) vs late (more than 2 days) EN and norepinephrine at low (<0.1 µg/kg/min), medium (0.1-0.3 µg/kg/min), or high dose (>0.3 µg/kg/min). Mortality was significantly lower in the low- and medium-dose norepinephrine groups, with no difference in mortality between the high-dose pressor groups. While this was a national inpatient database study and not a prospective randomized clinical trial, it does demonstrate safety with a low incidence of bowel necrosis in both the early and late groups (0.2% vs 0.3%, respectively) and lower mortality in patients receiving early EN. A randomized study in intubated patients on pressors was conducted by Reignier et al., the NUTRIREA-2 trial, which compared outcomes in patients receiving EN vs PN. Although no difference in mortality was demonstrated, there was a significant increase in bowel ischemia in patients receiving EN. Importantly, these patients were receiving high doses of vasopressors (mean 0.53 µg/kg/min).

Monitoring Nutrition Support

While the measurement of albumin and prealbumin in the ambulatory setting has been correlated with surgical outcomes, the use of these markers as a measure of nutrition adequacy is not reliable in the critical care setting. Similarly, measurement of transferrin and retinol-binding protein are not useful markers in the critically ill patient as these are all negative acute phase reactants, which are reduced in the inflammatory state. More appropriate nutrition indicators include the urine urea nitrogen (UUN) measurement demonstrating a positive nitrogen balance, progress toward ventilator liberation, maintenance of dry weight and muscle mass, and evidence of wound healing. Nitrogen balance is calculated using 24-hour UUN and 24-hour nutrition delivery:

$$\text{Nitrogen intake (g/day)} - [(\text{UUN (g/day)} \div 0.85) + 2]$$

where 2 is a standard factor for insensible losses from stool, hair, sweat, and skin desquamation. Nitrogen balance results are less reliable in patients with unquantifiable nitrogen losses, such as from draining wounds or renal replacement therapy.

Indirect calorimetry (IC) can be used in patients for whom UUN is not available or in patients not responding to nutrition as anticipated. It measures oxygen consumed (VO_2) and carbon dioxide produced (VCO_2) to calculate energy expenditure and respiratory quotient (RQ). The ASPEN/SCCM guidelines recommend using IC, if available, to assess energy needs in critically ill adults. RQ correlates with the different substrates being metabolized with the physiological range being 0.67-1.3. IC can help determine differences in nutrition delivery vs expenditure, substrate utilization, and tailor nutrition to the individual patient.

The Convalescent Phase of Recovery

After the acute phase of critical illness, consideration should be given to the advancement of nutrition via the oral route. A bedside swallow test can be completed to assess for gross signs of aspiration, which is not uncommon after a prolonged course on the ventilator. If there are signs of aspiration or dysphagia, such as a wet voice, a cough, or gagging, a formal evaluation by a trained speech therapist (ST) should ensue. Based on the formal recommendations of the ST, an oral diet may be ordered. Traditionally, a clear liquid diet has been used first, advancing to full liquids and finally a general diet. However, clear, thin liquids carry the highest aspiration risk of all oral intake and provide essentially no nutritional value, as the broth and juice most commonly available on these menus are high in sugar and salt. Some patients even find clear liquid diets to promote nausea and emesis. No robust data support the notion that an initial clear liquid diet is protective for a new anastomosis or that patients tolerate it better than full liquids. As such, it is becoming increasingly more common to initiate an oral diet with full liquids. This has been well studied with Enhanced Recovery After Surgery (ERAS) protocols, is well tolerated, and has no increased risk or untoward outcomes for patients. Patients with inadequate oral intake can have supplemental enteral feedings. Once 60%-70% of volitional oral intake goals are being met, the supplemental feedings can be discontinued.

Following transfer out of the ICU, data have shown that patients significantly fail to achieve nutritional needs. The recent *E*ffect of early nutritional support on *F*railty, *F*unctional *O*utcomes, and *R*ecovery of malnourished medical inpatients *T*rial (EFFORT) demonstrated in non-ICU medical patients that individualized nutritional support to reach protein and caloric goals vs the standard hospital food group reduced both adverse clinical outcomes and mortality, suggesting that attention to nutrition should not end with the ICU.

Enhanced Recovery After Surgery

Implications for Emergency General Surgery ERAS is a multidisciplinary multimodal approach to improve the care of the surgical patient. It involves preoperative, perioperative, intraoperative, and postoperative elements, which have been shown to improve outcomes and reduce costs in several surgical populations. A number of these have direct and indirect nutrition implications aimed to minimize catabolism and insulin resistance and are outlined in **Table 7.2**. Additionally, the American Society for Enhanced Recovery and Perioperative Quality has generated a consensus statement focusing on nutrition, which expands on traditional ERAS recommendations to include a high-protein diet with the elimination of traditional clear and full liquids. They stress the importance of protein over calories in the postoperative period and further recommend oral protein supplements in the posthospital period, especially for high nutrition risk patients.

TABLE 7.2 ■ Benefits of Nutrition-Related Elements of ERAS

Direct	Indirect
Reduce catabolism and insulin resistance	Mitigate postoperative ileus
Preoperative nutrition screening and with assessment in high-risk patients	Intraoperative avoidance of long-acting opioids
Preoperative carbohydrate treatment	Intraoperative minimization of fluids
Postoperative institution of oral fluids and solids	
Postoperative administration of protein and energy-rich oral supplements	

The American College of Surgeons (ACS) has an Agency for Healthcare Research and Quality (AHRQ)-funded initiative to roll out ERAS initiatives in colorectal, orthopedic, bariatric, gynecology, and emergency general surgery patients (https://bulletin.facs.org/2017/03/acs-launches-ahrq-safety-program-eras/). Results are pending but will have important implications for how the emergency surgery patient is cared for in the postoperative care period.

SUMMARY

Emergency general surgery patients with abdominal catastrophes present the clinician with a situation requiring complex decision-making. Optimal outcomes are achieved with a multidisciplinary team approach and the daily, attentive care of the changing nutritional needs of the patients throughout their hospital stay and into the post-discharge period.

SUGGESTED READINGS

Braga M, Ljungqvist O, Soeters P, Fearon K, Weimann A, Bozzetti F; ESPEN. E.S.P.E.N. guidelines on parenteral nutrition: surgery. *Clin Nutr*. 2009;28:378-386.

Cederholm T, Jensen GL, Correia MITD, et al. GLIM criteria for the diagnosis of malnutrition—a consensus report from the global clinical nutrition community. *J Cachexia Sarcopenia Muscle*. 2019;10(1):207-217.

Chabot E, Nirula R. Open abdomen critical care management principles: resuscitation, fluid balance, nutrition, and ventilator management. *Trauma Surg Acute Care Open*. 2017;2(1):e000063.

Galindo Martín CA, Aportela Vázquez VA, Becerril Hernández F, et al. The GLIM criteria for adult malnutrition and its relation with adverse outcomes, a prospective observational study. *Clin Nutr ESPEN*. 2020;38:67-73.

Hedrick TL, McEvoy MD, Mythen MMG, et al. American Society for Enhanced Recovery and Perioperative Quality Initiative Joint Consensus Statement on postoperative gastrointestinal dysfunction within an enhanced recovery pathway for elective colorectal surgery [published correction appears in Anesth Analg. 2018 Sep;127(3):e53] [published correction appears in Anesth Analg. 2018 Nov;127(5):e94]. *Anesth Analg*. 2018;126(6):1896-1907.

Heidegger CP, Berger MM, Graf S, et al. Optimisation of energy provision with supplemental parenteral nutrition in critically ill patients: a randomised controlled clinical trial. *Lancet*. 2013;381(9864):385-393.

Herbert G, Perry R, Andersen HK, et al. Early enteral nutrition within 24 hours of lower gastrointestinal surgery vs later commencement for length of hospital stay and postoperative complications. *Cochrane Database Syst Rev*. 2018;10(10):CD004080.

Herbert GS, Steele SR. Acute and chronic mesenteric ischemia. *Surg Clin North Am*. 2007;87(5):1115-1134.

Heyland DK, Dhaliwal R, Jiang X, Day AG. Identifying critically ill patients who benefit the most from nutrition therapy: the development and initial validation of a novel risk assessment tool. *Crit Care*. 2011;15(6):R268.

Heyland DK, van Zanten ARH, Grau-Carmona T, et al. A multicenter, randomized, double-blind study of ulimorelin and metoclopramide in the treatment of critically ill patients with enteral feeding intolerance: PROMOTE trial. *Intensive Care Med*. 2019;45(5):647-656.

Lee JC, Williams GW, Kozar RA, et al. Multitargeted feeding strategies improve nutrition outcome and are associated with reduced pneumonia in a level 1 trauma intensive care unit. *JPEN J Parenter Enteral Nutr*. 2018;42(3):529-537.

Lewis K, Algahtani Z, Mcintyre L, et al. The efficacy and safety of prokinetic agents in critically ill patients receiving enteral nutrition: a meta-analysis of randomize trials. *Critical Care*. 2016;20(259):2-12.

Ljungqvist O, Scott M, Fearon KC. Enhanced recovery after surgery: a review. *JAMA Surg*. 2017;152(3):292-298.

Marik PE, Zaloga GP. Early enteral nutrition in acutely ill patients: a systematic review [published correction appears in Crit Care Med 2002 Mar;30(3):725]. *Crit Care Med*. 2001;29(12):2264-2270.

Marvin RG, McKinley BA, McQuiggan M, et al. Nonocclusive bowel necrosis occurring in critically ill trauma patients receiving enteral nutrition manifests no reliable clinical signs for early detection. *Am J Surg*. 2000;179(1):7-12.

Montomoli J, Donati A, Ince C. Acute kidney injury and fluid resuscitation in septic patients: are we protecting the kidney? *Nephron Clin Pract*. 2019;143(3):170-173.

Ohbe H, Jo T, Matsui H, Fushimi K, Yasunaga H. Differences in effect of early enteral nutrition on mortality among ventilated adults with shock requiring low-, medium-, and high-dose noradrenaline: a propensity-matched analysis. *Clin Nutr*. 2020;39(2):460-467.

Olson MC, Fletcher JG, Nagpal P, Froemming AT, Khandelwal A. Mesenteric ischemia: what the radiologist needs to know. *Cardiovasc Diagn Ther*. 2019;9(Suppl 1):S74-S87.

Ortiz-Reyes LA, Chang Y, Quraishi SA, et al. Early enteral nutrition mitigates the neutrophil-lymphocyte ratio improving clinical outcomes in critically ill surgical patients. *Nutr Clin Pract*. 2019;34(1):148-155.

Osland E, Yunus RM, Khan S, Memon MA. Early versus traditional postoperative feeding in patients undergoing resectional gastrointestinal surgery: a meta-analysis. *JPEN J Parenter Enteral Nutr*. 2011;35(4):473-487.

Peterson SJ, Tsai AA, Scala CM, Sowa DC, Sheean PM, Braunschweig CL. Adequacy of oral intake in critically ill patients 1 week after extubation. *J Am Diet Assoc*. 2010;110(3):427-433. doi:10.1016/j.jada.2009.11.020

Pourhassan M, Rommersbach N, Lueg G, et al. The impact of malnutrition on acute muscle wasting in frail older hospitalized patients. *Nutrients*. 2020;12(5):1387.

Pradelli L, Mayer K, Klek S, et al. ω-3 fatty-acid enriched parenteral nutrition in hospitalized patients: systematic review with meta-analysis and trial sequential analysis. *JPEN J Parenter Enteral Nutr*. 2020;44(1):44-57.

Rahman A, Hasan RM, Agarwala R, Martin C, Day AG, Heyland DK. Identifying critically-ill patients who will benefit most from nutritional therapy: further validation of the "modified N.U.T.R.I.C." nutritional risk assessment tool. *Clin Nutr*. 2016;35(1):158-162.

Reignier J, Boisramé-Helms J, Brisard L, et al. Enteral versus parenteral early nutrition in ventilated adults with shock: a randomised, controlled, multicentre, open-label, parallel-group study (NUTRIREA-2). *Lancet*. 2018;391(10116):133-143.

Reignier J, Mercier E, Le Gouge A, et al. Effect of not monitoring residual gastric volume on risk of ventilator associated pneumonia in adults receiving mechanical ventilation and early enteral feeding: a randomized controlled trial. *JAMA*. 2013;309(3):249-256.

Schuetz P, Fehr R, Baechli V, et al. Individualised nutritional support in medical inpatients at nutritional risk: a randomised clinical trial. *Lancet*. 2019;393(10188):2312-2321. doi:10.1016/S0140-6736(18)32776-4

Skeie E, Tangvik RJ, Nymo LS, Harthug S, Lassen K, Viste A. Weight loss and B.M.I. criteria in GLIM's definition of malnutrition is associated with postoperative complications following abdominal resections—results from a National Quality Registry. *Clin Nutr.* 2020;39(5):1593-1599.

Taylor BE, McClave SA, Martindale RG, et al. Guidelines for the provision and assessment of nutrition support therapy in the adult critically ill patient: Society of Critical Care Medicine (S.C.C.M.) and American Society for Parenteral and Enteral Nutrition (A.S.P.E.N.). *Crit Care Med.* 2016;44(2):390-438.

van den Heijkant T, Aerts BAC, Teijink J, Buurman WA, Luyer MDP. Challenges in diagnosing mesenteric ischemia. *World J Gastroenterol.* 2013;19(9):1338-1341.

Wadnling M. ERAS Implementation in Emergency General Surgery—A.C.S. reports.nsqip.facs.org › nsqippublicdocs › service. 2019.

White JV, Guenter P, Jensen G, Malone A, Schofield M; The Academy Malnutrition Work Group; The A.S.P.E.N. Malnutrition Task Force; and the A.S.P.E.N. Board of Directors. Consensus Statement: Academy of Nutrition and Dietetics and American Society for Parenteral and Enteral Nutrition: Characteristics Recommended for the Identification and Documentation of Adult Malnutrition (Undernutrition). *JPEN J Parenter Enteral Nutr.* 2012;36:275-283.

Williams DGA, Molinger J, Wischmeyer PE. The malnourished surgery patient: a silent epidemic in perioperative outcomes? *Curr Opin Anaesthesiol.* 2019;32(3):405-411.

Wischmeyer PE, Carli F, Evans DC, et al. American Society for Enhanced Recovery and Perioperative Quality Initiative Joint Consensus Statement on Nutrition Screening and Therapy Within a Surgical Enhanced Recovery Pathway [published correction appears in Anesth Analg. 2018 Nov;127(5):e95]. *Anesth Analg.* 2018;126(6):1883-1895.

Wischmeyer PE, Hasselmann M, Kummerlen C, et al. A randomized trial of supplemental parenteral nutrition in underweight and overweight critically ill patients: the TOP-UP pilot trial. *Crit Care.* 2017;21(1):142.

Yeh DD, Ortiz LA, Lee JM, et al. PEP uP (Enhanced Protein-Energy Provision via the Enteral Route Feeding Protocol) in surgical patients—a multicenter pilot randomized controlled trial. *JPEN J Parenter Enteral Nutr.* 2020;44(2):197-204. doi:10.1002/jpen.1521

CHAPTER

8 Operating Room (General Setup, Approaches, and Incisions)

Fernando Ferreira, Eva Barbosa, and Emanuel Guerreiro

William Stewart Halsted (1852–1922), British-American, considered the Father of Modern Surgery, stated wisely, that "*Every important hospital should have on its staff of surgeons at least one who is able to deal with any emergency that may arise.*"

CASE PRESENTATION

A 23-year-old male was involved in a motor vehicle crash on a Friday afternoon. He complained of right ankle pain and was normal hemodynamically, without any past medical history. He was on weekend leave from the Army. Physical examination revealed only his right ankle fracture. Laboratory tests and full imaging including pan CT revealed no additional injury. Hemoglobin/Hematocrit were 15.5/46.0.

The following morning, orthopedic surgery was in the operating room, repairing his ankle fracture. The operation was proceeding uneventfully, with a stable patient. Two hours into the operation, the anesthesia team called because his heart rate was 132/min, his systolic blood pressure 80 mm Hg, and H/H now 7.6/24.0 with a base deficit of 9. He was transfused a unit of red blood cells.

Question: *On your way to the operating room, what are you thinking, and what do you plan to do?*

Answer: *The patient has been hemodynamically normal for 2 hours. The patient has lost <100 mL of blood in the operative field. No central lines were placed. A chest radiograph is requested while you are rushing to the operating room. On arrival to the OR, you view the normal CXR, without hemothorax or pneumothorax. Unanticipated blood loss must be interrogated. His CXR is normal, he has no pelvic or long bone fracture, and he has no external blood loss. Even in review, his chest/abdomen/pelvic CT is normal. His abdomen is mildly distended. With all other sources of blood loss excluded, his abdomen is prepped and draped. A minilaparotomy reveals a 2-L hemoperitoneum. At full exploration, a splenectomy is performed for a ruptured subcapsular hematoma of the spleen (**Figure 8.1**). His recovery is uneventful. The teaching point in this case is—prepare for the expected; anticipate the unexpected.*

INTRODUCTION

In treating the emergency general surgical or trauma patient, the operating room must be prepared to deal with pathology in all body regions. Preparation for immediate operative intervention for "any emergency that may arise" is vital, as is the ability to rapidly change operative plans, open other body cavities, or engage multiple surgical services simultaneously in care of the patient.

Surgical safety for the patient is paramount in this discussion of the operating room. Basic principles and routines must be followed rigorously to avoid patient harm. The World Health Organization has generated a checklist of 10 essential objectives for safe surgery (**Table 8.1**) as well as a Surgical Safety Checklist (**Table 8.2**).

It is intuitive that an OR is one of the costliest sectors in a hospital; administration and the surgical teams should be "synchronized" to achieve the best care possible. Balance must be maintained between workflow issues and emotional and physical fatigue of the health care professionals who frequently deal with many potentially contaminated, unpredictable, and untimely high-risk emergency surgical situations.

THE "IDEAL" OR THAT OPTIMIZES INFRASTRUCTURE AND RESOURCE USE

Acute care surgery incorporates trauma, emergency general surgery (EGS), and surgical critical care with the goal to reduce mortality, morbidity, and length of stay (LOS) in these patient groups. A dedicated acute care surgery service provides shorter LOS and decreased time to operation for common emergency surgical procedures.

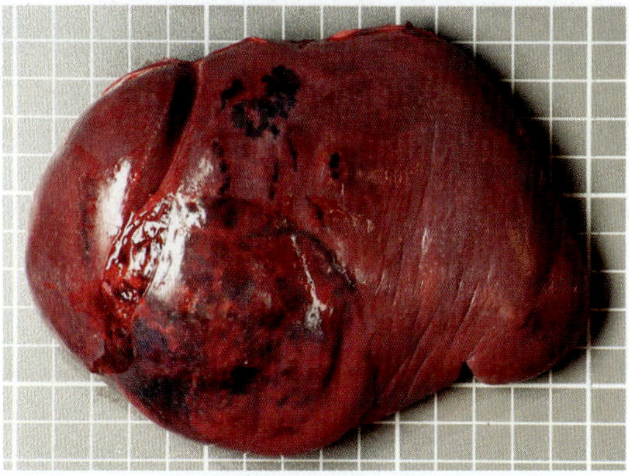

Figure 8.1 Despite the normal admission CT imaging, the patient ruptured this subcapsular splenic hematoma 18 hours after admission. Fortunately, this occurred in the operating room and was promptly diagnosed and treated.

Access to the operating room must be immediate for the patient requiring emergent operation for life- or limb-threatening hemorrhage. Urgent cases are seen more frequently on the EGS service, with more time to prepare and setup the OR. Balancing the emergent or urgent need for operating room availability with an already busy elective operating schedule is challenging. These unscheduled patients require prompt operative intervention without major disruption to the elective operating room schedule (delay or canceling of elective cases). Hospitals must balance the trade-off between planned elective operations and the unexpected need to accommodate the EGS case expeditiously. Following an elective OR schedule without ex-ante preparation for unexpected arrivals will fail to provide timely OR access for the emergent/urgent EGS case. Thus, the daily OR schedule must proactively account for the unplanned add-on cases. This conflict for resources has been studied with some recommending a vacant, available OR for the emergent EGS patient. Others support evenly allocating capacity to all elective ORs, leaving deliberate gaps between cases, thus creating a virtual emergency OR team. The former model assures access to the OR for the EGS patient with less disruption of the elective schedule, accepting potential operational expense when vacant.

Delay in access to the operating room for life-threatening EGS operations increases mortality in these patients. Thus, immediate access to an operating room with appropriate surgeon, anesthesiology, and nurse staffing is vital. To expand on this, an evidence-based care bundle for emergency laparotomy has been reported to decrease mortality (Aggarwal). A six-point bundle was used:

1. Prompt measurement of blood lactate levels
2. Early review and treatment of sepsis, including early broad-spectrum antibiotics as recommended by the Surviving Sepsis Campaign (see Chapters 2 and 5)
3. Prompt patient transfer to the operating room defined after the decision to operate
4. Use of goal-directed fluid therapy
5. Admission of all patients to the ICU after a surgical procedure
6. Involvement of senior clinicians in the decision to proceed to the operating room and throughout the surgical procedure

TABLE 8.1 ■ Ten Essentials for Safe Surgery (World Health Organization)

1. The operating team must ensure that the correct surgical procedure is to be carried out on the correct patient.
2. The operating personnel should have adequate knowledge regarding the anesthesia, its methods of administration as well as its effects so that minimum pain is experienced by the patient.
3. The operating personnel should be well prepared for any life-threatening conditions like loss of airway or respiratory function.
4. The operating team should be prepared for risk of high loss of blood.
5. The operating team should be well versed with the history of the patient in order to prevent or induce any allergic or adverse drug reactions that can cause a significant risk for the patient.
6. Care must be taken to minimize the formation of surgical site infections by using proper measures.
7. Proper care must be taken to not leave any instrument or any foreign material at the surgical site.
8. All specimens should be carefully identified and secured for further investigation.
9. Proper communication must be present among the operating team personnel for the safe conduct of the surgical procedure.
10. A routine surveillance of the surgical volume, safety protocols, capacities, and the outcomes must be carried out by all the hospitals and the health care systems.

Adapted from WHO Guidelines for Safe Surgery 2009: Safe Surgery Saves Lives. *N Engl J Med*. 2009;360(5):10.

TABLE 8.2 ■ Surgical Safety Checklist (World Health Organization)

Before Induction of Anesthesia	Before Skin Incision	Before Patient Leaves Operating Room
Sign in	Time out	Sign out
Patient has confirmed: • Identity • Site • Procedure • Consent	Confirm all team members have introduced themselves by name and role.	Nurse verbally confirms with the team: • The name of the procedure recorded. • The instrument, sponge, and needle counts are correct (or not applicable). • How the specimen is labeled (including patient name). • Whether there are any equipment problems to be addressed.
Site marked/not applicable.	Surgeon, anesthesia professional, and nurse verbally confirm: • Patient • Site • Procedure	
Anesthesia safety check completed.	Anticipated critical events • Surgeon reviews: What are the critical or unexpected steps, operative duration, anticipated blood loss? • Anesthesia team reviews: Are there any patient-specific concerns? • Nursing team reviews: Has sterility (including indicator results) been confirmed? • Are there equipment issues or any concerns?	Surgeon, anesthesia professional, and nurse review the key concerns for recovery and management of this patient.
Pulse oximeter on patient and functioning.	Has antibiotic prophylaxis been given in the last 60 min? • Yes/not applicable Is essential imaging displayed? • Yes/no applicable	
Does the patient have a known allergy • No/yes Difficult airway/aspiration risk • No • Yes, and equipment/assistance available Risk of >500 mL blood loss (7 mL/kg in children) • No • Yes and adequate intravenous access and fluids planned		

Adapted from Elements of surgical safety checklist. In: WHO Guidelines for Safe Surgery 2009: Safe Surgery Saves Lives. *N Engl J Med*. 2009;360(5):111.

EFFICIENT WORKFLOW AND OR SETUP

Emergency general surgery operations may require a large volume of equipment, as well as numerous surgical staff. The operating room must be large enough to accommodate all necessary equipment, while providing adequate space for staff. Care providers in the anesthesia and surgery departments should agree on a standardized setup of equipment to minimize waste, increase efficiency, and increase patient safety.

- The dedicated needs of anesthesia should be considered separately from those of the surgeon, including the positioning requirements to support equipment and monitors in multiple locations. Anesthesia requires dedicated services (medical gas, fluids, communications, power outlets, data, and phone) delivered to a key target separate from the surgeon. Consider adding a separate flat-panel display arm to the ceiling mounted structure for anesthesia. This could also be activated through voice command serving as an access to fully integrated audiovisual OR control. These ideal options would provide surgeons with the necessary information for each operation—all in real time.
- Monitor all patients with electrocardiography, pulse oximetry, and blood pressure. Consider arterial line and central venous access for patients with hemodynamic compromise or requiring transfusion of blood products.
- Blood gas and point of care electrolyte testing must be available.
- Legs supports, arm boards, head rings.
- Trays/carts must be prepackaged, clearly labeled, and available.
- A laparotomy tray with an aortic clamp and/or compressor.
- A thoracotomy tray with an Allison lung retractor, Finochietto rib spreader, Lietchke knife and Duvall clamps, sternal saw.
- A vascular instrument tray/set.
- Multiple suction canisters and tubing.
- Tubing and device for blood salvage.
- Stapling devices.
- Commonly used sutures and ties.
- Drapes, sterile towels, lap sponges.
- OR table with fluoroscopic capabilities.
- Video towers and equipment for laparoscopy, endoscopy, or bronchoscopy.
- Monitors for viewing radiologic studies.
- Rapid transfusion apparatus, fluid warmers.
- Underbody external patient warming device.
- Multiple suction setups.
- Energy devices for dividing the mesentery.
- Topical hemostatic agents.
- Head lights.

The integrated OR is not easily attainable. Although many equipment choices, floor plans, and solutions are available, having a clear understanding of your own facility's future goals is a big step toward arriving at the best solution to meet your facility's growth requirements. The key for the future OR is to integrate multiple devices allowing hub and user interfaces. The result may signify changes of workflow and requires the creation of a nursing command station within each OR to facilitate quick turnover, which is vital to any productive operating room.

Assembling a qualified, multidisciplinary hospital team in guiding decisions pays big dividends later, when clinical staff and other team members actually begin using or supporting activities in the OR suite. Trusted representatives from your key support staff are essential to your decision-making team. Examples include, but are not limited to, surgeons; nurse managers; hospital administrators; purchasing, anesthesia, and nursing team leaders; and scrub and circulating nurses. A well-coordinated team approach to planning your OR suite will deliver the highest probability for success and acceptance, including expeditious implementation once the planning is completed.

With extensive resources, a hybrid OR provides the maximum technology and versatility as an OR. The surgical table features have intraoperative imaging capabilities, including optional radiotranslucent carbon components, C-Arm access, and head-to-toe x-ray channels for unrestricted imaging not only for surgeons but also for the anesthesia team. Monitors are flatter and wider, to handle advances in more precise formatting capabilities and the quality of images surgeons need for minimally invasive surgery, picture archiving communication systems (PACS), vascular, orthopedic, biliary, and digestive fluoroscopic images.

If available, the hybrid operating room may be used in situations where a multidisciplinary approach to hemorrhage control or operative management concomitantly with vascular surgery, orthopedics, and/or interventional radiology is anticipated. The design of a hybrid operating room should ensure that all disciplines utilizing the space agree on the layout and equipment.

Physicians and staff who will be involved in these cases should have training on the equipment. Desire to use the hybrid room should never delay operative intervention.

COVID-19 (AS OF 12.2021)

The COVID-19 pandemic has disrupted multiple aspects of patient care. First, the initial wave of COVID-19 patients overwhelmed so many of our hospitals. With this wave came personal risk to health care workers and the disruption of care to non-COVID patients. With repeated waves of COVID globally, as well as better understanding of the epidemiology and management of the COVID infections over the past 2 years, it continues to have a major impact on our daily lives and our ability to provide patient care. In reviewing the setup of the operating room, we must discuss COVID.

The greatest risk of exposure to health care workers is during an aerosol-generating procedure. Four factors explain the transmission risk during medical procedures. The first is forced air. Air forced over moist respiratory mucosa generates more virus-laden respiratory particles. High-risk conditions include positive-pressure ventilation, CPR, or heavy coughing. The second factor is disease severity and viral load in the exposure. Symptomatic patients are 10-20 times more likely to infect than asymptomatic patients. The third factor is distance. Respiratory emissions are most concentrated close to the source, especially in closed spaces. The fourth factor is duration of exposure; the longer the exposure, the greater the risk. Obviously, the presence of several of these risk factors in an exposure will increase risk of transmission.

Procedures to be Followed for an Operation on the COVID+ Patient

- Zones of the COVID operating room:
  - Zone 1: Entry dressing room where basic PPE is donned
  - Zone 2: Anteroom for disinfection and surgical dressing
  - Zone 3: COVID-19 operating room
  - Zone 4: Exit room for removal of PPE
  - Zone 5: Exit dressing room where staff showers
- The intubation and procedure should be performed by the most experienced team member. Neither intubation nor the operation should be treated as a teaching opportunity.
- Intubation should be by rapid sequence induction, avoiding bag-valve mask ventilation. A videolaryngoscope is recommended to separate the patient and intubator.
- Procedures/operations on the COVID+ patient should be performed in a negative pressure OR or in an airborne isolation room.
- The OR must have a high-efficiency particulate air filter (HEPA) with an air exchange cycle >25 cycles/hour.
- An OR should be designated as the COVID room.
- No one enters or leaves the OR during the operation on the COVID patient.
- Only essential personnel should be in the OR.
- PPE is mandatory for all OR personnel:
  - N99 or N95 (US) FFP3 or FFP2 (Europe) mask
  - Disposable, longsleeve, waterproof gowns/suits
  - Double glove
  - Goggles or visors
  - Disposable head covers
  - Disposable shoe covers
  - Alcohol hand hygiene solution
- Masks and shields must be worn by all personnel.
- A smoke evacuation system is mandatory.
- Local/regional anesthesia is preferred over general anesthesia if appropriate.
- Scalpels are preferred over energy-utilizing devices.
- Avoid the use of pressure-irrigating devices, power drills, oscillating saws.
- If the procedure is laparoscopic—minimize insufflation pressure, do not vent ports, use high particulate filters, reduce surgical smoke formation, closed/active evacuation of the pneumoperitoneum at conclusion of the procedure.

Protection against COVID by masks in decreasing order: powered air-purifying respirator (PAPR) > FFP3 (N99) > N95 > 3-ply surgical masks

CONDUCT IN THE OPERATING ROOM

Several key principles are vital to facilitate dealing with complex operative pathology while minimizing collateral and iatrogenic injury. *Plan for what you expect; anticipate and prepare for the unexpected.*

The conduct and comportment of the lead surgeon sets the tone for the operating team, resulting in optimal communication and performance. The surgeon on entry must quickly assess the OR. Obtain a concise report from the other team members on entering the OR. Control the room; maintain composure, communicate calmly, and do not shout. Request necessary actions or equipment in sequence, rather than issuing multiple requests at once. Be explicit to whom each request is made. Insist on closed-loop communication; expect feedback acknowledgement on all requests or statements.

Operative maneuvers must be deliberate, progressive, without wasted moves. Control bleeding rapidly; reconstruct deliberately. Control bleeding digitally; do not clamp or suture haphazardly. Repair correctly on the first attempt.

TRAINING TO MAINTAIN TOP STANDARDS

Team Training

Perioperative care of the EGS patient requires a multidisciplinary approach between surgeons, anesthesiologist, nursing, operating room staff, emergency department personnel, and the post-anesthesia receiving unit.

Simulation training focused on team performance allows understanding role assignments, teaching communication skills, identifying operational challenges, and building trust between team members.

Didactic and hands-on training of OR surgical teams increases knowledge of procedures, equipment, and troubleshooting skills.

Training Surgical Residents

Adequate training of surgical residents has become increasingly challenging due to numerous factors such as technological evolution, pressure from hospital administration for shorter operative time, and less availability of experienced surgeons.

Patient management and decision-making have the added difficulty of greater numbers of older patients with more comorbidity and frailty. Perioperative morbidity and mortality of EGS procedures are higher for these frail, elderly patients.

It is necessary to develop a structured program of teaching excellence that promotes the safe, progressive autonomy of surgical residents within the acute care surgery environment. The resident involvement begins in the emergency department with accurate patient assessment and appropriate surgical planning. The residency program must provide the training and skills to effectively develop this early patient care. Patient safety is paramount in this process.

There are several ways to achieve this through training:

1. Mentoring from the most experienced to the less experienced of the team, and promoting progressive autonomy both outside and in the OR.
2. Discussion of clinical cases, and review of the literature.
3. Review of results through morbidity and mortality conferences, and discussion of clinical cases or review of performance videos. It is essential that the discussion of complications be rigorous and constructive, yet avoiding blame, to allow room for professional growth and learning.
4. "Hands-on" courses such as ESC, ETC, ATLS, DSTC, MUSEC, Open, and Laparoscopic courses. These courses have proven to be effective for learning and systematizing concepts, providing greater confidence in surgical decisions and maneuvers. Even though some courses are focused on trauma, many of the clinical principles also apply to nontrauma patients (damage control and truncated operations for source-control). Thus, these courses are useful beyond the original design.
5. Simulation training, which has become an increasingly effective teaching instrument. Through simulation, the resident can practice movements repeatedly, developing the dexterity and confidence needed when performing these for the first time on a patient. This simulation of events training need not always be associated with technology and high costs, such as virtual reality. The aim of training through simulation is to provide experience, education, and the acquisition of skills through simulated environments and is applied a more global way than solely technological simulation. In the operating room, a brief pre- and postdiscussion of the clinical case, possible scenarios, and concordant action is important to establish goals and communication within the team. In the case of emergency surgery, the operating room is often a frantic and confusing situation. The resident must learn "skills" related to expeditious decision-making and strong and efficient team leadership, fundamental to better outcomes in any clinical situation.

In EGS, asking for help may be confused with insecurity by some. An environment where all, including the residents, are expected and encouraged to solicit help is critical for both patient safety and resident learning. We strongly believe this philosophy leads to the best patient outcomes.

BEFORE YOU START: *THE BASICS OF APPROACHES AND INCISIONS*

The hemodynamic status and physiological reserve will dictate the timing of surgical intervention: emergent, urgent, or urgent-elective. If the patient remains unstable, the most prudent surgical approach should be an immediate open procedure. If hemodynamically stable, a laparoscopic procedure is preferable, as long as technical proficiency is available and a possibly longer duration of surgery does not compromise patient outcome.

Once you decide that you need to operate on a patient, plan and anticipate, so surgery is efficiently and safely completed. Please consider the following:

- Early, before entrance into theater, confirm that the respective OR table is appropriate for fluoroscopic imaging; if x-rays are required, confirm that the radiology technician is also available. If a perineal approach is considered, request appropriate leg supports.
- Need for any IV fluids, analgesia, blood or blood products, microbiology cultures, and broad-spectrum antibiotics.
- Need to inform the ICU of a potential patient.
- Preoperative imaging displayed on a screen in the OR, if critical for approach.

In the OR, it is essential to apply an antiseptic solution extensively to the exposed area of surgical approach. Drape widely, to facilitate any possible need for placement of drains, extended or additional incisions. At our institution, if major septic contamination is expected, we also place a second water protective drape (a c-section drape kit) to facilitate management of fluid overflow of bodily fluids or peritoneal lavage with the intent to keep the patient and surgical staff as dry as possible (**Figure 8.2**).

In open surgery, surgeons need training in the simplest aspects, from decision to operate, to basic foot positioning (**Figures 8.3** to **8.5**) to efficient use of surgical instruments. In laparoscopic surgery, one cannot easily move about the patient, and the camera view and triangulation of trocars for coordinated movements of traction, countertraction, and tissue dissection is dependent on optimal and ergonomic trocar placement.

The skin incision should be planned and easy to extend to obtain adequate exposure and avoid from scars that have probable bowel adhesions to

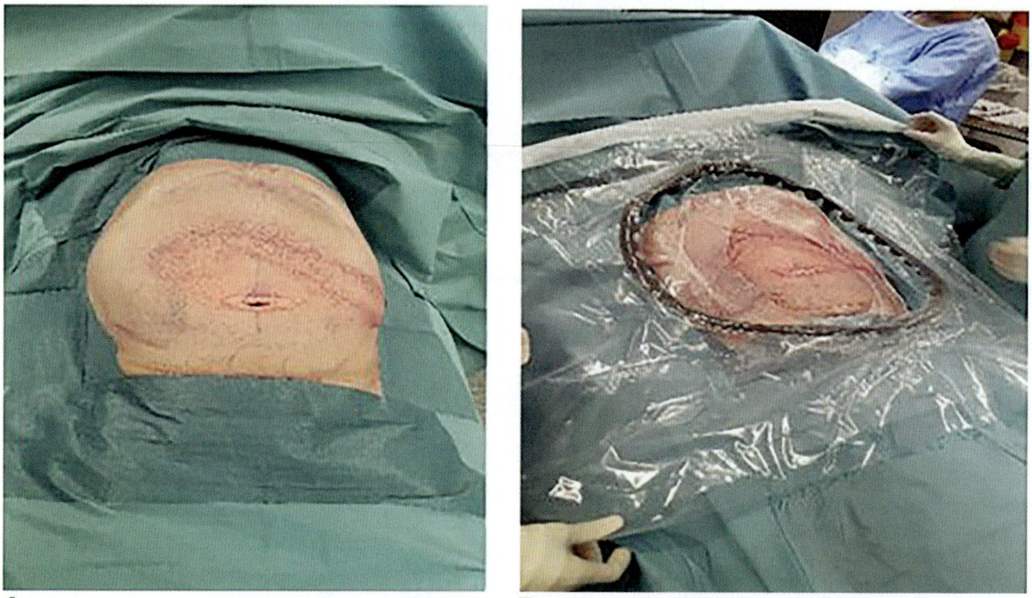

A **B**

Figure 8.2 Wide draping further reinforced with a c-section kit used to keep outside field dry. **A.** Wide draping. **B.** C-section kit reinforcement. (Authorized patient photos from Pedro Hispano Hospital, Matosinhos-Porto, Portugal.)

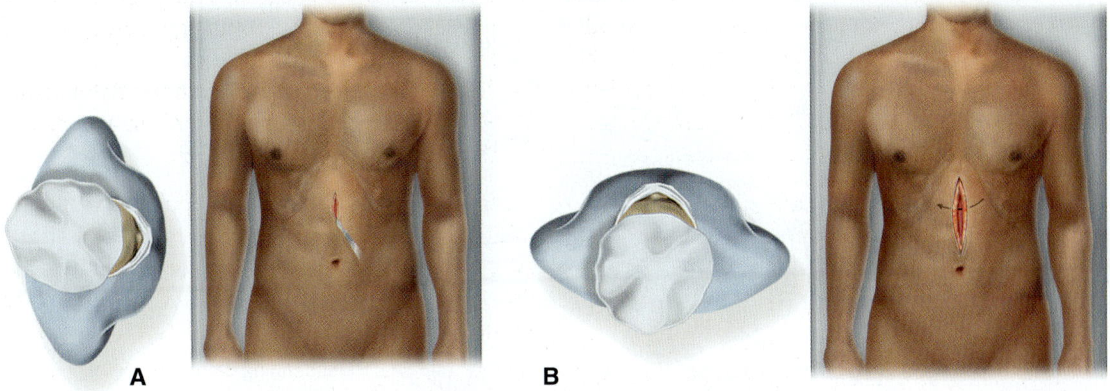

Figure 8.3 **A, B.** Basic foot position for laparotomy opening and closure.

the abdominal wall. Also critical in laparoscopy, incisions to place trocars should take into account previous operations to achieve exposure with ease for safer surgery.

In open surgery, we prefer a precise midline longitudinal incision placed above and/or below the umbilicus according to expected pathology and body habitus and folds. Midline incisions interfere less with future reoperations, and if a ventral hernia develops, it will be easier to repair than incisions that divide the rectus muscles, potentially resulting in muscle denervation and atrophy. We believe that the rectus muscles are so crucial that if we need to perform an open cholecystectomy, we favor a midline over a subcostal incision, which in theory would allow a more direct approach. Gallbladder exposure through a midline access is facili-

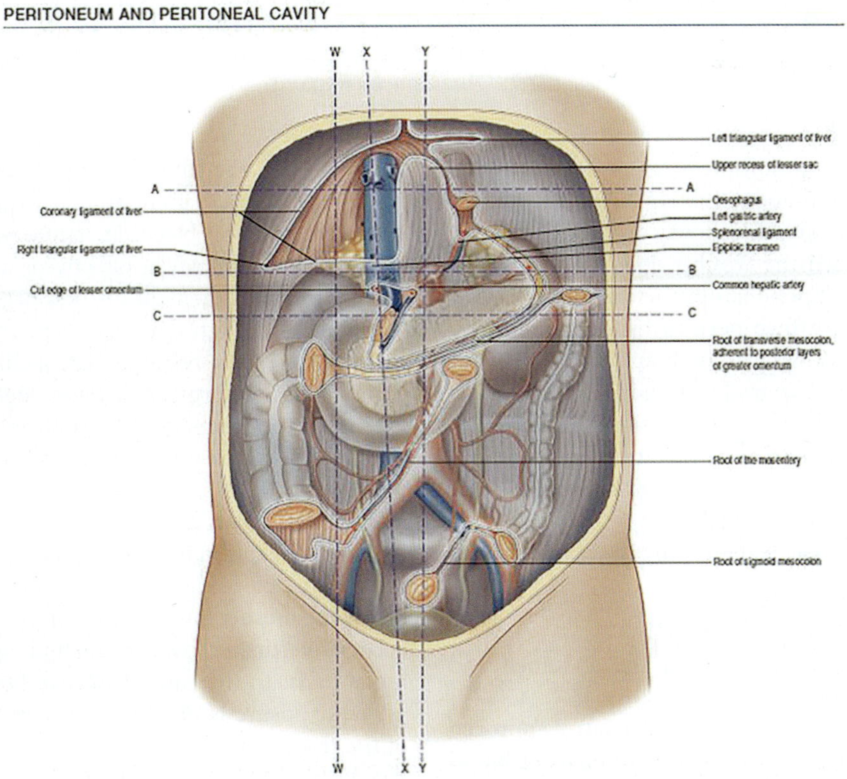

Figure 8.4 Peritoneal attachments that permit better peritoneal exposure when divided. (From Rohen JW, Yokochi C, Lutjen-Drecoll E. *Photographic Atlas of Anatomy*. 9th ed. Wolters Kluwer; 2022. Figure 6.64.)

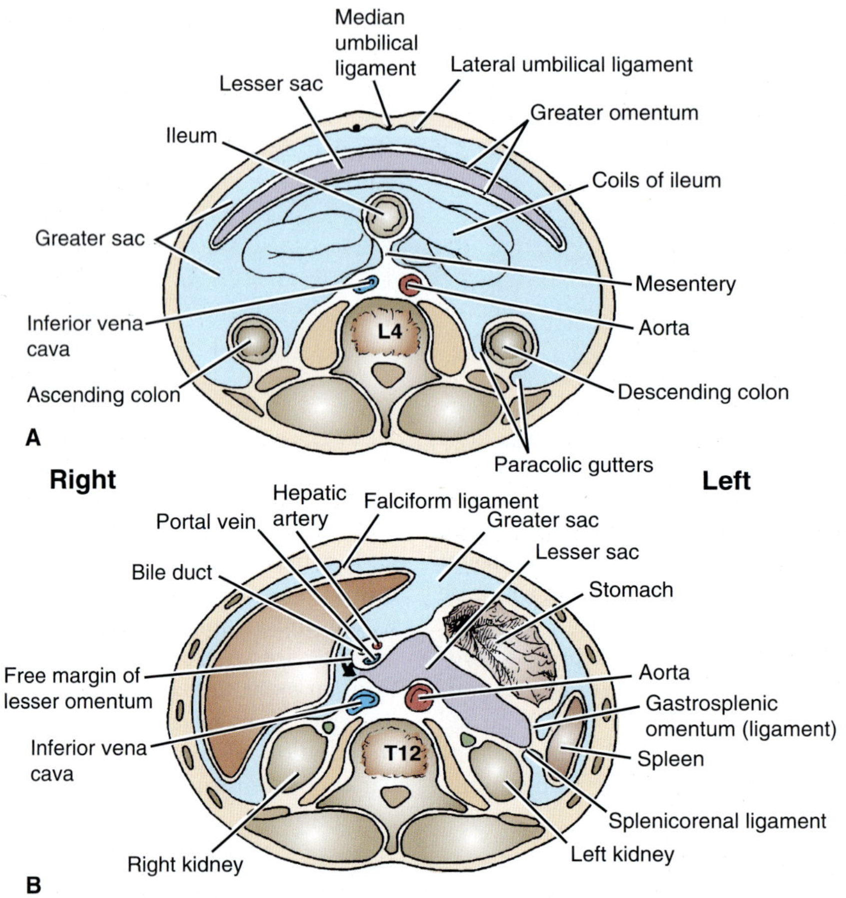

Figure 8.5 Peritoneal attachments that allow better liver retraction to the right and better gastric exposure when divided. (From Wineski LE. Snell's. *Clinical Anatomy by Regions*. 10th ed. Wolters Kluwer; 2019. Figure 7.6.)

tated by placing multiple large moist large pads to the right and above the right hepatic lobe to project the gallbladder away from the subcostal area toward the wound opening. We rarely perform an appendectomy as an open operation, even if diffuse peritonitis exists and give preference to a laparoscopic approach owing to the high risk of wound infection and decreased complexity of resultant incisional hernias. If conversion to open appendectomy is inevitable, we prefer peritoneal access through a midline infraumbilical incision.

The sequence of laparotomy is:

1. control active bleeding,
2. control GI contamination,
3. systematic exploration of the abdomen and retroperitoneum, and
4. decision to invoke a damage control approach or to proceed with definitive repair of blood vessels/restoration of GI continuity and definitive closure.

Approach the most life-threatening problem first; stabilize the patient applying the least invasive strategy. For bleeding, apply well-directed pressure. Packing may be effective intially or damage control management of solid organ or pelvic bleeding. Although definitive repairs are tempting, hasty moves result in iatrogenic injury or complicate the surgical challenge before the full extent of the problem is recognized. If simple maneuvers fail to control the problem, proceed with stepwise escalation to more complicated approaches. Upon entry into the abdominal cavity, quickly explore the peritoneal cavity to determine if the bleeding or septic source is above or below the mesocolon. If above, one can gain more access by further liver retraction with applied moist pads. In the case of relative hepatomegaly, added exposure is obtained through the division of the triangular and falciform hepatic ligaments. If a gastric perforation is suspected, dividing the gastrocolic ligament to open the lesser sac will allow direct observation of the posterior gastric wall. If the pancreas is the source of the patient's problem, opening the lesser sac is the safest way to obtain the anterior view of the pancreas. The duodenum is best approached with a generous Kocher maneuver, which also provides inferior vena cava exposure, if needed.

If contamination is most likely below the mesocolon, start by examining the small bowel from the cecum and progress to the ligament of Treitz. Sometimes, owing to major bowel distension, more visceral space is needed. A useful trick is to carefully "milk" the bowel contents retrograde toward the stomach. The bowel should be longitudinally aligned in front of the surgeon to allow complete visualization of the bowel, never disregarding the mesenteric aspect. If a larger diameter NG tube is not sufficient for evacuation of gastric contents, an optimal option is to temporarily place an orogastric 36 Fr Faucher tube. After this, observe and palpate the colon from the cecum to the rectum. If a retrocolic septic source is suspected, facilitate exposure through right/left colic visceral rotation, as required (**Figures 8.6 and 8.7**). If exposure of retroperitoneal genitourinary structure is necessary, a respective right or left visceral rotation exposes the kidney and the ureter as it crosses the bifurcation of the iliac vessels. A delicate tap with the forceps will show minor peristalsis of the ureter and then proceed proximally or distally as required.

As shown above, peritoneal exposure is dependent upon dividing peritoneal attachments. An important second step, many times underappreciated, is to properly pack away the small bowel into a bundle with large moist gauze sheets to safely displace it from the area of operation. You may further need to mobilize the cecum when dealing with a source of sepsis in the pelvis.

Protect and retract the wound edges. We favor atraumatic wound protector-retractors. If necessary, we create more exposure by adding a Balfour retractor, which can be further augmented by adding a chain (**Figure 8.8**). A self-retaining retractor

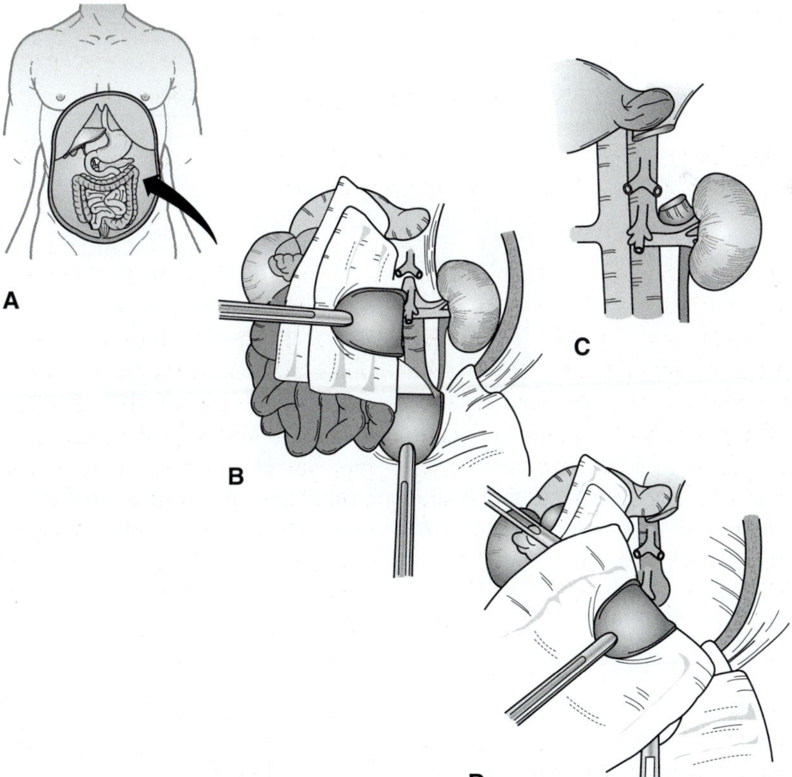

Figure 8.6 Left-sided medial visceral rotation. **A.** The open abdomen. **B, C.** Left to right mobilization of the left colon, pancreas, kidney, and stomach; left kidney remains *in situ*. **D.** Further mobilization, elevating the left kidney from its fossa; the retroperitoneal aorta and its branches are exposed. (From Peitzman AB, Yealy DM, Fabian TC, C. W Schwab CW, Guyette FX, Seamon MJ, Zuckerbraun BS. *The Trauma Manual*. 5th ed. Wolters Kluwer; 2020. Figure 38.4.)

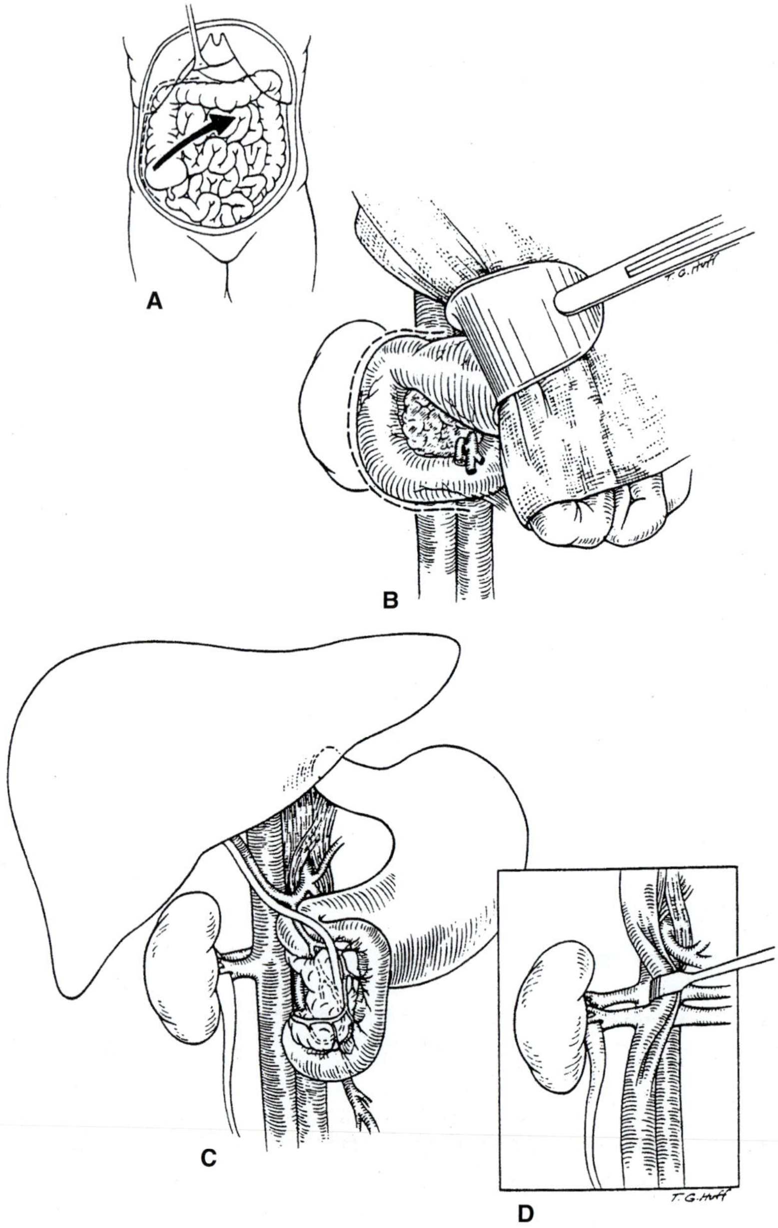

Figure 8.7 Right-sided medial visceral rotation. **A.** The open abdomen. **B.** The right colon and small bowel after fully mobilized from the retroperitoneum. **C.** The duodenum is widely kocherized. **D.** The IVC has been encircled with a loop. (Used with permission of Georg Thieme Verlag KG, from Frey W. Abdominal arterial trauma. In: Blaisdell FW, Trunkey DD, eds. Trauma Management-Abdominal Trauma. 2nd ed. New York, NY: Thieme Medical Publishers; 1993:345; permission conveyed through Copyright Clearance Center, Inc.)

such as the Omni, upper hand, or Bookwalter retractor is also useful.

In the presence of patient stability, where time is not of the essence, we consider an optimal primary fascia closure favoring whenever possible 5-mm bites of fascia using a slowly absorbed 2/0 continuous monofilament suture. Closure of adipose tissue in layers as necessary is performed to minimize possible dead space, which can be a location for potential fluid to infect, concluded with skin sutures or clips. There is also evidence for topical negative wound pressure therapy as an adjunct to decrease superficial wound infections.

Please note that patients who are at risk of being hypocoagulable, hypothermic, or acidotic need abbreviated procedures with the intent to increase survival by allowing source control with minimal possible surgical insult. (See Chapter 9.) The concept is to serve as a bridge to definite

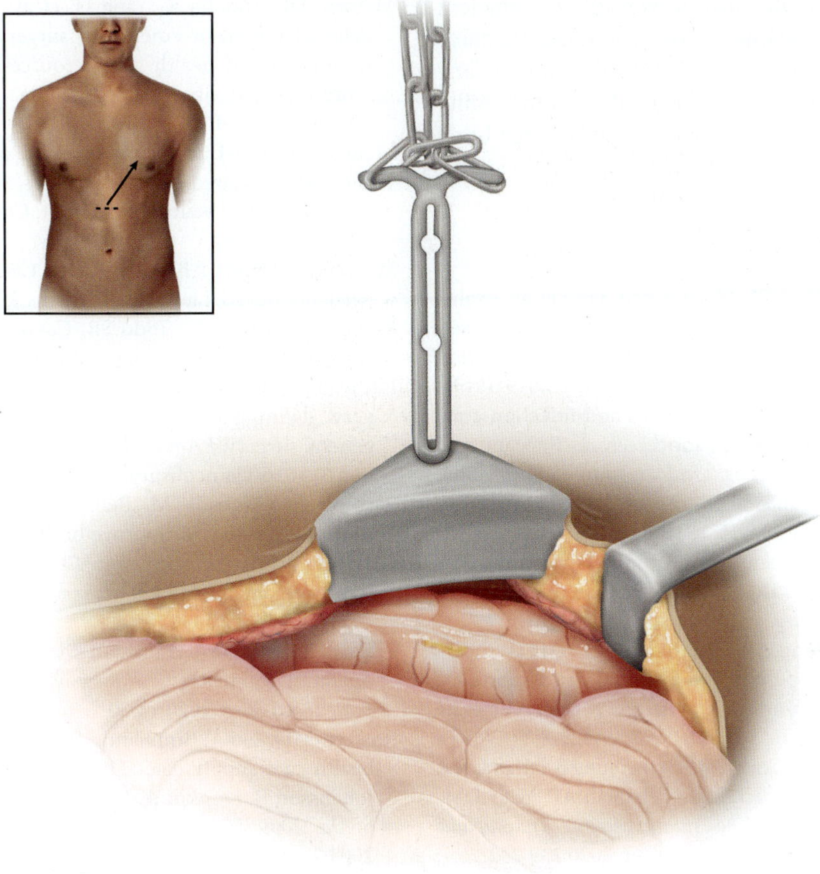

Figure 8.8 Balfour retractor augmented by adding an ordinary chain.

repair once the patient is physiologically restored. Do not truncate the operation until *surgical bleeding* is controlled. Temporize quickly and transfer the patient to the ICU to avoid the "deadly triad" of acidosis, hypothermia, and coagulopathy. Keep track of operative time, physiologic metrics (blood transfused, temperature, pH, and thromboelastography), and clinical indicators of physiology such as "oozing" from the operative field (*medical bleeding*). In abbreviated procedures, we usually cut the falciform ligament to ease initial abdominal access and at the end of the procedure the placement of a plastic fenestrated sheet over the liver to avoid abdominal fixation, which can compromise subsequent fascial closure. Bowel lacerations should be temporarily clamped expeditiously with Babcock forceps and then stapled or sutured. Bowel segments should be resected and left without anastomosis and an NG tube placed past the pylorus for proximal bowel decompression.

When dealing with liver, bile ducts, pancreas, or duodenum, and if surgical repair is not advisable, good sense may guide us toward external diversion with tube drainage.

In an abbreviated surgery, the abdomen is temporarily closed, and first a disposable plastic fenestrated sheet (interface) is applied for bowel protection from the applied foam with negative wound pressure therapy (NPWT). Return to operating theater should be within 24-48 hours to decrease complications.

SUMMARY

The emergency surgical patient often requires emergent or urgent surgery. Delay to control bleeding or source control results in preventable morbidity and mortality. Operations for these patients cannot simply be added to the end of the day, when all elective cases are completed. Conversely, routinely canceling or delaying elective cases to accommodate these emergency cases is disruptive for the patient and surgeon. Thus, an operative schedule must preemptively include an open room or sufficient flexibility to manage the competing needs.

The designated OR must be versatile yet efficient without overcrowding or overstocking. Preparation for immediate operative intervention for "any emergency that may arise" is vital, as is the ability to rapidly change operative plans, open other body cavities, or engage multiple surgical services simultaneously in care of the patient.

SUGGESTED READINGS

Aggarwal G, Peden CJ, Mohammed MA, et al. Evaluation of the collaborative use of an evidence-based care bundle in emergency laparotomy. *JAMA Surg.* 2019;154:e190145. doi:10.1001/jamasurg.2019.0145

Bali RK. Operating room protocols and infection control. In: Bonanthaya K, Panneerselvam E, Manuel S, Kumar VV, Rai A, eds. *Oral and Maxillofacial Surgery for the Clinician.* Springer; 2021. https://doi.org/10.1007/978-981-15-1346-6_9

Christie SA, Peitzman AB. Trauma laparotomy. In: Hawn MT, Albo D, Brown K, et al., eds. *Operative Techniques in Surgery.* Wolters Kluwer; 2022.

Daniel VT, Rushing AP, Ingraham AM, et al. Association between operating room access and mortality for life-threatening general surgery emergencies. *J Trauma Acute Care Surg.* 2019;87:35-42.

Dauer E, Sjoholm L, Goldberg A. Operating room practice and operative approaches. In: Peitzman AB, Yealy DM, Fabian TC, et al., eds. *The Trauma Manual: Trauma and Acute Care Surgery.* Wolters Kluwer; 2020:239-242.

El Boghdady M, Ewalds-Kvist BM. Laparoscopic surgery and the debate on its safety during the COVID-19 pandemic: a systematic review of recommendations. *Surgeon.* 2021;19:e29-e39.

Jung KS, Pinedo M, Sriskandarajah C, et al. Scheduling elective surgeries with emergency patients in shared operating rooms. *Product Operat Manag.* 2019;28:1407-1430.

Kirkpatrick AW, et al. The evolution of a purpose designed hybrid trauma operating room from the trauma service perspective: the RAPTOR (resuscitation with angiography percutaneous treatments and operative resuscitations). *Injury.* 2014;45:1413-1421. http://dx.doi.org/10.1016/j.injury.2014.01.021

Klompas M, Baker M, Rhee C. What is an aerosol-generating procedure? *JAMA Surg.* 2020;156:113-114.

McIsaac DI, Abdulla K, Yang H, et al. Association of delay of urgent or emergency surgery with mortality and use of health care resources: a propensity score-matched observational cohort study. *CMAJ.* 2017;189:E905-E912.

Miao H, Wang J-J. Scheduling elective and emergency surgeries at shared operating rooms with emergency uncertainty and waiting time limit. *Comp Indust Eng.* 2021;160:107551.

Moore KL, Dalley AF, Agur AMR. *Clinically Oriented Anatomy.* 6th ed. Lippincott Williams & Wilkins; 2010.

Moore LJ, Turner KL, Todd SR. *Common Problems in Acute Care Surgery.* Springer-Verlag; 2013.

Narayan M, Bruns B, Tesoriero R, et al. Acute care surgery: defining the economic burden of emergency general surgery. *J Am Coll Surg.* 2016;222(4):691-699. doi:10.1016/j.jamcollsurg.2016.01.054

Perrone G, Giuffrida M, Bellini V, et al. Operating room setup: how to improve health care professionals safety during pandemic COVID-19—a quality improvement study. *J Laparoendosc Adv Surg Tech A.* 2021;31:85-89.

Prakash L, Dhar SA, Mushtaq M. COVID-19 in the operating room: a review of evolving safety protocols. *Patient Saf Surg.* 2020;14:30.

Rossetti MD, Liu Y. Simulating SKU proliferation in a health care supply chain. In: Rossetti MD, Hill RR, Johansson B, Dunkin A, Ingalls RG, eds. *Proceedings of the 2009 Winter Simulation Conference.* Austin; 2009:2365–2374.

Scott-Conner CEH, ed. *Chassin's Operative Strategy in General Surgery.*© Springer Science & Business Media New York; 2014. doi:10.1007/978-1-4614-1393-6_2

Søreide K. Trauma and the acute care surgery model—should it embrace or replace general surgery? *Scand J Trauma Resusc Emerg Med.* 2009;17:4. http://www.sjtrem.com/content/17/1/4

Stoner R. The impact of COVID-19 on surgical practice—a summary. *World J Surg Surg Res.* 2021;4:1272.

van Veen-Berkx E, Elkhuizen SG, Kuijper B, et al. Dedicated operating room for emergency surgery generates more utilization, less overtime and less cancellations. *Am J Surg.* 2016;211:122-128.

WHO Guidelines for Safe Surgery 2009. World Health Organization; 2009.

CHAPTER

9 Damage Control in Emergency General Surgery

Andrea Spota, Stefania Cimbanassi, and Osvaldo Chiara

CASE PRESENTATION

A 63-year-old man with a history of arterial hypertension and diverticular disease was referred to the emergency department (ED) complaining of severe abdominal pain, fever, and vomiting for 2 days.

Physical examination revealed a distended abdomen with signs of peritonitis. The NEWS (National Early Warning Score) score was 6. Blood tests showed: WBC 12 000/mm^3, CRP 28 mg/dL, procalcitonin 39 ng/mL, bilirubin 1.5 mg/dL, INR 1.8, pH 7.34, and lactate 3.1 mmol/L.

The patient underwent a CT scan, which showed pneumoperitoneum in the presence of sigmoid thickening and pneumatosis. Moreover, a perisigmoid and a peritransverse colon fluid collection were found (**Figure 9.1**).

Emergency surgery was scheduled with the diagnosis of colonic perforation.

Upon opening the abdomen, diffuse fecal peritonitis was found.

A left colectomy extended to the proximal transverse colon was performed; the left colon was ischemic with several perforations. The abdomen was irrigated.

The septic shock, need for inotropic support, abdominal contamination, and extensive colonic involvement led us to opt for damage control surgery (DCS). The stapled colonic stumps were left in discontinuity, and a temporary abdominal closure (TAC) using a Barker type vacuum pack was placed.

The patient was admitted to the intensive care unit (ICU), after 48-hour resuscitation, hemodynamics improved and the patient no longer required inotropes. The patient returned to the operating room (OR) where reexploration revealed that intraoperative contamination was controlled with healthy, well-vascularized colonic ends (**Figure 9.2**).

We proceeded with definitive surgery: after extensive mobilization of the right colon, a stapled anastomosis between the proximal transverse colon and the distal sigmoid was performed. At the conclusion of the operation, after fascial approximation, the intra-abdominal pressure, measured through intravesical assessment, was 8 mm Hg. The abdominal wall was closed (double layer with absorbable sutures). Two Jackson-Pratt drains were placed.

The patient was discharged from the ICU to the emergency general surgery department on postoperative day 4.

On day 4, the patient had signs of severe inflammation on blood tests and the abdominal drains evacuated purulent fluid. A CT scan revealed minimal fluid in the paracolic gutters and a large pleural effusion **(Figure 9.3)**; blood cultures were positive for Klebsiella.

After chest drainage and antibiogram-driven antibiotics, the patient's condition improved.

The remaining hospital stay was uneventful with progressive return to normal physiological functions.

Question: *What are the factors to be considered in the decision-making process to undertake a damage control and open abdomen strategy in this patient?*

Answer: *Septic shock with need for vasopressor support, diffuse fecal contamination, and high risk of postoperative abdominal compartment syndrome.*

This patient is in severe septic shock with need of inotropes to maintain an adequate hemodynamic state. Furthermore, perioperative high-volume fluid infusion would expose the patient to a high risk of abdominal compartment syndrome in the setting of fascial closure.

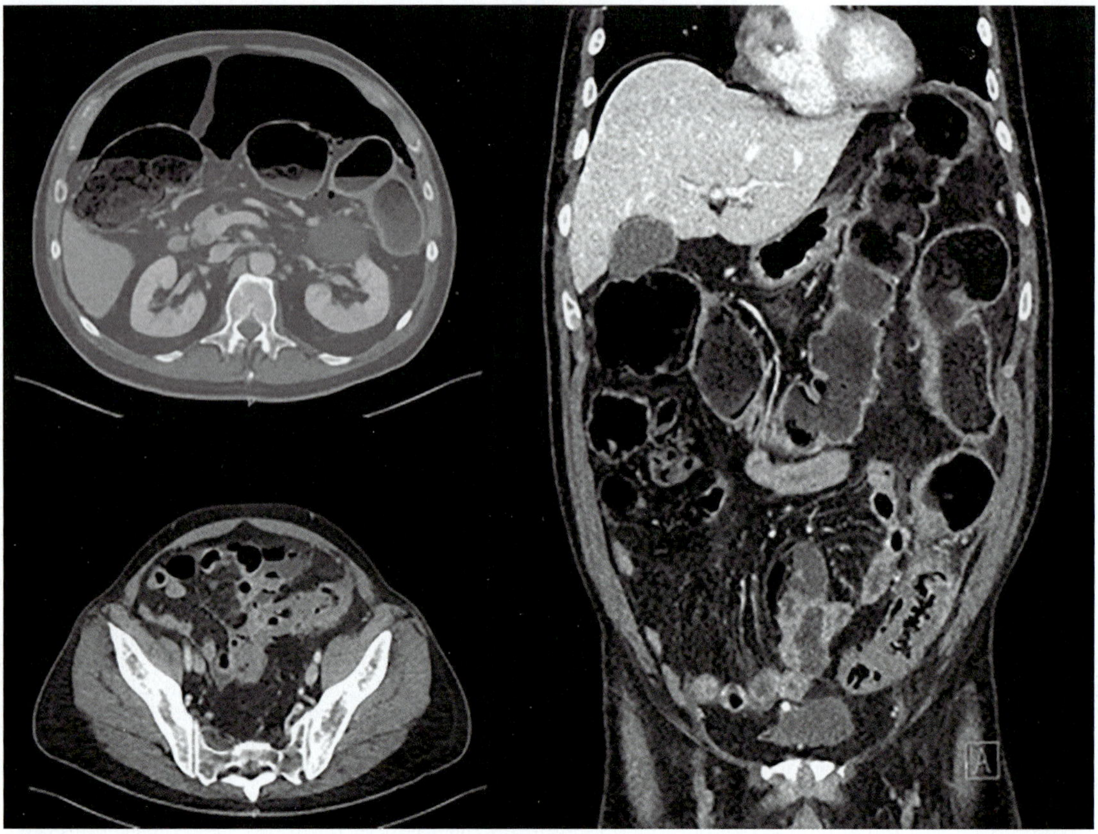

Figure 9.1 Emergency department CT scan: colonic perforation.

INTRODUCTION

Over the last three decades, damage control surgery (DCS) has become the standard of care in the treatment of critically trauma patients requiring surgery. DCS is not a procedure in itself but part of an overall damage control (DC) strategy, which also includes DC resuscitation.

The principles of DCS include abbreviated surgery and delayed definitive surgical management, only after restoration of normal physiology. Primary definitive repair should not be attempted in patients who are unfit for complex surgery. The patient with deranged physiology needs a surgical strategy that prioritizes physiology over anatomy.

Caring for patients with severe physiological derangement (due to mechanisms different from traumatic bleeding, ie, nontraumatic bleeding and sepsis) has led acute care surgeons to extend the use of DCS from trauma to selected nontrauma emergency general surgery (EGS).

Thus, DC consists of a staged management requiring teamwork (ie, surgeons working together with anesthesiologists) to treat these patients by prioritizing intensive care and then definitive surgery, usually following a staged approach (**Figure 9.4**).

Patient Selection

Pathophysiology

The management of critically ill patients with severe physiologic derangement involves several intensive care cornerstones such as volume

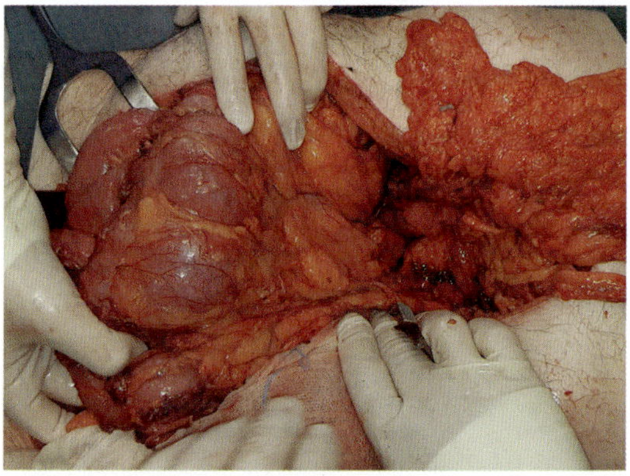

Figure 9.2 Surgical reexploration at 48 hours from the index operation: healthy colon with good vascularization, the abdominal cavity is clean.

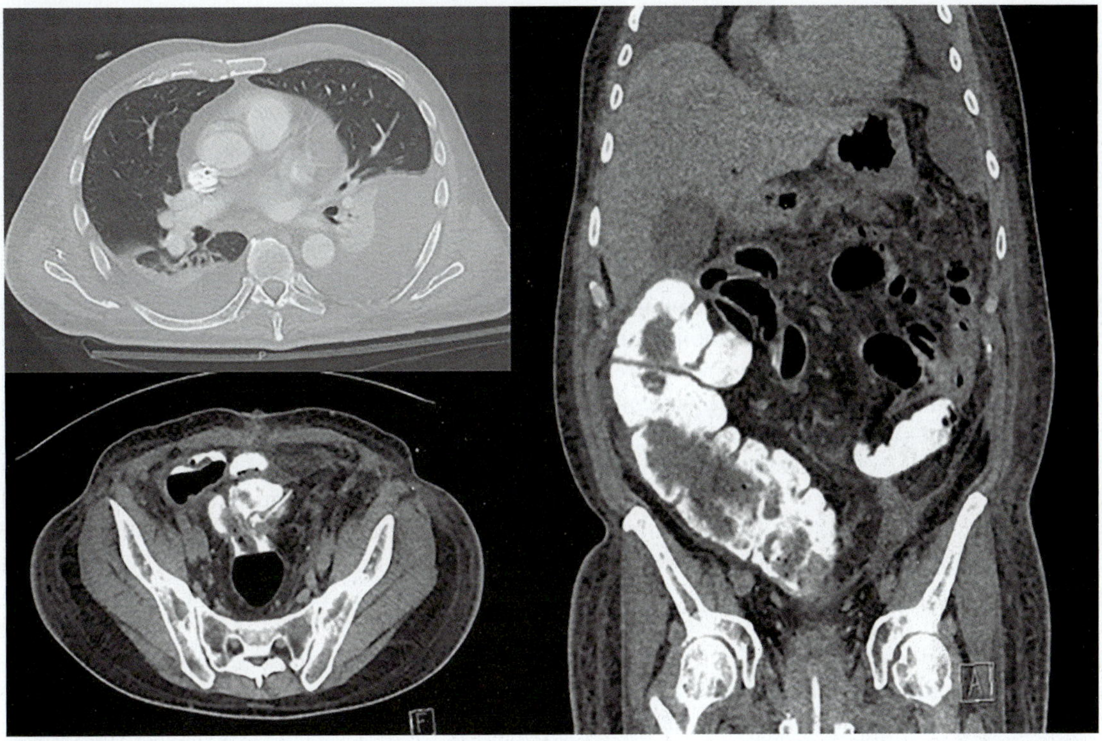

Figure 9.3 Postoperative CT scan: minimal fluid in the paracolic gutters and a large pleural effusion; the intraluminal contrast injection showed no anastomotic leak.

resuscitation, coagulopathy reversal, correction of hypothermia, and acidosis. The "lethal triad" (hypothermia, acidosis, and coagulopathy) should be promptly interrupted as done with severely injured patients.

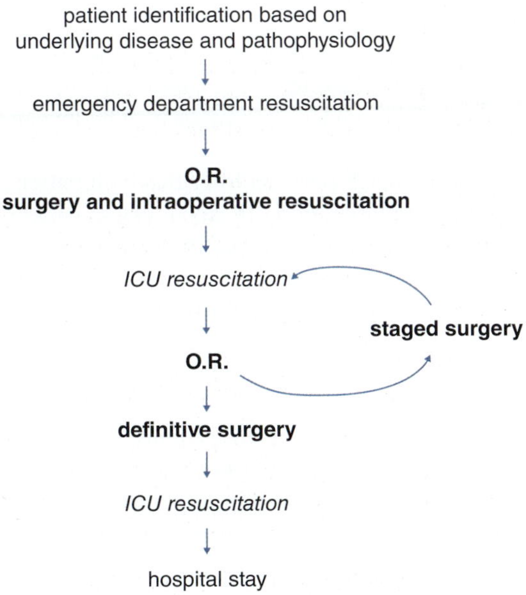

Figure 9.4 Algorithm: staged approach for damage control strategy.

However, trauma and nontrauma patients represent two different populations with different types of physiological derangement. While traumatic shock is usually caused by major bleeding, nontraumatic shock can be either hemorrhagic without tissue injury (eg, abdominal aortic aneurysm [AAA]) or septic (driven by several anatomical conditions, eg, complicated diverticulitis, peptic ulcer perforation). Frequently, due to failure to identify and intervene early on a septic source, the patient's condition may rapidly worsen with a poor outcome.

Specific triggers for DC in EGS still need to be clearly defined.

In the case of bleeding of nontraumatic origin, Girard et al. tested criteria similar to those used in traumatic bleeding by evaluating the outcome of DCS. These included hypothermia (<35 °C), arterial hypotension (systolic <70 mm Hg), acidosis (pH < 7.25), elevation of the international normalized ratio (INR > 1.7), and massive blood transfusion (more than 5 packed red blood cells). The increasing number of the aforementioned criteria resulted in greater operative mortality: 1 criterion (24% mortality), 2 (48%), or 3 (62%).

In the setting of sepsis, the same study proposed different triggers for DC such as advanced age (≥70 years), male gender, acidosis (pH < 7.25), elevated lactate (>3.0 mmol/L), and multiple comorbidities (more than 3) (see also Chapter 5: Abdominal Sepsis). However, the study did not prove a statistically significant association of these triggers with patient outcome.

Furthermore, several ICU scoring systems have been applied to identify patients at high risk of poor outcome. They consist of combinations of several items in cardiovascular, respiratory, renal, hepatic, coagulation, and neurological systems, to readily document multiorgan failure.

The APACHE II (acute physiology and chronic health evaluation II) score evaluates the chronic health through 12 physiologic factors, although not routinely measured universally. Similarly, the MODS (multiorgan dysfunction score) includes the measurement of central venous pressure that is not consistently measured. The P-POSSUM score (Portsmouth physiological and operative severity score for the enumeration of mortality) contains 12 physiological and 6 operative variables but provides incomplete preoperative information and has led to overprediction of mortality in both high- and low-risk patients. The SAPS II (simplified acute physiology score II) is based on the worst values of 12 physiological variables measured during the first 24 hours of ICU admission and estimates the mortality risk for a group of patients but does not predict the individual chance of survival.

The aforementioned scores estimate the risk of prolonged ICU stay and mortality and are used primarily in ICU units and are rarely collected in the emergency department (ED); therefore, their usefulness is controversial.

In the above-mentioned Girard's study, 164 patients who underwent DCS for nontraumatic abdominal emergencies were analyzed. Patient outcome was compared to several previously described scores (ie, APACHE II, POSSUM, P-POSSUM, SAPS II) to evaluate the usefulness in DCS. At 30 days, the observed mortality was lower than that expected by the scores. Also, the overall observed morbidity was lower than predicted by the POSSUM score, specifically in case of bleeding or peritonitis.

In the case of sepsis, two simplified scores may be applied in day-to-day ED activity: the quick-SOFA (sequential organ failure assessment) and the NEWS 2 (national early warning score) scores.

The quick-SOFA represents a simplified version of SOFA score, which includes only three values: arterial hypotension (systolic pressure <100 mm Hg), high respiratory rate (>22 breaths/min), and altered mentation (GCS < 15). This score is easy to use and can be repeated serially. The score ranges from 0 to 3; two or more points in patients with infection is associated with need for prolonged ICU stay and higher risk of death.

The NEWS 2, including eight easy-to-collect parameters, determines the degree of illness of a patient and the need for prompt critical care intervention when the results are higher than 5.

Given the handiness of the included parameters, these two scores could have potential application to help recognize patients with reduced physiological reserve who could be considered for DC. Thus, none of the previous scores has been validated yet for use in selection of patients to undergo DC.

In 2017, the World Society of Emergency Surgery (WSES) listed five triggers to define an unstable patient, potentially amenable for DC: pH < 7.2; core temperature <35 °C; base excess < −8; laboratory/clinical evidence of coagulopathy; and any sign of sepsis/septic shock (the necessity for inotropic support is included). Documenting at least one of these items is considered significant.

Finally, currently the choice of performing DCS in EGS can be supported from several physiological triggers but is most often, still left to surgeons' clinical judgment.

Indications

Depending on the underlying condition, DCS can be planned before laparotomy or may be invoked as a bail out strategy.

Planned DCS pertains to critically ill patients requiring an operation. In such cases, patients requiring procedures such as cholecystectomy or bowel resection-anastomosis may be unfit for primary definitive surgery and undergo gallbladder percutaneous drainage or intestinal resection leaving bowel in discontinuity and deferred anastomosis, respectively.

Bail out DCS refers to patients undergoing elective (or emergency) surgery with intraoperative adverse events causing rapid physiological deterioration. Conditions such as intraoperative bleeding or a complex, time-consuming surgical reconstruction could require an unplanned need for DCS.

Damage Control Surgery: What Is and How to Do It

DCS encompasses all surgical strategies required to treat patients whose physiological reserves are near exhaustion. These techniques are described in following paragraphs according to organ/pathology.

By Organ/Pathology

Once in the operating room (OR), DCS aims to control the source of bleeding/sepsis, while the reconstructive phase and abdominal wall closure represent a secondary goal, postponed until after physiological improvement, postoperatively, in the ICU.

The specific surgical procedure used to achieve damage source control varies depending on the underlying disease.

BLEEDING PEPTIC ULCERS

The role of surgery in control of bleeding ulcers has been minimized with the promulgation of endoscopic techniques (see also Chapter 13: Gastrointestinal Hemorrhage in Emergency Surgery). However, endoscopic treatment is not always effective, and, in the presence of uncontrolled bleeding, the surgeon should consider other therapeutic alternatives, that is, angiography and surgery.

According to a recent meta-analysis, predictors of recurrent bleeding include fresh blood at endoscopy, ulcers larger than 2 cm or localized on the lesser gastric curvature or posterior wall of the duodenal bulb (because of their proximity to gastric and gastroduodenal arteries, respectively).

Angiography and surgery should be immediately considered after failure of the first hemostatic endoscopic attempt. However, angiographic embolization is less effective in case of impaired coagulation, which is a common condition in case of deeply debilitated patients.

If the patient remains in hemorrhagic shock despite vigorous resuscitation, emergency surgery and DC may become mandatory. A DC approach is planned, with the goal to stop hemorrhage, not to definitively treat the peptic ulcer disease on the OR.

Surgical procedures depend on ulcer location and extension and on the type of bleeding vessel. Oversewing of the ulcer or resection can be performed in case of gastric ulcer. If a Dieulafoy lesion is found (ie, erosion of a large tortuous arteriole in the gastric submucosal), a wedge resection of the stomach may be required. On the other hand, posterior duodenal ulcers require duodenotomy and oversewing of the bleeding vessel on the floor of the ulcer. If the bleeding site is difficult to recognize, an extension of the incision through the pylorus may be performed to inspect the duodenal bulb and the gastric antrum. Then, four sutures (cardinal points around the bleeding point) can complete vessel ligature (see also Chapter 13: Gastrointestinal Hemorrhage in Emergency Surgery). The modified Weinberg procedure (elective ligation of the gastroduodenal artery above and below the bleeding point without pyloroplasty and vagotomy) is another alternative.

It should also be mentioned that these procedures are associated with high mortality rates (up to 36%).

More time-consuming procedures such as formal gastric resections can be performed in a second procedure in an elective setting.

PERFORATED PEPTIC ULCER

Although perforation of the upper GI tract usually produces less severe contamination compared to the lower GI tract, patients can still present with severe sepsis when the peritoneal spillage is diffuse, or diagnosis is delayed (see also Chapter 16: Peptic Ulcer Disease). As discussed above, in the unstable patient, the operation should be approached in a DC mode, with the goal to obtain source control, not to perform a definitive ulcer operation.

Small (<2 cm) ulcers are easily treated by suturing, while larger ulcers require different procedures depending on the location.

Gastric ulcers uncommonly require a DC strategy.

Duodenal ulcers become progressively more challenging as they are near the ampullary region. In patients who otherwise would require pancreatic head resection but are physiologically unfit for such a procedure, consider pyloric exclusion with oversew/stapling of the pylorus and gastric decompression through nasogastric tube/gastrostomy or gastrojejunostomy. (Some authors recommend external biliary and pancreatic diversion as well.) (See also Chapter16: Peptic Ulcer Disease.)

ACUTE MESENTERIC ISCHEMIA

Acute mesenteric ischemia (AMI) frequently represents as a dramatic condition since in most cases when symptoms appear, bowel ischemia has already occurred and survival is closely related to patient's general conditions and comorbidities (see also Chapter 12: Mesenteric Ischemia). Surgery must be performed without delay with resection of ischemic bowel, preservation of viable bowel, and restoration of blood supply. These key points are essential for optimal outcome: unrecognized ischemic bowel leads to multiorgan dysfunction; viable bowel is essential to ensure a healthy anastomosis and can affect the outcome depending on the remaining visceral length; blood supply is essential to guarantee adequate vascularization.

The vascular restoration depends on the etiology of the AMI: occlusive (arterial embolism/thrombosis or venous thrombosis) and nonocclusive (NOMI) (due to vasoconstriction in the presence of low splanchnic blood flow). If the bowel is not yet necrotic, venous thrombosis does not need revascularization, only anticoagulation, while nonocclusive ischemia (NOMI) requires adequate volume restoration and treatment of the precipitating cause. Arterial revascularization can require various procedures based on the site of occlusion. If proximal, embolectomy or angioplasty are well-established definitive treatment alternatives.

These procedures are time demanding and high risk in patients with arterial hypotension requiring high doses of vasopressors. In addition, suboptimal vascularization jeopardizes the anastomosis; restoration of intestinal continuity needs to be deferred. DCS includes resection of nonviable bowel leaving the bowel in discontinuity with temporary abdominal closure (TAC). Revascularization can be optimized as intraoperative or postoperative endovascular treatment.

After blood flow restoration and ICU resuscitation, a second look is planned to check bowel viability and eventually complete the surgical procedure with an anastomosis. Often at the second look operation, the surgeon is faced with the inability to close the abdomen due to bowel edema caused by fluid derangement and ischemic-reperfusion injury; this condition requires a continued open abdomen (OA) strategy. Thus, in case of AMI, the OA has a dual purpose: bowel reevaluation with deferred anastomosis and abdominal compartment syndrome (ACS) prevention. At times, surgeons perform a TAC after definitive bowel reconstruction at the index procedure with the intent to reexamine the anastomosis at a second operation. This strategy should be avoided because of the morbidity associated with OA and the advantages of a relaparotomy on-demand strategy for such cases.

COLORECTAL OBSTRUCTION/PERFORATION

Patients presenting with obstruction or perforation from either colorectal cancer or acute diverticulitis can be unstable due to the association of preexisting comorbidities, as well as fluid and electrolyte imbalance, bacterial translocation, and peritonitis (see also Chapter 18: Gastrointestinal Inflammatory Diseases).

If the disease in the colon is *right sided*, a right colectomy with terminal ileostomy represents a viable surgical option.

In presence of a clean field and satisfactory bowel vascularization, an ileocolic anastomosis can be fashioned, without excessive operative time.

In presence of a severely contaminated field, the anastomosis and the ileostomy should be postponed and the operation is abbreviated by means of TAC. At second look, after physiologic restoration, an ileostomy and/or anastomosis represent the definitive surgical options.

If the disease in the colon is *left sided*, Hartmann procedure should be considered as the first choice. This avoids time-consuming procedures, and the surgeon then can choose either a two- or three-stage strategy for elective intestinal restoration.

In uncommon, selected cases of obstruction, a loop colostomy can be a safe alternative. However, the Hartmann procedure has been found to have comparable morbidity while ensuring a shorter hospital stay. Thus, a loop colostomy should be limited to unresectable tumors or if neoadjuvant therapy is planned.

In case of perforation with a severely contaminated abdominal field, colostomy creation should be deferred and relaparotomy is planned after TAC.

When the underlying disease is cancer, whatever its localization, the tumor should be preferentially resected at the index surgery; certainly, DCS, if necessary, can jeopardize this timing.

It should be emphasized that standard colonic resections may require some modification due to the invasion of adjacent structures by the colorectal cancer.

As an alternative to emergency surgery for obstruction, the endoscopic positioning of self-expandable metal stents (SEMS) represents a controversial option as a bridge-to-surgery strategy. Initial promising results (clinical success over 90%) have been adjusted as studies have demonstrated a lower clinical success rate (around 70%) in the presence of comparable complications (50%-60%). Moreover, in case of cancer, SEMS placement may induce hematogenous spread of malignant cells; the oncologic impact remains uncertain.

On the other hand, SEMS are associated with lower rate of stoma creation and higher rate of subsequent laparoscopic elective procedure, defining a sort of "endolaparoscopic approach."

The potential advantages of SEMS are counterbalanced by frequent adverse events such as stent migration and colonic perforation, which can cause significant delays to surgery.

Finally, adequate patient selection through risk stratification is paramount.

ACUTE CHOLECYSTITIS

The decision to perform simple gallbladder drainage (cholecystostomy) in patients with acute cholecystitis who are deemed unfit for cholecystectomy because of general physiological derangement is a typical DCS application (see also Chapter 15: Biliary Tract Disease). In the OR, subtotal cholecystectomy as a bailout technique is a form of DC.

The Tokyo guidelines originally recommended the use of percutaneous gallbladder drainage as the first alternative to cholecystectomy for this type of patient (grade III acute cholecystitis). Since those publications, innovative endoscopic solutions have developed including (not yet standard practice):

1. Transpapillary drainage up to the gallbladder under endoscopic retrograde cholangiography. Then, either a nasogallbladder tube is positioned or gallbladder stenting is performed, and the bile is drained across the papilla. This approach is preferred in case of altered coagulation or inability to reach the anatomical window adequate for the second option.
2. The transmural approach consists of an endoscopic ultrasound-guided drainage: positioning of double pigtail stents or SEMS or lumen-apposing metal stents (LAMS) between the gallbladder and duodenum (some cases of gallbladder-gastric stents have been described but with worse outcomes). This technique affords the advantage of effective drainage even in case of difficulty of biliary tract exploration and precludes the need for tubes.

Both endoscopic methods are associated with less abdominal pain compared to percutaneous drainage; however, they are currently not standard techniques because they require high-skilled endoscopists and high-volume centers.

SEVERE ACUTE PANCREATITIS

Patients with severe acute pancreatitis unresponsive to medical management should undergo a step-up approach where percutaneous/endoscopic drainage represents the first-line operative treatment for infected pancreatic necrosis (see also Chapter 14: Acute Pancreatitis).

Percutaneous drainage is preferred for lateral collections, while endoscopic transgastric necrosectomy (ETN) is indicated for central, retrogastric collections. Of note, ETN should be preferably performed for infected pancreatic necrosis, at least 4 weeks after onset of disease; this timing is associated with a decrease in mortality.

This strategy allows complete resolution of infected necrosis in 25%-60% of cases and delays surgical treatment to a more favorable time.

Moreover, the two strategies can be combined and potentially include mini-invasive surgery (ie, VARD—video-assisted retroperitoneal debridement) to tailor the most appropriate treatment for each case.

On occasion, when the step-up approach fails, patients with severe acute pancreatitis can develop intra-abdominal hypertension (IAH), potentially leading to ACS (see also Chapter 10: Abdominal Compartment Syndrome, Open Abdomen). In this case, DCS includes abdominal decompression as an OA procedure. OA represents the last resort after failure of the conservative management.

When DCS for ACS is necessary, surgical drainage/necrosectomy is not routinely recommended. A decompressive laparotomy is performed but the lesser omental sac, and the retroperitoneal space should not be opened to reduce the risk of infection of pancreatic and peripancreatic necrosis.

OA reexploration should be planned 24-48 hours after the index laparotomy; the interval may be shortened in case of patient deterioration.

ABDOMINAL COMPARTMENT SYNDROME

The World Society of the Abdominal Compartment Syndrome (WSACS) defines IAH as an IAP higher than 12 mm Hg and ACS as an IAP > 20 mm Hg in conjunction with new-onset organ dysfunction/failure (see also Chapter 10: Abdominal Compartment Syndrome, Open Abdomen).

In patients at risk of developing IAH or ACS, repeated clinical examination and continuous abdominal pressure measurement (at least every 12 hours until diagnosis and every 6 hours after diagnosis) are essential.

A typical condition leading to ACS is rupture of an AAA. ACS occurs in up to 20% of ruptured AAA, whose mortality (30%-50%) is doubled in case of ACS. ACS also can occur after endovascular repair of the aorta (EVAR) due to massive resuscitation or simply the presence of the associated large retroperitoneal hematoma.

The use of OA reduces the incidence of ACS, but no formal indications exist. Relative indications include massive resuscitation, deranged physiology, blood loss >5 L, use of resuscitative endovascular balloon of the aorta (REBOA), and abdominal hypertension at closure.

IAH/ACS ideally should be prevented and thus managed without surgery. Surgical decompression should be the last resort but remains an effective option to avoid the vicious circle leading to multiorgan failure.

OPEN ABDOMEN AND TEMPORARY ABDOMINAL CLOSURE

The majority of procedures in DCS result in an OA and TAC (see also Chapter 10: Abdominal Compartment Syndrome, Open Abdomen).

The aims of the OA are to

- Facilitate abdominal wall reopening
- Protect the skin and fascia for definitive closure
- Protect the abdominal viscera from contamination, heat loss, and evaporation
- Drain abdominal fluid collections
- Minimize acute visceral adhesions
- Prevent ACS

Conditions requiring its use in EGS patients are listed in **Table 9.1**.

Although the OA is used to treat patients with severely deranged physiology, it must be stressed that it represents a nonanatomic condition with potential life-threatening morbidity.

TABLE 9.1 ■ Indications for the Open Abdomen

In emergency general surgery patients, the open abdomen should be considered in following conditions:

- Persistence of the sepsis source (failure of source control)
- Presence of hemodynamic instability, including on-going fluid resuscitation or vasopressor support
- Gastrointestinal resection, which planned deferred anastomosis
- Need for a second look in case of ischemic bowel
- High risk of abdominal compartment syndrome

Due to the lack of strong data supporting the OA strategy in abdominal EGS, the decision-making process to leave an abdomen open after laparotomy should be carefully considered. OA should be performed in highly selected cases as it is associated with a 30% mortality, essentially due to multiorgan failure and enteroatmospheric fistulae.

Technique

OA consists of intentionally leaving the abdominal fascia and rectus abdominis muscles separated. Several techniques of TAC can be applied to provide protection of the abdominal viscera (**Table 9.2**).

Three categories of TAC have been proposed:

1. *Loose technique*: This is the easiest solution that consists of covering the abdominal viscera, guaranteeing simple access to the cavity. Examples are the Bogota bag ("father" of all OA techniques), loose packing, and skin approximation. The main limitations of this techniques include fascial retraction and not providing extensibility in case of visceral swelling.
2. *Tension technique*: Tension is maintained on the fascia to progressively approximate fascial edges, while allowing easy access to the abdominal cavity. Examples are dynamic retention sutures, the Wittmann Patch, mesh/sheet, and zipper techniques. The main disadvantage of this alternative is that it results more often in enteroatmospheric fistula (EAF). This method can be combined with vacuum techniques to provide fluid evacuation.
3. *Vacuum technique*: A sponge device connected to a negative pressure pump provides constant tension on the abdominal wall while suctioning excess abdominal fluids. There are commercial negative pressure wound therapy (NPWT) systems (eg, RENASYS, VAC, ABTHERA) as well as noncommercial NPWT systems (eg, Barker vacuum pack).

The choice of the specific technique of TAC includes commercial and noncommercial NPWT systems with related costs and outcome comparisons.

For example, hypothermia represents one of the key issues in the OA management, and noncommercial cheaper systems are fraught with a reduced capacity for heat preservation.

In addition, the recent introduction of NPWT with instillation and dwell time (eg, V.A.C. ULTA) consists of a negative pressure system with

TABLE 9.2 ■ Techniques of Temporary Abdominal Closure (TAC)

	Technique	Description	Characteristics	Closure	EAF Development	Mortality
Loose technique	Bogota bag	A sterile x-ray film cassette bag or a bag for organ insulation is sutured between skin or fascial edges	It can be opened in the middle for rapid access to the abdominal cavity By reducing the size of the bag, it is possible to approximate the skin or fascial edges	++	+++	+++++
	Loose packing	Only standard wound dressing is applied to cover the abdominal defect	Easily obtained but does not prevent fascial retraction	+	+++	++++
	Skin approximation	The fascial defect is covered only by skin	Easy and natural coverage but does not prevent fascial retraction	++	+++	++++
Tension technique	Dynamic retention sutures	The viscera are covered with a mesh (eg, ISODrape), and horizontal plastic tubes are inserted through the skin and the fascial edges across the abdominal defect. The tubes are attached to the skin on both sides of the wound by button anchors	The tubes provide continuous tension on the fascia and may be tightened to approximate the fascial edges This technique can be applied with a vacuum system	++++	++++	+++
	Wittmann Patch	Two opposite velcro sheets are sutured to the fascial edge and closed in the middle	Easy repeatable access to the abdominal wall by opening and closing the velcro sheets	++++	+	++
	Mesh, sheet, zipper suture	A mesh or a sheet is sutured between the fascial edges. In the middle, a sterile zipper can be inserted	Easy repeatable access to the abdominal wall. By reducing the size of the mesh, it is possible to approximate the fascial edges. At the end of the open treatment, absorbable or nonresorbable mesh may be removed or left in place	++	++/+++	+++
Vacuum technique	Commercially available vacuum-assisted closure systems (eg, VAC)	Viscera are covered by a perforated sheet; a sponge is placed over that and between the fascial edges. A sealed wound dressing connected to a suction pump is placed over the wound	The continuous aspiration provides a constant tension to the fascial edge and removes exudate excess. The aspiration is adjustable depending on the amount of the peritoneal fluids reducing the edema	+++	+	++
	Noncommercially available vacuum-assisted closure systems (eg, Barker vacuum pack)	The viscera are covered by a perforated sheet, damp surgical towel is placed over that and between the fascial edges, and a surgical drain is placed on the towels. A sealed wound dressing is placed over the wound and negative pressure is applied to the drains	The continuous aspiration provides a constant tension to the fascial edge and removes exudate excess	+++	++	+++

associated controlled saline wound irrigation to dilute the local cytokines, improves both local and systemic immune response.

Furthermore, a recent meta-analysis on TAC techniques in the nontraumatic setting showed an overall fistula rate of 12.1%, ranging from 17.2% for mesh placement to 5.7% with concurrent application of NPWT and fascial traction. An associated fistula doubles the mortality.

The availability and preference for different techniques has changed over the last 30 years; vacuum-assisted solutions are utilized in 85% of OA.

ICU Management

With the OA, fastidious intensive care management is essential to limit associated morbidity.

Thus, several factors, also impacting the surgical strategy, should be carefully scrutinized.

Fluid balance potentially impacting IAP requires close monitoring of

- Cardiac output, to avoid vasopressor excess and fluid overload
- Resuscitation fluids, avoiding high-rate maintenance infusions and preferring small-volume boluses
- Urinary output, as an end point for evaluation of response to ongoing resuscitation
- Routine, scheduled measurement of bladder pressure

Appropriate antimicrobial therapy must be chosen to supplement surgical lavage and debridement. As recommended in Chapter 4: General Surgery Issues in the MICU and CTICU, initial antibiotic coverage should be broad and modified or deescalated based on subsequent culture results.

Abdominal closure should be planned as early as possible since prolonged OA is associated with fascial retraction and consequent inability to close the abdomen, development of a frozen abdomen and EAF. Furthermore, severe fluid and protein loss negatively impacts the patient's electrolyte balance and nutritional state.

Nutritional support is key in OA management (see also Chapter 7: Nutrition). The hypermetabolic condition associated with OA requires starting enteral nutrition as soon as possible. The OA is associated with a nitrogen loss of around 2 g/L of abdominal fluid. Therefore, quantification of abdominal fluid loss is paramount to balance nutritional support. Nutrition should be started as soon as possible, and oral feeding can be restarted as soon as the patient is able to eat.

Initiation of enteral nutrition within the first 24-48 hours decreases catabolism and the pneumonia and fistula rates.

Indeed, enteral nutrition enhances mucosal barrier function, decreases systemic inflammation and oxidative injury, facilitates wound healing, and consequently reduces complications, ICU and hospital stay, and overall costs.

Enteral nutrition is preferred over parenteral nutrition. The only relative contraindication to full enteral nutrition is the presence of viable bowel shorter than 75 cm.

Nitrogen loss is greater in case of EAF, but enteral nutrition should not be neglected. On the contrary, as soon as possible, the patient should be encouraged to *per os* feeding to reach a metabolic state necessary for successive surgical steps.

OA Closure

Regardless of the technique used, international societies such as the WSES and Trauma Association of Canada recommend return to the OR 24 to 72 hours after the index surgery. In general, during this interval, failure of improvement should raise the suspicion of ongoing intra-abdominal problems and lead to consideration of early return to the OR.

One of the main objectives in patients with OA should be to achieve primary fascial closure as soon as patient physiology permits (fascia-to-fascia closure within the index hospitalization and ideally within 7 days from the index surgery).

However, differences in TAC techniques result in different primary fascial closure and EAF rates (see **Table 9.2**).

To achieve a delayed fascial closure within an acceptable time, a dynamic temporary closure through negative pressure in conjunction with a mesh-mediated fascial traction is supported by high success rates.

Successful primary fascial closure is more likely to occur at the first reexploration compared to later laparotomies. Indeed, fascial closure rates correlate with fewer reexplorations and shorter duration of OA management.

Primary fascial closure rates seem to have a bimodal distribution, early closure being related to ICU management and late closure related to the selected TAC technique. The importance of early closure (within 4-7 days from index surgery) is demonstrated by the significant association with lower complications and mortality.

Furthermore, the underlying disease influences patient outcome. Fascial closure during the index hospitalization is less likely in the EGS patient than the trauma patient. Patients with pancreatitis have the lowest fascial closure rate, probably due to the higher number of operations precluding an early closure. Moreover, pancreatitis was associated with greater mortality, suggesting that patient outcome may be related more to the underlying disease than the DCS technique.

As mentioned, this hypothesis is in line with lower rate of fascial closure with nontraumatic OA compared to traumatic OA. Peritonitis is an independent predictor of failure for fascial closure.

In certain settings, primary fascial closure simply cannot be achieved. In case of persistent visceral edema and loss of domain, and/or fascial retraction, surgeons may choose to close the wound through skin grafting on granulation tissue with/without mesh. A planned ventral hernia is created, with the objective to prevent complications by covering the viscera as soon as possible and shorten the duration of OA. (Rarely, depending on center facilities, the wall defect can be covered through pedicled or free flaps.)

Thus, at the conclusion of the OA management, the abdominal wall may be totally closed, closed with a planned ventral hernia or still open with inability to approximate the skin edges.

The different abdominal wall closure techniques after OA are summarized as follows:

- Nonabsorbable synthetic meshes (eg, polypropylene mesh) are not recommended in contaminated fields.
- Nonabsorbable synthetic mesh used to bridge a fascial defect without native tissue protecting the viscera enhances adhesions, erosions, and fistula formation.
- Non–cross-linked biological meshes are well integrated and have lower infection rates.
- Cross-linked biological meshes are preferred if a bridge between fascial edges is needed.
- Biological prostheses tolerate the addition of NPWT to enhance wound healing.
- In case of a planned ventral hernia, after patient recovery and scar maturation, the abdominal wall reconstruction can be planned as an elective procedure with up to 75% of successful fascial closure rates.
- The use of component separation in the acute setting is discouraged because it entails high morbidity and represents a "one-shot" solution, therefore hindering future applications.

Of note, these closed techniques have a high rate of ventral hernia, and therefore, the mesh should be placed as a sublay (ie, with the closure of linea alba).

DCS: CLOSED vs OPEN ABDOMEN

The concept of DCS is often confused with OA: OA is not DCS but indeed an integral part of it.

When abbreviated surgery is chosen, the surgeon must choose between two strategies: close the abdomen or perform a TAC.

If abdominal closure is chosen, a delayed relaparotomy (months) can be planned after restoration of physiological reserve, as happens when a Hartmann procedure is performed and a two- or three-stage strategy is chosen. However, this strategy accounts for the possibility that during patient's index hospitalization, an abdominal adverse event makes it necessary to resort to a "relaparotomy on demand."

In case of OA, reexploration of the abdominal cavity is usually planned between 24 and 72 hours from the previous one. However, even in OA, an on-demand reexploration can be required if patient's condition deteriorates.

In EGS and especially in patients with peritonitis, the choice between abdominal closure (AC) and OA is critical.

The aim of AC is to avoid unnecessary reexploration in an already critical patient and consider relaparotomy only when patient condition demands. Indeed, multiple OA reexplorations amplify the systemic inflammatory response, increasing the risk of multiorgan failure and, ultimately, mortality.

In one randomized trial, OA was compared to AC in patients with severe secondary peritonitis (APACHE II score >10). The AC group showed significantly shorter mechanical ventilation duration, ICU stay, hospital stay, and a significant reduction of relaparotomies. However, no difference in morbidity and mortality was found. In presence of comparable efficacy, with a substantial increase in health care costs in the case of OA, the authors concluded that AC should be preferred under strict patient monitoring to avoid potentially harmful delay in reintervention.

Of note, patients with peritonitis caused by pancreatitis and conditions requiring reexploration (ie, stapled in discontinuity or abdominal gauze packing) were excluded from this study.

In conclusion, the choice of the most appropriate strategy (AC vs OA) boils down to limit use of the OA to cases characterized by the inability to close the abdominal wall; peritoneal contamination should not mandate OA by itself.

Unlike the trauma patient, the World Society for Abdominal Compartment Syndrome suggests avoiding the OA routinely for septic cases. This position is based on data showing greater risks of intra-abdominal abscesses, EAF, and frozen abdomen, along with lower rates of definitive fascial closure.

Patients with hemodynamic instability and life-threatening conditions are most likely to derive potential survival benefits from the DCS approach.

FUTURE PERSPECTIVES

Direct Peritoneal Resuscitation

The current resuscitative standard for severely unstable patients aims for restoration of the physiological reserve through the recovery of central hemodynamic parameters (heart rate, blood pressure, central venous pressure, cardiac output). However, increasing evidence suggests that this strategy reduces but does not completely eliminate cellular hypoxia, microcirculatory hypoperfusion, and inflammation. Thus, constant efforts are needed to improve DC with new effective techniques.

Direct peritoneal perfusion (DPR) is not new; however, now is approached with renewed interest and under evaluation.

Direct peritoneal perfusion consists of intravenous resuscitation concurrent with the irrigation of the peritoneal cavity with a hypertonic glucose-based peritoneal dialysis solution.

In the OA, a Jackson-Pratt drain is inserted into the abdominal cavity, the tip positioned near the base of the mesentery. A TAC is then created; available studies cite the use of a Barker vacuum pack with two suction drains. Eight hundred milliliters of peritoneal dialysis fluid are infused through the Jackson-Pratt drain over the first hour and then a continuous flow of 400 mL/h is maintained and suctioned out through the TAC setup (**Figure 9.5**).

The process is based on the theory that visceral exposure to hypertonic fluids may improve the microcirculation, reducing organ injury, edema, and inflammation.

Conventional resuscitation is associated with high production of the proinflammatory mediators (eg, TNF-α and IL-6), while DPR has been shown to down-regulate their secretion and to increase the production of the anti-inflammatory cytokine IL-10. The inflammatory response modulation reverses the endothelial cell dysfunction

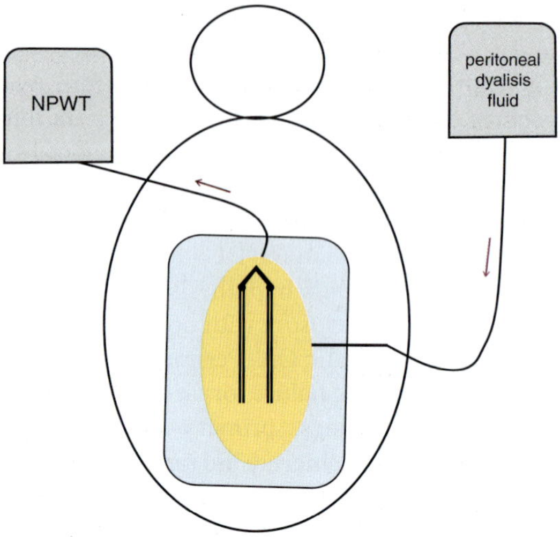

Figure 9.5 Direct peritoneal resuscitation setup. NPWT, negative pressure wound therapy.

with progressive normalization of systemic water compartments. Moreover, the irrigation with a hyperosmotic solution results in dilation of the microcirculation, which improves the blood flow, decreasing tissue edema. Finally, the reduced organ edema preserves cellular structure and limits the tissue damage.

The first human studies were on trauma patients, with the technique extended to nontraumatic cases. Both groups showed improved clinical outcomes.

Direct peritoneal perfusion was found to accelerate the restoration of physiological reserve and significantly reduce number of relaparotomies, time to AC, primary fascial closure, EAF rate, and ICU stay.

SUMMARY

DCS in EGS is a recent extension of DCS for trauma.

Compared to the trauma setting, nontraumatic emergency surgery seems to be more challenging because of the greater number of involved factors; more specifically, sepsis and systemic immune response playing a pivotal role in defining patient outcome. Nevertheless, at the present time, most of the international scientific community endorses DCS with caution in the nontrauma setting.

Many questions remain unanswered, including the real benefit of staged laparotomies vs on-demand strategies, the effect of mechanical abdominal irrigation on the immune response, as well as the correct selection of patients who ultimately benefit from DCS.

SUGGESTED READINGS

Arezzo A, et al. Colonic stenting as a bridge to surgery versus emergency surgery for malignant colonic obstruction: results of a multicentre randomised controlled trial (ESCO trial). *Surg Endosc.* 2017;31:3297-3305.

Atema JJ, Gans SL, Boermeester MA. Systematic review and meta-analysis of the open abdomen and temporary abdominal closure techniques in non-trauma patients. *World J Surg.* 2015;39:912-925.

Bala M, et al. Acute mesenteric ischemia: guidelines of the World Society of Emergency Surgery. *World J Emerg Surg.* 2017;12:38.

Becher RD, et al. Damage control operations in non-trauma patients: defining criteria for the staged rapid source control laparotomy in emergency general surgery. *World J Emerg Surg.* 2016;11:10.

Boele van Hensbroek P, Wind J, Dijkgraaf MGW, Busch ORC, Goslings JC. Temporary closure of the open abdomen: a systematic review on delayed primary fascial closure in patients with an open abdomen. *World J Surg.* 2009;33:199-207.

Coccolini F, et al. The open abdomen in trauma and non-trauma patients: WSES guidelines. *World J Emerg Surg.* 2018;13:7.

Coccolini F, et al. The role of open abdomen in non-trauma patient: WSES Consensus Paper. *World J Emerg Surg.* 2017;12:39.

Elmunzer BJ, Young SD, Inadomi JM, Schoenfeld P, Laine L. Systematic review of the predictors of recurrent hemorrhage after endoscopic hemostatic therapy for bleeding peptic ulcers. *Am J Gastroenterol.* 2008;103:2625-2632; quiz 2633.

Garrison RN, Conn AA, Harris PD, Zakaria ER. Direct peritoneal resuscitation as adjunct to conventional resuscitation from hemorrhagic shock: a better outcome. *Surgery.* 2004;136:900-908.

Girard E, et al. Damage control surgery for non-traumatic abdominal emergencies. *World J Surg.* 2018;42:965-973.

Kirkpatrick AW, et al. Intra-abdominal hypertension and the abdominal compartment syndrome: updated consensus definitions and clinical practice guidelines from the World Society of the Abdominal Compartment Syndrome. *Intensive Care Med.* 2013;39:1190-1206.

Leppäniemi A, et al. 2019 WSES guidelines for the management of severe acute pancreatitis. *World J Emerg Surg.* 2019;14:27.

Mori Y, et al. Tokyo Guidelines 2018: management strategies for gallbladder drainage in patients with acute cholecystitis (with videos). *J Hepatobiliary Pancreat Sci.* 2018;25:87-95.

Pisano M, et al. 2017 WSES guidelines on colon and rectal cancer emergencies: obstruction and perforation. *World J Emerg Surg.* 2018;13:36.

Sorrentino L, et al. Combined totally mini-invasive approach in necrotizing pancreatitis: a case report and systematic literature review. *World J Emerg Surg.* 2017;12:16.

Tarasconi A, et al. Perforated and bleeding peptic ulcer: WSES guidelines. *World J Emerg Surg.* 2020;15:3.

Tsuei BJ, Skinner JC, Bernard AC, Kearney PA, Boulanger BR. The open peritoneal cavity: etiology correlates with the likelihood of fascial closure. *Am Surg.* 2004;70:652-656.

van Ruler O, et al. Comparison of on-demand vs planned relaparotomy strategy in patients with severe peritonitis: a randomized trial. *JAMA.* 2007;298:865-872.

Weaver JL, Smith JW. Direct peritoneal resuscitation: a review. *Int J Surg.* 2016;33:237-241.

Weber DG, Bendinelli C, Balogh ZJ. Damage control surgery for abdominal emergencies. *Br J Surg.* 2014;101:e109-e118.

CHAPTER

10 Abdominal Compartment Syndrome and the Open Abdomen

Bruno M. Pereira, Nathália Sampaio, and Michael Sugrue

CASE PRESENTATION

The relationship between severe acute pancreatitis (SAP) and abdominal compartment syndrome (ACS) is well established and described by some authors as its most lethal complication. Since acute pancreatitis is a well-established risk factor for ACS, the most recent guidelines from the World Society of the Abdominal Compartment (WSACS) recommend routine measurement of intra-abdominal pressure (IAP) in this specific group of patients presenting with SAP. Diagnosis of ACS in SAP is especially difficult in this setting because symptoms can resemble those of other complications such as systemic inflammatory response syndrome, acute respiratory distress syndrome, infected necrosis, and multiple organ dysfunction syndrome. It is for this reason that the measurement of IAP should be performed based on risk factors for ACS, on patients' admission, every four or six hours. Delay in revealing the diagnosis of ACS in the presence of SAP undoubtedly increases the mortality of these patients since low tissue perfusion is perpetuated.

In current practice, the best treatment for ACS is its prevention by intensive monitoring to avoid excessive fluid administration and the exaggerated effects of severe inflammation. Once the ACS-SAP binomial is present, the first-line treatment of the disease must be conservative, following the clinical treatment flow proposed by the WSACS however, surgical decompression is necessary and recommended when conservative methods are insufficient, proven by 3 consecutive and sustained measurements during the application of the recommended clinical treatment.

Literature has demonstrated that surgical decompression considerably reduces IAP, however, it is not possible to relate this decrease in IAP to clinical evolution from the available evidence. Therefore, it remains unknown when and whether invasive intervention should be performed and by what method (percutaneous catheter drainage or various surgical decompression techniques). Given the morbidity of open abdominal decompression, non-invasive means of lowering IAP are indeed an attractive alternative and these include sedation, neuromuscular blockade, nasogastric decompression, correction of a positive cumulative fluid balance and perhaps even continuous hemodiafiltration if available. In addition to the non-invasive treatment strategies, another promising alternative for surgical decompression is percutaneous catheter drainage, but little is known about the best decompression method, time to perform the procedure, and operative technique to use.

Evidence shows that early ACS decompression in SAP is associated with lower mortality. There is no doubt that surgical decompression is effective in decreasing IAP and improves respiratory and renal functions in more than half of patients, however, open abdomen in patients with SAP is associated with significant morbidity, high rate of reoperation, intestinal fistulas and low rate of primary fascial closure. Among SAP patients, those with early MODS and SCA appear to be good candidates for surgical decompression.

In patients with PAS and organ function deterioration, the degree to which IAH contributes to the progression of MODS is unknown. Although the IAP was correlated with the Acute Physiology and Chronic Health Evaluation II score in patients with SAP, a causal relationship between ACS and MODS in SAP has not been proven. According to the current literature, the development of MODS is multifactorial and the inflammatory response plays an important role in the pathogenesis. In experimental models, IAH has been shown to increase the release of pro-inflammatory cytokines into the circulation and cause acute lung and liver injury in the presence of activated circulating neutrophils. In patients with SAP, activation of circulating neutrophils and monocytes is an early event and precedes ICU admission. Considering these factors, the development of ACS could further increase a pro-inflammatory stimulus that contributes to the development of organ failure in SAP. Therefore, early recognition of ACS and its appropriate and timely treatment can prevent the progression of MODS until the patient's death.

Unfortunately, the optimal IAP threshold that would require surgical decompression is unknown. In addition, the optimal timing for intervention is unclear. Recent evidence demonstrates that patients with an IAP greater than 25 mmHg in the first 4 days after disease onset may be good candidates for surgical decompression.

Most studies on the subject agree that early treatment should be instituted as well as surgical decompression in case of failure of clinical or less invasive treatments, and in case of clinical worsening of patients with SAP. Decompression via midline laparotomy, bilateral subcostal laparotomy or subcutaneous linea alba fasciotomy have already been described as technical options, but further studies are needed to effectively compare the proposed methods for surgical decompression.

A 68-year-old Caucasian male is admitted to the emergency department with abdominal pain. His specific complaints are diffuse abdominal pain radiating to the back and vomiting for the last 4 hours. His past medical history includes primary arterial hypertension, type II diabetes mellitus, and previous episodes of acute alcoholic pancreatitis. He has no additional surgical history and no known allergies.

At primary survey in the emergency department, the patient is drowsy and confused. The initial clinical examination reveals a distended abdomen, a small umbilical hernia, and signs of diffuse peritonitis. His temperature is 37.8 °C, blood pressure 102/78 mm Hg, pulse 92 beats/min, respiratory rate 23, and oxygen saturation 92% on ambient air. He appears uncomfortable and diaphoretic.

Secondary survey demonstrates a mildly obese patient with a body mass index of 31 kg/m^2. Initial laboratory tests reveal white blood cell count 22.600 cells/mm^3, hemoglobin 13.9 g/dL, platelets 158 000 cells/mL, sodium 132 milliequivalents per liter (mEq/L), potassium 4.4 mEq/L, blood urea nitrogen (BUN) 23 mg/dL, creatinine 1.3 mg/dL, serum amylase 1050 U/L, serum lipase 644 U/L, AST 15 U/L, ALT 25 U/L, GGT 783 U/L, FALC 1010 U/L, and C-reactive protein (CRP) 112 mg/dL.

The qSOFA score is 2 (respiratory rate and altered mental status). High-flow oxygen (12 L/min) is started, and a peripheral i.v. line is inserted. After 1000 mL of i.v. crystalloid administration, the patient's systolic blood pressure increases to 110 mm Hg. The arterial blood gas analysis reveals a lactate level of 5.1 mmol/L.

Acute alcoholic pancreatitis is suspected, and a nasogastric tube is inserted. 1200 mL of gastric fluid are evacuated promptly. Blood cultures are obtained, and ICU admission is requested. As recommended by recent guidelines, NPO is started, and no antibiotics are prescribed.

Despite fluid resuscitation, the patient's clinical picture worsens, and he requires endotracheal intubation and vasoactive drugs. A contrast-enhanced computed tomography scan of the abdomen is performed and reveals acute pancreatitis (Balthazar-Ranson score of 8). The clinical scenario deteriorates, and abdominal compartment syndrome (ACS) is suspected. After three consecutive intra-abdominal pressure measurements, sustained grade IV intra-abdominal hypertension is observed, and ACS is confirmed as concomitant new organ failure is detected. The surgical team and intensivist agree that decompressive laparotomy (DL) is indicated. The anesthesiologist is informed, and the patient taken to the operating room.

On DL, the surgical team observes full-blown ACS, with free inflammatory fluid in all abdominal quadrants and "candle wax" saponification throughout the upper abdomen. The decision is made to not touch the pancreas but aspirate the free abdominal fluid and leave the cavity open applying mesh-mediated negative pressure wound therapy. After surgery, the patient's clinical picture steadily improves with the intra-abdominal pressure and fluid balance well controlled. Abdominal closure is performed in 2 steps and closed after 72 hours. The patient is discharged after a hospital stay of 28 days and is currently being followed up in clinic.

Question: *What are the indications for surgical decompression in intra-abdominal hypertension in patients with severe acute pancreatitis?*

Answer: *Acute pancreatitis is relatively present in medical practice and contemporary society due to several factors. Its incidence can vary by up to 80 cases/year per 1000,000 inhabitants, as is the case in the United States and Finland. The severe course of the disease is among 20% of this population, associated with mortality of up to 49%.*

ABDOMINAL COMPARTMENT SYNDROME

Abdominal compartment syndrome (ACS) is a potentially lethal condition resulting from an acute and sustained increase in intra-abdominal pressure (IAP), causing significant morbidity and mortality. Intra-abdominal hypertension (IAH) is defined as an IAP above 12 mm Hg in two consecutive measurements within 4-6 hours. **Table 10.1** shows the definitions coined by the World Society of the Abdominal Compartment Syndrome. Rapid progression of IAH leads to ACS, which is defined as an IAP > 20 mm Hg associated with new organ dysfunction. ACS is the end result of a progressive increase in the IAP that if uncorrected will result in dysfunction or failure of multiple organs. However, the harmful effects of IAH occur long before the manifestation of ACS occurs.

Abdominal compartment syndrome is not a problem exclusive to trauma or surgical patients. Its pathophysiological effects are comprehensive and predispose patients to multiple organ failure if no urgent action is taken. Hemodynamic, renal, respiratory, and neurological abnormalities are common.

Etiology and Pathophysiology

Potential causes of IAH in the surgical population include acute pancreatitis, abdominal aortic

TABLE 10.1 ■ WSACS Definitions

1.	IAP is the steady-state pressure concealed within the abdominal cavity
2.	The reference standard for intermittent IAP measurements is via the bladder with a maximal instillation volume of 25 mL of sterile saline
3.	IAP should be expressed in mm Hg and measured at end expiration in the supine position after ensuring that abdominal muscle contractions are absent and with the transducer zeroed at the level of the midaxillary line
4.	Normal IAP is ~5-7 mm Hg in critically ill adults
5.	IAH is defined by a sustained or repeated pathological elevation in IAP ≥ 12 mm Hg
6.	ACS is defined as a sustained IAP > 20 mm Hg (with or without an APP < 60 mm Hg) that is associated with new organ dysfunction/failure
7.	IAH is graded as follows: Grade I, IAP 12-15 mm Hg Grade II, IAP 16-20 mm Hg Grade III, IAP 21-25 mm Hg Grade IV, IAP > 25 mm Hg
8.	Primary IAH or ACS is a condition associated with injury or disease in the abdominopelvic region that frequently requires early surgical or interventional radiological intervention
9.	Secondary IAH or ACS refers to conditions that do not originate from the abdominopelvic region
10.	Recurrent IAH or ACS refers to the condition in which IAH or ACS redevelops following previous surgical or medical treatment of primary or secondary IAH or ACS
11.	APP = MAP – IAP
12.	A polycompartment syndrome is a condition where two or more anatomical compartments have elevated compartmental pressures
13.	Abdominal compliance is a measure of the ease of abdominal expansion, which is determined by the elasticity of the abdominal wall and diaphragm. It should be expressed as the change in intra-abdominal volume per change in IAP
14.	The open abdomen is one that requires a temporary abdominal closure due to the skin and fascia not being closed after laparotomy
15.	Lateralization of the abdominal wall is the phenomenon where the musculature and fascia of the abdominal wall, most exemplified by the rectus abdominis muscles and their enveloping fascia, move laterally away from the midline with time

Based on Pereira BM. Abdominal compartment syndrome and intra-abdominal hypertension. *Curr Opin Crit Care*. 2019;25(6):688-696.

aneurysms, abdominal and retroperitoneal tumors, metabolic ileus, mechanical bowel obstruction, and sepsis. In addition, trauma with intra-abdominal hemorrhage, hypovolemic shock, exacerbated volume replacement, and massive transfusion are important causes of IAH.

In patients with hypovolemic shock, vasoconstriction, mediated by the sympathetic nervous system, decreases blood flow to the skin, muscles, kidneys, and gastrointestinal tract in favor of the heart and brain. Marked reduction of splanchnic circulation leads to intestinal tissue hypoxia. This is frequently associated with three critical factors in the pathogenesis of IAH: cytokine release, oxygen free radical formation, and decreased production of cellular ATP.

Cytokine release promotes vasodilation and increased capillary permeability leading to edema formation. After cell reperfusion, free oxygen radicals are generated and have a toxic effect on cell membranes. The presence of cytokines stimulates the release of more free radicals. Tissue hypoxia limits the production of ATP impairing all dependent cellular energy activities, particularly the sodium and potassium (Na^+/K^+) pumps. The effective operation of the Na^+/K^+ pumps is essential for regulating intracellular electrolytes. When these pumps fail, sodium and water influx into the cells. With cellular edema, the membranes lose their integrity, spilling intracellular content into the extracellular environment. This promotes tissue irritation and inflammation. Inflammation quickly leads to edema, as a result of increased capillary fragility, promoting bowel edema and increased IAP. With increased IAP, abdominal perfusion decreases further, and the cycle of hypoxia, cell death, inflammation, and edema are perpetuated (**Figure 10.1**).

Clinical Manifestations

As shown in **Figure 10.2**, a rise in IAP has important systemic effects. The increase in IAP forces the diaphragm upward, thereby decreasing the volume of the thoracic cavity and increasing the intrathoracic pressure (ITP). Increased ITP leads to increased central venous pressure, which impairs the venous return from the brain, thereby increasing intracranial pressure (ICP) and consequently decreasing cerebral blood flow.

High ITP also raises pulmonary artery pressure (PAP) which increases the afterload on the right ventricle. This can cause right ventricular failure and dilatation with consequent deviation of the cardiac septum to the left, making it difficult to fill the left ventricle. Clinically, the patient presents with low cardiac output, high filling pressures, and high peripheral vascular resistance.

Elevation of IAP can also decrease chest compliance, such that greater pressures are required for adequate mechanical ventilation. Functional residual capacity is also reduced, and ventilation:perfusion ratio increased causing difficulty in gas exchange

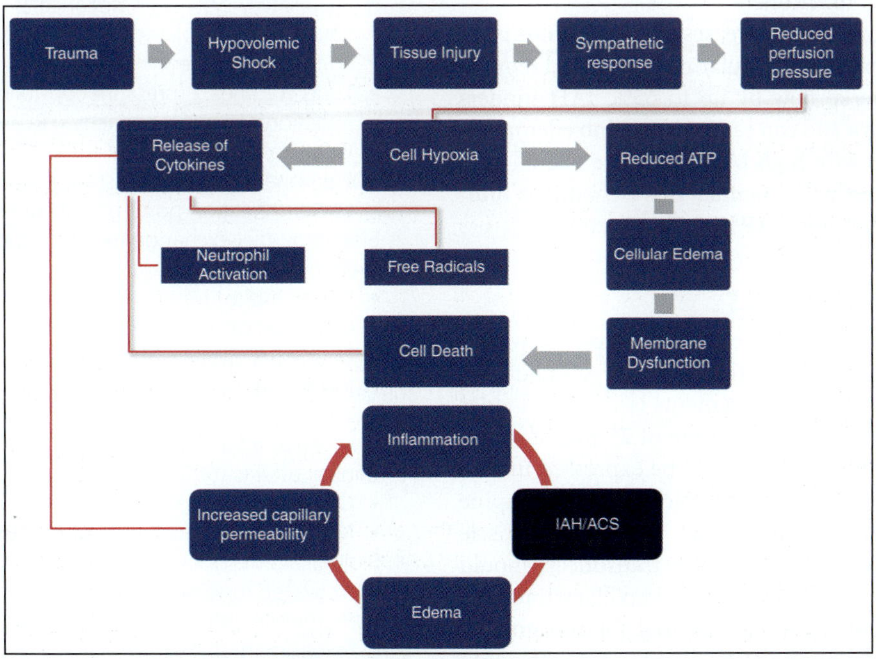

Figure 10.1 Etiology of IAH/ACS.

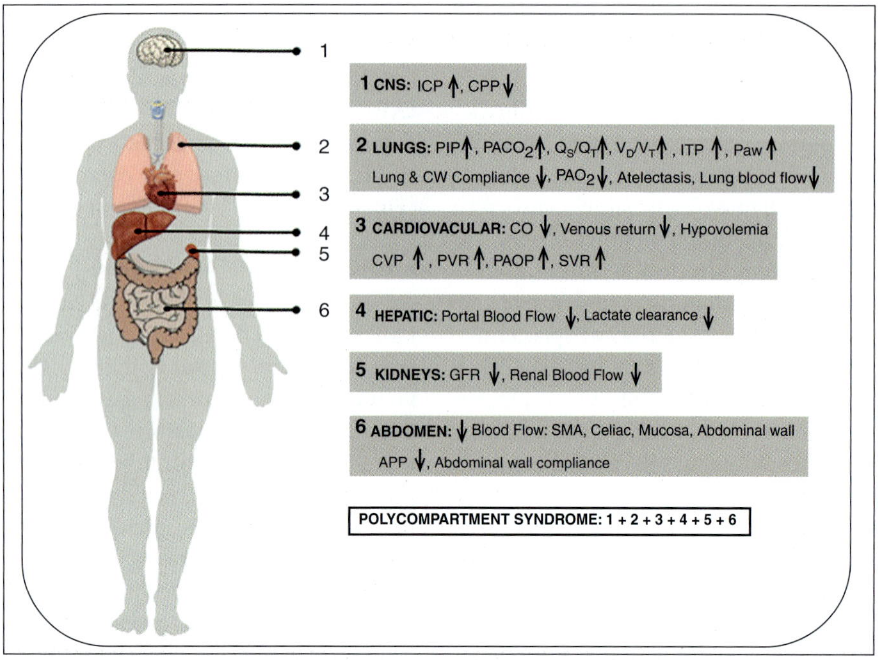

Figure 10.2 Clinical consequences of ACS.

and oxygenation. **Table 10.2** shows the respiratory effects related to increased IAP.

Oliguria or anuria despite aggressive volume replacement is a typical early sign of ACS. It is often the first clinical sign to appear in IAH. Direct compression of the renal parenchyma, decreased renal perfusion due to decreased cardiac output, and water and sodium retention caused by the activation of the renin–angiotensin system will reduce renal function.

Elevation of IAP increases femoral venous pressure and peripheral vascular resistance and reduces femoral arterial flow by up to 65%. IAH hinders venous return and can cause lower limb edema.

Patients with high IAP and tissue edema may develop intestinal ischemia. This ischemia is multifactorial, but high IAP is the key factor.

Diagnosis of IAH/ACS

IAP is defined as the steady-state pressure within the abdominal cavity. The reference standard for intermittent IAP measurements is via the bladder into which a maximal volume of 25 mL of sterile saline is instilled. IAP should be expressed in mm Hg and measured at end expiration in the supine position after ensuring that abdominal muscle contractions are absent. The transducer should be zeroed at the level of the midaxillary line. The measurement of IAP is essential for recognizing IAH. Physical examination alone is not sufficient.

TABLE 10.2 ■ Respiratory Effects Related to Increased IAP

1. Effects on respiratory mechanics (diaphragm elevation)
   - Intrathoracic pressure ↑
   - Pleural pressure ↑
   - Peak airway pressure ↑ (volume controlled)
   - Mean airway pressure ↑
   - Plateau airway pressure ↑
   - Respiratory system compliance ↓
   - Chest wall compliance ↓
   - Lung compliance =
   - Lung volumes ↓ (pressure controlled)
   - Functional residual capacity (FRC) ↓
   - Compression atelectasis ↑
   - Pulmonary vascular resistance ↑
   - Lower inflection point on PV curve ↑
2. Effects on gas exchange (reduced gas exchange)
   - Hypercarbia ↑
   - Oxygenation ↓
   - Dead-space ventilation ↑
   - Intrapulmonary shunt ↑
   - Ventilation perfusion mismatch ↑
   - Alveolar edema ↑
3. Clinical effects (difficult weaning)
   - Oxygen consumption ↑
   - Metabolic cost and work of breathing ↑
4. Biological effects
   - Activated lung neutrophils (experimental) ↑
   - Pulmonary inflammatory infiltration (experimental) ↑

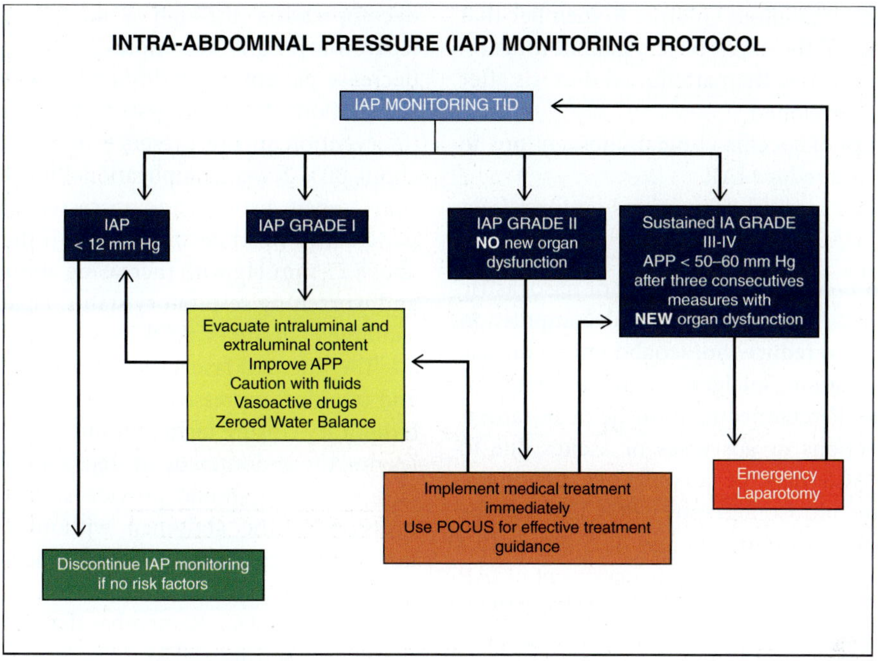

Figure 10.3 Suggested protocol for intra-abdominal pressure monitoring.

The value of IAP that induces multiple organ failure is variable. Abdominal perfusion pressure (APP) is the most reliable parameter for determining the degree of perfusion of the abdominal organs. It is calculated by the formula APP = MAP – IAP (where MAP is mean arterial pressure). The aim should be to maintain APP above 60 mm Hg to improve patient prognosis. **Figure 10.3** shows our suggestion for an IAP monitoring protocol.

Classification of IAH/ACS

Table 10.3 shows the IAH/ACS classification to grade intraabdominal hypertension (IAH) recommended by the *WSACS*. ACS is classified into primary, secondary, tertiary (or recurrent), and quaternary. *Primary ACS* is the condition associated with abdominopelvic disease or trauma. *Secondary ACS* refers to conditions that do not originate in the abdomen or pelvic cavity, such as sepsis, massive volume resuscitation, reperfusion injury, or large burns. *Tertiary ACS* refers to the condition in which ACS recurs after treatment of primary or secondary ACS. *Quaternary ACS* is seen in patients undergoing abdominal wall reconstruction.

TABLE 10.3 ■ IAH/ACS Classification

Grade I	12-15 mm Hg
Grade II	16-20 mm Hg
Grade III	21-25 mm Hg
Grade IV	>25 mm Hg

Risk factors associated with the development of IAH include the following:

- Trauma/lethal triad (hypothermia, coagulopathy, and acidosis)
- Massive transfusion/high infusion volume (>3.5 L/24 h)
- Sepsis
- Changes in intra-abdominal volume
- Pulmonary, renal, or hepatic dysfunction
- Metabolic ileus
- Recent laparotomy with fascial closure

The IAP should be measured if two or more risk factors are present. In the presence of IAH (IAP above 12 mm Hg), 4-6 hourly (or continuous) measurement of the IAP should be performed while steps are taken to treat it expediently. **Figure 10.3** presents a protocol for monitoring the IAP.

Management of IAH/ACS

The basic principles for the management of IAH and ACS are as follows:

- Continuous or repeated monitoring of IAP.
- Optimization of systemic perfusion and organ function.

- Minimize crystalloid volume. Remember that avoidance of the excessive crystalloid infusion is more effective than attempted diuresis after IAH has developed.
- Institution of specific clinical interventions to control and reduce IAP.
- Immediate surgical decompression for refractory IAH/ACS.

IAP can be reduced by the use of nasogastric tubes, enemas, and endoscopic decompression and measures to reduce thoracoabdominal muscle tone with sedation, analgesia, and neuromuscular blockade. Percutaneous drainage of intraperitoneal collections or abscesses or ascites due to secondary ACS may be an effective treatment. Point-of-care ultrasonography (POCUS) can be used to improve care in IAH and ACS. **Figure 10.4** shows a stepwise protocol for management of IAP and POCUS use and probe positions (**Figure 10.5**).

If nonoperative management fails, the gold standard treatment for primary ACS is surgical decompression through a median xipho-pubic laparotomy. Early decompressive laparotomy may decrease patient morbidity and mortality. Recent publications have suggested that early surgical intervention in the presence of ACS resulted in about 80% fewer complications, including infections, sepsis, fistulae, and abscesses. Patients with pancreatitis need decompression if they have IAP above 25 mm Hg with increasing abdominal signs and worsening respiratory status. **Figure 10.6** is an example of grade IV ACS.

The skin and fascia should not be closed at the end of a decompressive laparotomy, but instead a temporary closure technique employed, effectively leaving the abdomen open. Temporary abdominal closure (TAC) should provide sufficient decompression of the abdomen without significantly impairing the fascia or skin to facilitate subsequent approximation of the abdominal wall (see **Figure 10.6B and C**). Remember that ACS can recur even in the setting of TAC.

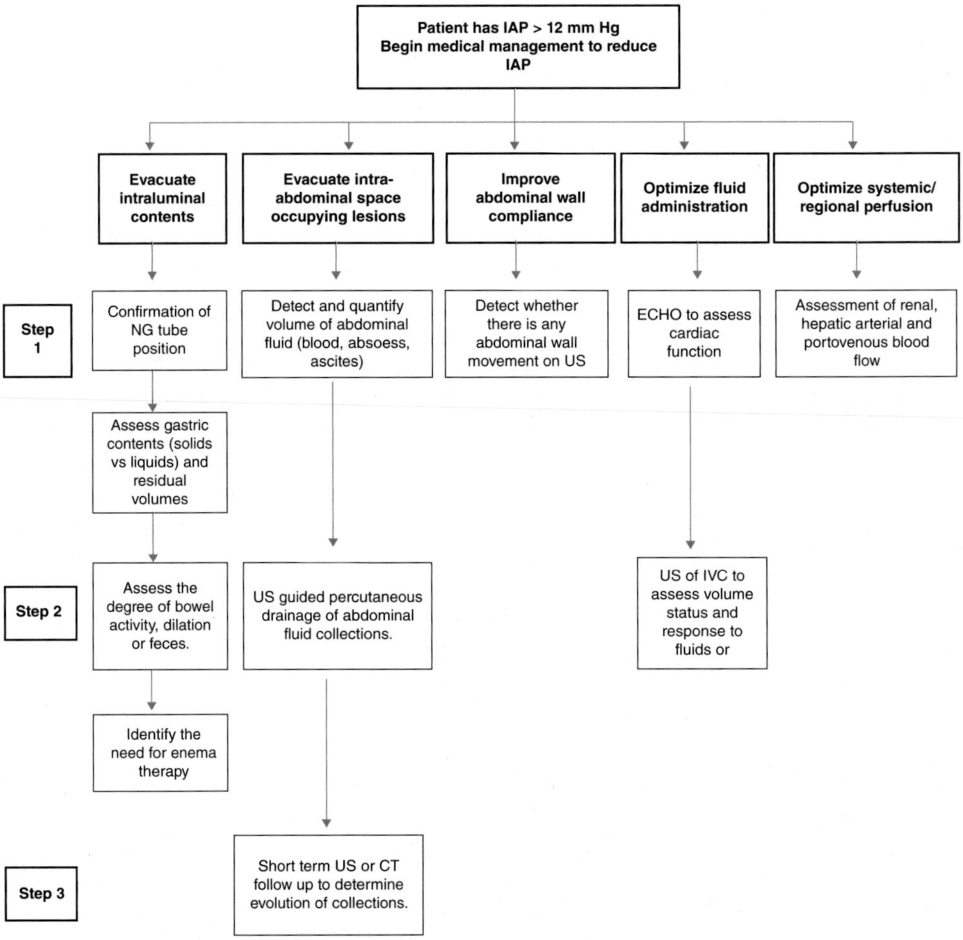

Figure 10.4 Stepwise approach for medical management of IAH.

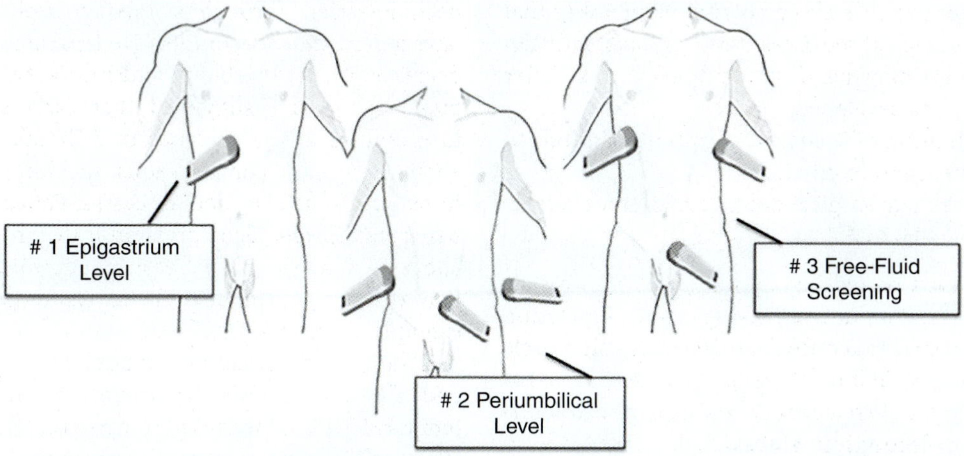

Figure 10.5 Diagnosis and treatment POCUS probe positions for IAH/ACS management.

Open Abdomen

The open abdomen technique (OA) is a surgical strategy used in the prevention or treatment of IAH and other life-threatening conditions such as those related to intra-abdominal bleeding and treatment of intra-abdominal sepsis. It is a temporary measure to stabilize patients with the goal of correcting metabolic and physiologic disorders, besides facilitating access to the abdominal cavity.

The indications for the use of the OA technique in nontrauma patients are not well elucidated. Prophylactic decompression should be considered in patients with high volume fluid resuscitation prior to or during laparotomy, hemodynamic instability from severe abdominal sepsis, mesenteric ischemia with bowel resection, abdominal wall loss, or use of double strength inotropes. Patients with purulent or fecal peritonitis do not routinely need an OA unless they require large doses of inotropes intraoperatively to maintain adequate blood pressure, planned deferred anastomosis, or failure of source control.

Patients with intestinal ischemia will benefit from leaving the abdomen open, not only to facilitate reinspection and further resection, but also from the positive effects of negative pressure wound therapy (NPWT).

When planning an OA, anastomoses should be avoided. A lateral stoma will avoid potential seal issues particularly with a NPWT dressing. An entero-atmospheric fistula can be diverted to the lateral abdominal wall using the technique of migration described by Pereira *et al.* in 2020 (see **Figure 10.6C**). Jejunostomy should be avoided if possible as this may leak due to the lack of adhesions from multiple repeat operations. Abdominal drains are generally not required where an effective NPWT system is used.

Evolution of this concept has led to greater use of the damage-control staged laparotomy and the avoidance of primary closure of the fascia. However, overuse of this technique for damage control may result in an increase in hospital mortality, ileus, enteric suture line failure, fascial dehiscence, and superficial surgical site infection. A classification of the grades of the open abdomen helps to understand the progression and risks of the OA (see **Table 10.4**). Therefore, a cautious approach to OA is important. It is a life-saving procedure in the right patient but can be a source of unnecessary morbidity and mortality if misapplied.

Complications of OA include stimulation of a hypercatabolic state and protein loss via removal of peritoneal fluid, entero-atmospheric or other intestinal fistulae, retraction of the abdominal wall and development of large ventral hernias, hemorrhage, and reperfusion syndrome (**Figure 10.7**). Bacterial colonization of wounds is common and can lead to long-term infectious complications particularly in patients who have undergone decompressive surgery for ACS after aortic repair with a synthetic graft. The risk of fistulae, ventral hernias, and bacterial colonization increases the longer an OA is maintained. New devices such as the Veraflo can be applied on these scenarios and be used either for direct peritoneal resuscitation (DPR) (see below) and/or continuous wash out saline flow (**Figure 10.8**).

It is important to stress that that IAH and tertiary ACS may still occur in an open abdomen. Temporary abdominal closure methods may not always have the capacity to increase the abdominal volume sufficiently to prevent an increase in IAP.

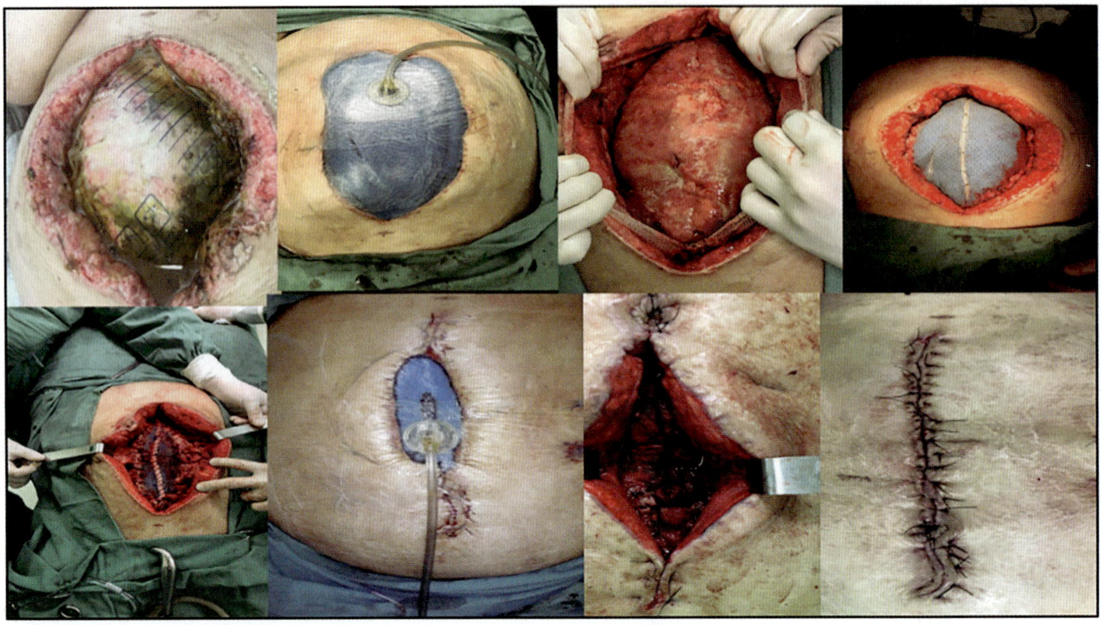

Figure 10.6 Temporary abdominal closure with mesh-mediated closure. The polypropylene mesh is cut into two halves and sutured to the abdominal fascia. The two halves are then sutured together over the abdominal part of the negative pressure wound therapy device to maintain medial traction on the fascia. The mesh can be tightened when the device is changed. Literature has demonstrated that surgical decompression considerably reduces IAP, however, it is not possible to relate this decrease in IAP to clinical evolution from the available evidence. Therefore, it remains unknown when and whether invasive intervention should be performed and by what method (percutaneous catheter drainage or various surgical decompression techniques). Given the morbidity of open abdominal decompression, non-invasive means of lowering IAP are indeed an attractive alternative and these include sedation, neuromuscular blockade, nasogastric decompression, correction of a positive cumulative fluid balance and perhaps even continuous hemodiafiltration if available. In addition to the non-invasive treatment strategies, another promising alternative for surgical decompression is percutaneous catheter drainage, but little is known about the best decompression method, time to perform the procedure, and operative technique to use.

Evidence shows that early ACS decompression in SAP is associated with lower mortality. There is no doubt that surgical decompression is effective in decreasing IAP and improves respiratory and renal functions in more than half of patients, however, open abdomen in patients with SAP is associated with significant morbidity, high rate of reoperation, intestinal fistulas and low rate of primary fascial closure. Among SAP patients, those with early MODS and SCA appear to be good candidates for surgical decompression.

In patients with PAS and organ function deterioration, the degree to which IAH contributes to the progression of MODS is unknown. Although the IAP was correlated with the Acute Physiology and Chronic Health Evaluation II score in patients with SAP, a causal relationship between ACS and MODS in SAP has not been proven. According to the current literature, the development of MODS is multifactorial and the inflammatory response plays an important role in the pathogenesis. In experimental models, IAH has been shown to increase the release of pro-inflammatory cytokines into the circulation and cause acute lung and liver injury in the presence of activated circulating neutrophils. In patients with SAP, activation of circulating neutrophils and monocytes is an early event and precedes ICU admission. Considering these factors, the development of ACS could further increase a pro-inflammatory stimulus that contributes to the development of organ failure in SAP. Therefore, early recognition of ACS and its appropriate and timely treatment can prevent the progression of MODS until the patient's death. Unfortunately, the optimal IAP threshold that would require surgical decompression is unknown. In addition, the optimal timing for intervention is unclear. Recent evidence demonstrates that patients with an IAP greater than 25 mmHg in the first 4 days after disease onset may be good candidates for surgical decompression.

TABLE 10.4 ■ Classification of the Open Abdomen

Grade	Description
1	No fixation
1A	Clean, no fixation
1B	Contaminated, no fixation
1C	Enteric leak, no fixation
2	Developing fixation
2A	Clean, developing fixation
2B	Contaminated, no fixation
2C	Enteric leak, no fixation
3	Frozen abdomen
3A	Clean, frozen abdomen
3B	Contaminated, frozen abdomen
4	Established enteroatmospheric fistula

Derived from Pereira BM, Duchesne JC, Concon-Filho A, Leppãniemi A. Entero-atmospheric fistula migration: a new management alternative for complex septic open abdomen. *Anaesthesiol Intensive Ther*. 2020;52(1):56-62. doi:https://doi.org/10.5114/ait.2020.92748.

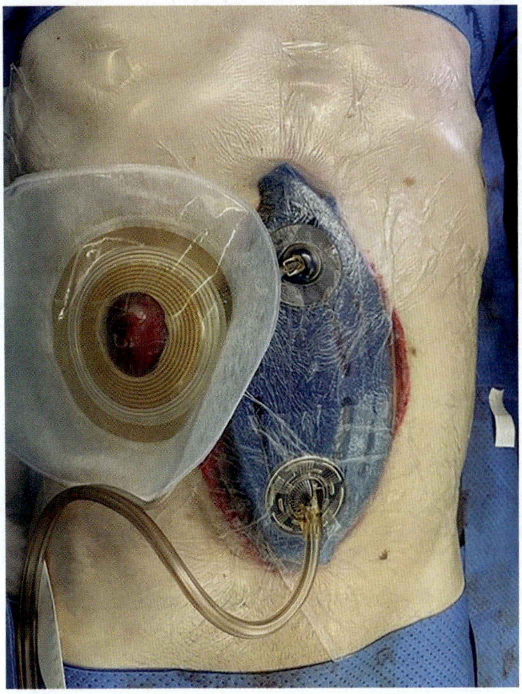

Figure 10.8 Dressing system allows peritoneal resuscitation or continuous saline flow.

Recurrent ACS from persistent bleeding, sepsis, or tissue edema has been reported to occur in up to 20% of decompressed patients. Thus, continued monitoring for ACS is required even after surgical decompression.

Abdominal Closure

Whenever an abdomen is left open, a plan for definitive closure should be made. Recent key performance indicators recommend abdominal closure after 1 day following resection for ischemia, 2 days for posttrauma packing, and 7 days for pancreatitis. If the abdomen is not closed within 7 days, the complication rate increases dramatically. Thus, plan repeated operations over the first week with progressive closure of the abdominal wall. However, up to 15% will need reexploring either due to tertiary or quaternary ACS or wound dehiscence. Abdominal wall closure will generally need to be delayed where there is a fistula. On returns to the operating room, it is critical that the nonadherent plastic placed between the viscera and abdominal wall be placed laterally to both posterolateral gutters and as far cephalad and caudally as possible. This helps avoid adherence of the abdominal visceral to the posterior abdominal wall, which if it develops, will impede closure of the fascia. Both this adherence and retraction of the muscles laterally must be prevented with the open abdomen.

Management of the open abdomen can be facilitated by the use of a NPWT device, which can reduce the morbidity and mortality of patients

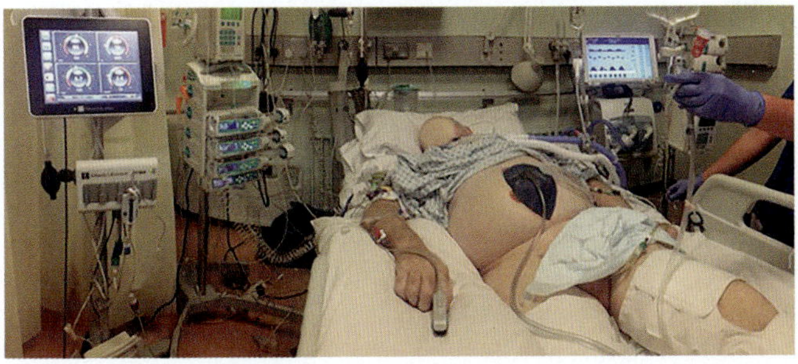

Figure 10.7 ICU care of a patient with NPWT TAC.

with ACS. Negative pressure therapy will also reduce the risk of tertiary ACS. The combination of NPWT with continuous suture or mesh-mediated fascial traction (see **Figure 10.6B and C**) has been shown to significantly reduce the fistula rate compared with the use of NPWT alone. These techniques can be instituted at the first operation and will help prevent lateralization of the abdominal wall. This is the phenomenon where the musculature and fascia, most exemplified by the rectus abdominis muscles and their enveloping fascia, move laterally away from the midline with time.

However, management of the open abdomen with NPWT does not always prevent the development of ACS.

To facilitate closure, a number of novel techniques have been proposed. Intravenous hypertonic saline has been used in the past. One of the most promising technique is DPR (DIRECT PERITONEAL RESUSCITATION) with hyperosmolar renal dialysis fluid. This is infused into the peritoneal cavity to reduce tissue edema. DPR can be combined with NPWT and is a potential adjunct in facilitating the control of sepsis (see **Figure 10.8**).

When closing the abdomen, up to 15% will dehisce. A prophylactic on-lay mesh or retention sutures can be used to reinforce the closure (**Figure 10.9**). The skin should not be left open unless there is significant contamination. The use of wound bundles has resulted in less contamination and fewer wound complications. The combination of NPWT and a closed incision negative pressure therapy system can enable the wounds to be closed primarily with a subcuticular stitch. Overt infection is rare due mainly to effective NPWT. If there is frank pus, a negative pressure superficial wound system will facilitate management, and skin edges will heal by secondary intention.

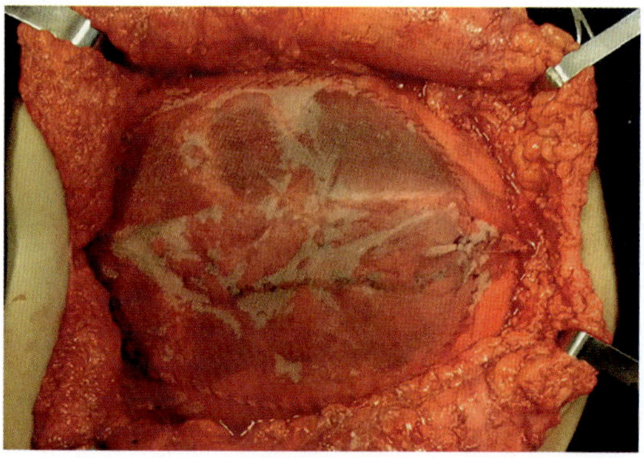

Figure 10.9 Definitive abdominal closure with prophylactic on-lay mesh.

SUMMARY

Abdominal compartment syndrome is a potentially lethal condition resulting from an acute and sustained increase in IAP, causing significant morbidity and mortality. IAH is defined as an IAP above 12 mm Hg in two consecutive measurements within a range of 4-6 hours. Rapid progression of IAH leads to ACS, which is defined as an IAP > 20 mm Hg associated with new organ dysfunction. ACS is the end result of a progressive increase in the IAP that if uncorrected will result in dysfunction or failure of multiple organs. However, the harmful effects of IAH occur long before the manifestation of ACS occurs.

ACS is not a problem exclusive to trauma or surgical patients. Its pathophysiological effects are comprehensive and predispose patients to multiple organ failure if no urgent action is taken. Hemodynamic, renal, respiratory, and neurological abnormalities are common.

The open abdomen technique (OA) is a surgical strategy used in the prevention or treatment of IAH and other life-threatening conditions, such as those related to intra-abdominal bleeding and treatment of intra-abdominal sepsis. It is a temporary measure to stabilize patients with the goal of correcting metabolic and physiologic disorders, besides facilitating access to the abdominal cavity.

In this chapter, authors brought important and up-to-date points regarding ACS and the OA.

SUGGESTED READINGS

Atema J, Gans S, Boermeester M. Systematic review and meta-analysis of the open abdomen and temporary abdominal closure techniques in non trauma patients. *World J Surg.* 2015;39:912-925.

Bjork M, Kirkpatrick AW, Cheatham M, et al. Amended classification of the open abdomen. *Scand J Surg.* 2016;105:5-10.

Coccolini F, Montori G, Ceresoli M, et al. The role of the open abdomen in non-trauma patient: WSES consensus paper. *World J Emerg Surg.* 2017;12:39.

Coccolini F, Roberts R, Ansolini L, et al. The open abdomen in trauma and nontrauma patients: WSES guidelines. *World J Emerg Surg.* 2018;13:7.

Fietsam Jr R, Villalba M, Glover JL, Clark K. Intra-abdominal compartment syndrome as a complication of ruptured abdominal aortic aneurysm repair. *Am Surg.* 1989;55:396-402.

Frazee RC, Abernathy SW, Jupiter DC, et al. Are commercial negative pressure systems worth the cost in open abdomen management? *J Am Coll Surg.* 2013; 216:730-735.

Kirkpatrick AW, Coccolini F, Ansaloni L, et al. Closed or open after source control laparotomy for severe complicated intra-abdominal sepsis (the COOL trial): study protocol for a randomized controlled trial. *World J Emerg Surg.* 2018;13:26.

Kirkpatrick AW, Nickerson D, Roberts D, et al. Intra-abdominal hypertension and abdominal compartment syndrome after abdominal wall reconstruction: quaternary syndromes? *Scand J Surg.* 2017;106:97-106.

Kirkpatrick A, Roberts D, Faris P, et al. Active negative pressure peritoneal therapy after abbreviated laparotomy: the intraperitoneal vacuum randomized controlled trial. *Ann Surg.* 2015;262:38-46.

Malbrain MLNG, De Laet I. A new concept: the polycompartment syndrome—Part 2. *Int J Intensive Care.* 2009;Spring:19-25.

Pereira BM. Abdominal compartment syndrome and intra-abdominal hypertension. *Curr Opin Crit Care.* 2019;25(6):688-696.

Pereira BM. Abdominal compartment syndrome: immeasurable relevance. *Rev Col Bras Cir.* 2019;46:e2001.

Pereira BM, Duchesne JC, Concon-Filho A, Leppãniemi A. Entero-atmospheric fistula migration: a new management alternative for complex septic open abdomen. *Anaesthesiol Intensive Ther.* 2020;52(1):56-62. doi:10.5114/ait.2020.92748

Pereira BM, Pereira RG, Wise R, et al. The role of point-of-care ultrasound in intra-abdominal hypertension management. *Anaesthesiol Intensive Ther.* 2017;49:373-381.

Rasilainen S, Mentula P, Salminen P, et al. Superior primary fascial closure rate and lower mortality after open abdomen using negative pressure wound therapy with continuous traction. *J Trauma Acute Care Surg.* 2020;89:1136-1142.

Reintam Blaser A, Regli A, De Keulenaer B, et al. Incidence, risk factors, and outcomes of intra-abdominal hypertension in critically ill patients-a prospective multicenter study (IROI study). *Crit Care Med.* 2019;47:535-542.

Sugrue M. Abdominal compartment syndrome and the open abdomen: any unresolved issues? *Curr Opin Crit Care.* 2017;23:73-78.

Sugrue M, Catena F, Coccolini F, Kluger Y, Maier R, Moore E. *Resources for Optimal Care of Emergency Surgery.* 1st ed. Springer International Publishing; 2020.

Sugrue M, Maier R, eds. Emergency surgery performance, quality and outcome consensus summit-resource for optimal care of emergency surgery. Donegal, Ireland. 2016. ISBN: 978-0-9926109-9-9.

CHAPTER

11 Bowel Obstruction

Andrea Costanzi, Michela Monteleone, Alan Biloslavo, and Marina Troian

CASE PRESENTATION

A 52-year-old woman presented to the emergency department with severe epigastric pain, bloating, failure to pass stool and flatus, nausea, and significant weight loss (more than 10 kg in 1 month). The patient had a previous hospitalization for suspected adhesive small bowel obstruction (SBO) treated nonoperatively 3 months earlier. Her medical history was significant for laparoscopic hysterectomy and Rendu-Osler-Weber syndrome, with multiple hepatic hemangiomas and a right hepatic artery aneurysm. The patient complained of vomiting and anorexia for 2 months.

In the emergency department, the patient underwent blood tests: normal WBC and CRP, with abnormal electrolytes (Na 128 mmol/L and K 3.2 mmol/L). An erect abdominal plain radiograph showed air-fluid levels with multiple dilated small bowel loops, duodenum, and jejunum, without radiographic evidence of pneumoperitoneum. The abdominal CT and the abdominal MRI (performed for the multiple liver hemangiomas) revealed dilated loops consistent with adhesions from previous surgery, which led to the diagnosis of SBO. Diagnostic imaging also identified duodenal malrotation to the right, not passing behind the superior mesenteric vessels, and displacement of the duodenojejunal flexure inferiorly and to the right (**Figure 11.1**).

The patient was initially managed conservatively with fluid and electrolyte resuscitation, nasogastric decompression, and fasting for 48-72 hours. The patient did not improve, vomiting and nausea persisted, and she was scheduled for surgery. A diagnostic laparoscopy confirmed the picture of duodenal malrotation with massive distension, making further progress with a minimally invasive approach impossible. At laparotomy, a large radiologically unappreciated tumor of the jejunum was identified, infiltrating the mesentery with a single lesion of carcinoma in the sigmoid mesocolon. The small bowel was atonic and distended, without peristalsis.

A jejunal resection about 60 cm from the pylorus was performed with a side-to-side stapled jejunojejunal anastomosis (**Figure 11.2**). A sigmoid resection with a side-to-side colonic anastomosis was also completed. The pathologic examination demonstrated a high-grade mucinous adenocarcinoma of the jejunum with nodal involvement and distant metastasis to the sigmoid mesocolon (pT4, pN2, pM1 TNM AJCC 2017) and lymphovascular invasion. The postoperative course was slow but uneventful. The patient underwent adjuvant chemotherapy with oxaliplatin and with 5-fluorouracil.

Question: *What is the first approach in uncomplicated small bowel obstruction?*

Answer: *Blood test, radiological imaging, conservative management with fluid and electrolyte resuscitation, nasogastric decompression, and fasting for 48-72 hours.*

INTRODUCTION

Acute intestinal obstruction is a common presentation in emergency settings and a significant cause for admission to emergency surgical departments. Small bowel obstruction (SBO) is the most frequent form of intestinal obstruction (76%), with adhesions following surgery as the most common etiology (65%). One in 10 patients develops at least one episode of SBO within 3 years of colectomy. Other causes of SBO include hernia, cancer or peritoneal carcinomatosis, inflammatory bowel disease, radiation, endometriosis, infection, and foreign bodies (including gallstone ileus). In patients without previous surgery, strangulated hernias represent the most frequent cause of obstruction; meticulous inspection of all potential sites of herniation is required. Large bowel obstruction (LBO) accounts for 10%-15% of cases of bowel obstruction. Cancer is the most common etiology. Other causes of LBO include volvulus, diverticulitis, hernia, and ischemic colitis.

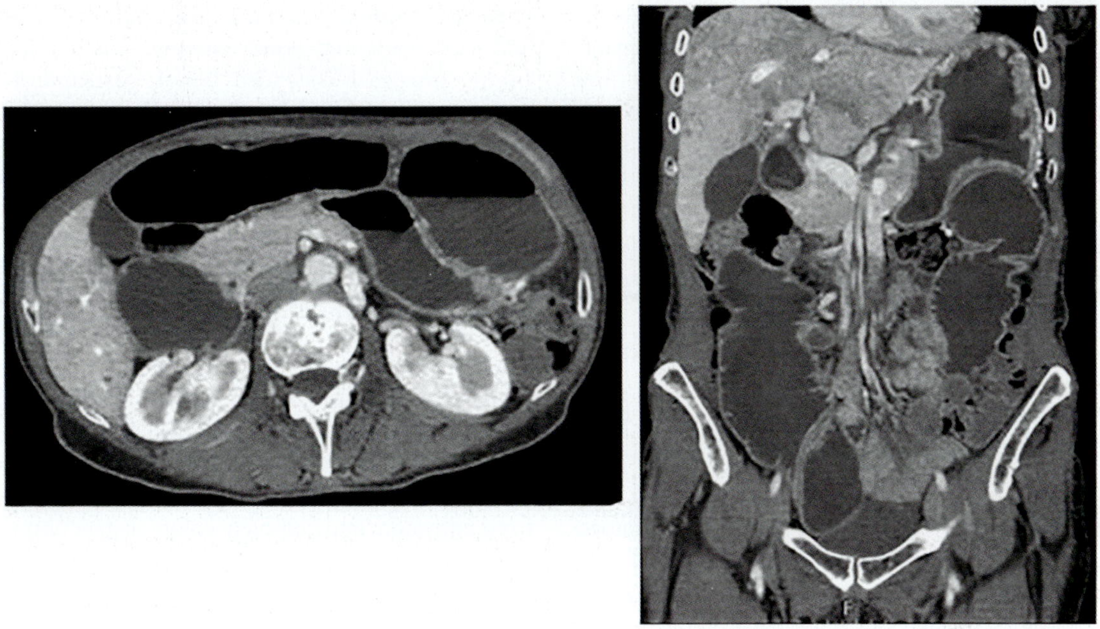

Figure 11.1 Abdominal CT on axial (*left*) and coronal (*right*) planes, showing dilated bowel loops and duodenal malrotation.

Motility disorders of the intestine produce a functional, nonmechanical "obstruction." These present as a paralytic ileus (nonmechanical decrease or stoppage of the flow of intestinal contents) or colonic pseudo-obstruction (Ogilvie syndrome). The cause of postoperative ileus has yet to be clearly defined, with an incidence of 10%-20% depending on the initial surgical procedure. These factors include prolonged abdominal/pelvic surgery, retroperitoneal spinal surgery, opioid use, peritonitis, perioperative complications (pneumonia, abscess), blood loss, hypokalemia, delayed enteral nutrition, or nasogastric tube placement. Distension and vomiting are characteristic of ileus. Adynamic ileus is due to paralysis of the bowel musculature. Hypokalemia leads to intracellular reduction of potassium that is replaced by sodium and consequently depolarization of electric potentials of muscle and nerve cell membranes, which aggravates intestinal paralysis. Distension is associated with altered bowel motility. Initially, intestinal distension stimulates peristalsis, but when functional obstruction results with increasing distension, peristalsis stops. The accumulation of fluid and gas is accompanied by altered intestinal mucosal function.

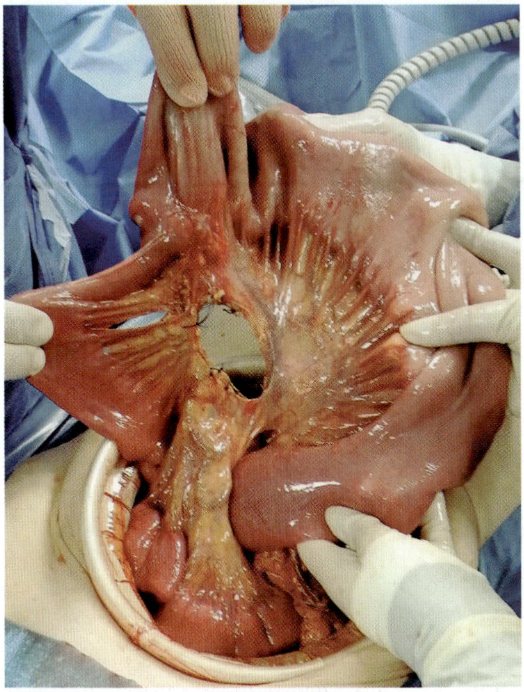

Figure 11.2 Surgical specimen showing the tumor of the jejunum infiltrating the mesentery.

Clinical presentation of adynamic ileus is usually less severe than mechanical obstruction. Clinical findings are abdominal distension, the absence of flatus and bowel movement, and vomiting. There is neither colicky pain nor peristaltic movement because of intestinal paralysis. Plain radiographs show intestinal distension and some air-fluid levels. Abdominal scout films detect air in the colon and rectum, and on abdominal computed tomography (CT), no mechanical obstruction is demonstrated.

Normally, the intestinal mucosa absorbs nutrients but provides a highly efficient barrier to luminal bacteria and their products. Epithelial cells prevent transepithelial migration of microorganisms, and maintenance of the tight junctions between cells limits movement along the paracellular channels. This physical barrier is enhanced by several immunologic mechanisms. Three basic mechanisms of bacterial translocation across the intestinal barrier have been suggested:

1. Permeability of the mucosa may be reduced, in hemorrhage or sepsis
2. The host defense may be impaired by steroids or hypoproteinemia.
3. Bacterial load within the intestine may overwhelm host defenses.

Such factors may occur together, and their effects may become synergistic and, therefore, increase the susceptibility of the patient. Under certain circumstances, however, the barrier function is lost. In such cases, the bacteria most likely to translocate include *Pseudomonas aeruginosa*, *Escherichia coli*, *Klebsiella pneumoniae*, *Staphylococcus epidermidis*, *Candida Albicans*, and enterococci. Although anaerobic bacteria are present in greater numbers than aerobic bacteria, they rarely translocate and may have an important role in preventing aerobic bacterial translocation. Simple intestinal obstruction induces bacterial translocation across the viable intestinal wall and leads to systemic infection.

SMALL BOWEL OBSTRUCTION

Clinical Presentation and Radiological Findings of Small Bowel Obstruction

The clinical presentation of SBO is usually a combination of signs and symptoms with different grades of intensity, including abdominal pain and distension, diffuse tenderness, nausea, vomiting, and failure to pass stool and flatus. As obstruction develops, the bowel becomes congested, and intestinal contents fail to be absorbed. This results in vomiting and anorexia. The combination of decreased absorption, vomiting, and reduced intake leads to volume depletion with hemoconcentration and electrolyte imbalance and may lead to renal failure or shock.

Bowel distension often accompanies mechanical obstruction. Distension is due to the accumulation of fluid in the bowel lumen, an increase in intraluminal pressure with enhanced peristaltic contractions, and air swallowing. When intraluminal pressure exceeds capillary and venous pressure in the bowel wall, absorption and lymphatic drainage decrease, the bowel becomes ischemic, and septicemia and bowel necrosis can develop. In the proximal distended bowel, gastrointestinal secretions accumulate in large amounts. This occurs for two reasons: deprivation of the absorptive activity of the intestine beyond the obstruction and derangement of fluid and electrolyte exchange in the wall of the obstructed and distended gut. Shock ensues rapidly. Mortality approaches 70% if bowel obstruction has progressed to this degree. For these reasons, nasogastric aspiration in patients with intestinal distension is useful. This sequence of events occurs more rapidly in a closed loop obstruction with no proximal escape for bowel contents. Examples of closed loop obstruction include an incarcerated hernia, volvulus on a fixed adhesion, and complete colon obstruction in the presence of a competent ileocecal valve. The "whirl sign" of the mesenteric vessels highly suggests a volvulus. The clinical presentation is associated with specific radiological findings of air/fluid levels on abdominal films (**Figure 11.3**).

Abnormal gastric distension associated with sparse air in the remaining abdomen is an indication of proximal bowel obstruction. Diffuse air/fluid levels are indicative of a more distal intestinal obstruction. In the case of complete SBO, air may not be visible in the colon or rectum, contrary to

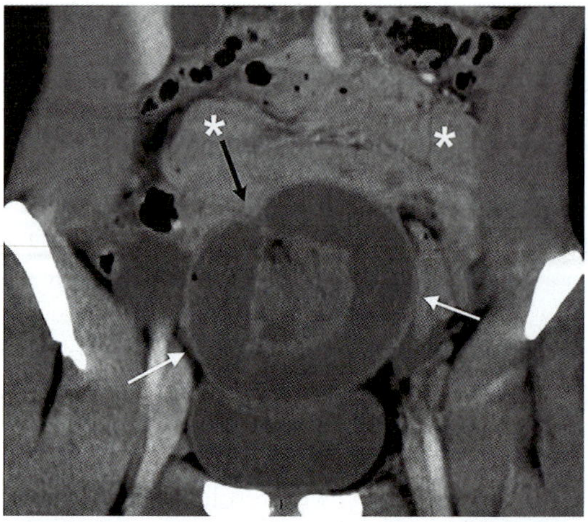

Figure 11.3 Flat belly closed loop obstruction. Venous phase contrast-enhanced CT shows a U-shaped closed loop (*white arrows*) converging to the transition zones (*black arrow*). The afferent intestinal loops are collapsed (*). Hemorrhagic necrosis of the closed loop small bowel segment was resected. (From Zins M, Millet I, Taourek P. Adhesive small bowel obstruction: predictive radiology to improve patient management. *Radiology*. 2020;296:480-492. Copyright ©2022 Radiological Society of North America, Inc. (RSNA), All Rights Reserved.)

the appearance in paralytic ileus where both large and small bowel are often dilated. Oral administration of 100 mL of the water-soluble contrast Gastrografin, followed by abdominal radiographs may help in diagnosis and due to its high osmotic load, may sometimes be therapeutic. If the contrast arrives at the cecum within 24 hours, the obstruction is incomplete, and it will most often resolve without surgery. Oral and intravenous contrast-enhanced CT scan is the gold standard investigation and can be helpful in deciding on nonoperative management (NOM). CT images can show signs suggestive of bowel distress, such as mesenteric edema, free intraperitoneal fluid, torsion of the mesentery, intussusception, pneumatosis intestinalis, and portal venous gas.

Laboratory Findings

Patients with SBO present with a volume deficit because of vomiting, ascites, and "third spacing." Typical laboratory findings include hemoconcentration with elevated values of hematocrit/hemoglobin, white blood cell (WBC) count, and C-reactive protein (CRP), although the sensitivity and specificity of these tests are relatively low. Leukocytosis >20 000/mL suggests perforation or bowel compromise. Metabolic acidosis is a common finding, due to loss of electrolytes. Hypokalemia is the most common electrolyte abnormality. Urea nitrogen, creatinine, and lactate levels are often increased, due to low renal perfusion, but generally improve with fluid resuscitation.

Management of Small Bowel Obstruction

Nonoperative Management

The management of adhesive SBO is based on clinical, biochemical, and radiological evaluation and the patient's clinical course. The decision for initial operative or nonoperative treatment of SBO depends on several factors. For patients presenting with acute adhesive SBO, without signs of strangulation, peritonitis, or intestinal impairment, evidence supports NOM with resolution rates as high as 70%. NOM is based on early nasogastric tube decompression, fluid resuscitation, and correction of electrolyte imbalance and is especially indicated for paralytic ileus. Several studies have investigated the diagnostic-therapeutic role of the water-soluble contrast agent Gastrografin. It promotes movement of water into the small bowel lumen, decreases edema of the intestinal wall, and may also enhance smooth muscle contractility that can generate effective peristalsis and overcome the obstruction.

Twenty to thirty percent of patients with adhesive SBO require operation with an average hospitalization after operative treatment of 16 days, compared to 5 days following NOM. There are no absolute criteria that identify those patients who are likely to respond to conservative treatment. Some studies have proposed models to predict the need for surgical intervention. The most accurate model was based on a score composed of radiological findings, sepsis criteria, and comorbidity index.

Nonoperative management of an incomplete SBO with nasogastric decompression, fluid-electrolyte replacement, and careful clinical reassessment can have a considerable success rate. Conversely, failure or late recognition of strangulation increases morbidity and mortality. In this complicated setting, appropriate patient selection is critical. Criteria have been proposed to identify patients with suspected SBO requiring immediate operative treatment. Clinical appearance of rapid onset of abdominal pain, continuous, not colicky, or abdominal tenderness (localized or diffuse) on physical examination, suggests the need for immediate surgery. Free intraperitoneal fluid, closed loop obstruction, mesenteric edema, thickened wall, or lack of enhancement of the bowel wall should also prompt an operation. Fecalization of the small bowel (gas bubbles and debris within the lumen of obstructed small bowel) on abdominal CT, identification of a transition point, and high-grade obstruction are more likely to fail observation. Although pneumatosis intestinalis (PI) previously was an absolute indication for operation, recent studies suggest otherwise. The PIPES trial of 500 patients with pneumatosis intestinalis reported that 60% had benign disease, not requiring an operation. Regression analysis revealed a lactate ≥2.0 mmol/L, and vasopressors or hypotension correctly predicted the need for operation in 92% of cases. Pathologic PI was more likely with peritonitis, the presence of portal vein gas, and greater extent of PI. A more recent study identified 5 factors associated with pathologic pneumatosis intestinalis: small bowel PI, age ≥70 years, heart rate ≥110 beats/min, lactate ≥2.0 mmol/L, and neutrophil-lymphocyte ratio ≥10.

On the other hand, NOM can be entertained in the patient with normal vital signs, in the absence of abdominal wall hernias as the cause of the obstruction, and absence of abdominal tenderness or peritoneal irritation on clinical assessment. For patients with partial SBO, there is no consensus for the optimal duration of nonoperative approach, but most authors consider a 72-hour period as safe and appropriate. Delaying operation beyond 72 hours of observation increases the risk of complications with significant decrease in the likelihood that the obstruction will resolve. No agreement exists about the ability to predict the risk of recurrence.

In addition, the choice of operative management within the first 24-48 hours from the onset of symptoms can be followed by nontherapeutic laparotomy with the potential risk of future adhesions and postoperative morbidity.

Operative Management

Surgical treatment is usually straight forward: release of obstruction by lysis of adhesions; intestinal resection of any tumor responsible for the obstruction usually followed by immediate restoration of continuity. Resection is also indicated for segments with vascular compromise resulting from the obstruction.

Along with the traditional approach *via* laparotomy, laparoscopic surgery has been introduced in recent years and may decrease morbidity in subgroups of patients undergoing surgery for SBO. Patient selection is still controversial, and the surgeon should carefully select patients for laparoscopy.

Ideally, a minimally invasive approach can be proposed in patients with a first episode of SBO and/or anticipated single-band adhesions (eg, SBO after appendectomy or hysterectomy). Markedly distended bowel loops and multiple complex adhesions increase the risk of severe complications (ie, enterotomy, delayed diagnosis of perforation).

The potential benefits of laparoscopy include less extensive adhesion (re)formation, earlier return of bowel function, reduced postoperative pain, earlier return to full activity, fewer wound complications, and shorter length of stay. Laparoscopic treatment of SBO is not associated with significant difference in operative time, rates of reoperation within 30 days, or mortality. According to recent trials, predictors for successful laparoscopic treatment of SBO include $\leq$2 previous laparotomies, appendectomy, no previous median laparotomy incision, and a suspected single adhesive band. In a recent trial, a panel of experts recommended that absolute exclusion criteria for laparoscopic adhesiolysis in SBO are those related to the pneumoperitoneum (hemodynamic instability or cardiopulmonary impairment); all other contraindications should be judged on a case-to-case basis, depending on the laparoscopic skills of the surgeon. Radiotherapy is also an exclusion criterion for laparoscopic adhesiolysis, due to the risk of fragile small bowel. One study found that the number of previous laparotomies, anatomical site of the operation, presence of bowel fistula, and laparotomy *via* a preexisting median scar were independent predictors of bowel perforation associated with the laparoscopic approach for SBO. Maintain a low threshold to convert from laparoscopy to laparotomy with failure to identify the point of obstruction or if adhesiolysis is overly difficult or unsafe. Preemptive conversion to laparotomy with a difficult dissection is highly preferred to reactive conversion after an iatrogenic enterotomy has occurred.

Prevention

The recent guidelines of management of SBO include recommendations on prevention. Laparoscopy and antiadhesion barriers are the main current methods of adhesion prevention. A recent systematic review and meta-analysis showed a lower incidence of adhesions from laparoscopy and not closing the peritoneum. The incidence of reoperation for SBO was 1.4% (95% CI 1.0%-1.8%) after laparoscopy and 3.8% (95% CI 3.1%-4.4%) after open surgery. The bias was in the type and indications for surgery. In a recent meta-analysis of SBO after colorectal operations, the incidence of SBO after laparoscopic surgery was lower than after open colorectal procedures (OR 0.62, 95% CI 0.54-0.72). However, no significant difference was found in other randomized trials.

Adhesion barriers (solid membranes, gels, and liquids) introduced into the peritoneal cavity are adjuvant methods that can effectively reduce adhesion formation. The aim of these barriers is to separate injured peritoneal and serosal surfaces until complete adhesion-free healing has occurred. The efficacy of adhesion barriers has been established for reducing the incidence of adhesion formation in open surgery. In a recent trial, patients were randomized to either receive a liquid adhesion barrier or not. The SBO recurrence rate was 2.19% (2/91) in the barrier groups vs 11.11% (10/90) in the control group after a mean follow-up period of 41.4 months ($P < .05$). In this study, the barrier was applied in patients treated for SBO by laparotomy. However, some adhesion barriers (such as icodextrin 4%) can also be used in laparoscopic surgery.

Gallstone Ileus

Gallstone ileus results when an impacted stone in the gallbladder fistulizes to the intestine, most commonly as a cholecystoduodenal fistula (85%). (See Chapter 15: Biliary Tree Disease.) The intraintestinal gallstone travels within the small bowel to produce a SBO, most commonly at the ileocecal valve or in the terminal ileum. The patient presents as a SBO, with nausea, vomiting, and dilated small bowel loops. Pneumobilia may be noted on imaging. CT imaging is the test of choice. The impacted stone may be approached via laparoscopy or laparotomy. The stone is milked proximally from the point of obstruction and an enterotomy created on the antimesenteric small intestine. Open the enterotomy longitudinally and close it transversely (**Figures 11.4** and **11.5**). Be certain to run the remainder of the GI tract for other stones. The decision to perform a concomitant cholecystectomy depends on the patient's overall status and the perceived difficulty of the cholecystectomy. Cholecystectomy in this setting can be extremely difficult and generally is not indicated. Consider delayed cholecystectomy in the patient with recurrent symptoms, if they can be medically optimized.

Small Bowel Obstruction in the Virgin Abdomen

Due to the high risk of cancer as the etiology of the SBO, the classic teaching has been that any SBO in a virgin abdomen required urgent operation. Recent studies have questioned this approach, as the most common etiology for the SBO is reported to be adhesions (>50%). The current reported risk of cancer with an SBO in the virgin abdomen is 7%-14%. These observations have led several authors to recommend approaching the SBO in the setting of a virgin abdomen as we would the patient with previous abdominal surgery, meaning attempted NOM. However, long-term follow-up was not available in published studies, suggesting the risk of cancer in this setting is clearly higher than 14%. If a nonoperative approach is taken, the patient must be

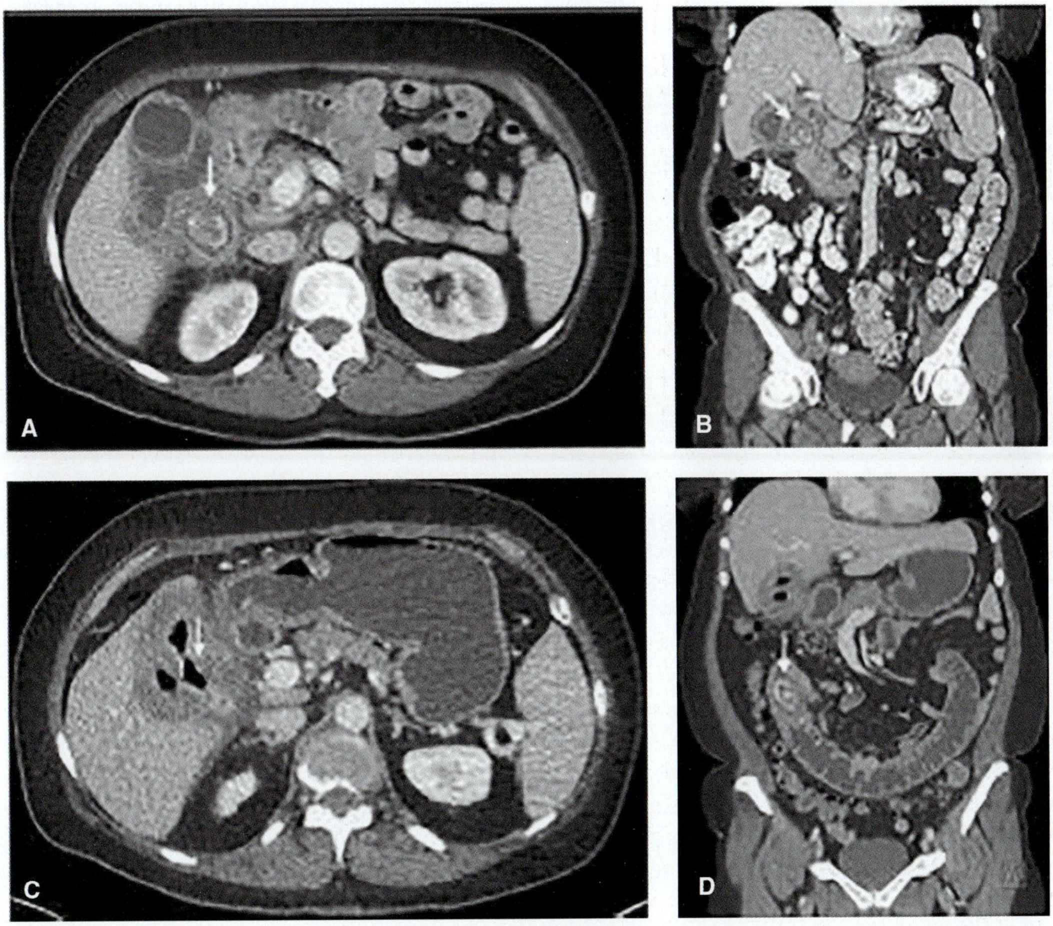

Figure 11.4 Gallstone ileus. **(A)** Axial and **(B)** coronal images show a loculated mass in the gallbladder fossa and a large, calcified stone in the gallbladder neck (*white arrow*). Repeat CT shows **(C)** air in the gallbladder and **(D)** migration of the gallstone into the small intestine. (Reprinted by permission from Springer: Springer Nature. Panda N, Cauley C, Qadan M. Gallstone ileus. *J Gastrointest Surg*. 2018;22:1990.)

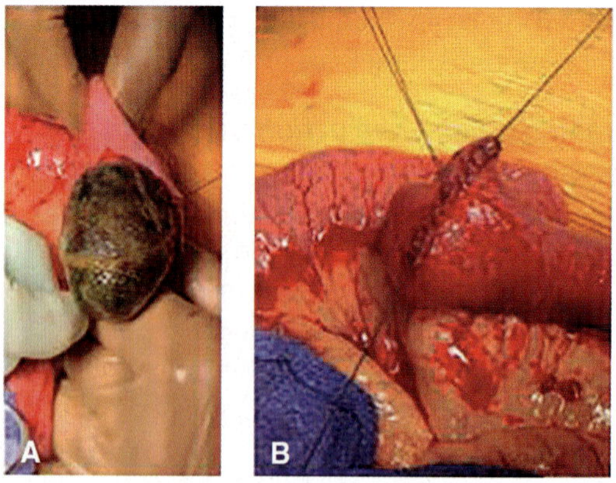

Figure 11.5 Gallstone ileus, operative findings. **A.** Enterolithotomy with evacuation of large gallstone from the distal small intestine. **B.** Enterotomy opened longitudinally and closed transversely without narrowing the lumen of the small intestine. (Reprinted by permission from Springer: Springer Nature. Panda N, Cauley C, Qadan M. Gallstone ileus. *J Gastrointest Surg*. 2018;22:1990.)

thoroughly evaluated after discharge with colonoscopy and CT or MR enterography for SBO patients. A conservative approach to avoid missing a cancer would be laparoscopy at the index admission or after resolution of the SBO, as an outpatient.

Intussusception

Intussusception is an invagination of a segment of intestine into the lumen of an adjacent segment. Unlike in children, intussusception in the adult is usually not suspected, accounting for <5% of SBO in adults. Asymptomatic intussusception (incidental finding on CT) rarely requires treatment. On the other hand, a pathologic lead is present in 70%-90% of symptomatic cases in adults. CT findings may include mesenteric vessels within a bowel lumen or the "target sign," which is caused by the image of bowel within bowel (**Figure 11.6**).

Small bowel intussusception is generally due to a benign lead point: Meckel diverticulum, strictures, or benign neoplasms (lipoma, adenoma, polyp). A cancer is the lead point in ~30% of small bowel intussusception, generally from metastatic disease. Adult colonic intussusception is due to a primary carcinoma in 60%-70% of cases. The probability that lead point in an intussusception is malignant is as follows: colo-colonic intussusception (highest risk) > ileocolonic intussusception (medium risk) > enteroenteric intussusception (lowest risk). Operate on the patient with intussusception for a likely anatomic etiology with signs of gut ischemia, chronic symptoms, intussusception resulting in bowel obstruction, palpable abdominal mass (high risk of cancer), anemia or GI bleeding (high risk of cancer), lead point or "target sign" on CT, or a lesion length >3.5 cm. In the operating room, if a benign etiology is firmly established, the intussusception may be milked out to limit the extent of the bowel resection. If the etiology is unknown or the patient has a history of cancer, resect the intussusception en bloc—do not reduce it.

LARGE BOWEL OBSTRUCTION

CASE PRESENTATION

A 66-year-old male, with a medical history of non-Hodgkin lymphoma, presented to the emergency department with a distended abdomen without abdominal pain, tenderness on palpation, or guarding. He presented with abundant diarrhea and failure to pass flatus within the last few hours without overt signs of blood per rectum. Body temperature was 38 °C, blood pressure was 130/70 mm Hg, and pulse rate was 89 bpm. Overnight, CRP levels rose from 20 to 50 mg/L and WBC from 11.06 to 12.45 g/L. A plain abdominal x-ray demonstrated a clearly distended left colon with coffee bean sign suggesting a sigmoid volvulus.

A CT scan of the abdomen revealed a LBO with a massively dilated, elongated, and twisted loop of sigmoid colon without signs of perforation (**Figure 11.7**).

Emergent decompressive colonoscopy and repositioning of the sigmoid colon was successfully achieved. The patient's postendoscopy course was uncomplicated, and he was discharged after 3 days. One month after discharge, the patient presented to our department with symptoms of subacute bowel obstruction without signs of inflammation or perforation. An elective sigmoidectomy was performed to prevent recurrence. The postoperative course was uneventful, and the patient was discharged on day 7 after surgery.

Question: *What are the possible causes of large bowel obstruction?*

Answer: *Large bowel obstruction can be mechanical or functional. The main cause for obstruction in the adult is cancer (60% of cases), followed by volvulus and diverticular disease (30%).*

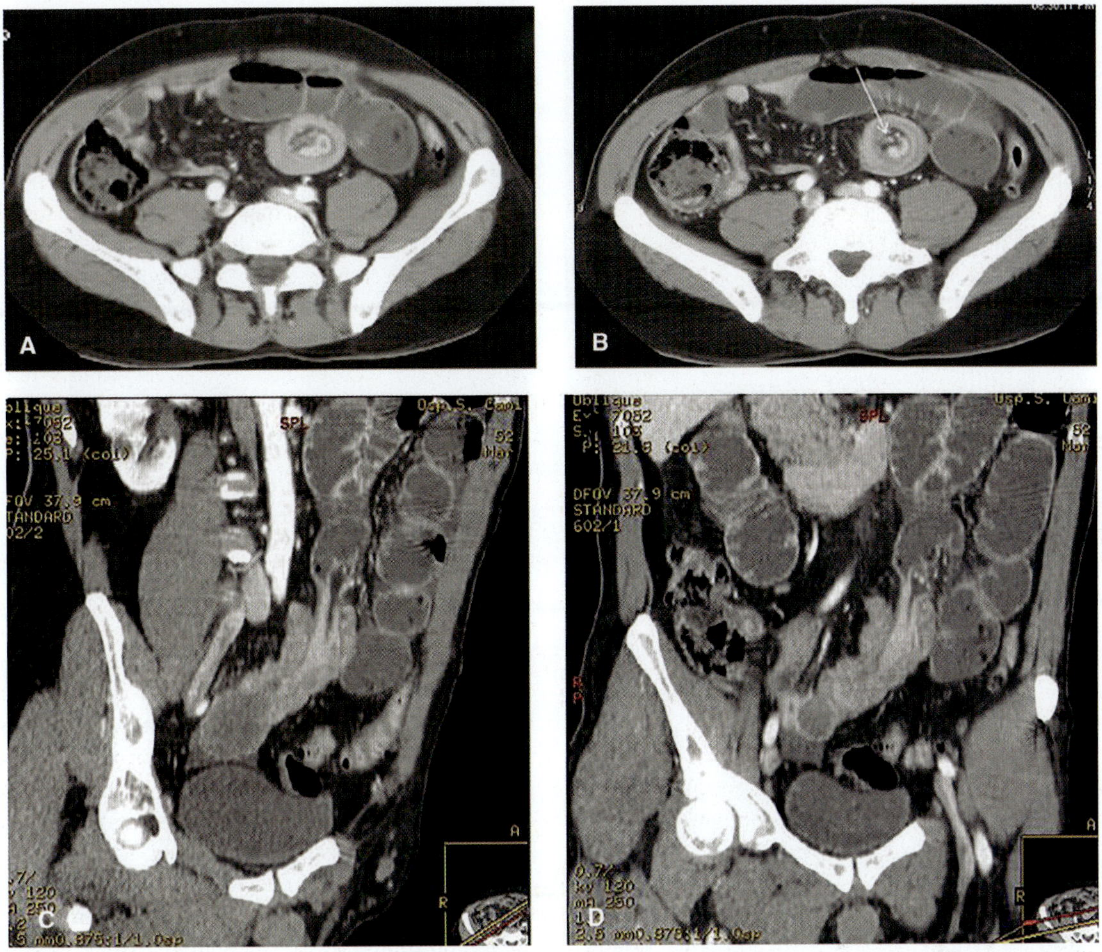

Figure 11.6 Enteroenteric intussusception. **A, B.** Demonstrate a "target sign" and central hypodense area of mesenteric fat in which vessels are seen. **C, D.** Depict the intussusception of a large sausage-shaped mass, showing the length of involvement. The dilated small bowel loops indicate the SBO. (From Valentini V, Buquicchio GL, Galluzzo M, et al. Intussusception in adults: the role of MDCT in the identification of the site and cause of obstruction. *Gastroenterol Res Pract*. 2016;2016. doi:10.1155/2016/5623718.)

INTRODUCTION

Approximately 20% of bowel obstructions present in the large bowel. Because of the potential life-threatening complications, timely recognition and management are crucial. LBO includes any physical or mechanical obstruction to the flow of intraluminal contents through the colon or rectum. It is well recognized that not all obstructions are completely mechanical; some can be functional (acute colonic pseudo-obstruction or Ogilvie syndrome, presenting with dilatation usually confined to the cecum and ascending colon with transition near the splenic flexure). Ogilvie syndrome is common in older adults with comorbidities but may develop in healthy patients after trauma or following a surgical procedure. Mechanical vs functional LBO should be recognized in the differential diagnosis. LBO is caused by colorectal cancer in about 60% of cases; volvulus and diverticular disease are responsible for another 30%. Other causes (carcinomatosis, endometriosis, inflammatory bowel disease stenosis) are responsible for LBO for the remaining 10% of cases.

Clinical Presentation and Radiological Findings

The signs and symptoms of LBO vary greatly and depend on the cause, chronicity, and location of the obstruction. Patients with LBO usually present with generalized abdominal pain, abdominal distension, and failure to pass stool or flatus. Unlike SBO, nausea and vomiting are not common presenting symptoms. Symptoms may present in an acute or chronic setting. If LBO is suspected,

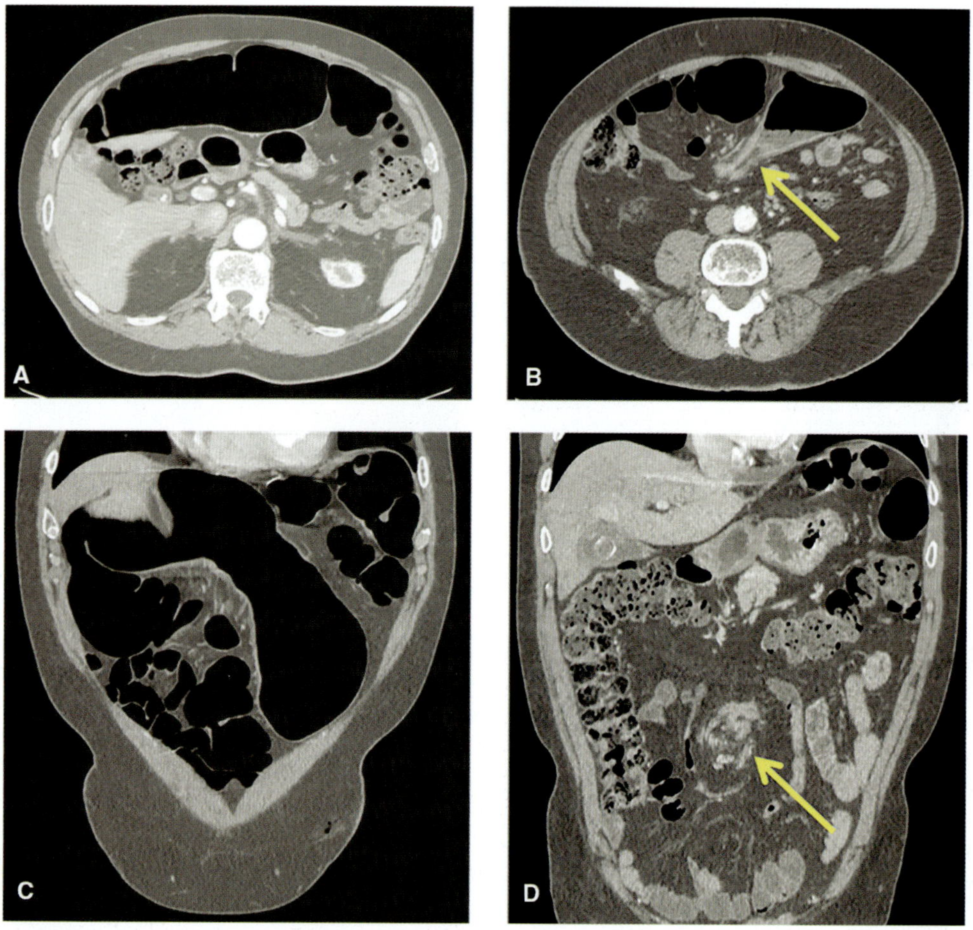

Figure 11.7 Large bowel obstruction on CT imaging: axial **(A** and **B)** and coronal **(C** and **D)** images. Note the elongated and twisted loop of sigmoid colon (*yellow arrows*).

attention to the vital signs is fundamental. Severe bowel obstruction can cause hypovolemic shock or, in cases of perforation, septic shock with tachycardia, tachypnea, cool extremities, mottled or cyanotic skin, slow capillary refill, and oliguria. While patients with untreated LBO may have signs of significant dehydration, sepsis, abdominal distension, and a palpable mass, in most chronic cases of LBO, the symptoms of dehydration are less severe. In the early stages, the colon retains the capacity to absorb fluid and electrolytes. In the obstructed colon, distension increases intracolonic and intramural pressure; the latter can lead to mucosal ischemia, localized bowel wall edema, transudation of fluid, and bowel perforation; in the majority of cases, of the cecum. Impairment of the blood flow in the visceral vessels occurs earlier and affects the vascular supply more severely than in small bowel because the colon has the lowest blood flow of all the abdominal viscera. As ischemia involves the mucosa early in its evolution, the intraoperative evaluation of colonic blood perfusion cannot be based only on an external examination of the serous membrane. The blockage of intestinal contents increases the growth of bacterial flora, and the altered intestinal wall function allows the absorption of septic-toxic fluid. Initially, only the colon is distended, but the ileocecal valve usually becomes incompetent and allows the dilatation to progress proximally into the small bowel. The presentation of the clinical picture of "closed loop obstruction" without the distension of small bowel that preserves its functions for a short period is unusual. This condition is due to a competent ileocecal valve with a double obstruction: the valve and colonic obstruction. The risk in the closed loop with an increase in intraluminal pressure and obstruction of its blood supply is gangrene, perforation, and peritonitis.

Abdominal radiography is usually the first-line diagnostic investigation in patients suspected of a LBO, sometimes in association with a water-soluble contrast enema (96% sensitivity and 98% specificity in diagnosing LBO). These imaging methods provide information on the degree and anatomic location of the obstruction, but usually cannot identify the cause. CT imaging with the addition of intravenous contrast, which improves the ability to identify the presence of a mass, inflammation, or bowel wall ischemia, is the modality of choice, with a reported sensitivity of 93% and a specificity of 96%. CT leads to more precise management and better preoperative planning. Colonoscopy is a second-level diagnostic tool. The goal is to define the cause of obstruction. Biopsy should be performed in cases of suspected malignancy when emergency surgery has not been indicated or endoscopic stent placement is envisioned.

Laboratory Findings

Initially, a complete blood count, renal function tests and electrolytes (to detect prerenal acute renal failure), liver function tests, amylase, and blood gas analysis are recommended. Marked leukocytosis with hyperamylasemia suggests possible ischemia or perforation. The basic metabolic panel helps determine the degree of dehydration and aids in the correction of electrolyte and acid-base abnormalities. Low serum bicarbonate levels, low arterial blood pH, and high lactic acid levels are common findings. Lactate levels may be helpful in identifying colonic ischemia; however, elevated lactate is a late sign. If malignancy is suspected, a carcinoembryonic antigen (CEA) level can be considered as a baseline for longitudinal oncologic follow-up.

Management

The definitive management of LBO depends on the underlying etiology. NOM consists of fluid resuscitation, nasogastric decompression, and bladder catheterization to allow measurement of urine output and guide resuscitation.

Operative Management

The operative management of LBO is dictated by patient physiology, the cause and location of the LBO in the colon/rectum.

The operative management of volvulus can be divided into two broad categories: resective vs nonresective procedures. Colonic volvulus may occur in any segment of the colon, which is mobile and attached to a long mesentery that is fixed to the retroperitoneum by a narrow base. Volvulus may also involve sigmoid colon (most commonly), the right colon and terminal ileum (cecal volvulus), the cecum alone (cecal bascule), and, rarely, the transverse colon. In 60%-90% of cases, plain abdominal radiographs alone are sufficient to establish the diagnosis of sigmoid volvulus, but only 20% of cecal volvuli can be diagnosed on a plain radiograph. Cecal volvulus and sigmoid volvulus exhibit different patient demographics. While sigmoid volvulus presents more commonly in older men, the majority of patients with cecal volvulus are younger women.

Cecal volvulus

Cecal volvulus occurs when the cecum is poorly fixed and highly mobile or when there is anomalous fixation of the right colon to the retroperitoneum. Factors such as previous abdominal operations, chronic constipation, high fiber diets, ileus, distal colon obstruction, and late-term pregnancy have been identified as predisposing factors in the development of cecal volvulus. The typical presentation of the patient with cecal volvulus is the acute onset of abdominal pain and distension. Depending on the acuity of symptoms, the patient may be able to identify the exact time of onset. Cecal volvulus may resolve spontaneously (**Figure 11.8**). Many patients complain of chronic, intermittent symptoms. Cecal volvulus may involve both the cecum and terminal ileum; symptoms of SBO may be present. Plane radiographs are diagnostic in only 20% of cases of cecal volvulus. Findings on

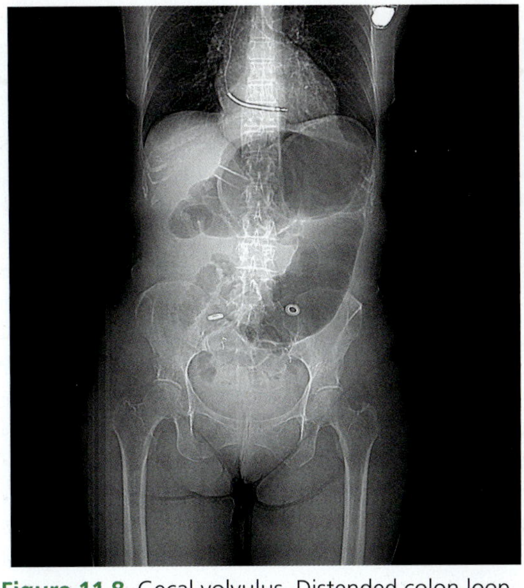

Figure 11.8 Cecal volvulus. Distended colon loop centered in the left upper quadrant.

CT include whirl sign, ileocecal twisting, decompression of the distal colon, a misplaced appendix, and cecal apex in the left upper quadrant. The "X marks the spot" sign is convergent, crossing transition points. The "split-wall sign" demonstrates mesenteric fat between two loops of bowel, giving the impression of a split in a single twisted loop of bowel. In patients with cecal volvulus, surgical resection remains the mainstay of treatment. In addition, cecopexy as an option often fails as a long-term solution for cecal volvulus. Colonoscopic decompression, while commonly used for sigmoid volvulus, has not shown long-term efficacy as the sole treatment for cecal volvulus but allows the surgical intervention to be performed on an elective or semi-elective basis. In case of ischemic volvulus or failed derotation, surgery should be performed as soon as possible. At operation, untwisting of the cecum is not recommended, as septic shock may result from rapid intravascular influx of toxins from the gangrenous segment.

Sigmoid Volvulus. The volvulus of the sigmoid colon is the most common form of volvulus. It occurs when the sigmoid colon is significantly elongated (dolichosigmoid), and the mesocolon is narrow at its base. Other factors include chronic constipation and the use of psychotropic medications, as evidenced by the high incidence among chronically institutionalized, elderly patients, with inadequate intake of fluids and dietary fiber. The clinical presentation depends on the duration and degree of colonic torsion; the main symptoms are abdominal pain, cramping, distension, and obstipation. If the obstruction is incomplete, liquid stools can pass, and paradoxical diarrhea may be a presenting feature. In 60%-90% of cases, plain abdominal radiographs alone are sufficient to establish the diagnosis. The distended ahaustral sigmoid loop will be oriented with its apex in the right upper quadrant, "omega" or "coffee bean" sign (**Figure 11.9**). Unlike cecal volvulus, the primary strategy for treating sigmoid volvulus, without signs of perforation or ischemia, is early sigmoidoscopic or colonoscopic decompression followed by elective surgery. The recurrence rate following decompression approaches 90%. Definitive surgery should be performed within 2-7 days following decompression. During surgery, detorsion alone should be avoided as it carries an unacceptable recurrence rate. Sigmoid resection and anastomosis are the preferred operative treatment.

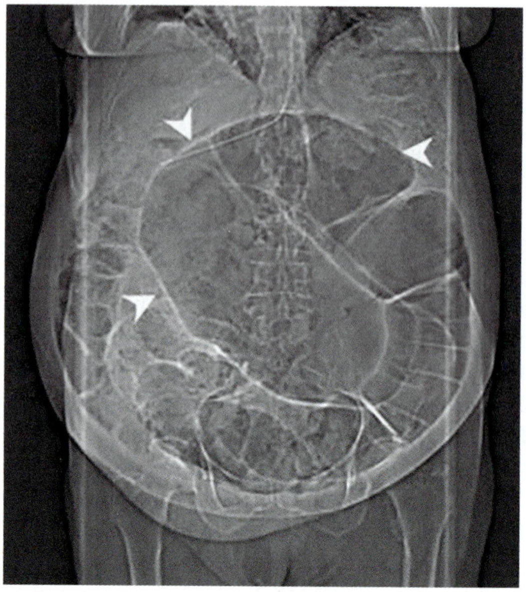

Figure 11.9 Sigmoid volvulus. AP film shows sigmoid distension (*arrowheads*) with an inverted "U" pointing to the right upper quadrant. (From Lepage-Saucier M, Tang A, Billiard J-S, et al. Small and large bowel volvulus: clues to early recognition and complications. *Eur J Radiol*. 2010;72:60-66. With permission.)

LBO From Diverticular Disease

Laparoscopic resection with anastomosis is the gold standard for diverticular LBO, ideally performed after successful conservative treatment. A loop ileostomy should be considered in frail patients, and a Hartmann procedure may be more appropriate for high-risk patients.

Ogilvie Syndrome

Ogilvie syndrome or acute colonic pseudo-obstruction is a condition characterized by massive colonic distension in the absence of mechanical obstruction. It can be described as a functional disturbance of colonic motility often observed in hospitalized patients as a result of hemodynamic, metabolic, pharmacologic, inflammatory, or postoperative conditions. Common predisposing conditions associated with Ogilvie syndrome are trauma (11%), infection (10%), and cardiac disease (10%); severe metabolic disorders; sepsis; gastrointestinal infection; medications; and spinal cord injury. Plain abdominal radiographs may show colonic dilatation, but air is noted in the rectum. It is important to exclude a mechanical obstruction of the distal colon when considering the diagnosis of Ogilvie syndrome. Symptoms and signs of the disease usually manifest over 3-5 days but may develop more acutely, sometimes within 48 hours. Ogilvie syndrome can be complicated by bowel ischemia, peritonitis, or perforation. The risk of complications increases with increasing cecal diameter and duration of illness. In uncomplicated cases, supportive care with close observation remains the primary treatment, although early pharmacologic intervention is increasingly encouraged (intravenous neostigmine). Initial medical management should also focus on correcting the underlying illness and electrolyte abnormalities, bowel test, and minimizing medications associated with pseudo-obstruction. Success of conservative management is variable, ranging from 20% to 92%. In patients for whom medical management has failed, perform colonoscopic decompression. Surgical management is rarely necessary and should be reserved for patients who have failed pharmacologic and endoscopic management or those who have clinical signs of colonic ischemia or perforation.

Malignant Etiology of LBO

Resection and anastomosis are the best options for malignant LBO in the absence of significant risk factors, carcinomatosis, or perforation. For obstructing right colon cancers, the majority can be resected with standard right hemicolectomy with extension to the left if needed. If the obstructing right colon cancer is nonresectable, options include ileotransverse colon bypass or diverting loop ileostomy.

The risk of anastomotic leak after resection and primary anastomosis for left colon cancer in patients with LBO ranges from 2.2% to 12%, comparable to the 2%-8% rate after elective surgical procedures. Patients with high surgical risk can be treated with a staged procedure or a temporary protective loop ileostomy (**Figure 11.10**).

In cases of rectal cancer, resection of the primary tumor should be postponed and a stoma fashioned to permit correct staging and appropriate oncological neoadjuvant treatment, as indicated.

Endoscopic Management

In the setting of operable patients, the temporary placement of colonic self-expanding metal stents, allowing colonic decompression, may avoid the need for emergency surgery, avoiding colostomy and provide the possibility of subsequently performing an elective segmental resection with primary anastomosis. Preoperative neoadjuvant therapy can be administered with the stent in place after relief of obstruction. Scientific studies on advantages and limitations of colorectal self-expanding metal stents are still ongoing. Current indications for colorectal stent placement include palliation for colonic obstruction by a primary colorectal cancer or extracolonic malignancy with placement of the stent, as a bridge to radical surgery. This approach is appropriate in those patients at high surgical risk, such as those with an ASA classification ≥ III or elderly patients aged over 70 years.

SUMMARY

Acute bowel obstruction is a common and significant cause of admissions to emergency surgical departments. Bowel obstruction can be due to either mechanical (intrinsic luminal obstruction or extrinsic compression) or functional obstruction of the small or large intestine. Obstruction frequently causes abdominal pain, nausea,

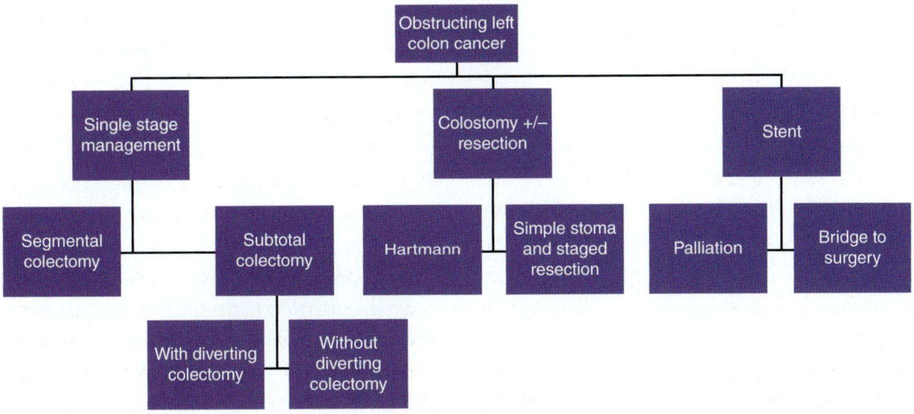

Figure 11.10 Operative options for the obstructing left colon cancer.

vomiting, constipation-to-obstipation, and distension. In the diagnostic work up, it is crucial to determine if the bowel obstruction involves the small or the large bowel, as the medical and surgical treatments are different. The most common causes of SBO are adhesions or hernia, but other causes must be considered (benign tumors, cancer, inflammatory bowel disease, radiation therapy, endometriosis, infections, and foreign bodies—eg, bezoars or stones).

In SBO, conservative management is successful in 40%-70% of clinically stable patients, with a higher success rate in those with partial obstruction. With conservative management, resolution generally occurs within 48-72 hours. Beyond this time frame, the risk of complications, including vascular compromise, increases. If intestinal obstruction is not resolved with conservative management, surgical intervention is required.

The most common cause of LBO is an underlying colorectal malignancy. Approximately 40% of colorectal cancers present as emergencies, and LBO is the most common presentation. Other causes of LBO are strictures secondary to diverticular disease or inflammatory bowel diseases, as well as volvulus, most commonly of the sigmoid colon. Occasionally, the sigmoid colon can be obstructed in a left inguinal hernia. LBO usually presents as an emergency, and patients can potentially be very ill, septic, dehydrated, and hemodynamically compromised. The treatment of LBO depends on the etiology, and when surgery is indicated, the patient needs to be adequately resuscitated with intravenous fluids and correction of electrolyte disturbances. The critical issue is the delay before treatment; in most cases, early treatment results in better outcomes.

SUGGESTED READINGS

Ayman M, Hassanien MD, Sarwat M. Laparoscopic adhesiolysis for recurrent small bowel obstruction with ultrasonically activated shears. *Egypt J Surg.* 2004;23:67-73.

Bellows CF, Webber LS, Albo D, Awad S, Berger DH. Early predictors of anastomotic leaks after colectomy. *Tech Coloproctol.* 2009;13(1):41-47.

Bower KL, Lollar DI, Williams SL, et al. Small bowel obstruction. *Surg Clin N Am.* 2018;98:945-971.

Catena F, Ansaloni L, Di Saverio S, Pinna AD. POPA study: prevention of postoperative abdominal adhesions by icodextrin 4% solution after laparotomy for adhesive small bowel obstruction. A prospective randomized controlled trial. *J Gastrointest Surg.* 2012;16(2):382-388.

Catena F, De Simone B, Coccolini F, Di Saverio S, Sartelli M, Ansaloni L. Bowel obstruction: a narrative review for all physicians. *World J Emerg Surg.* 2019;14:20.

Choi J, Fisher AT, Mulaney B, et al. Safety of foregoing operation for small bowel obstruction in the virgin abdomen: systematic review and meta-analysis. *J Am Coll Surg.* 2020;231:368-375.

Coccolini F, Ansaloni L, Manfredi R, et al. Peritoneal adhesion index (PAI): proposal of a score for the "ignored iceberg" of medicine and surgery. *World J Emerg Surg.* 2013;8(1):6.

Conner S, Nassereddin A, Mitchell C. Ogilvie syndrome. In: *StatPearls*. StatPearls Publishing; 2020.

Di Saverio S, Catena F, Kelly MD, Tugnoli G, Ansaloni L. Severe adhesive small bowel obstruction. *Front Med.* 2012;6(4):436-439.

Di Saverio S, Coccolini F, Galati M, et al. Bologna guidelines for diagnosis and management of adhesive small bowel obstruction (ASBO): 2013 update of the evidence-based guidelines from the World Society of Emergency Surgery ASBO working group. *World J Emerg Surg.* 2013;8(1):42.

Diamond M, Lee J, LeBedis CA. Small bowel obstruction and ischemia. *Radiol Clin N Am.* 2019;57:689-703.

Dindo D, Schafer M, Muller MK, et al. Laparoscopy for small bowel obstruction: the reason for conversion matters. *Surg Endosc.* 2010;24:792-797.

DuBose JJ, Lissauer M, Maung AA, et al. Pneumatosis intestinalis predictive evaluation study (PIPES): a multicenter epidemiologic study of the Eastern Association for the Surgery of Trauma. *J Trauma Acute Care Surg.* 2013;75:15-23.

Frager D. Intestinal obstruction role of CT. *Gastroenterol Clin North Am.* 2002;31(3):777-799.

Halabi WJ, Jafari MD, Kang CY, et al. Colonic volvulus in the United States: trends, outcomes, and predictors of mortality. *Ann Surg.* 2014;259(2):293-301.

Krielen P, van den Beukel BA, Stommel MW, Van GH, Strik C, Ten Broek RP. In-hospital costs of an admission for adhesive small bowel obstruction. *World J Emerg Surg.* 2016;11:49.

Loftus T, Moore F, VanZant E, et al. A protocol for the management of adhesive small bowel obstruction. *J Trauma Acute Care Surg.* 2015;78(1):13-21.

Makar RA, Bashir MR, Haystead CM, et al. Diagnostic performance of MDCT in identifying closed loop small bowel obstruction. *Abdomin Radiol.* 2016;41:1253-1260.

Millet I, Ruyer A, Alili C, et al. Adhesive small-bowel obstruction: value of CT in identifying findings associated with the effectiveness of nonsurgical treatment. *Radiology.* 2014;273(2):425-432.

Mir SA, Hussain Z, Davey CA, et al. Management and outcome of recurrent gallstone ileus: a systematic review. *World J Gastrointest Surg.* 2015;7:152-159.

Mosley JG, Shoaib A. Operative versus conservative management of adhesional intestinal obstruction. *Br J Surg.* 2000;87:362-373.

Nazzani S, Bandini M, Preisser F, et al. Postoperative paralytic ileus after major oncological procedures in the enhanced recovery after surgery era: a population based analysis. *Surg Oncol.* 2019;28:201-207.

Panda N, Cauley C, Qadan M. Gallstone ileus. *J Gastrointest Surg.* 2018;22:1989-1991.

Rieser CJ, Dadashzadeh ER, Handzel RM, et al. Development and validation of a five factor score for prediction of pathologic pneumatosis. *J Trauma Acute Care Surg.* 2021;90:477-483.

Sallinen V, DiSaverio S, Haukijarvi E, et al. Laparoscopic versus open adhesiolysis for adhesive small bowel obstruction (LASSO): an international, multicentre randomized, open-label trial. *Lancet Gastroenterol Hepatol.* 2019;4:278-286. doi:10.1016/S2468-1253(19)300160

Shahin H, Nilanjan P, Rao MAK, et al. Operative versus non-operative management of adhesive small bowel obstruction: a systematic review and meta-analysis. *Int J Surg.* 2017;45:58-66.

Ten Broek R, Issa Y, van Santbrink E, et al. Burden of adhesions in abdominal and pelvic surgery: systematic review and metanalysis. *Br Med J.* 2013; 347:f5588.

Ten Broek RP, Strik C, Van GH. Preoperative nomogram to predict risk of bowel injury during adhesiolysis. *Br J Surg.* 2014;101(6):720-727.

Ten Broek RPG, Krielen P, Di Saverio S, et al. Bologna guidelines for diagnosis and management of adhesive small bowel obstruction (ASBO): 2017 update of the evidence-based guidelines from the world society of emergency surgery ASBO working group. *World J Emerg Surg.* 2018;13:24.

Valentini V, Buquicchio GL, Galluzzo M, et al. Intussusception in adults: the role of MDCT in the identification of the site and cause of obstruction. *Gastroenterol Res Pract.* 2016;2016. doi:10.1155/2016/5623718

Yamada T, Okabayashi K, Hasegawa H, et al. Meta-analysis of the risk of small bowel obstruction following open or laparoscopic colorectal surgery. *Br J Surg.* 2016;103(5):493-503.

Yeo HL, Lee SW. Colorectal emergencies: review and controversies in the management of large bowel obstruction. *J Gastrointest Surg.* 2013;17(11):2007-2012.

CHAPTER

12 Mesenteric Ischemia

Hayato Kurihara, Enrico Marrano, and Martina Ceolin

CASE PRESENTATION

A 45-year-old man with previous history of pulmonary thrombosis presents to the emergency department reporting 3 hours of acute abdominal pain, localized mainly in the right lower quadrant. The patient describes episodes of diarrhea a few days before the onset of acute abdominal pain. He has no additional past medical or surgical history and he is not taking any medication. He has no significant family history and works as company manager. He does not smoke and drinks a glass of wine occasionally. His temperature is 36.8 °C, blood pressure 110/80 mm Hg, pulse 84 beats/min, respiratory rate 20, and oxygen saturation 99% on ambient air. He appears uncomfortable and diaphoretic and his abdomen is mildly distended and diffusely tender. In the right lower quadrant are local signs of peritonitis. Initial laboratory tests reveal white blood cell count 34 800 cells per microliter (cells/μL), hemoglobin 13.9 g/dL, platelets 432 cells/μL, sodium 132 milliequivalent per liter (mEq/L), potassium 4.4 mEq/L, blood urea nitrogen (BUN) 23 mg/dL, creatinine 1.3 mg/dL, serum amylase 93 U/L, serum lipase 64 U/L, AST 15 U/L, ALT 25 U/L, GGT 36 U/L, D-dimer 8500 μg/mL, and C-reactive protein (CRP) 18.8 mg/dL.

CT angiography (CTA) was performed and identified acute mesenteric venous ischemia with portomesenteric thrombosis and a portal cavernoma. Diffuse intraperitoneal fluid was present in all abdominal quadrants.

Question: *What is the best next step for this patient?*

Answer: *Although in most cases acute venous mesenteric ischemia can be initially treated with a nonoperative approach using anticoagulant therapy, this patient has signs of peritonitis and surgical exploration is mandatory. If bowel necrosis is confirmed, resection is the treatment of choice, but anticoagulation with a continuous infusion of unfractionated or low molecular weight heparin should be started immediately upon diagnosis.*

Furthermore, an open abdomen strategy for a second look may be considered in order to spare viable bowel.

PRINCIPLES OF MANAGEMENT

Diagnosis

Acute mesenteric ischemia (AMI) accounts for 1:1000 acute hospital admissions in the USA and Europe. AMI is defined as a sudden interruption of blood supply to a segment of intestine leading to bowel ischemia, necrosis, and, if left untreated, death.

Twenty-five percent of the cardiac output flows to the splanchnic circulation at rest and it increases to 35% in the postprandial phase. Although the gut can survive a 75% reduction in blood flow for up to 12 hours without significant injury, its viability drops to 54% between 12 and 24 hours and to 18% after 24 hours. On the other hand, microscopic changes occur in the bowel within 5 minutes of vascular occlusion. Irreversible damage to the bowel results with <6 hours of total ischemia.

The diagnosis is difficult and failure to recognize ischemic bowel is responsible for the high mortality of the disease. The incidence appears to be due to the increasing aging (with comorbidities) of the general population. These preexisting conditions worsen the prognosis of the patient with intestinal necrosis. Although mortality rates have declined over the last 50 years, it remains high at 50%-69%. AMI mortality is related to treatment timing, ranging from 11% in patients undergoing surgery within 24 hours of symptom onset to 73% if operated after 24 hours. Only 26% of people admitted to hospital with AMI will be alive 1 year later.

There is no current level 1 evidence to guide the evaluation and treatment of patients with suspected AMI.

The etiology of AMI can be divided into four categories:

- EAMI—embolic arterial AMI
- TAMI—thrombotic arterial AMI
- VAMI—venous AMI
- NOMI—nonocclusive mesenteric ischemia

Clinical Presentation

The key to early diagnosis is a high level of clinical suspicion. The clinical scenario of a patient complaining of excruciating abdominal pain with an unrevealing abdominal examination is classic for early AMI. If the clinical examination reveals signs of peritonitis, irreversible intestinal necrosis is likely. In large case studies, 95% of patients present with abdominal pain, 44% with nausea, 35% with vomiting, 35% with diarrhea, and 16% with blood per rectum. In early stages, patients may present with the triad of abdominal pain, fever, and hemoccult-positive stools. Later, the scenario will progress to sepsis and septic shock.

The symptoms reported by the patient may be different according to the etiology.

Embolic Arterial Acute Mesenteric Ischemia

Arterial embolism is the most frequent cause of AMI (45%). It is characterized by a sudden onset of pain, frequently associated with atrial fibrillation. Other comorbidities often associated are ischemic heart disease, cardiomyopathy, recent myocardial infarction with intramural thrombus, hypertension, diabetes mellitus, and renal insufficiency. Approximately 33% of patients present with a history of recent embolism and the absence of proper anticoagulant therapy should raise suspicion for EAMI. The association between the sudden onset of abdominal pain and spontaneous bowel emptying (vomiting and/or diarrhea) with no significant findings on clinical examination is a classic presentation of EAMI. The majority of emboli lodge 3-10 cm distal to the origin of the superior mesenteric artery (SMA) (**Figure 12.1**).

Thrombotic Arterial Acute Mesenteric Ischemia

Arterial thrombosis (**Figure 12.2**) is responsible for ~25% of AMI. It has a more indolent course and is often associated with a history of abdominal angina and weight loss suggestive of undiagnosed chronic mesenteric ischemia. Patients may report fear of eating due to the pain caused by digestion. The main risk factors for TAMI are atherosclerotic disease and dyslipidemia. Patients might also report previous vascular events or vascular surgery. Thrombosis occurs at the origin of visceral arteries, and an underlying plaque in the SMA usually progresses to a critical stenosis over years, resulting in the development of collateral vessels. The involvement of the ileocolic artery will result in necrosis of the proximal colon.

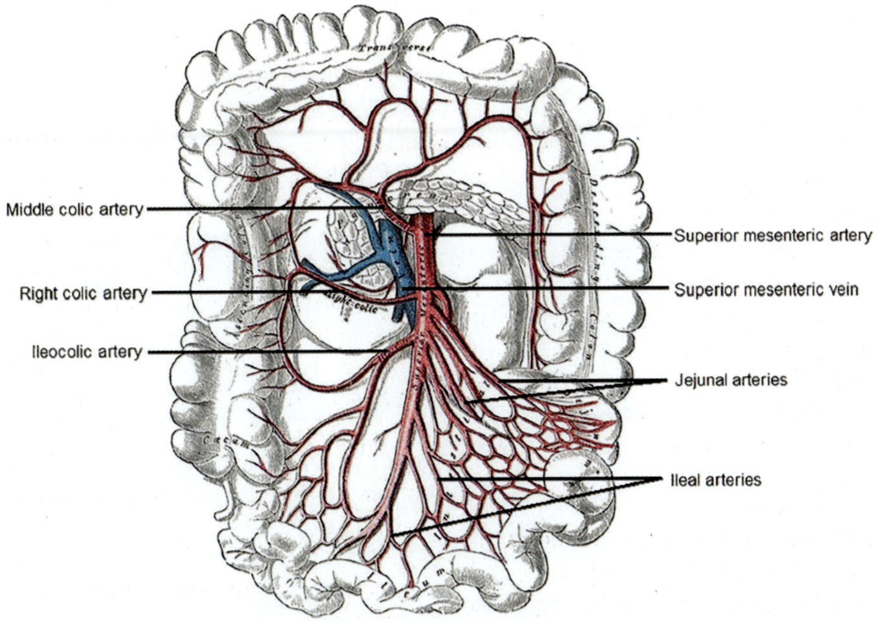

Figure 12.1 Branches of the superior mesenteric artery. (From Gray H, Lewis WH, eds. *Anatomy of the Human Body*. 20th ed. Lea & Febiger; Public domain, 1918.)

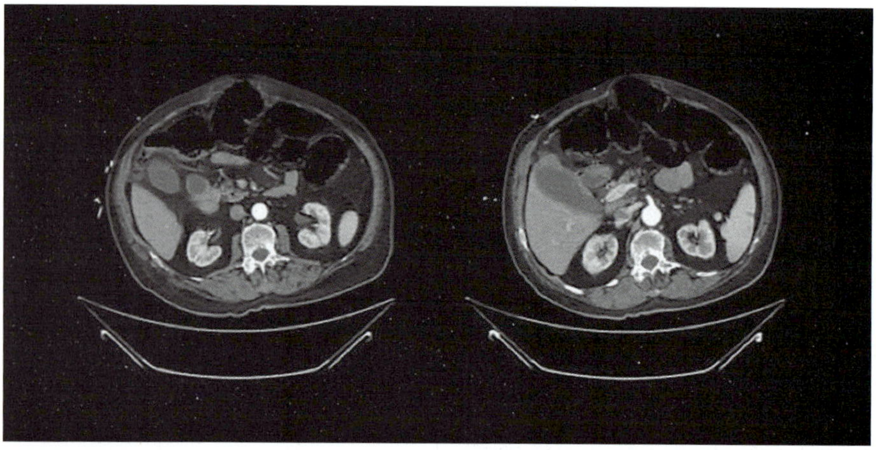

Figure 12.2 TAMI of the SMA.

Venous Acute Mesenteric Ischemia

Venous thrombosis (**Figure 12.3**) represents 10% of patients with AMI and usually occurs in a younger population (40-60 years old). It is frequently associated with hypercoagulable states (protein C and S deficiency, polycythemia, Leiden factor V mutation, cirrhosis or portal hypertension, severe pancreatitis, nephrotic syndrome, abdominal trauma, or advanced malignancy), although it may be idiopathic (20%). Oral contraceptives, pregnancy, and puerperium are risk factors in young women. Up to 50% of the patients report a previous deep thrombosis or pulmonary embolism. The onset of VAMI is characterized by vague subacute abdominal pain that may develop over a period up to 2 weeks. Half of the patients will complain of nausea and vomiting. Classical CT signs of VAMI are typically demonstrated by bowel thickening, venous engorgement, and mesenteric haziness with ascites. The associated venous engorgement may produce splenomegaly.

Nonocclusive Mesenteric Ischemia

Nonocclusive mesenteric ischemia accounts for ~20% of cases of mesenteric ischemia. It is often silent as it occurs as a secondary event in critically ill patients often sedated and ventilated in ICU (intensive care unit). The pathophysiology is poorly understood, but it can be explained by a combination of low cardiac output and vasoconstriction. Hypovolemia and the use of vasoconstrictive agents may precipitate NOMI. Risk factors for NOMI are age over 50, history of acute myocardial infarction, congestive heart failure, aortic insufficiency, cardiopulmonary bypass, kidney or liver diseases, or major abdominal surgery. It should be suspected in patients with mesenteric hypoperfusion secondary to circulatory shock or vasoactive drugs. Acute or insidious pain, bloating, abdominal distension, the presence of blood in the stools, or difficult defecation are all consistent with NOMI in critically ill patients. Most patients will display evidence of abdominal sepsis associated with distension as a late clinical sign.

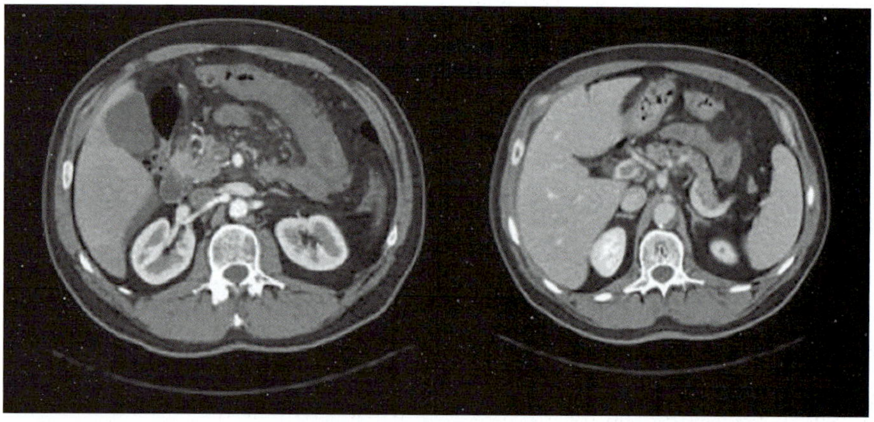

Figure 12.3 VAMI of the portal vein.

Laboratory Tests

There are no specific laboratory tests that routinely detect AMI early, although there are promising plasma biomarkers, such as the intestinal fatty acid-binding protein (I-FABP), α-glutathione S-transferase (GST), and D-lactate that might be helpful for an early diagnosis. They are not routinely used in clinical practice.

Most patients present with laboratory abnormalities such as hemoconcentration, leukocytosis, and metabolic acidosis with a high level of lactate, serum amylase, aspartate aminotransferase, lactate dehydrogenase, and creatine phosphokinase, but none of these tests are sufficiently sensitive or specific to diagnose AMI. An elevated WBC is reported in more than 90% of patients, while elevated levels of serum L-lactate are reported in 88% of patients with AMI. Serum L-lactate is a specific marker of tissue hypoperfusion, but since the liver can clear large quantities of L-lactate through the portomesenteric circulation, high levels of lactate might not be present in the initial stage of bowel ischemia. Lactic acidosis develops later after extended transmural infarction, tissue hypoperfusion, and sepsis. In a patient with acute abdominal pain, a normal serum lactate level does not rule out AMI, while a lactate level >2 mmol/L is generally associated with irreversible intestinal ischemia and high mortality.

Due to the thrombotic etiology of AMI, the laboratory tests related to clot formation, such as D-dimer and fibrinogen, will usually be elevated, but these are not specific. The level of D-dimer does not help differentiate VAMI from EAMI or TAMI.

Imaging

Unless there is high suspicion for pneumoperitoneum, the use of plain abdominal x-rays should be abandoned since radiographic signs are not specific and may delay a prompt diagnosis.

Abdominal point of care ultrasound (POCUS) might be used as a primary diagnostic tool in the emergency department as an extension of physical examination but should not delay carrying out computed tomography angiography (CTA). POCUS might help differentiate a small bowel obstruction, where bowel spasms and a sonographic *"to-and-fro"* motion of the bowel can be recognized from an AMI where signs of intestinal mobility might be absent due to extended necrosis. Moreover, intraperitoneal fluid is often detected by ultrasound and a sample of the fluid can be obtained through a US-guided diagnostic peritoneal aspiration (DPA). This method represents a powerful tool in the decision-making process since the presence of serosanguineous fluid detected by US-DPA strongly suggests bowel infarction and can guide the next steps of the diagnostic and therapeutic pathway.

Color Doppler US can show stenosis, embolism, or thrombosis at the celiac trunk or SMA level and assess intestinal wall perfusion. However, its sensitivity is low when compared to CTA. Furthermore, patient body habitus, excessive bowel distension, and the need for advanced ultrasound skills limit the routine use of this procedure.

Computed tomography angiography is the first-line imaging method, and it should be obtained as soon as possible when AMI is suspected since the most favorable outcome is strictly related to time to intervention. A delay in initiating proper treatment in fact accounts for mortality rates as high as 30%-70% despite clinical experience and recognition of the acute disease. CTA should be performed even in patients with renal failure, as the consequences of a delayed or incorrect diagnosis are far more detrimental to the kidneys and the patient than exposure to contrast media. CTA plays an important role not only because of its high diagnostic accuracy but also to identify other causes of acute abdominal pain. It is fundamental to distinguish the causes of AMI such as embolic, thrombotic, nonocclusive, or venous etiologies.

Oral contrast administration is not recommended for two reasons: Firstly, the associated clinical conditions such as vomiting and ileus, and secondly, the prolonged transit time of the oral contrast through the bowel can further delay definitive treatment.

Computed tomography angiography images should be acquired before intravenous contrast is given since precontrast scans can detect vascular calcification, hyperattenuating intravascular thrombus, or intramural hemorrhage, while contrast-enhanced CT allows the identification of thrombus in the mesenteric vessels, abnormal enhancement of the bowel wall, and the presence of embolism or infarction of other organs. Sagittal and 3D reconstructions are used to assess the origin and patterns of emboli and/or thrombus within the mesenteric arteries.

Features of AMI include the following:

- Appearance of bowel wall thickening
- Bowel dilation
- Occlusion of mesenteric vessels

- Mesenteric haziness
- Intestinal pneumatosis and portal venous gas
- Intraperitoneal fluid

Computed tomography angiography scan requires a high spatial resolution achieved with a collimation of 1.25-2.5 mm in the arterial or the portal venous phase to identify intestinal pneumatosis as gas bubbles may be no larger than 1-2 mm.

Nonocclusive mesenteric ischemia represents the most difficult diagnostic challenge and diagnosis may need to rely primarily on clinical suspicion. In these critically ill patients, transfer to the radiology department might not be safe due to severe hemodynamic instability. On CTA, the bowel wall of the involved segments may be normal or thickened and the pattern of enhancement is variable ranging from absent or diminished to increased, while fat stranding of the mesentery and ascites are usually visible. With strong suspicion of NOMI, the diagnosis can also be confirmed by selective catheter angiography. Findings include patent vessels with "pruning" of peripheral vessels, the arteries appearing as a "string of sausages," and loss of submucosal blush.

Mesenteric vessel evaluation by CTA is critically important to plan the subsequent surgical strategy and patient management since the therapeutic options might require angiography and endovascular intervention.

In general, CTA findings related to irreversible ischemia are intestinal dilatation and wall thickening, reduction or absence of visceral enhancement, pneumatosis intestinalis, portal venous gas, or free intraperitoneal air. These findings, associated with the clinical presentation, patient's frailty, age, and comorbidities, might guide the surgeon to consider palliative treatment.

The radiological features of AMI are listed in **Table 12.1**.

Pneumatosis intestinalis (**Figure 12.4**) is seen as the presence of air within the bowel wall as an expression of AMI-related bowel transmural

TABLE 12.1 ■ CTA of Mesenteric Ischemia Presentation

CTA Characteristics of Mesenteric Ischemia in Various Conditions			
Characteristic	**Arterial Occlusion**	**Venous Occlusion**	**No Occlusion**
Bowel wall thickness	Thinning, unchanged, or thickening (thickening may be seen with reperfusion)	Thickening	Thinning, unchanged, or thickening (thickening may be seen with reperfusion)
Involved site and location	Peripheral region of the occlusion, which is broader in mesenteric artery thrombosis (MAT) (owing to a more proximal occlusion) than in mesenteric artery embolism (MAE)	Peripheral region of the venous occlusion	Changes occur discontinuously and segmentally
Bowel wall attenuation on nonenhanced CT	Not a characteristic finding or has high attenuation in hemorrhagic infarction	Low with edema and high with intramural hemorrhage or hemorrhagic infarction	Not a characteristic finding or has high attenuation in hemorrhagic infarction
Bowel wall enhancement on contrast enhanced CT	Diminished or absent, target appearance or high signal intensity with reperfusion	Diminished or absent, or increased; target appearance	Diminished or absent, target appearance or high signal intensity with reperfusion
Bowel dilatation	Not apparent or is seen as hypotonic dilatation	Moderate to prominent, with fluid retention	Not apparent or is seen as hypotonic dilatation
Appearance of the mesenteric vessels	Defects in the arteries; stenosis with or without calcification in MAT; the diameter of the SMA is greater than that of the superior mesenteric vein (SMV)	Defects in the portomesenteric veins; venous engorgement	No defect in the vessels; arterial constriction and a smaller diameter of the SMV
Appearance of the mesentery	Not hazy until mesenteric infarction occurs	Hazy with ascites	Not hazy until mesenteric infarction occurs

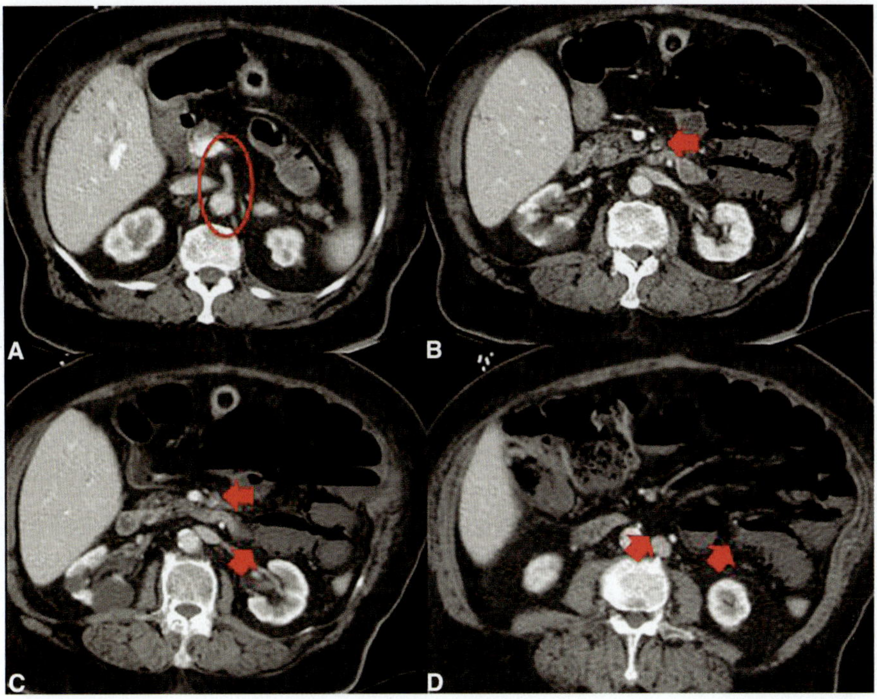

Figure 12.4 TAMI: CTA scan images of occlusion of mesenteric vessels and intestinal pneumatosis. **A:** In the circle the superior mesenteric artery. **B:** Arrow indicates a trombus in the superior mesenteric artery. **C:** Superior arrow indicates the trombus in the superior mesenteric artery; inferior arrow indicates intestinal pneumatosis. **D:** Left arrow indicates the trombus in the superior mesenteric artery and right arrow indicates the intestinal pneumatosis.

infarction. In end-stage cases, it is frequently associated with portomesenteric venous gas. However, although pneumatosis intestinalis (PI) strongly suggests bowel infarction or ischemia, it is not specific and, according to clinical features of the patient, pneumatosis as an isolated finding does not always require surgery. Sixty-percent of patients with pneumatosis intestinalis have benign disease, not requiring an operation. The PIPES trial reported that lactate ≥2.0 mmol/L and vasopressors or hypotension correctly predicted the need for operation in 92% of cases. Peritonitis mandates exploration. The findings of small bowel vs colonic pneumatosis, extent of pneumatosis, and portal venous gas are more likely to be pathologic pneumatosis. A more recent study identified five factors associated with pathologic pneumatosis intestinalis: small bowel PI, age ≥70 years, heart rate ≥110 beats/min, lactate ≥2.0 mmol/L and neutrophil-lymphocyte ratio ≥10.

Treatment

Once the diagnosis of AMI is suspected, the basic principles of patient support must be initiated. One of the main goals of resuscitation is the restoration of adequate tissue/organ perfusion. In the context of AMI, this can be summarized in the six Rs: Resuscitation, Rapid diagnosis, Revascularization, Resection, Relook and Restoration of GI continuity.

Resuscitation
Rapid diagnosis
Revascularization
Resection
Relook
Restoration of GI continuity

Resuscitation requires the administration of supplemental oxygen and intravenous fluids to ensure adequate blood volume and oxygenation. Fluid resuscitation and blood products are essential for the management of a patient with suspected AMI. To guide effective resuscitation, early hemodynamic monitoring should be implemented. A recent Cochrane Review showed no advantages of colloids over crystalloids in reducing mortality. Moreover, evidence suggests that the use of hydroxyethyl starch might increase mortality and should be avoided until further proof of safety can be provided.

Start systemic anticoagulation promptly, planning to continue it perioperatively. Assess electrolyte levels and metabolic status. Any metabolic acidosis or hyperkalemia should be corrected; nasogastric decompression should also be considered.

Vasopressors reduce splanchnic perfusion and avoid it whenever possible. When required, consideration should be given to drugs that have less effect on mesenteric blood flow such as dobutamine, low-dose dopamine, or milrinone.

A rapid diagnosis followed by prompt treatment is mandatory for the optimal outcome for the patient; a complete vascular occlusion of the bowel for more than 6 hours in fact leads to an irreversible damage with bowel necrosis and, in general, a delay of more than 24 hours is associated with a mortality increase to 80%. Early revascularization, when possible, is therefore a crucial key point of AMI treatment.

Resection of nonviable bowel is the only therapeutic option. But a relook strategy is frequently needed in association with an open abdomen strategy in order to reassess viability after resuscitation and or other therapeutical strategies such as bowel perfusion optimization after interventional radiology procedures. The use of a second look (or even multiple surgical explorations) is associated with a significant reduction in morbidity and mortality.

The final step before closing the abdomen is restoration of viable GI tract continuity; the length of remaining bowel should always be measured to help plan appropriate nutritional support.

Broad-spectrum antibiotics should be given since intestinal ischemia leads to early loss of the mucosal barrier, which facilitates bacterial translocation and the risk of septic complications.

Specific treatments should be taken in account for each different etiology (a proposed management flowchart is shown in **Figure 12.5**).

Arterial Embolism (EAMI)

Open embolectomy is still widely performed via a midline incision approaching the SMA just below the pancreas and the mesenteric root. A transverse arteriotomy is made after proximal and distal clamping and embolectomy catheters (No 2 or 3 Fogarty balloon catheters) are used to clear the artery proximally and distally. High-pressure proximal flushing should be avoided, so as not to dislodge any thrombus in the aorta and produce further emboli. After completing the thrombectomy, the artery should be flushed gently with heparinized saline. The arteriotomy is then closed in a standard fashion.

Endovascular embolectomy has become more common with the development of dedicated catheters. It is achieved by percutaneous mechanical aspiration or thrombolysis and permits percutaneous transluminal angioplasty (PTA), if necessary, with or without stenting. There is a risk of distal embolization of thrombus.

The caveat accompanying the endovascular treatment first strategy is avoiding delay to laparotomy if symptoms do not resolve after successful embolus aspiration. If irreversible bowel necrosis has already developed, surgical exploration and resection of necrotic tissue are mandatory. It is not unusual that occlusive AMI is followed by NOMI after revascularization.

Arterial Thrombosis (TAMI)

Endovascular treatment should be the first choice for TAMI whenever possible and should be accomplished as soon as possible. It should be performed before intestinal infarction occurs and when ischemia is still potentially reversible. The commonest interventions are PTA and stenting. Other endovascular techniques include percutaneous aspiration thrombectomy, local fibrinolysis, or intra-arterial drug perfusion (such as heparin or papaverine).

If surgery (**Figure 12.6**) is needed to resect ischemic bowel before vascular intervention, or when percutaneous treatment has failed, options for revascularization are thromboendarterectomy, reimplantation of the SMA, SMA bypass, and retrograde open mesenteric stenting (ROMS). Among these options, ROMS is generally indicated but requires technical expertise. When the patient is in extremis, the operative time should be kept to a minimum.

Retrograde open mesenteric stenting is a hybrid approach during laparotomy. The SMA is exposed and punctured in its main trunk and the proximal SMA lesion is crossed in a retrograde direction with a long hydrophilic guidewire. The guidewire is then snared in the aorta to establish a through-and-through access from the femoral or brachial artery. The stenting can then be performed in the normal antegrade fashion. The advantage of the hybrid technique over conventional stenting is that the recanalization can be done over a short distance, avoiding the trouble of getting enough support for the guidewire to pass through the lesion. The operation is less invasive than surgical bypass, and the risk of infection of the implant is minimal even with abdominal contamination. Further advantages of the hybrid technique are that any fresh thrombus can be removed via open arteriotomy and the SMA can be clamped distally to the puncture site prior to the stenting to avoid distal embolization.

An antegrade bypass from the supraceliac aorta to the superior mesenteric trunk using an endogenous vein graft will give the best result for

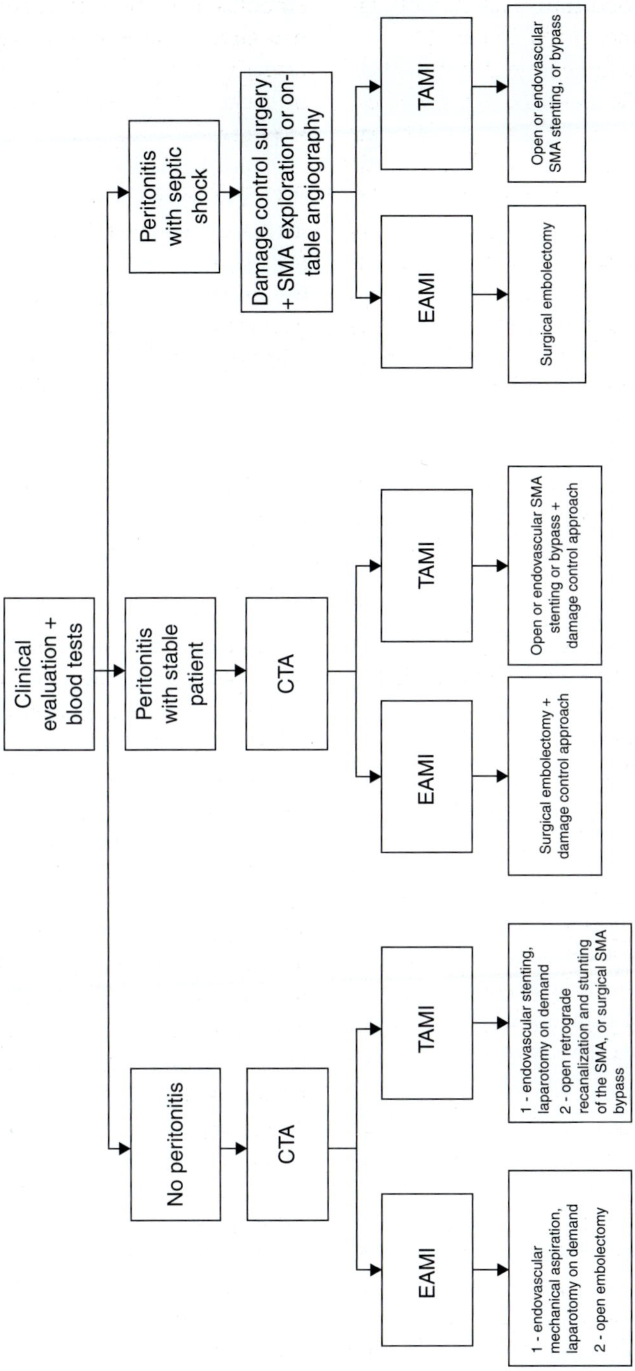

Figure 12.5 Decision-making flowchart.

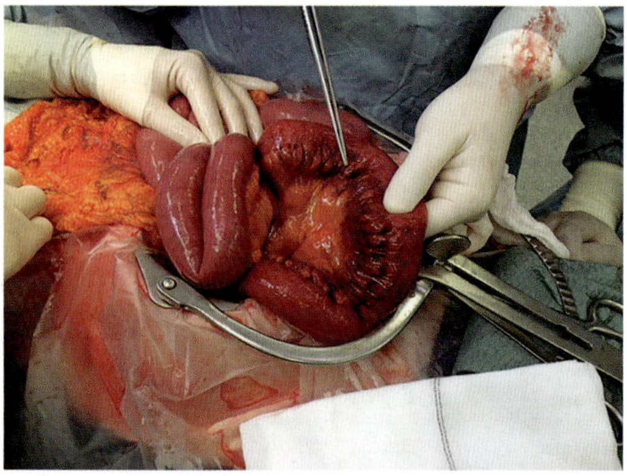

Figure 12.6 VAMI: intraoperative findings.

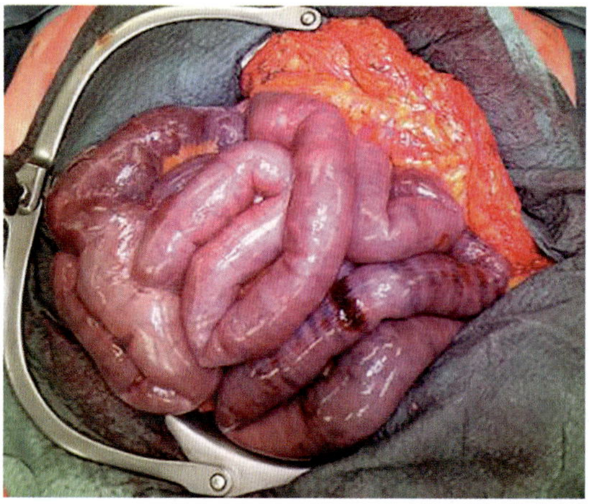

Figure 12.7 TAMI: aspect of the small bowel wall in TAMI before performing open arteriotomy.

open bypass. An alternative approach would be a renal-mesenteric bypass. However, the most practical option for proximal mesenteric atherosclerotic occlusive disease is a retrograde bypass from the common iliac artery with a synthetic graft.

Where vascular expertise is not available, it may be reasonable to resect the necrotic bowel first and then transfer the patient for urgent interventional angiography or vascular surgery.

The choice of open, endovascular, or hybrid technique must be based on the long-term patency of the arterial supply, lower after stenting than after open surgical procedures. Approximately 30% of patients treated with endovascular techniques require a second angioplasty during the following 2 years.

Venous Ischemia (VAMI)

Venous AMI is usually managed without surgery. Anticoagulation with a continuous infusion of unfractionated or low molecular weight heparin (LMWH) is the first-line treatment for VAMI and should also be started in the setting of intraoperative diagnosis. Isolated thrombosis of the superior mesenteric vein is usually compensated by the collateral circulation. However, additional complete thrombosis of the portal vein leads to venous infarction of segments of small intestine of varying severity and may require laparotomy (**Figure 12.7**).

The approaches differ due to the patient's clinical symptoms and CTA findings:

- If the symptoms are mild and no CTA signs of compromised bowel perfusion (such as bowel wall edema or ascites), simple anticoagulation starting with LMWH and continued with warfarin is usually sufficient.
- If the initial symptoms are more severe and CTA shows edematous bowel, continuous infusion of unfractionated heparin should be started instead of LMWH. The advantages of continuous heparin infusion are that the efficacy of the treatment can be monitored with blood tests (activated partial thromboplastin time) and the anticoagulation can be reversed quickly with protamine if surgery is required.
- The second step is endovascular treatment, which includes mechanical thrombectomy and/or catheter-directed thrombolysis via transhepatic or transjugular portosystemic access. Intra-arterial administration of a thrombolytic agent through a catheter inserted to the SMA via endovascular access has also been used as an adjunctive therapy, or as first-line thrombolytic therapy in cases of acute mesenteric venous thrombosis where the portal vein is chronically occluded. Contraindications to thrombolytic treatment are well established and can be divided into absolute (central nervous system tumors, recent hemorrhagic stroke, gastrointestinal [GI] bleed, and uncontrolled hypertension) and relative (pregnancy, remote history of GI bleeding, and recent major surgery).
- Surgery is required when bowel necrosis is suspected, or the patient develops abdominal compartment syndrome. Damage control principles can be applied in venous mesenteric ischemia, and open abdomen therapy with vacuum dressings is used in abdominal compartment syndrome caused by extensive bowel edema. Rarely, open venous thrombectomy may need to be considered in extreme cases.

Nonocclusive Mesenteric Ischemia

The treatment of NOMI is based on correcting the clinical or pharmacological conditions that induced the splanchnic vasoconstriction, as well as improving mesenteric perfusion together with early recognition and resection of infarcted bowel.

The main factor in improving mesenteric perfusion is restoration of circulatory volume and hemodynamic stability coupled with the use of vasodilators administered directly into the SMA to reverse the intestinal vasospasm that causes ischemia.

The diagnosis of NOMI should be confirmed by selective mesenteric angiography and, if no contraindications, the infusion of vasodilators directly into the SMA can be started. The best vasodilator drug appears to be prostaglandin E1 (alprostadil) given as a 20-μg bolus followed by 60-80 μg/24 h infusion; papaverine (30-60 mg/h) has been shown to reduce the mortality rate for NOMI from 70% to 50%-55% and is an acceptable alternative.

The decision to intervene surgically is based on the presence of peritonitis, perforation, or overall worsening of the patient's condition.

Role for Laparoscopy

A minimally invasive approach should be entertained when facing uncertain scenarios. It may avoid a laparotomy yet lead to a diagnosis. Use laparoscopy in patients with normal hemodynamic status where there is a clinical suspicion of abdominal pathology, but laboratory tests and imaging are not diagnostic. One limitation would be the inability to fully explore the abdomen and visualize the whole bowel, although this risk can be mitigated by the surgeon's experience and skill.

To increase the sensitivity and specificity of the procedure, vascular assessment by indocyanine green fluorescence (ICG) can be used.

Another use of laparoscopy should be in unstable patients where the extent of ischemic bowel may lead to either a damage control or a palliative approach. A bedside laparoscopy may be performed in ICU to help clinical decision-making.

Indocyanine Green Fluorescence

Indocyanine green fluorescence is a near infrared fluorophore. It has been used extensively in fluorescence angiography in the elective surgical setting. The fluorescence can be seen using special laparoscopic cameras as the dye passes through the circulation. It can identify and color the areas where a constant and adequate blood flow is present and also allows visualization of areas where the blood supply is inadequate, before macroscopic changes develop on the serosa. ICG utilization in the emergent setting, particularly in AMI, has not been well investigated to date, although early animal models and isolated case and cohort studies show promise.

The technique can be used in open or laparoscopic surgery.

Open Abdomen Strategy and Damage Control Surgery (DCS)

Patients with AMI who have severe sepsis or septic shock and undergo life-saving surgery should have a damage control approach. (See Chapter 9.) The decision to implement the DCS modality should be made early during the laparotomy, or even before. It should be based on the response to resuscitation and ongoing physiology of the patient. Advanced age is not a contraindication to DCS as good outcomes have been observed in the elderly.

A bowel anastomosis should be performed only in the adequately resuscitated and stable patient where there is no doubt about the viability of the bowel. During the first operation, only the clearly necrotic areas should be resected. A second-look strategy should then be considered in every situation where the physiology of the patient is unstable (damage control surgery), when the viability of the bowel is uncertain (eg, after an SMA bypass) or when the patient may need an angiographic procedure after a laparotomy. In each scenario, it is useful to recheck bowel viability after adequate resuscitation. The timing of the second look should be within 48 hours, but not before 24 hours. If during a second-look procedure there is still doubt about the viability of the bowel, a further relook should be planned.

The use of second-look procedures in selected patients is associated with a significant reduction in morbidity and mortality with resection of ischemic bowel during the relook laparotomy in 31%-71% of the cases.

When leaving the abdomen open, recent evidence suggests that the use of peritoneal resuscitation may aid restoration of normal bowel physiology before the second look.

Futile Care

Resection of all ischemic bowel may result in short bowel syndrome (SBS) with serious associated consequences. This may not be a preferable state, particularly in elderly and infirm patients, who may not tolerate long-term parenteral nutrition.

APACHE-II and P-POSSUM are not accurate scoring systems for outcomes after emergency surgery; moreover, P-POSSUM may underpredict mortality.

In this particular and challenging decision-making process, the use of a clinical frailty scale might also be helpful in discussion of the clinical scenario with patients' relatives and avoid misleading expectations.

An SBS requiring total parenteral nutrition has been reported in 13%-31% of long-term survivors of AMI and weight loss has been documented in 38%. SBS usually occurs when <200 cm of functioning bowel remains. *Intestinal failure* is defined as insufficient intestinal length or function to maintain health without parenteral nutrition. The risk of intestinal failure depends upon the amount of small bowel resected and the portion of small bowel resected. Jejunal resection of ~50% is usually well tolerated. Ileal resection >30% is usually poorly tolerated. It is important to refer to remaining bowel length at surgery in your operative note. Some degree of intestinal failure occurs with residual small bowel length of 100-150 cm. Short gut syndrome results when the postoperative anatomy is <100 cm of small bowel without an ileocecal valve or <65 cm of small bowel with an intact ileocecal valve and colon. In young patients, remember that small bowel transplantation is an option. When this limit cannot be respected, careful consideration should be given to the significant risk of resection.

The benefit of extensive small bowel resection should be balanced against the resultant quality of life, morbidity, and mortality especially in elderly patients.

ISCHEMIC COLITIS

Diagnosis

Ischemic colitis (IC) is a totally separate entity from small bowel ischemia. Colonic ischemia is more common than small bowel ischemia. The natural history and overall outcome are generally less severe than small bowel ischemia. The incidence of IC has been estimated to range from 4.5 to 44 per 100 000 population but generally occurs in the elderly population (80%).

Its etiology is related to a gradual decrease of colonic perfusion with an acute ischemic insult of the colonic wall. It is usually a segmental disease with a typical sharp demarcation between the normal mucosa and the affected areas. The left colon and sigmoid colon are most frequently involved. Watershed areas are the splenic flexure (Griffiths point) and rectosigmoid junction (Sudek point). Isolated right colon ischemia should be managed differently than other ischemic colitis because of the high likelihood of transmural infarction and need to operate.

Predisposing factors are generally divided into two categories: vascular factors and intrinsic bowel factors.

Any condition that causes a reduction in the blood supply to the colon can potentially induce IC including vasospasm of the colonic vessel, a hypercoagulable state, or vasculitis (**Figure 12.8**).

Bowel factors that can precipitate IC include constipation, irritable bowel syndrome, fecal impaction, colonic obstruction, and any condition that increases the colonic intraluminal pressure.

The pathologic spectrum of IC includes transient ischemia, chronic ischemia, and gangrene. The mucosa is the layer of the colon that is most vulnerable to ischemia. Ischemia limited to the mucosa may be transient and recovery complete.

When IC involves the muscularis, it can result in scarring and possibly to a chronic stricture. Ischemia involving the full thickness of the colonic wall may lead to gangrene or perforation. Colonic ischemia is generally nonocclusive, with good prognosis. It can be seen with a hypercoagulable state, pancreatitis, portal hypertension, or congestive heart failure. Occlusive colonic ischemia may occur with arterial embolism, dissection, or arteritis. Ischemic colitis must be distinguished from C diff colitis, other infectious colitis, or inflammatory bowel disease.

Clinical Presentation

The initial presentation of ischemic colitis may have some overlap with small bowel ischemia, with nonspecific abdominal pain, vague GI symptoms, or pain out of proportion to physical examination. The classic presentation of IC includes abdominal pain, hematochezia, diarrhea, and leukocytosis. Symptoms are mainly related to the degree of the ischemia and the length and thickness of affected colon: Ischemia limited to a small segment of the mucosa may cause crampy abdominal pain, fecal urgency, and minimal rectal bleeding. Fresh bleeding usually occurs when the left colon is involved. Right-sided colonic ischemia often will not present with blood per rectum. More severe and extensive intestinal ischemia will result in acute abdominal pain, bacterial translocation with septic signs, and acidosis.

The clinical patterns of IC are still based on the *Classification of Brandt and Boley* and depend on the degree of the histopathological damage of the colonic wall: (1) reversible colitis (submucosal or intramural bleeding), (2) transient colitis, (3) chronic segmental ischemia, (4) gangrenous colitis, and (5) fulminant pancolitis.

The nongangrenous types account for 80%-85% of cases (and will not require operation); gangrene occurs in 15% of cases; fulminant pancolitis is rare (1%).

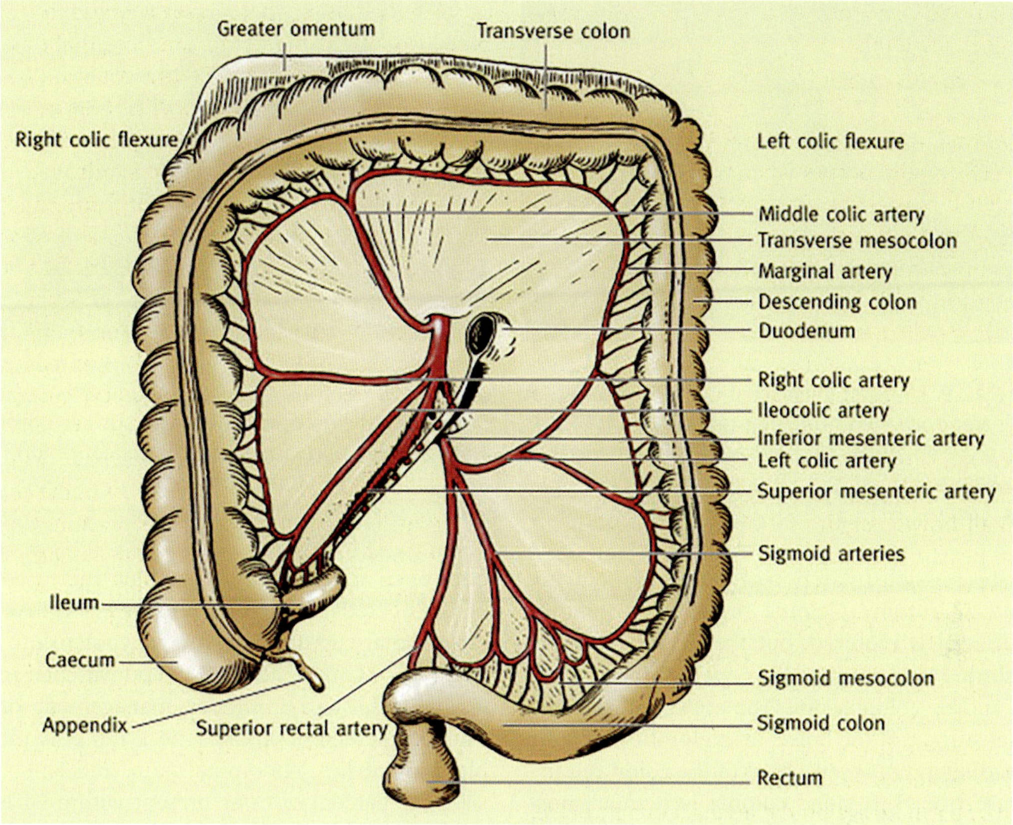

Figure 12.8 Arterial blood supply to the colon. (Reprinted from Ellis H, Mahadevan V. Anatomy of the caecum, appendix and colon. *Surgery*. 2014;32:4. Elsevier. https://doi.org/10.1016/j.mpsur.2014.02.001)

Laboratory Tests

Laboratory studies are usually nonspecific for IC. A complete blood count, metabolic panel, and liver function tests are required to assess the physiological status of the patient. Leukocytosis and elevated tissue injury markers (lactate, amylase, lactate dehydrogenase, and creatine kinase) are the most common findings. However, the lactate level may not be elevated. Check stool cultures and C diff toxins if a clinical possibility. A thrombophilia workup may be indicated.

Imaging

Ileus is the most common finding on abdominal plain films. Abdominal CTA is the most helpful imaging examination for the patient with suspicion of IC. CTA can exclude other causes of an acute abdomen, identify the site, extent, and source of ischemia, and detect complications associated with severe disease. In the mild form of disease, CTA may appear normal; in more advanced but nongangrenous forms, the CTA will often show colonic wall thickening, thumbprinting, colonic dilatation, and pericolic fat stranding.

In the absence of peritonitis, a flexible endoscopy with minimal insufflation can assess the degree of mucosal ischemia: The *colon single stripe sign* is suggestive of ischemic injury and is seen as a single line of erythema with erosion or ulceration placed along the longitudinal axis of the large bowel (**Figure 12.9**). More severe findings include loss of haustral markings, cyanosis, and gangrene of the colonic wall. Bowel preparation prior to colonoscopy is not indicated to avoid toxic dilation or perforation.

Treatment

Initial treatment is usually conservative with good prognosis. The use of broad-spectrum antibiotics (a third-generation cephalosporin in combination with metronidazole) to cover both aerobic and anaerobic bacteria is recommended. Start systemic anticoagulation, rest the bowel, and volume resuscitate the patient.

In cases with no clinical improvement within 24-48 hours (moderate disease), repetition of colonoscopy or imaging might be necessary to re-evaluate the severity of the disease, and, in the case of clinical deterioration, a surgical approach might be needed.

Increasing abdominal tenderness, fever, uncontrollable bleeding, or paralytic ileus

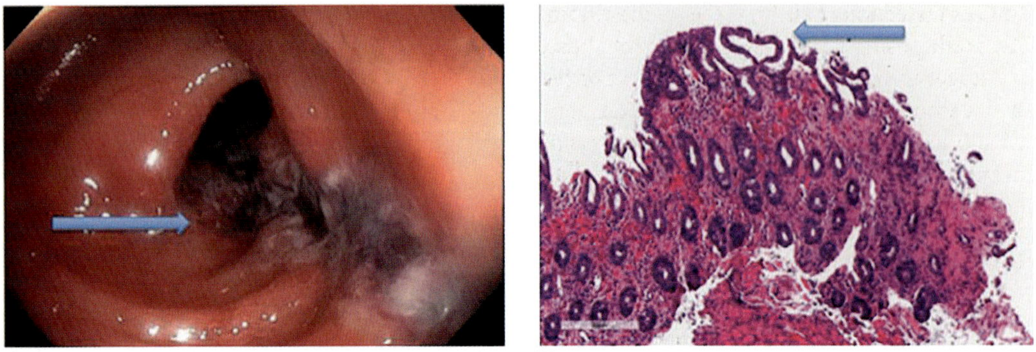

A B

Figure 12.9 Single stripe sign of colonic ischemia. **A:** Colonoscopy demonstrates a longitudinal nonbleeding ulcer without stigmata of recent bleeding (arrow). **B:** Microscopic evaluation: surface epithelial injury, crypt epithelial atrophy, crypt loss, lamina propria hemorrhage, and lamina propria hyalinization. (From Parikh MP, Satiya J, Berger-Saunderson M, et al. The colonic single stripe sign: a case of ischemic colitis. *Cureus*. 2019;11:e4622. doi:10.7759/cureus.4622.)

indicates possible infarction of the colon requiring urgent laparotomy. Colonic resection of gangrenous bowel is required, but the extent of resection should be determined preoperatively through CTA and/or colonoscopy. The appearance of the serosal surface of the bowel at exploration may be misleading as far as the extent of the colon requiring resection. Left-sided colonic ischemia (most common) is managed with resection, proximal colostomy, and closure of the distal colon. In carefully selected cases, a primary anastomosis with or without proximal loop ileostomy may be possible.

Right-sided colonic ischemia is more likely to result in colonic necrosis. Right-sided colonic compared to transverse or left-sided ischemia may present with only abdominal pain and nonbloody diarrhea. These patients are more likely to require resection and have higher mortality. Be certain to assess SMA patency with right-sided ischemia. In uncomplicated right colon ischemia in a stable patient with no signs of perforation or peritonitis, resection with primary anastomosis is generally advised. Some authors recommend a cholecystectomy as part of the operation to avoid postoperative acalculous cholecystitis. If a severe case of ischemic colitis responds to medical management, the sloughed cast of colonic mucosa may be replaced by fibrosis and result in colonic stricture, which may need subsequent resection for obstructive symptoms.

Colonic Ischemia After Abdominal Aortic Surgery

Ischemic colitis may occur after 7% of elective operations on the abdominal aorta. Up to 60% of patients will develop ischemic colitis after surgery for a ruptured aortic aneurysm, occurring after both open and endovascular repair. Increased risk of postoperative ischemic colitis is associated with aneurysmal rupture (5%-20%), hypotension, prolong cross-clamp time, open vs endovascular repair, arrhythmias, and improper management of the inferior mesenteric artery. The symptoms include bloody diarrhea, abdominal pain, and leukocytosis. Fifty percent of cases present within 24 hours postoperatively, nearly all within 7 days. Prompt flexible sigmoidoscopy is recommended when ischemic colitis is suspected. The findings will confirm (or exclude) the diagnosis and guide management. The finding of normal mucosa at *sigmoidoscopy* has 100% negative predictive value. If moderate to severe mucosal ischemia is seen, the positive predictive value for transmural necrosis is 55%-73%. This means endoscopy cannot differentiate severe mucosal ischemia alone from transmural necrosis—only a laparotomy/laparoscopy can do this.

Nontransmural colonic ischemia is treated with hydration, antibiotics, close clinical follow-up, and at times repeat endoscopy.

Gastric Pneumatosis

Gastric pneumatosis is a rare finding and may be associated with a benign condition—gastric emphysema (GE)—or a life-threatening condition—emphysematous gastritis (EG). Benign gastric emphysema is far more common. Both conditions have different postulated etiologies with disruption in gastric mucosa in GE due to dissection of air into the gastric wall, while EG occurs secondary to gas production by bacteria with resultant necrosis and sloughing of the gastric wall. Various predisposing conditions for GE are raised intragastric pressure (commonly secondary to gastric outlet obstruction), postgastroscopy, severe vomiting, or dissection of air from the mediastinum. For EG, predisposing conditions are alcohol abuse, gastric surgery, recent gastroenteritis, corrosive ingestion, chronic consumption of nonsteroidal anti-inflammatories (NSAIDs)/steroids, diabetes mellitus, chronic obstructive pulmonary disease (COPD), and immunosuppression.

Differentiating GE from EG is difficult based on CT findings alone. However, in GE, the air in the stomach wall is usually seen as loculated round air bubbles, while in EG, the air has a streaky and linear consistency with associated gastric wall thickening. Portal venous air may be seen in GE or EG.

Lactate levels are important as markers of 30-day mortality. A lactate level lower than 2 mmol/L is associated with higher chances of survival and lower probability of surgical exploration.

In the GE scenario, the patient is usually asymptomatic and the gastric pneumatosis is an incidental finding. On the other hand, EG often is associated with abdominal pain, fever, nausea and vomiting, leukocytosis, and signs of generalized infection.

Treatment is still not completely clarified even though some authors claim that gastric pneumatosis should be treated as per intestinal pneumatosis with conservative treatment first, involving operative exploration when signs of peritonitis or hemodynamic instability arise.

SUMMARY

Mesenteric ischemia is a rare condition with misleading clinical scenarios of presentation. If the clinical suspicion is high and the physiology of the patient allows, a contrast-enhanced CTA scan is the gold standard for the diagnosis and the following treatment. In general, the treatment can be summarized in 6Rs: Resuscitation, Rapid diagnosis, Revascularization, Resection, Relook, and Restoration of GI continuity. A CT allows a correct diagnosis differentiating EAMI, TAMI, VAMI, and NOMI, leading to the correct treatment for each cause. When the patient is physiologically abnormal during a laparotomy, consider a damage control approach with an open abdomen. Balance the amount of "damage" you are creating with the operation in a frail patient (is your act futile?).

For ischemic colitis, the first-line treatment is usually conservative; if it fails, a surgical resection may be needed.

SUGGESTED READINGS

Acosta S, Kärkkäinen J. Open abdomen in acute mesenteric ischemia. *Anaesthesiol Intensive Ther.* 2019;51(2):159-162.

Bala M, Kashuk J, Moore EE, et al. Acute mesenteric ischemia: guidelines of the World Society of Emergency Surgery. *World J Emerg Surg.* 2017;12:38.

Bryski MG, Frenzel Sulyok LG, Kaplan L, Singhal S, Keating JJ. Techniques for intraoperative evaluation of bowel viability in mesenteric ischemia: a review. *Am J Surg.* 2020;220(2):309-315.

DuBose JJ, Lissauer M, Maung AA, et al. Pneumatosis intestinalis predictive evaluation study (PIPES): a multicenter epidemiologic study of the Eastern Association for the Surgery of Trauma. *J Trauma Acute Care Surg.* 2013;75:15-23.

Furukawa A, Kanasaki S, Kono N, et al. CT diagnosis of acute mesenteric ischemia from various causes. *Am J Roentgenol.* 2009;192(2):408-416.

Garzelli L, Nuzzo A, Copin P, et al. Contrast-enhanced CT for the diagnosis of acute mesenteric ischemia. *Am J Roentgenol.* 2020;215(1):29-38.

Jalalzadeh H, van Schaik TG, Duin JJ, et al. The value of sigmoidoscopy to detect colonic ischemia after ruptured aortic aneurysm repair. *Eur J Vasc Endovasc Surg.* 2019;57:229-237.

Kanasaki S, Furukawa A, Fumoto K, et al. Acute mesenteric ischemia: multidetector CT findings and endovascular management. *Radiographics.* 2018;38(3):945-961.

Kärkkäinen JM, Acosta S. Acute mesenteric ischemia (Part II)—vascular and endovascular surgical approaches. *Best Pract Res Clin Gastroenterol.* 2017;31(1):27-38.

Lee MJ, Daniels SL, Drake TM, et al. Risk factors for ischaemic colitis after surgery fpr abdominal aortic aneurysm: a systematic review and observational meta-analysis. *Int J Colorectal Dis.* 2016;31:1273-1281.

Misiakos EP, Tsapralis D, Karatzas T, et al. Advents in the diagnosis and management of ischemic colitis. *Front Surg.* 2017;4:47. https://www.frontiersin.org/articles/10.3389/fsurg.2017.00047/full

Naseer M, Gandhi J, Chams N, Kulairi Z. Stercoral colitis complicated with ischemic colitis: a double-edge sword. *BMC Gastroenterol.* 2017;17(1):129.

O'Keefe SJD, Buchman AL, Fishbein TM, et al. Short bowel syndrome and intestinal failure: consensus, definitions and overview. *Clin Gastroenterol Hepatol.* 2006;4:6-8.

Pironi L, Arends J, Baxter J, et al. ESPEN endorsed recommendations. Definition and classification of intestinal failure in adults. *Clin Nutr.* 2015;34:171-180.

Reginelli A, Genovese E, Cappabianca S, et al. Intestinal ischemia: US-CT findings correlations. *Crit Ultrasound J.* 2013;5(1):S7.

Rieser CJ, Dadashzadeh ER, Handzel RM, et al. Development and validation of a five factor score for prediction of pathologic pneumatosis. *J Trauma Acute Care Surg.* 2021;90:477-483.

Theodoropoulou A, Koutroubakis IE. Ischemic colitis: clinical practice in diagnosis and treatment. *World J Gastroenterol.* 2008;14(48):7302-7308.

Tilsed JVT, Casamassima A, Kurihara H, et al. ESTES guidelines: acute mesenteric ischaemia. *Eur J Trauma Emerg Surg.* 2016;42(2):253-270.

CHAPTER

13 Gastrointestinal Hemorrhage in Emergency Surgery

Nicole A. Stassen and Linda Ding

CASE PRESENTATION

A 61-year-old male presents to the emergency department with fatigue, upper abdominal pain, and several episodes of dark tarry stool for the last day. His past medical history includes end-stage renal disease on hemodialysis (last dialyzed the day prior to presentation), coronary artery disease, atrial fibrillation on anticoagulation with warfarin, and obstructive sleep apnea. His past surgical history includes a laparoscopic cholecystectomy and an open right inguinal hernia repair. He is afebrile, heart rate was 110 beats/min, and a blood pressure of 90/45 mm Hg. On examination, he is pale with mild upper abdominal tenderness and melena on rectal examination. Labs are notable for a hemoglobin of 6.5 g/dL and an INR of 4.1. Intravenous access is obtained with two large-bore peripheral intravenous lines, and resuscitation is initiated with isotonic fluid with some improvement in his hemodynamics.

Question: *What is the most simple next step to help identify the source of this patient's gastrointestinal hemorrhage?*

Answer: *Placement of a nasogastric tube to determine if there is a higher probability of an upper tract source.*

INTRODUCTION

Acute gastrointestinal (GI) bleeding is a common medical emergency that acute care surgeons are called on to manage. GI bleeding is not a singular disease but a symptom and clinical manifestation of a broad range of diseases of the GI tract. The definition of GI bleeding can be conceptualized by an anatomic division relative to the ligament of Treitz. Upper GI bleeds (UGIB) encompass sources proximal to the ligament of Treitz including the esophagus, stomach, and duodenum, while lower GI bleeds (LGIB) encompass sources distal to the ligament of Treitz including the small bowel, colon, and rectum. The approach to the treatment and management of GI bleeding is variable and depends on the site and rate of bleeding as well as the clinical presentation. Fortunately, the vast majority of patients with GI bleeding will stop bleeding spontaneously or with initial treatment (80%-85%). There is an increase in incidence of GI bleed with increasing age, with 70% of patients with acute GI bleeding being older than 65 years.

PRINCIPLES OF MANAGEMENT

In the case of overt upper or lower GI bleeding with hemorrhagic shock, initial resuscitation principles from posttraumatic hemorrhagic shock should be applied. Attention to airway protection and restoration of circulating volume in the form of massive transfusion protocols are of utmost importance in stabilizing such patients. Coagulopathies must be corrected, and antagonists of novel oral anticoagulants may be necessary. Thromboelastographic data may be a useful adjunct in correcting coagulopathies. Transfuse platelets to maintain a platelet count of $>50 \times 10^9$/L. As in trauma patients, the efficacy and safety of a restrictive transfusion target (Hb > 7 g/dL) in acute GI bleed patients has also been demonstrated.

Once the patient is stabilized clinically, efforts to localize the source of hemorrhage should be undertaken expeditiously as the anatomic localization of the hemorrhage is paramount in guiding the priority and choice of diagnostic and therapeutic strategies. Differentiation of an upper vs a lower GI bleed starts with the clinical assessment. Classically, patients with an UGIB present with coffee-ground hematemesis, bright red hematemesis, melena, or even hematochezia. Whereas LGIB patients typically present with melena or hematochezia. Place a nasogastric tube to help elucidate if there is an upper tract source. Return of nonbloody but bilious nasogastric tube effluent makes an upper tract source much less

TABLE 13.1 ■ Sources of Upper GI Bleeding

Nonvariceal Bleeding (90%)		Portal Hypertensive Bleeding	
Peptic ulcer bleeding	30%-50%	Gastroesophageal varices	>90%
Mallory-Weiss tear	15%-20%	Hypertensive portal gastropathy	<5%
Gastritis and duodenitis	5%-10%	Isolated gastric varices	Rare
Esophagitis	5%-10%		
AVM	5%		
Tumors	2%		
Other	5%		

likely. The remainder of the chapter will be divided into upper and lower GI hemorrhage, its workup, and management.

UPPER GASTROINTESTINAL HEMORRHAGE

Etiology

UGIB can be characterized as variceal or nonvariceal bleeding. Approximately 90% of UGIB result from nonvariceal sources including peptic ulcer disease, Mallory-Weiss syndrome, erosive gastritis, duodenitis, esophagitis, malignancy, angiodysplasias, and Dieulafoy lesion (**Table 13.1**). Nonvariceal bleeding is most commonly caused by peptic ulcer disease where ulcers can occur in multiple locations (**Figure 13.1**). Younger patients are more likely to have upper GI bleeding. Bleeding in older patients is generally lower GI bleeding.

Peptic ulcers can form in the duodenum or the stomach as a result of NSAID use or *Helicobacter pylori* infection. The incidence of peptic ulcer disease has decreased over time with the prevalence of proton pump inhibitor (PPI) therapy and the recognition of NSAIDs as a cause of ulcers via the effects of prostaglandin inhibition. However, peptic ulcer disease remains a significant burden on the health care system, with 10%-20% of patients experiencing complications.

Mallory-Weiss tears are longitudinal mucosal disruptions at the gastroesophageal junction due to vomiting or severe retching, causing sudden

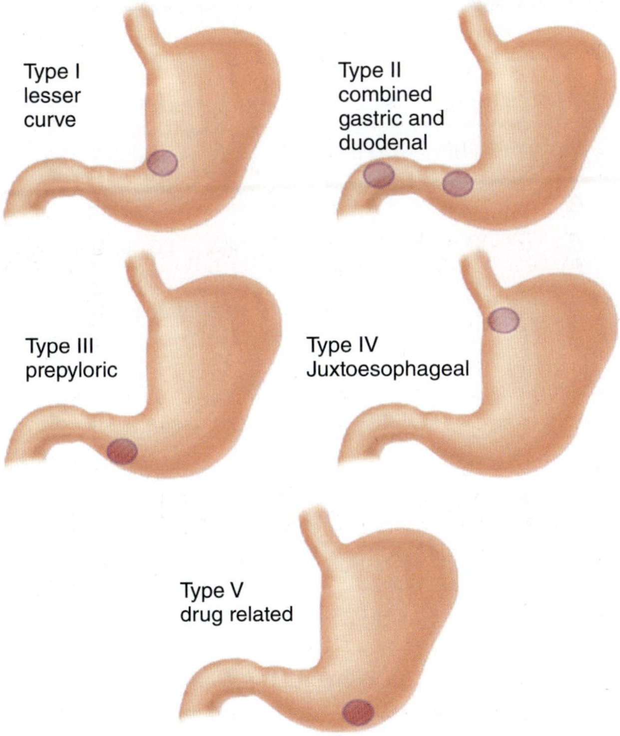

Figure 13.1 Type and location of peptic ulcers. (From Britt LD, et al. *Acute Care Surgery*. Wolters Kluwer, 2019.)

rapid increases in intra-abdominal pressures. A *Dieulafoy lesion* is a rare cause of GI bleeding due to submucosal artery that has ulcerated. Although it can occur anywhere along the GI tract, it is most commonly found in the proximal stomach. The pathophysiology is poorly understood, but associated risk factors include male sex, cardiovascular disease, hypertension, chronic kidney disease, and alcoholism.

Stress-related mucosal damage (SRMD) is a clinical entity seen in critically ill patients, with an incidence of overt bleeding in up to 8.5%. The major risk factors for overt GI bleed in this population are mechanical ventilation for more than 48 hours or coagulopathy (platelets $<50 \times 10^9$/L and/or INR > 1.5).

Variceal bleeding results from portal hypertension, a sequelae of end-stage liver disease. Cirrhosis leads to obstruction of the portal venous outflow, and varices develop to decompress the portal system and return blood to the systemic circulation. This most commonly manifests as gastroesophageal varices. Each episode of variceal hemorrhage carries a 6-week mortality rate of 15%-25% with a high late rebleeding rate (60%-70%) without prophylaxis. Prophylaxis is the mainstay of management in patients who have gastroesophageal varices including β-blockade, endoscopic band ligation, or portosystemic shunts. The following discussion focuses on the evaluation and management of nonvariceal bleeding.

Evaluation and Management

After resuscitation and stabilization of a patient with acute upper GI bleed, prepare the patient for endoscopic evaluation. It should be noted that the sensitivity of gastric lavage is only about 44% in distinguishing between upper and lower GI bleed and does not improve endoscopic visualization or rebleeding risk. There are a number of scoring systems for predicting the need for endoscopy or surgery: Rockall score (**Table 13.2**), Glasgow-Blatchford Score (GBS), and AIMS65 score. **Table 13.3** outlines the GBS, which is particularly useful for determining patients who are at very low risk (GBS 0-1), who can be safely discharged from the emergency room without endoscopy and can be followed as an outpatient. The remainder of patients who undergo endoscopy evaluation during the same admission should be started on intravenous erythromycin as well as high-dose IV PPI therapy (80-mg bolus followed by 8 mg/h infusion). Endoscopic findings of the source of bleeding can be stratified according to the Forrest classification system to guide choice of intervention and predict

TABLE 13.2 ■ Rockall Risk Score

	Score			
Variable	**0**	**1**	**2**	**3**
Age	<60	60-79	>80	
Shock	"No shock"	SBP > 100 mm Hg HR < 100 BPM	SBP > 100 mm Hg HR > 100 BPM	SBP < 100 mm Hg
Comorbidity	No major Comorbidity		CHF, IHD	Renal failure, hepatic failure, disseminated malignancy
Diagnosis	Mallory-Weiss tear, no lesion identified, no SRH	All other diagnoses		
Major SRH	None or dark spot only		Blood in upper GI tract, adherent clot, visible/spurting vessel	
Age, shock, comorbidity = initial score criteria (maximum additive score before diagnosis = 7). Diagnosis, major stigmata of recent hemorrhage =additional criteria (maximum additive score after diagnosis = 11).				

CHF, congestive heart failure; IHD, ischemic heart disease; SBP, systolic blood pressure; SRH, stigmata of recent hemorrhage.
Adapted from Rockall TA, Logan RFA, Devlin HB, Northfield TC. Risk assessment after acute upper gastrointestinal hemorrhage. *Gut.* 1996;38:316-321.

TABLE 13.3 ■ Glasgow-Blatchford Score

BUN (mg/dL)	<18.2	0
	18.2-22.3	+2
	22.4-28	+3
	28-70	+4
	>70	+6
Hemoglobin (g/dL) for men	>13	0
	12-12	+1
	10-12	+3
	<10	+6
Hemoglobin (g/dL) for women	>12	0
	10-12	+1
	<10	+6
Systolic blood pressure (mm Hg)	>110	0
	100-109	+1
	90-99	+2
	<90	+3
Other criteria	Pulse ≥ 100 (per min)	+1
	Melena present	+1
	Presentation with syncope	+2
	Liver disease history	+2
	Cardiac failure present	+2

Low risk = score of 0. Any score higher than 0 is high risk for needing intervention: transfusion, endoscopy, or surgery.

Reprinted from The Lancet, Blatchford O, Murray WR, Blatchford M. A risk score to predict need for treatment for upper-gastrointestinal hemorrhage. *Lancet*. 2000;356:1318, with permission from Elsevier.

risk of rebleeding **(Table 13.4)**. There are a variety of endoscopic interventions at the endoscopist's disposal: epinephrine injection, hemoclips, thermal coagulation, argon plasma coagulation (APC), or hemospray. In high-risk lesions, endoscopic therapy should be performed. In low-risk lesions such as ulcers with flat pigmented spots and clean bases, endoscopic therapy should be deferred. Epinephrine injection should always be used in conjunction with a second modality.

Following successful intervention, patients who have high-risk lesions should be continued on an infusion of IV PPI for 72 hours. (Continued orally as an outpatient.) Low-risk lesions can receive standard oral once-daily PPI therapy. In general, routine second-look endoscopy is not necessary in the absence of clinical evidence of rebleed. Perform repeat endoscopy with intervention if there is evidence or suspicion of rebleed or high-risk stigmata. If patients are refractory to two therapeutic endoscopic interventions, consider surgical or endovascular therapy. **Figure 13.2** summarizes an algorithmic approach to UGI bleeding.

All patients with a bleeding peptic ulcer should undergo *H pylori* testing. Eradication of *H pylori* is recommended to avoid rick of recurrent bleeding. One-year risk of rebleeding among patients with *H pylori*–associated bleeding peptic ulcers who did not receive treatment was 26%.

Although gastroscopy is the first-line evaluation of suspected upper GI bleed, when it is negative or not possible due to clinical factors, computed tomographic (CT) scanning is a useful tool to detect the source of bleeding as well as determining the severity of bleed. In fact, CT angiography (CTA) may be first line in the undifferentiated GI hemorrhage as it is highly sensitive, detecting bleeding as low as 0.3 mL/h. However, CTA lacks therapeutic capabilities. On the other hand, catheter-directed angiography is of both diagnostic and therapeutic value.

Transcatheter arterial embolization (TAE) is a technique that has been in use for GI bleeding for nearly 50 years. Historically, percutaneous access and selective angiography was performed for continuous infusion of vasopressin to achieve hemostasis by way of its vasoconstrictive effects. This was extremely time consuming as it required 18-24 hours of infusion time. Advances in the field of interventional radiology in both technique and availability of a variety of embolic agents have allowed TAE to become a mainstay of the treatment algorithm, often replacing surgery as the first-line treatment for endoscopically refractory bleeding.

With the rise of therapeutic effectiveness of endoscopy and angiography, surgery has had a diminishing role in the acute upper GI bleed. Clear indications remain the cases in which hemorrhage continues despite aforementioned therapies, or in high-risk patients to prevent future rebleed. Surgical approaches to bleeding peptic ulcer disease include more minimal approaches aimed at hemostasis and more definitive operations with the additional goal of future acid reduction for ulcer prevention.

In general, ulcer location dictates operative decision-making. For gastric ulcers, a gastrotomy should be made at the greater curvature to avoid denervating the stomach. Hemostasis can be achieved by oversewing the ulcer or resection. Biopsy should be undertaken when resection is not performed to exclude neoplasm. For duodenal

TABLE 13.4 ■ Forrest Classification

	Clinical Finding		Rebleed Risk
Grade: Ia	Arterial spurting bleeding	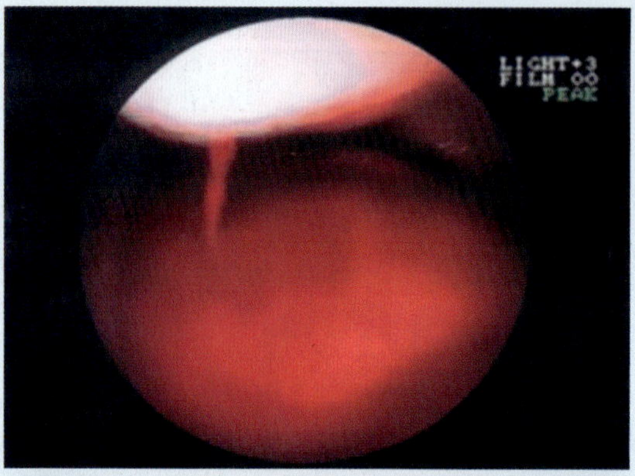	**High**
Grade: Ib	Arterial oozing/ bleeding	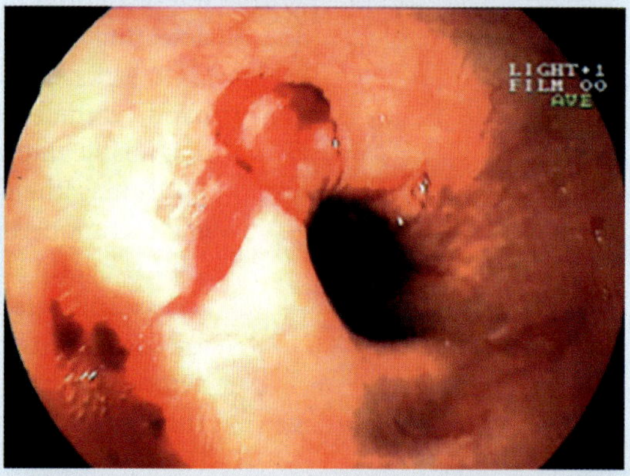	**High**
Grade: IIa	Nonbleeding visible vessel	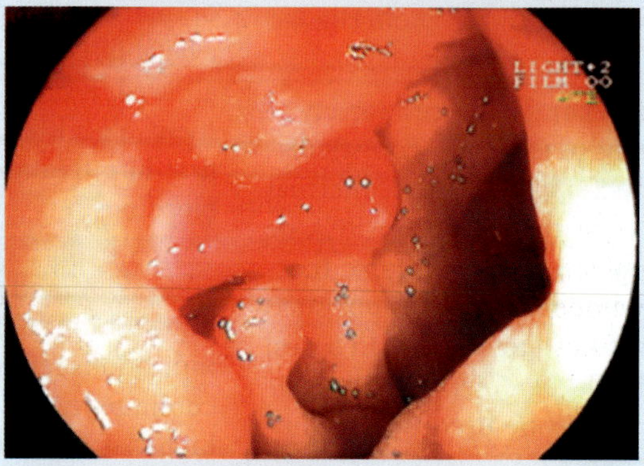	**High**
Grade: IIb	Sentinel clot, adherent	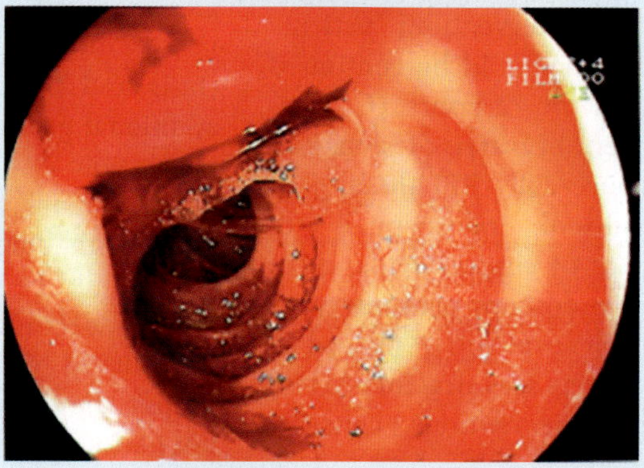	**Medium**

(Continued)

TABLE 13.4 ■ Forrest Classification *(Continued)*

	Clinical Finding		Rebleed Risk
Grade: IIc	Dark base, hematin-covered lesion	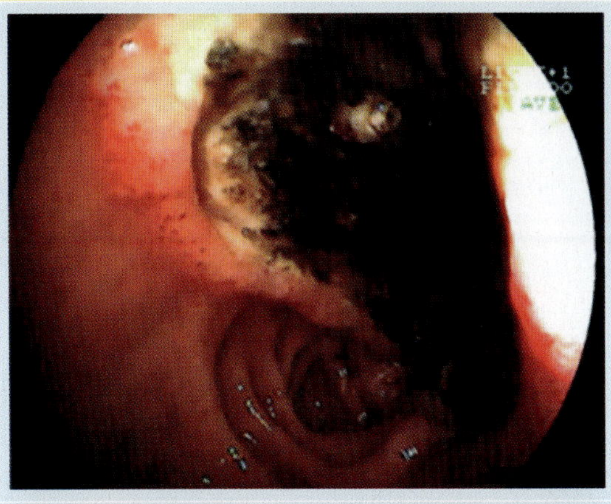	**Low**
Grade: III	No signs of recent hemorrhage	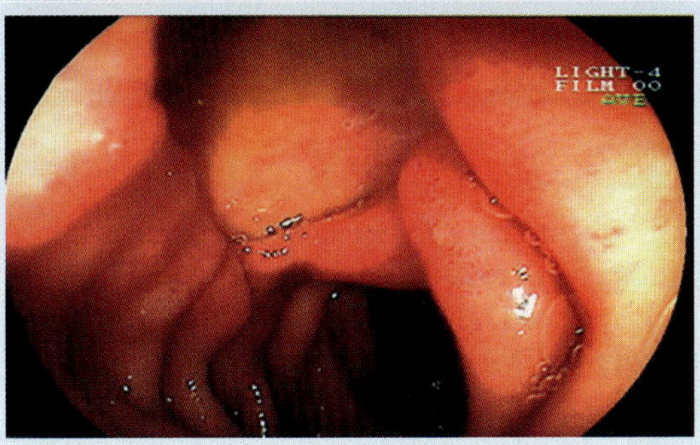	**Low**

Reprinted from The Lancet, Forrest JA, Finlayson ND, Shearman DJ. Endoscopy in gastrointestinal bleeding. *Lancet*. 1974;2:394-397, with permission from Elsevier.

ulcers, the lesion is often large and posterior with bleeding usually from gastroduodenal artery. **Figure 13.3** illustrates the surgical approach. A longitudinal incision is made across the pylorus. Two stay sutures are placed to expose the ulcer bed. Once the gastroduodenal artery is exposed and dissected, three sutures are placed to control hemorrhage. Take care to avoid injury to the common bile duct. Finally, the pylorus is closed in a transverse fashion to minimize luminal narrowing. Truncal vagotomy should be considered in the patient who has failed medical therapy, has had previous *H pylori* treatment, or needs long-term ulcerogenic medications.

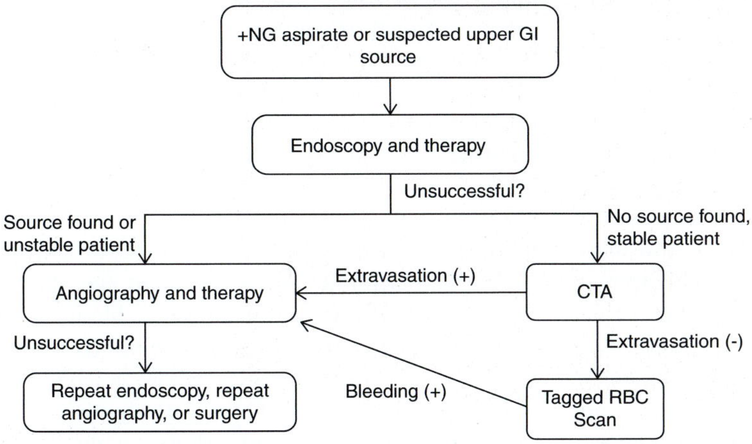

Figure 13.2 Upper GI bleed algorithm. (Adapted from British Institute of Radiology, from Wortman JR, Landman W, Fulwadhva UP, et al. CT angiography for acute gastrointestinal bleeding: what the radiologist needs to know. *Br J Radiol.* 2017;90; permission conveyed through Copyright Clearance Center, Inc.)

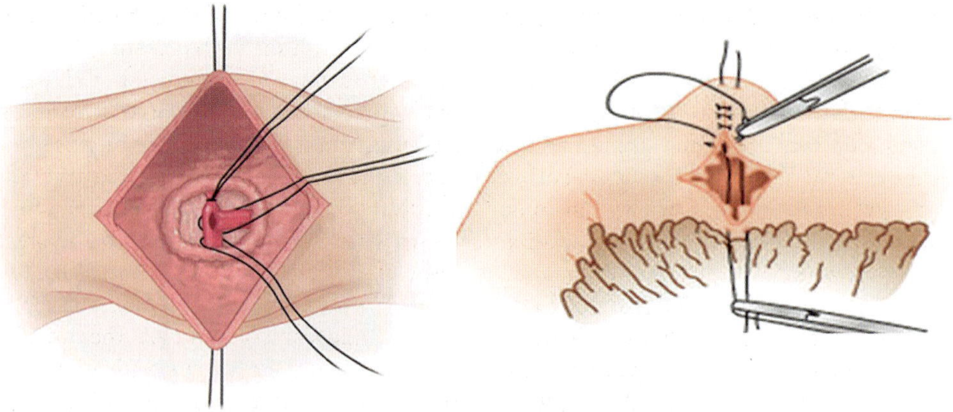

Figure 13.3 Exposure and ligation of the gastroduodenal artery. (Modified from Peitzman AB, Yealy DM, Fabian TC, C. W Schwab CW, Guyette FX, Seamon MJ, Zuckerbraun BS. *The Trauma Manual*. 5th ed. Wolters Kluwer; 2020.)

LOWER GASTROINTESTINAL HEMORRHAGE

Etiology

Lower GI bleeding is a frequent cause for hospital admissions and accounts for ~10%-15% of all acute GI bleeds. The incidence of LGIB increases with age. The vast majority of LGI bleeds arise from the colon secondary to diverticular disease or angiodysplasia. Other LGIB etiologies include small bowel diverticuli, small bowel angiodysplasia, arteriovenous malformations, anorectal disease, tumors, inflammatory bowel disease, ischemia, and ulcers. Similar to UGI bleeds, bleeding from the lower GI tract generally ceases spontaneously. However, rebleeding is frequent, ranging from 14% to 38%. Approximately 15% of patients with presumed LGIB are ultimately found to have an upper GI source for their bleeding.

Evaluation and Management

The clinical presentation of LGIB patients dictates the order and urgency that the test/intervention is performed. LGIB can be categorized as massive, moderate, or occult. Massive bleeding is defined by the passage of profuse hematochezia with hemodynamic instability. Moderate bleeding reflects hematochezia in hemodynamically stable patients. Occult bleeding refers to the presence of a positive fecal-occult blood test or iron deficiency anemia without another identifiable source and without frank hematochezia. Remember that 6% of patients with an LGIB have an underlying GI cancer. Thus, follow-up endoscopy in high-risk patients is essential. This discussion will focus on the management of massive and moderate LGIB.

The main tools for evaluation of an LGIB include imaging with computed tomography angiography (CTA), nuclear scintigraphy, or angiography as well as direct visualization with colonoscopy. Although surgery was once a necessity for patients with ongoing lower GI bleed, advanced techniques in endoscopy and angiography have improved detection and treatment, with surgery now reserved for cases in which more conservative management has failed.

Triphasic (precontrast, arterial phase, and portal venous phase) CTA of the abdomen and pelvis has become the initial diagnostic test of choice for patients with LGIB as it is widely available, with fast acquisition and an overall accuracy of ~89% in patient with massive GI bleeding. Disadvantages of CTA include the relatively high radiation dose due to the scan being performed in multiple phases, the need for iodinated intravenous contrast, and the travel with a potentially labile patient to the radiology suite. CTA can detect bleeding rates as low as 0.3 mL/min and can provide both location and potential cause of the LGIB. Active GI bleeding is identified by contrast extravasation into the bowel lumen, appearing as a "blush" on arterial phase or contrast accumulation in the lumen on portal venous phase. If no active extravasation is identified, the presence of hyperdense material in the bowel lumen may represent an intraluminal thrombus. Although CTA has high accuracy in identifying a bleed, it has no therapeutic ability.

Nuclear scintigraphy with radiotracer technetium 99m–labeled autologous red blood cells is the most sensitive test to image GI bleeding, as it can detect bleeding rates as low as 0.05 mL/min. A positive nuclear bleeding study will show focal increased activity and radiotracer uptake at the site of the bleeding and then movement of the radiolabeled blood along the GI tract. Disadvantages include the prolonged time to complete the study, limited access in emergent situations, relative cost compared with CTA, and limited ability to localize the site and determine the specific cause of the bleed. Given the static and two-dimensional planar imaging of the gamma camera, bleeding sites may be localized inaccurately to large or small bowel. In addition, given the noncontinuous rate of imaging acquisition, extravasated radiolabeled blood may represent an origin of bleeding but may also represent the transit from peristalsis at a bleeding site upstream. Similar to CTA, nuclear scintigraphy has only diagnostic capability.

Visceral angiography is an invasive modality that provides accurate localization and the opportunity for potential therapy through embolization. Conventional mesenteric angiography is now generally reserved as a means of providing therapeutic intervention for previously diagnosed bleeding on CTA or nuclear scintigraphy. However, the detection of bleeding is significantly lower than nuclear scintigraphy, with bleeding rates perceptible at 0.5 mL/min. A positive result will demonstrate contrast extravasation outside the normal boundaries of a blood vessel that can increase over time provided the bleed is continuous. The main advantage of angiography revolves around the available interventions including embolization, compared with the purely diagnostic procedures such as CTA and nuclear scintigraphy. After embolization, an angiogram can be performed to confirm successful cessation of bleeding. Other advantages include the lack of need of bowel preparation. Disadvantages include need for the administration of iodinated contrast necessitating and radiation, much like CTA. The volume of dose as well as the radiation dose also varies depending on the complexity of the case. There is also the potential of bowel ischemia from embolization as well as angiographic access site complications.

Colonoscopy is a useful and widely available diagnostic modality for patients with LGIB. The advantage of colonoscopy is that it can be performed at bedside, has the ability to diagnose bleeding from the colon without the presence of active bleeding at the time of the examination, and has multiple therapeutic possibilities. Disadvantages include the requirement of bowel preparation, sedation, the logistical complexity of coordinating after-hours colonoscopy, and the low prevalence of stigmata of hemorrhage complicate the use of colonoscopy for LGIB, particularly in urgent situations. During the colonoscopy, the colonic mucosa should be carefully inspected during both colonoscope insertion and withdrawal, with aggressive attempts made to wash residual stool and blood to identify the bleeding site. Intubate the terminal ileum to exclude proximal blood suggestive of a small bowel lesion. Obscuration of the mucosa due to intraluminal blood and intestinal contents can limit the extent of evaluation of bowel lumen during endoscopic evaluation of an LGIB. Endoscopic hemostasis therapy should be provided to LGIB patients with high-risk endoscopic stigmata of bleeding including active bleeding, nonbleeding visible vessel, or adherent clot.

Obtain a focused history, physical examination, and laboratory evaluation at the time of patient presentation to assess the severity of bleeding and its possible location and etiology. Initial patient assessment and hemodynamic resuscitation should be performed simultaneously. Any patient with hemodynamic instability must be resuscitated with restoration of circulating volume in the form of massive transfusion protocols, correction of coagulopathies, and reversal of any novel oral anticoagulants in an intensive care unit. Once resuscitation is underway, localization of the site of bleeding as well as interventions to arrest the hemorrhage should be commenced. Physical examination is usually unremarkable in terms of localizing the source of the bleed. Digital rectal examination and proctoscopy are used to evaluate for anorectal sources of bleeding. As hematochezia can be present with UGIB, an upper source should be excluded with minimum nasogastric tube aspiration. There is no clear evidence for the benefit of colonoscopy vs CTA as the initial procedure for a patient with an LGIB. With the ease of access to CTA, it has become the initial diagnostic test of choice for the normotensive patient with an LGIB. If there is extravasation identified or the patient is unstable, the next step should be to proceed to visceral angiography with embolization. If unable to control hemorrhage angiographically, consider surgical intervention. If no extravasation is seen on CTA, the patient should undergo colonoscopy after bowel prep. The endoscopic hemostasis modality used (mechanical, thermal, injection, or combination) is most often guided by the etiology of bleeding, access to the bleeding site, and endoscopist experience with the various hemostasis modalities. If no bleeding site is identified on either CTA or colonoscopy, nuclear scintigraphy should be performed to assist with anatomic localization of the hemorrhage (**Figure 13.4**).

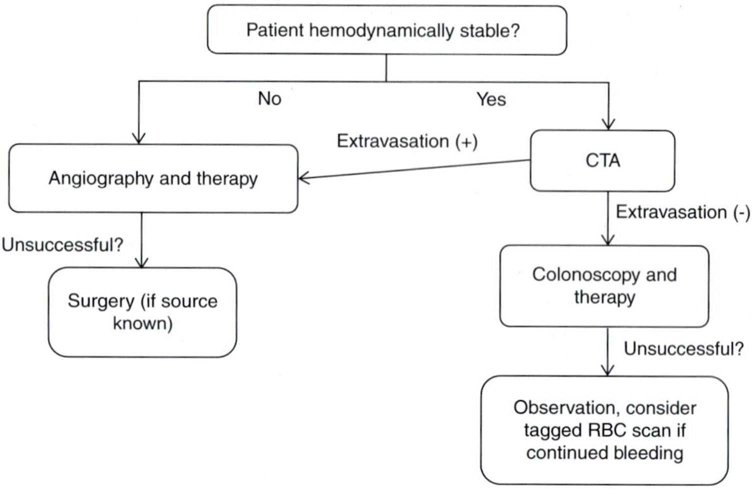

Figure 13.4 Lower GI bleed algorithm. (Adapted from British Institute of Radiology, Wortman JR, Landman W, Fulwadhva UP, et al. CT angiography for acute gastrointestinal bleeding: what the radiologist needs to know. *Br J Radiol*. 2017;90; permission conveyed through Copyright Clearance Center, Inc.)

In general, surgery for acute LGIB should be considered after other therapeutic options have failed and should take into consideration the extent and success of prior bleeding control measures, severity and source of bleeding, and the level of comorbid disease. It is important to very carefully localize the source of bleeding whenever possible before surgical resection to avoid continued or recurrent bleeding from an unresected culprit lesion. If the site of hemorrhage is definitively established, then standard colectomy (right or left) is the surgical intervention of choice. If site is definitely colon but cannot be localized, then subtotal colectomy with end ileostomy is preferred. It is essential that the anorectum and sigmoid colon are evaluated prior to total abdominal colectomy with rigid sigmoidoscopy in OR to exclude a stercoral ulcer or an anal canal source of bleeding.

Consider strategies to prevent recurrent bleeding. Avoid nonsteroidal anti-inflammatory drug use in patients with a history of acute lower GI bleeding, particularly if secondary to diverticulosis or angioectasia. Patients with established cardiovascular disease who require aspirin as secondary prophylaxis should generally resume aspirin as soon as possible after bleeding ceases and at least within 7 days. The exact timing depends on the severity of bleeding, perceived adequacy of hemostasis, and the risk of a thromboembolic event.

SMALL BOWEL BLEEDING

A source of small bowel bleeding should be considered in patients with GI bleeding after performance of a normal upper and lower endoscopic examination. Bleeding from the small intestine remains a relatively uncommon event, accounting for ~5% of all patients presenting with GI bleeding. Given advances in small bowel imaging with video capsule endoscopy (VCE), deep enteroscopy, and radiographic imaging, the cause of bleeding in the small bowel can now be identified in most patients. CT enterography should be performed in patients with suspected obstruction before VCE or after negative VCE examinations. If a source of bleeding is identified in the small bowel that is associated with significant ongoing anemia and/or active bleeding, the patient should be managed with endoscopic therapy. When there is acute overt hemorrhage in the unstable patient, angiography should be performed emergently to identify and treat the hemorrhagic site. Conservative management is recommended for patients without a source found after small bowel investigation, whereas repeat diagnostic investigations are recommended for patients with initial negative small bowel evaluations and ongoing overt or occult bleeding.

In summary, the workup of lower GI bleeding includes endoscopy, CTA, nuclear scintigraphy, conventional angiography, and surgery. The clinical presentation of patients dictates the order and urgency that the test/intervention is performed. Radiologic assessment of lower GI bleeding has come to the forefront of the workup, especially in patients with acute ongoing bleeding. Conventional angiography with embolization is now often the first-line treatment in patients who are unstable with surgery now reserved for cases in which more conservative management has failed.

SUMMARY

- Acute GI bleeding requires emergency resuscitation, investigation, and management.

- The GI tract is a more common and severe source of hemorrhage than the lower GI tract.
- Approximately 80% of GI bleeding stops spontaneously or with an initial intervention.
- Location of bleed matters both diagnostically and therapeutically.
- UGI bleed: EGD will likely identify source.
- LGI bleed: CTA and/or colonoscopy should localize the source.
- Capsule endoscopy or CT enterography may be needed to identify small bowel source.
- Endoscopic therapy is first-line treatment for GI bleeding, then angiography/embolization.
- Operative management is required in only 2%-5% of all patients with GI bleeding.
- Avoid operating without localization of source.

SUGGESTED READINGS

Abe N, Takeuchi H, Yanagida O, Sugiyama M, Atomi Y. Surgical indications and procedures for bleeding peptic ulcer: surgery for bleeding peptic ulcer. *Dig Endosc.* 2010;22:S35-S37. doi:10.1111/j.1443-1661.2010.00966.x

Barkun AN, Bardou M, Kuipers EJ, et al.; International Consensus Upper Gastrointestinal Bleeding Conference Group. International Consensus Recommendations on the Management of Patients With Nonvariceal Upper Gastrointestinal Bleeding. *Ann Intern Med.* 2010;152(2):101-113.

Blatchford O, et al. A risk score to predict need for treatment for upper gastrointestinal haemorrhage. *Lancet.* 2000;356(9238):1318-1321.

Carney BW, Khatri G, Shenoy-Bhangle AS. The role of imaging in gastrointestinal bleed. *Cardiovasc Diagn Ther.* 2019;9(S1):S88-S96. doi:10.21037/cdt.2018.12.07

Cirocchi R, Grassi V, Cavaliere D, et al. New trends in acute management of colonic diverticular bleeding: a systematic review. *Medicine* 2015;94:e1710.

D'Hondt A, Haentjens L, Brassart N, Flamme F, Preiser J-C. Uncontrolled bleeding of the gastrointestinal tract. *Curr Opin Crit Care.* 2017;23(6):549-555. doi:10.1097/MCC.0000000000000452

Gerson LB, Fidler JL, Cave DR, Leighton JA. ACG clinical guideline: diagnosis and management of small bowel bleeding. *Am J Gastroenterol.* 2015;110:1265-1287.

Gisbert JP, Khorrami S, Carballo F, et al. Meta-analysis: *Helicobacter pylori* eradication therapy vs. antisecretory non-eradication therapy for prevention of recurrent bleeding for peptic ulcer. *Aliment Pharmacol Ther.* 2004;19:617-629.

Gralnek I, Dumonceau J-M, Kuipers E, et al. Diagnosis and management of nonvariceal upper gastrointestinal hemorrhage: European Society of Gastrointestinal Endoscopy (ESGE) Guideline. *Endoscopy.* 2015;47(10):a1-a46. doi:10.1055/s-0034-1393172

Greco L, Zhang J, Ross H. Surgical options and approaches for lower gastrointestinal bleeding: when do we operate and what do we do? *Clin Colon Rectal Surg.* 2020;33:10-15.

He B, Yang J, Xiao J, Gu J, et al. Diagnosis of lower gastrointestinal bleeding by multi-slice CT angiography: a meta-analysis. *Eur J Radiol.* 2017;93:40-45.

Kim G, Soto JA, Morrison T. Radiologic assessment of gastrointestinal bleeding. *Gastroenterol Clin N Am.* 2018;47:501-514.

Laine L. Upper gastrointestinal bleeding due to a peptic ulcer. *N Engl J Med.* 2016;374:2367-2376.

Laine L, Jensen DM. Management of patients with ulcer bleeding. *Am J Gastroenterol.* 2012;107:345-360.

Lhewa DY, Strate LL. Pros and cons of colonoscopy in management of acute lower gastrointestinal bleeding. *World J Gastroenterol.* 2012;18:1185-1190.

Morrison TC, Wells M, Fidler JF, Soto JA. Imaging workup of acute and occult lower gastrointestinal bleeding. *Radiol Clin N Am.* 2018;56:791-804.

Oakland K, Chadwick G, East JE, et al. Diagnosis and management of acute lower gastrointestinal bleeding: guidelines from the British Society of Gastroenterology. *Gut.* 2019;68:776-789.

Pasha SF, Shergill A, Acosta RD, et al. The role of endoscopy in the patient with lower GI bleeding. *Gastrointest Endosc.* 2014;79(6):875-885. doi:10.1016/j.gie.2013.10.039

Rondonotti E, Marmo R, Petraccini M, deFranchis R, Pennazio M. The American Society for Gastrointestinal Endoscopy (ASGE) diagnostic algorithm for obscure gastrointestinal bleeding: eight burning questions from everyday clinical practice. *Dig Liver Dis.* 2013;45:179-185.

Samuel R, Bilal M, Tayyem O, Guturu P. Evaluation and management of non-variceal upper gastrointestinal bleeding. *Dis Mon* 2018;64:333-343.

Stanley AJ, Laine L, Dalton HR, et al. Comparison of risk scoring systems for patients presenting with upper gastrointestinal bleeding: international multicentre prospective study. *BMJ.* 2017;356:i6432. doi:10.1136/bmj.i6432

Strate LL, Gralnek IM. ACG clinical guideline: management of patients with acute lower gastrointestinal bleeding. *Am J Gastroenterol.* 2016;111(4):459-474. doi:10.1038/ajg.2016.4

Tarasconi A, Coccolini F, Biffl WL, et al. Perforated and bleeding peptic ulcer: WSES guidelines. *World J Emerg Surg.* 2020;15(1):3. doi:10.1186/s13017-019-0283-9

Weledji EP. Acute gastrointestinal bleeding: a review. *Int J Surg Global Health.* 2020;3:e18.

Wortman JR, Landman W, Fulwadhva UP, et al. CT angiography for acute gastrointestinal bleeding: what the radiologist needs to know. *Br J Radiol.* 2017;90. https://doi.org/10.1259/bjr.20170076

CHAPTER

14 Acute Pancreatitis

Mark H. Hoofnagle, Nathan T. Mowery, and Jose J. Diaz Jr

CASE PRESENTATION

A 49-year-old male with a history of SMA thrombosis/dissection, chronic anxiety, hypertension, and alcohol abuse presents to the emergency department complaining of abdominal pain with a lipase of 1800. He was admitted and managed with pain meds, and IV fluids resuscitation. A CT scan (**Figure 14.1**) demonstrated an inflamed edematous pancreas with minimal peripancreatic edema. He improved over 2 days and was discharged to home.

Four days later, the patient returned to the ED. He presented with abdominal pain and hematemesis. He had a syncopal event with EMS. He received two units of PRBCs and was transferred back to the tertiary medical center. On arrival, he was tachycardic to 110 bpm, BP 100/60 mm Hg, on room air, and on no vasopressors. His physical examination revealed tachycardia, and abdomen was distended and tender to palpation. His labs were WBC 25.7 × 10^3 μL, H/H—9.5 g/dL/26.2%, PTT 24 seconds, INR 1.1, Ca 8.4 mmol/L, glucose 185 mmol/L, and serum creatine of 0.71 mg/dL. CT scan (**Figure 14.2**) showed progression of acute pancreatitis with areas of pancreatic necrosis and increased peripancreatic stranding. He was admitted to the ICU for further resuscitation and pain management.

Twelve days after his second admission, he had a change in his clinical course with increased abdominal pain and fever. A stat CT scan (**Figures 14.3 and 14.4**) demonstrated emphysematous pancreatitis, increased size of the large rim-enhancing peripancreatic fluid collection and interval development of internal gas pockets. The patient was further resuscitated, and antibiotics started. He was not a good candidate for a percutaneous drainage due to bowel surrounding the collection. He was evaluated by GI for possible endoscopic internal drainage but was felt to be too early in his course to perform a transgastric drainage. His sepsis progressed and he went to the OR for an open transgastric necrosectomy. The patient did well and was discharged home in 10 days.

Question: *What is a decision point to "Step-Up" the management of acute pancreatitis from continued volume resuscitation?*

Answer: *CT scan evidence of retroperitoneal air that is concerning for infected pancreatic or peripancreatic necrosis.*

DIAGNOSIS OF PANCREATITIS

The yearly global incidence of acute pancreatitis (AP) is 34 cases per 100 000 people. However, there are regional differences with higher rates in North America and Western Pacific regions as defined by the World Health Organization. In 20% of cases of AP, patients will develop a recurrent episode of AP, and approximately a third of patients with a recurrent episode of pancreatitis will develop chronic pancreatitis. Approximately 20%-80% of AP patients that progress to chronic pancreatitis may develop diabetes. The disease affects men slightly more than women and the incidence increases with age. About 20% of pancreatitis cases are severe and 10%-30% will result in mortality.

Clinical diagnosis of AP is based on the Atlanta Classification, an international consensus guideline on diagnosis and severity scoring of AP first developed in 1992, revised in 2012, and generally accepted by all society diagnosis and management guidelines (**Table 14.1**). These diagnostic criteria require at least two of the three features of: (1) abdominal pain consistent with AP (epigastric, severe, persistent, often radiating to the back), (2) elevated serum lipase or amylase activity greater than three times the upper limit of normal, and (3) radiologic findings of AP on an IV contrast-enhanced CT or MRI/ultrasound. Imaging is not required or recommended in all presentations of pancreatitis if the laboratory and clinical examination findings correlate. Evidence of infective pancreatic necrosis is rare

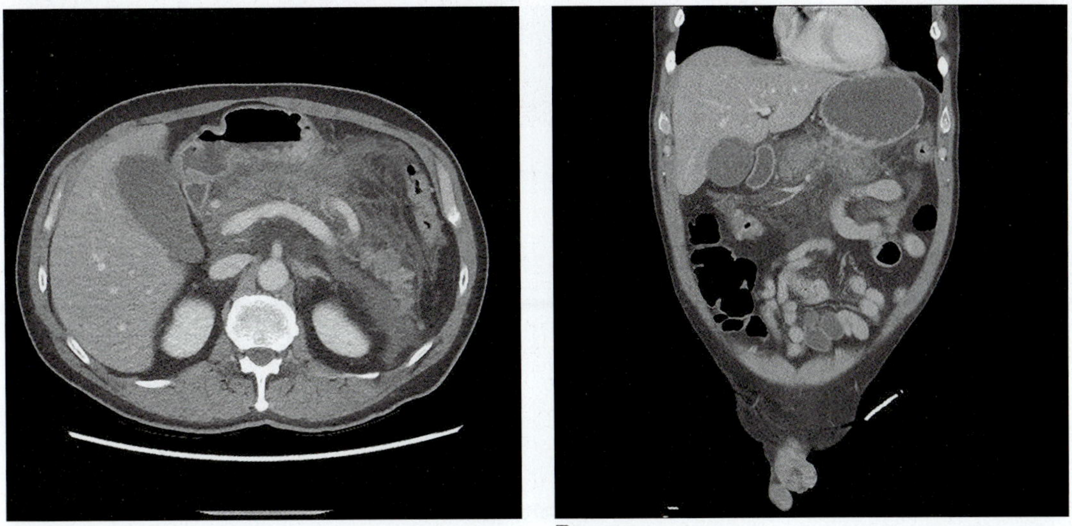

A B

Figure 14.1 A, B. Representative images from the initial CT of a 49-year-old male who presents with alcohol-induced pancreatitis showing classic necrosis of the body of the pancreas with a viable head and tail. There is significant stranding/edema but no defined fluid collection.

before day 7 since the onset of pain. An RUQ ultrasound is indicated to evaluate for possible gallstone etiology. CT imaging in patients with severe AP is recommended in a delayed fashion to evaluate for necrosis, pseudocysts, collections, or other complications of pancreatitis.

The Atlanta criteria further define AP as interstitial edematous pancreatitis or necrotizing pancreatitis based on whether there is radiologic evidence of necrosis on CT and its severity based on the presence of systemic inflammatory response and organ dysfunction using the modified Marshall Criteria to define organ failure and the SIRS criteria of systemic inflammatory response syndrome (**Table 14.2**).

PATHOPHYSIOLOGY AND INITIAL APPROACH TO THE PANCREATITIS PATIENT

The most frequent cause of pancreatitis is gallstone disease, then alcohol, and less commonly idiopathic or due to triglycerides, hypocalcemia,

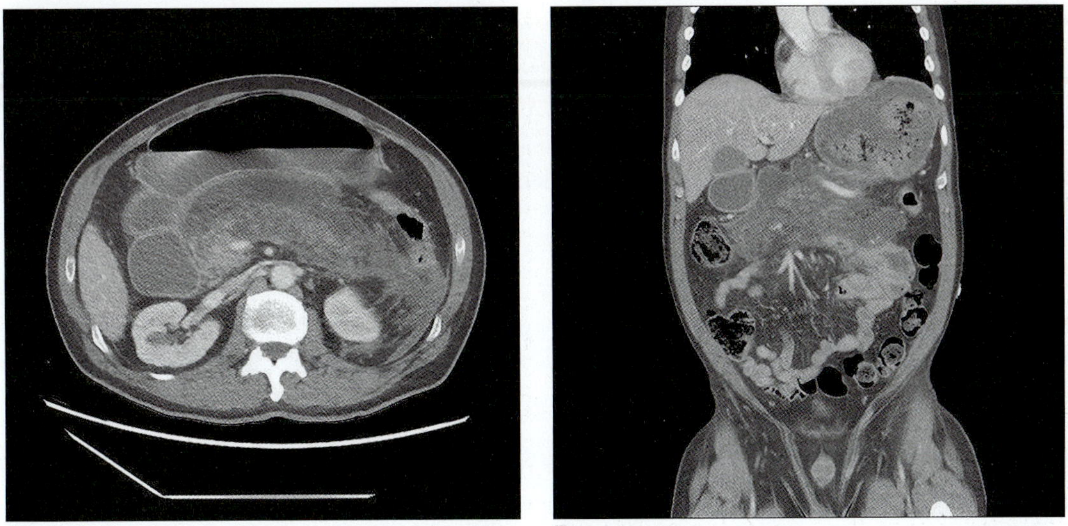

A B

Figure 14.2 A, B. Representative images from the same patient after presenting 4 days after discharge when he presents to the ED with signs of escalating inflammation and progression of disease. The pancreatitis has evolved and now has ill-defined fluid collections and the suggestion of delayed gastric emptying.

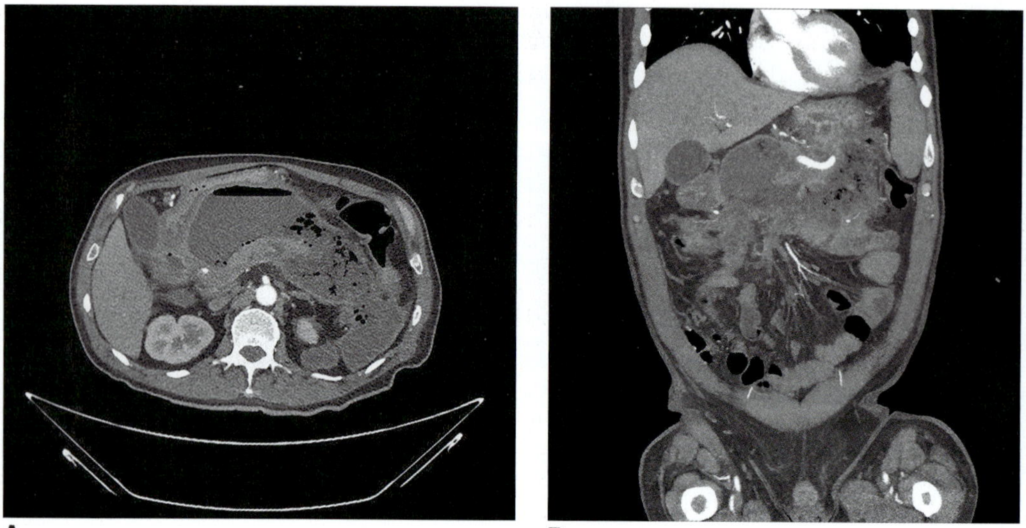

A B

Figure 14.3 A, B. Further imaging obtained 12 days later when the patient develops signs of sepsis shows emphysematous pancreatitis, increased size of the large rim-enhancing peripancreatic fluid collection, and interval development of gas within the collection. These findings are consistent with infected necrosis.

medications, toxins, trauma, post-ERCP, or other causes. Determination of the cause is important to guide therapy and prevent recurrence of disease. Recurrent pancreatitis is decreased by more than 50% in idiopathic pancreatitis when these patients undergo cholecystectomy suggesting subclinical stone disease (microlithiasis) or sludge may contribute to this process. Most international guidelines on management agree that patients should undergo laboratory testing with a complete blood count, comprehensive metabolic panel, lipase, amylase and triglycerides, as well as a right upper quadrant ultrasound to help determine etiology of the pancreatitis. C-reactive protein (CRP) or procalcitonin may be of additional value in assessing the severity of pancreatitis or presence of infected pancreatic necrosis.

Patients with gallstone pancreatitis, confirmed on RUQ ultrasound, with evidence of cholangitis should undergo MRCP (if needed to confirm stones, or more rarely a tumor, in the distal bile duct) and ERCP to relieve biliary obstruction within 24 hours of presentation to the hospital. All GI and surgical societies agree that patients with gallstone pancreatitis should undergo cholecystectomy prior to discharge from the hospital

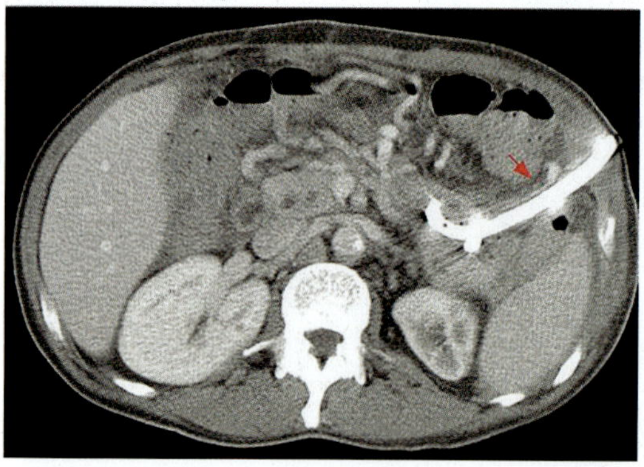

Figure 14.4 Imaging showing a large bore percutaneous drain (arrow shows drain) placed in the left flank, anterior to the spleen that is the ideal route to facilitate a later "step-up" procedure.

TABLE 14.1 ■ Revised Atlanta Classification

Mild AP
No organ failure
No local (effusions or collections) or systemic complications (SIRS)
Moderate AP
Transient organ failure (<48 h)
Local or systemic complications without persistent organ failure
Severe AP
Persistent single or multiple organ failure (>48 h)

From Foster BR, Jensen KK, Bakis G, Shaaban AM, Coakley FV. Revised Atlanta classification for acute pancreatitis: a pictorial essay. *Radiographics*. 2016;36: 675-687. Copyright ©2022 Radiological Society of North America, Inc. (RSNA), All Rights Reserved.

TABLE 14.2 ■ Modified Marshall Criteria

Marshall Criteria	Score >2 Is Organ Failure, >48 h Is Persistent				
Organ System	**0**	**1**	**2**	**3**	**4**
Respiratory (PaO_2/FiO_2 ratio)	>400	301-400	201-300	101-200	≤101
Renal (serum creatinine)	<1.4 mg/dL	1.4-1.8 mg/dL	1.9-3.6 mg/dL	3.6-4.9 mg/dL	>4.9 mg/dL
Cardiovascular (systolic blood pressure, pH)	>90 mm Hg	<90 mm Hg, fluid responsive	<90 mm Hg, not fluid responsive	<90 mm Hg, pH < 7.3	<90 mm Hg, pH < 7.2

to prevent recurrence and as the complication rate for same-admission surgery is not higher. Readmission with recurrent pancreatitis is common with delayed management. In patients with severe pancreatitis, a delay of 4-6+ weeks should be considered or until a pseudocyst matures so it may be addressed at the same time. Endoscopic stenting of the common bile duct may prevent recurrence in patients who are not surgical candidates. Diagnostic confusion may be resolved by measuring the ALT, which if elevated more than 3× in a patient without risk factors for alcoholic pancreatitis is 95% predictive for gallstone pancreatitis. Early MRCP/ERCP within 24 hours for biliary pancreatitis is recommended by all scientific societies if there is evidence of biliary obstruction causing cholangitis. The societies similarly agree that MRCP or EUS should follow RUQ ultrasound if choledocholithiasis is present or suspected without cholangitis, with timing determined by severity of illness or obstruction. They do not endorse routine ERCP in gallstone pancreatitis without obstruction.

Alcoholic pancreatitis is diagnosed primarily clinically and may be prevented by abstinence from alcohol. All clinical and social resources should be brought to bear to prevent relapse with alcohol intake, given the increasing morbidity and mortality of subsequent episodes. Calcium and triglyceride levels should also be measured when alcohol or gallstones are not the obvious causes. Triglyceride levels more than three times normal should be considered consistent with pancreatitis due to hypertriglyceridemia. Hypertriglyceridemia requires acute management with NPO, insulin drip, and dextrose source. Plasmapheresis is indicated if triglyceride levels do not return to less than three times normal within 48 hours. Chronically, triglyceride-lowering medications should be considered once they can be safely started. Management of recurrent AP is the subject of international guidelines, which guide the workup of idiopathic recurrent pancreatitis.

Recurrent idiopathic acute pancreatitis (IRAP) is diagnosed when exclusion of other common causes (biliary, alcoholic, triglycerides, etc.) by history, routine laboratory tests, conventional imaging, and workup does not yield the etiology of the episode. Certain medications should be considered and evaluated for risk of causing pancreatitis. Pancreas divisum is not a clear established cause of IRAP and should not be automatically considered the cause based on ERCP/EUS/MRCP findings. Genetic mutations and polymorphisms (*CFTR, SPINK1, PRSS1, CTRC*) may be investigated, as well as ampullary neoplasms, choledochal cysts, or other aberrant anatomy or consideration of multifactorial causes. Patients should be evaluated by EUS as a first-line test after conventional CT scan, MRCP (with secretin stimulation), and ultrasound. ERCP and sphincter of Oddi manometry and subsequent biliary sphincterotomy in patients without any anatomic abnormalities is a reasonable option. While empiric cholecystectomy without evidence of gallbladder disease and normal LFTs is not recommended by these guidelines, we disagree and believe it should be strongly considered as it is known to decrease recurrent episodes by >50%. Autoimmune pancreatitis is a rare cause and may benefit from serological testing for IgG4 and empiric steroids if there are imaging features suggestive of autoimmune disease on MRCP.

SCORING

There are at least 17 validated pancreatitis scoring systems developed since the original 11 Ranson criteria. Some scores may be more valuable in evaluation of the patient in the emergency room to determine disposition, including the Glasgow criteria, Acute Physiology and Chronic Health Evaluation II (APACHE II), computed tomography

TABLE 14.3 ■ Common Pancreatitis Prognostic Tools (Timing From Admission)

	Variables Included
Ranson criteria ≥3 Severe AP (0 and 48 h)	At admission, age >55 y, WBC > 16 000/mL, glucose >200 mg/dL, LDH >350 IU/mL, AST > 250 IU/mL; then at 48 h hematocrit decrease >10%, BUN increase >5 mg/dL, calcium <8 mg/dL, PaO_2 < 60 mm Hg, base deficit >4 mEq/L, fluid sequestration >6 L
APACHE II ≥8 Severe AP (0 and 48 h)	Alterations/abnormalities in temperature, MAP, heart rate, respiratory rate, PaO_2, arterial pH, HCO_3, sodium, potassium, creatinine, hematocrit, WBC, altered Glasgow Coma Score, age, chronic health points
BISAP ≥3 Severe AP (0 and 48 h)	BUN > 25 mg/dL, altered mental status GCS < 15, SIRS criteria ≥2, age >60 y, pleural effusion
Glasgow-Imrie score ≥3 Severe AP (0 and 48 h)	Age > 55 y, WBC > 15 000/mL, glucose >180 mg/dL, BUN > 45 mg/dL, PaO_2 < 60 mm Hg, calcium <8 g/dL, albumin <3.2 g/dL, LDH > 600 IU/L

imaging scoring systems, Bedside Index of Severity in AP (BISAP) score, Panc 3, Harmless AP Score (HAPS), and the Japanese Severity Score (**Table 14.3**). However, physicians should be aware that even at best (Glasgow criteria in this study), the scores only have moderate predictive value and continuous reassessment of patient status is indicated. Severity of pancreatitis may be defined as mild, moderate, or severe by several criteria, including Atlanta, based on presence or absence of organ failure (mild to moderate). The persistence of organ failure with or without pancreatic necrosis and infection defines moderate to severe and/or critical severity. We recommend choosing a score and using it consistently, as there is not a uniformly accepted prognostic system that performs consistently better and there is no consensus among societies of which is best.

MANAGEMENT

Resuscitation: Fluids—The Goldilocks Approach

A recent systematic review of fluid resuscitation strategies found equivalent numbers of studies across 15 trials to support either aggressive goal directed or nonaggressive fluid resuscitation in AP and general low quality of evidence on outcomes related to fluid therapy. Guiding much of the protocols on resuscitation in pancreatitis is early goal-directed fluid therapy (EGDT) strategies that have largely become standard of care in treatment of sepsis and septic shock. In Rivers follow-up 2008 review of EGDT, he reported over 50% RR reduction with sepsis improving on the initial findings of EGDT, and several subsequent meta-analyses have found EGDT may be lifesaving in severe septic shock. Complicating this are recent international, prospective randomized controlled trials such as ProMISe, ARISE, and ProCESS that have been equivocal on the value of rigid protocolization of care, which raise questions as to whether "usual care" has been so altered by Surviving Sepsis Campaign guidelines that it is no longer distinguishable from EGDT.

The sterile systemic inflammatory shock of pancreatitis and its pathophysiology may not directly translate from EGDT in sepsis, especially with the morbid risk of increased intra-abdominal hypertension, and abdominal compartment syndrome with fluid overload in these patients. Even in EGDT in sepsis, fluid overload is a known risk factor for mortality and multiple organ failure. There is evidence that protocolized practices such as goal-directed fluid resuscitation may cause fluid overload; those patients will experience higher end-organ damage and increased mortality.

Thus, in pancreatitis, it is not surprising that evidence for protocolized aggressive fluid resuscitation vs usual care has been persistently equivocal. Instead of pursuing the elusive optimal protocol for EGDT resuscitation, we suggest general critical care principles on fluid resuscitation, and intravascular fluid status assessed and reassessed often using multiple methods of clinical fluid responsiveness. This will change throughout each patient's clinical course. Pancreatitis patients often present clinically dehydrated and hemoconcentrated with an elevated hematocrit, BUN, and creatinine. Patients generally respond to fluids and benefit from aggressive early fluid resuscitation within the first 24 hours, especially within the initial 4-6 hours. We recommend a balanced salt solution such as Ringer lactate (LR). There is some evidence of benefit of

LR in AP relative to normal saline and is recommended by several society guidelines. After 24 hours, patients will encounter significant morbidity and mortality with excess fluid resuscitation, which can result in multiorgan failure (MOF) or abdominal compartment syndrome; this observation makes protocolization-based resuscitation on simple algorithms insufficient. There is additional evidence that in severe AP patients may not benefit even from early fluid resuscitation—especially when organ failure has already ensued.

Resuscitation based on CVP is a poor target, yet persistent in clinical practice. Assessing fluid resuscitation requires more than simple protocolized administration of fluids, or a single numeric target, and must rely on thoughtful critical care assessment of each patients' fluid status via multiple techniques. Assessments of end-organ perfusion include pulse-pressure variation, bedside echocardiography, ultrasound, and dynamic maneuvers such as the passive leg raise (although notably increased intra-abdominal hypertension may alter this test and stroke volume variation) and the end-expiratory occlusion test. Patients with severe systemic inflammatory response due to AP may manifest cardiac dysfunction. Clinicians should carefully avoid the morbidity of fluid overload with crystalloids and consider vasopressors and inotropes to raise systolic blood pressure in the fluid-unresponsive patients.

If patients do not respond to a test bolus with an increase of stroke volume >10% or fail to show evidence of fluid responsiveness using other bedside assessments, more fluid will only increase risk of organ injury and consequent mortality. Thus, after EGDT in the first 4-6 hours, we recommend a Goldilocks approach—avoidance of both fluid overload and hypovolemia as each extreme increases the possibility of MOF and mortality, with thoughtful consideration of each additional bolus of crystalloids based on serial bedside assessments after the first 24 hours.

Nutrition

In the 1970s, parenteral nutrition was originally shown to be an adjunct to the classic practice of making AP patients NPO. Subsequently, evidence from animal models suggested bacterial translocation may be part of the pathogenesis of infected pancreatic necrosis. Thus, enteral feeding was proposed to benefit in prevention of septic pancreatitis by improving mucosal barrier function and gut perfusion.

In 1993, the first trial comparing parenteral and nasojejunal (NJ) total parenteral nutrition (TPN) in 34 patients with lipase >1000 demonstrated improvement in clinical parameters and decreased ICU stay. Small subsequent trials showed enteral nutrition was more cost-effective and may result in faster resolution of inflammatory state and decreased mucosal permeability than parenteral nutrition.

Subsequent trials have failed to demonstrate a benefit of early nasoenteric tube feeding compared to oral diet initiated after 72 hours in reducing death or infections in pancreatitis patients at high risk for complications. However, many of the trials of enteral feeding may have diluted the benefit from studying patients with *predicted* severe AP based on criteria, rather than patients who had been diagnosed with severe AP. In this patient population with diagnosed AP, NJ enteral nutrition compared to TPN decreased the rate of infected pancreatic necrosis from 74% to 20%, similarly reduced multiorgan dysfunction (79% vs 31%) and death (35% vs 5%). This may explain why systematic meta-analysis including trials with more variable criteria for severe AP and confounding variables have not demonstrated a mortality benefit but have shown decreased necrosis and inflammatory markers. Subsequent trials have also compared TPN and NJ feeding to nasogastric feeding and found that nasogastric feeding is similar in terms of tolerance, mortality, and complications to NJ feeds but notably fail to replicate the same dramatic reduction in mortality from enteral feeding vs TPN. Other nutritional strategies of probiotics, immune-nutrition, vitamins, and prokinetics have failed to show significant benefit.

Thus, the likelihood is that early enteral feeding helps maintain mucosal barrier function and prevents the intestinal mucosa from ischemia, resulting in a benefit in preventing septic complications of pancreatitis, may decrease overall inflammatory state, and probably decreases mortality. It is strongly recommended by most societies' guidelines on pancreatitis (with the exception of the British Society of Gastroenterology Working Party on Pancreatitis, which finds the evidence inconclusive) as well as ASPEN. However, the clinician must be attuned to other factors impacting gut function including risk of gastric or duodenal outlet obstruction, high pressor requirements, ileus, or other factors preventing tolerance of enteric feeds. TPN, as a second-line therapy, should be instituted in cases in which enteral feeding is not tolerated, inadequate, or impossible.

Pain

Pain control with hydromorphone hydrochloride is preferred over morphine or fentanyl in the nonintubated patient. NSAIDs for risk of kidney injury and oversedation should be avoided. The ideal pain control regimen has not been discovered and multimodal pain control and adjuvant pain therapies such as epidural pain control may prevent excess narcotic use, which may aggravate ileus, low bowel motility, and risk of aspiration.

Triglycerides

Pancreatitis due to hypertriglyceridemia may have more severe symptoms and worse outcomes than alcoholic pancreatitis. In addition to usual care, the mainstay of treatment for triglyceride-induced pancreatitis is lowering triglycerides. Unlike other etiologies, most protocols emphasize a period of NPO to aid in decreasing triglyceride levels, which will decrease with fasting. Initiation of an insulin drip, with a dextrose source to prevent hypoglycemia, will help rapidly lower triglyceride levels with a target reduction of triglycerides to less than three times normal or 500 mg/dL. In patients with severe AP or inability to lower triglycerides, apheresis, or plasma exchange, should be considered early. Patients who would not tolerate these strategies may then benefit from continuous venovenous hemofiltration. Patients with pancreatitis due to hypertriglyceridemia should be counseled in prevention for recurrence with triglyceride-lowering medications such as gemfibrozil and niacin started once they tolerate PO and should also be counseled in abstinence from alcohol intake and diet and other risk factors for hypertriglyceridemia.

Continuous Hemofiltration, CVVH, CVVHD

Clinical and animal data suggest a role for high-volume continuous hemofiltration strategies in attenuating the sterile inflammation that results in MOF, preventing fluid overload, and decreasing intra-abdominal pressure in acute pancreatitis. However promising, high-quality data are lacking, but it may be considered as an adjunct in other goals of critical care, such as lowering fluid overload and intra-abdominal hypertension, rather than a routine component of care in severe AP, until future high-quality studies show conclusive benefit.

Ventilation

Severe AP frequently results in multiorgan failure including the adult respiratory distress syndrome (ARDS), likely due to a systemic inflammatory process and cytokine release resulting in pulmonary vascular permeability and inflammation. We recommend low stretch ventilation compatible with ARDSnet recommendations, even prior to onset of ARDS in ventilated patients as there are conclusive benefits of low stretch in patients without ARDS such as those undergoing surgery. The Berlin definition of ARDS is based on characteristic x-ray findings, not caused by other physiologic derangement such as cardiogenic edema and graded based on the severity of the hypoxia (**Table 14.4**). Severe and persistent organ dysfunction is ominous for early mortality in AP, and meticulous critical care is needed to avoid increasing mortality in severe pancreatitis-associated ARDS.

TABLE 14.4 ■ Berlin Criteria of ARDS Severity

Grade	PaO_2/FIO_2 (mm Hg) on PEEP > 5
Mild	≤201-300
Moderate	≤101-200
Severe	≤100

FIO_2, fraction of inspired oxygen; PaO_2, partial pressure of arterial oxygen; a decreased PaO_2/FiO_2 ratio indicates reduced arterial oxygenation from the available inhaled gas.

ECMO

Extracorporeal membrane oxygenation (ECMO) for severe ARDS complicating pancreatitis has been described since the 1990s. ECMO itself has long been known to increase inflammatory markers. However, VV ECMO should be considered an adjunct in critical care to bridge patients with ARDS through the inflammatory phase of pancreatitis until the lung injury resolves.

Prophylactic Antibiotics for Infected Pancreatic Necrosis

The routine use of antibiotics for prophylaxis in patients without other infection (eg, cholangitis) is not recommended except by the Japanese guidelines, which note a potential benefit early in acute necrotizing pancreatitis, and if used as prophylaxis, they should not extend beyond 14 days. Antibiotics are indicated for infected pancreatic necrosis diagnosed clinically from fevers, SIRS, elevated WBC, etc., positive blood cultures or by culture from fine needle aspiration, and CT scan with infected pancreatic necrosis (emphysematous pancreatitis). Antibiotic therapy should cover enteric and anaerobic organisms with regimens including expanded spectrum beta-lactamases or carbapenems and anaerobic coverage. In patients with penicillin allergies, quinolones are second-line antibiotics due to resistant organisms. Empiric fungal coverage is not recommended by expert consensus. Antibiotic guidance by routine fine needle aspiration is not universally recommended as it has high false negative rate (while a positive culture may guide therapy, a negative culture should not override clinical signs or suspicion for infection).

Hemorrhagic Conversion and Vascular Complications

Hemorrhagic pancreatitis is a rare (~1% of severe cases) but life-threatening complication of severe AP that usually occurs late within the index hospitalization or even years later, while hemorrhagic pancreatitis used to be treated exclusively operatively via celiac ligation and partial or total pancreatectomy at a mortality of 43%. Clinicians should be attuned to Cullen and Grey Turner signs, which may indicate retroperitoneal hemorrhage in unstable pancreatitis patients. Methods to treat this complication have improved significantly over the years. More recent methods of treatment via angioembolization of pseudoaneurysms of the celiac branches surrounding the pancreas have lowered the mortality to ~20%, as well as invasiveness of treatment. Surgery is now reserved for failure of endovascular approach.

Splanchnic venous thrombosis is seen in 20%-30% of severe AP. Splenic vein thrombosis is the most common and a potential cause of GI bleeding from gastric varices. Obstruction of drainage with or without pseudocyst compression of venous return increases left-sided portal pressures resulting in gastric variceal bleeding. Acute upper GI bleeding in the pancreatitis patient (acute or chronic) should result in investigations for possible variceal source and correction via banding, relief of obstruction, or even portal venous shunting. In the setting of sinistral portal hypertension due to splenic vein thrombosis, splenectomy is indicated. GI bleeding into the pancreatic duct itself is even more rare, but similarly treatable via interventional endovascular approaches.

Abdominal Compartment Syndrome

Have a high suspicion for increased abdominal hypertension. Patients with severe AP should be followed with serial abdominal examinations and bladder pressure monitoring, especially if the patient develops clinical decompensation, oliguria, or increased ventilatory peak pressures. If abdominal compartment pressure is >20 mm Hg as measured by bladder pressures, abdominal compartment syndrome (ACS) should be considered. ACS is associated with higher morbidity and mortality in AP, but when it develops, earlier decompression lowers mortality. If necessary, paralysis may be considered to lower intra-abdominal hypertension and temporize patients until they can undergo diuresis, dialysis, or paracentesis to drain at least 900-1000 mL of intra-abdominal ascites. If the classic triad of increased ventilatory peak pressures, abdominal hypertension, and oliguria develops, decompressive laparotomy for ACS should be strongly considered, especially if evidence of organ failure.

SURGICAL MANAGEMENT OF PANCREATIC NECROSIS: STEP-UP PROCEDURE

Background

Historically, open debridement was the surgery of choice for patients with infected pancreatic necrosis and, less commonly, in patients with symptomatic sterile necrosis. Although open surgical debridement has been the traditional treatment, it has been suspected that the physiologic stress of open surgical debridement increases complications. Efforts to minimize the stress of intervention have contributed significantly to the evolution of management of pancreatitis.

Over the last two decades, there have been substantial developments in the treatment of necrotizing pancreatitis. Most of this progress has been a result of the proliferation of minimally invasive treatment approaches for drainage and evacuation of pancreatic necrosis, including image-guided radiological, endoscopic transgastric, laparoscopic, and video-assisted retroperitoneal endoscopic techniques (VARD). Literature over the last 20 years has identified patient populations that have benefited from these new interventions further improving patient outcomes.

As the field of acute care surgery evolves, its practitioners are increasingly being called upon to be the primary service managing these complex patients. The timing and choice of intervention are decisions that often must be made outside of hours of optimal resource availability and are decisions that can result in increased complications.

Timing of Surgery in Acute Necrotizing Pancreatitis

- Traditionally, indications for intervention within weeks of the onset of acute pancreatitis included clearly infected acute necrotic collections associated with clinical deterioration and signs of sepsis. Infected pancreatic necrosis is the main indication for intervention currently. When needed, attempt to delay necrosectomy for 4 weeks.
- Patients with sterile necrosis who have clinical deterioration despite maximum medical support have not benefitted from surgical drainage or necrosectomy. Studies have looked at surgical intervention in these patients as a salvage operation and found it did not have the desired life-saving effect. Thus, sterile pancreatic necrosis is generally managed nonoperatively.

One exception would be addressing complications of pancreatitis such as abdominal compartment syndrome or ischemic bowel, where surgical management may be lifesaving.

In addition to the presence of multiorgan failure and a high APACHE II score, early surgery has been shown to be an independent predictor of poor outcome in acute necrotizing pancreatitis. Several case series have underscored that mortality decreases when interventions can be delayed. As advocated in guidelines by the International Association of Pancreatology in 2002, delay in open surgery for at least 3-4 weeks leads to lower morbidity and mortality. With delay in intervention, demarcation of necrotic from vital tissue occurs, so that if necrosectomy is performed, the operation is less difficult, risk of bleeding is less, and resection of vital viable tissue is minimized. This leads to better long-term endocrine and exocrine function and a reduction in postoperative adverse events. When emergency interventions are needed for perforated viscus, acute bleeding, fistula to or obstruction of a viscus, and abdominal compartment syndrome, drainage or debridement of necrosis is not required at the same setting.

While exactly how long to delay is in question, it would appear that delaying at least 14 days and potentially 30 days leads to additional decreases in mortality.

Adjuvant Therapy in Pancreatic Necrosis: Percutaneous or Endoscopic Drainage

In addition to the surgery for the treatment of pancreatic necrosis, a variety of nonsurgical methods have been described. The issues with these studies are that they involve heterogeneous patient populations, definitions of infected necrosis, and techniques. As a result, outcomes are not directly comparable outside of randomized control trials. The effect of nonsurgical methods when compared to surgery is variable and definitive mortality decreases have not been seen. Advantages of nonsurgical approaches include a reduction in systemic complications after intervention and a lower risk of developing new organ failure. Local adverse events including bleeding and fistula seem to be slightly increased in some retrospective studies when minimally invasive treatment regimens are used. However, this finding may reflect a difference in the definition of adverse events or represent a learning curve associated with early results.

The use of less invasive techniques allows surgical debridement to be deferred or avoided altogether. Antibiotics are the first-line therapy for infected pancreatic necrosis. Antibiotic therapy is most often a bridge to help delay intervention in these patients. As minimally invasive intervention replaces open necrosectomy, percutaneous intervention serves as the first interventional step in that algorithm. The two major adjuvant treatments for necrosectomy are percutaneous drainage and endoscopic drainage (DEN) or some combination of both (**Figure 14.5**).

Percutaneous Drain

Percutaneous catheter drainage (PCD) can be used as primary therapy, as an adjunct to other techniques, and as salvage management of residual necrotic or infected collections. Approaches include transperitoneal or retroperitoneal placement of 12- to 30-Fr catheters. Retroperitoneal approach is preferred because it avoids contamination and enteric leaks and facilitates planning for a step-up approach. Each collection should be drained separately, which can result in multiple catheters per patient. The optimal size, number of drains, and management of drains when PCD is used are unknown, but the larger the drain, the more effective the drainage of necrotic debris.

Percutaneous catheter drainage (PCD) originally played an adjuvant role in draining residual collections after open necrosectomy but is increasingly used in a step-up approach to defer or obviate the need for surgery or as an adjunct to endoscopic necrosectomy (see **Figures 14.3B and 14.4**). Placement of drains can delay surgery and decreases mortality. A systematic review of PCD as primary treatment for pancreatic necrosis

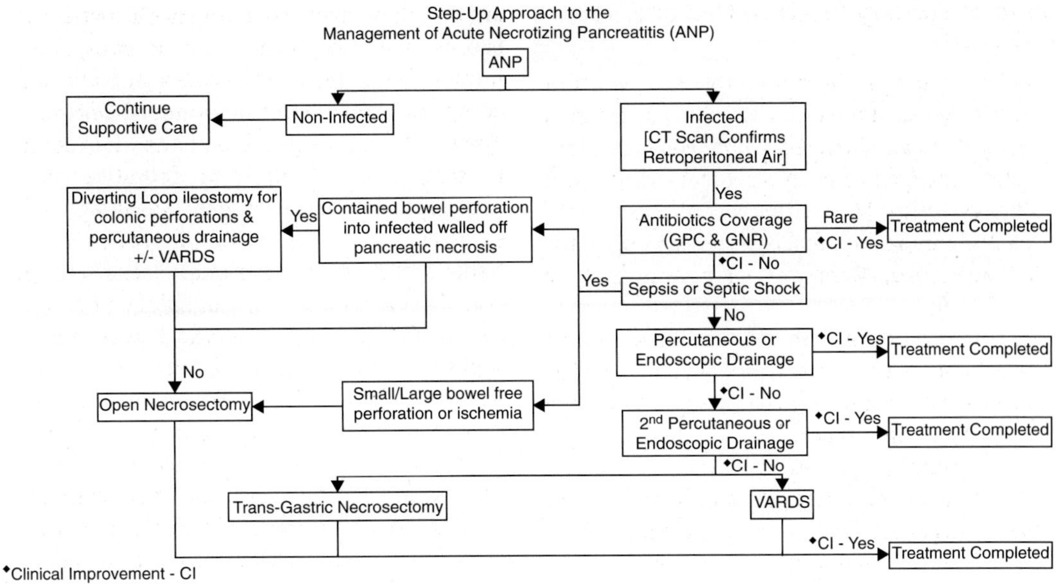

Figure 14.5 Diagram for the proposed treatment of acute necrotizing pancreatitis.

included 11 studies involving 384 patients. Seventy percent of patients had infected necrosis, and an average of two separate catheters was placed, with an overall success rate of 56%. In two prospective studies, the clinical success of PCD alone was 33% and 35%. Adverse events such as external fistulae occur in up to 27% of patients. In the EAST Practice Management Guideline for Pancreatic Necrosis, 10 studies that had comparison groups of primary PCD compared to primary surgical intervention. Although many of the studies were small and not powered to show a mortality difference, they did show safety with a significant percentage of patients having complete resolution of their process with PCD only.

Endoscopic vs Surgical Drainage

Direct endoscopic necrosectomy (DEN) is performed via upper endoscopy with gastric or transenteric entry into the necrotic cavity. Mechanical debridement and lavage are performed (**Figure 14.6**). DEN requires a collection to be located within 1-2 cm of the gastric or duodenal lumen. Typically, 3-6 sessions are necessary to completely debride the cavity.

While case series describe the safety of endoscopic drainage, little data compare it to other interventions. There are two prospective randomized trials with a small sample size comparing the two procedures. The Dutch Pancreatitis Study Group compared DEN with minimally invasive surgical necrosectomy or, if not feasible, open necrosectomy. Twenty patients completed randomization with 10 in each group. The study showed superiority of DEN over surgical necrosectomy with regard to inflammatory markers and a composite end point of major complications. New-onset organ failure occurred significantly less frequently with endoscopic necrosectomy (0% vs 50%, $P = .03$), as did pancreatic fistulas (10% vs 70%, $P = .02$). There was an insignificant trend toward lower mortality with DEN compared with surgery (10% vs 40%). The authors concluded that DEN was superior to surgical necrosectomy for infected necrosis. The drawback was that endoscopic patients required a median of three procedures to accomplish what a surgical necrosectomy did in one ($P = .007$).

The TENSION trial was a randomized controlled, multicenter trial that included 98 patients with infected necrosis comparing endoscopic surgery to step-up approach. Patients with (suspected) infected necrotizing pancreatitis with an indication for intervention and in whom both treatment modalities were deemed possible were randomized to either an endoscopic or a surgical step-up approach (drain followed by surgery if needed). It should be noted that roughly half the patients in each group were treated with a drain only with the key difference being the route, transgastric in the DEN group and percutaneous in the VARDS group. The primary endpoint was a composite of death and major complications within 6 months following randomization, which did not differ among the two groups. There were shorter

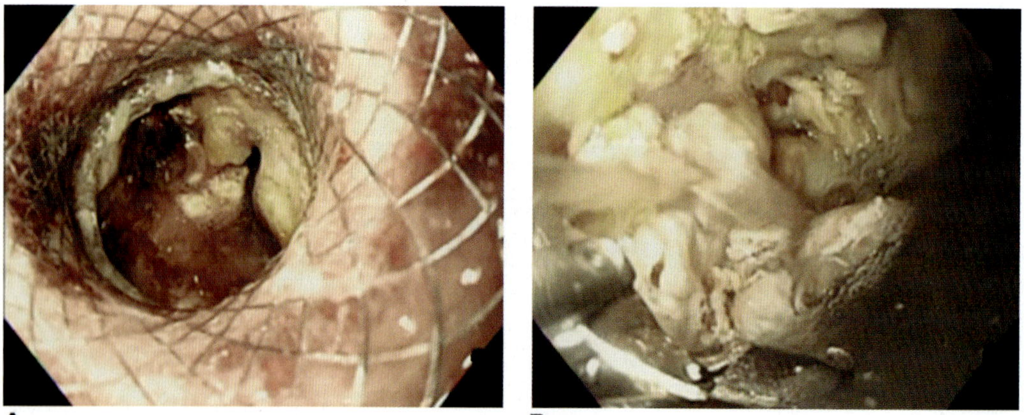

A B

Figure 14.6 A, B. Endoscopic images following the placement of a lumen-apposing transmural-covered metal stent to facilitate the endoscopic drainage and debridement of walled off pancreatic necrosis. (Reprinted from Lee A, Thompson CC. Direct endoscopic necrosectomy in retroflexion When using a lumen-apposing transmural covered metal stent. *Gastrointest Endosc.* 2016;83:255, with permission from Elsevier.)

hospital days and lower fistula in the endoscopy group. The number of interventions was not different in the two groups.

One of the limitations of the transgastric endoscopic approach is the location of the target collection. Central collections are generally accessible, but not left-sided and flank collections. As a result, the VARD procedure and the other percutaneous retroperitoneal approaches are likely to continue to have a significant role to play when there is no close abutment of the collection to the stomach or duodenum.

Combined Percutaneous and Endoscopic

Advantages of PCD include widespread availability with the presence of interventional radiology, access by transperitoneal and retroperitoneal approaches to the left and right sides of the abdomen and pelvis, ability to place multiple catheters, and the ability to flush catheters between procedures. However, 20% of patients developed pancreaticocutaneous fistulae; some of which do not close because of communication of the drain with an upstream disconnected pancreatic duct. Combining a percutaneous approach with endoscopic transmural drainage can prevent external fistulae and avoid repetitive endoscopic interventions to perform direct necrosectomy. Irrigation through the percutaneous approach with egress through the transmural fistula results in a form of debridement. In case-control series from a single center, the combined percutaneous-endoscopic approach increased the rate of nonsurgical resolution and resulted in a decrease in hospitalization, time to drain removal, number of CT scans, and number of drains compared to percutaneous drainage alone.

Role of Adjuvant Therapy

Percutaneous drainage and endoscopic debridement may have a role in the management of pancreatic necrosis at times as a definitive treatment. It certainly has value as a means to delay surgical intervention until a time that it is safe. Pursing PCD or DEN as primary therapy has a questionable effect on mortality but has been shown to increase the number of total procedures in at least one study. Numerous studies show equivalence in the different types of interventions suggesting health care teams have the ability to tailor care to the individual patient.

Open vs Laparoscopic Approach to Pancreatic Necrosis

Open surgical debridement historically has been the standard treatment for infected necrosis and for symptomatic sterile walled of necrosis with the aim of complete removal of necrotic tissue. The oldest and most established approach includes open laparotomy or retroperitoneal flank incision with manual debridement. After necrosectomy, the abdomen may be left open, or drains are placed for postoperative continuous lavage. The postoperative lavage technique was associated with fewer operations and a decrease in postoperative morbidity. The technique of closed packing is mainly advocated by a single group. In some cases of incomplete necrosectomy, percutaneous drains can be placed if needed to provide irrigation and to further debride postoperative collections

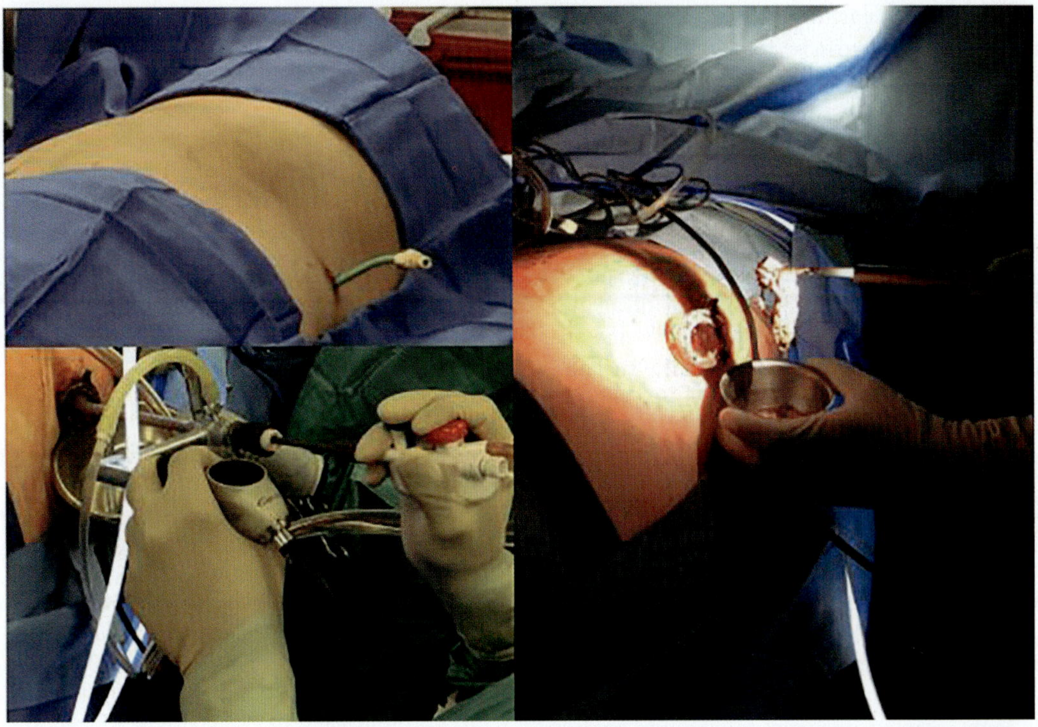

Figure 14.7 Positioning for the VARDs approach for pancreatic debridement. With the patient in full right lateral decubitus position, the percutaneous drain serves as the guide to the retroperitoneum. The operation can be performed with an irrigating cystoscope or laparoscope.

(step-down approach). Open necrosectomy is associated with relatively high morbidity (34%-95%) and mortality ranging from 6% to 25%.

An alternative to open initial necrosectomy is the step-up approach, using minimally invasive techniques to control necrosis, with definitive necrosectomy deferred or often avoided altogether. The first step is usually PCD, preferably into the retroperitoneum via the left flank (**Figure 14.7**). Alternative routes are percutaneous transabdominal or endoscopic transluminal. The objective is to postpone or obviate the need for surgery. If drainage fails to control sepsis, the next step is taken, and debridement accomplished via VARD, sinus tract endoscopy, or DEN. These approaches are thought to induce less stress than open surgery in already critically ill patients.

There is one randomized control trial (PANTER trial) evaluating if the step-up approach is superior to open necrosectomy as first-line treatment for necrosis. In this Dutch multi-institutional trial, 45 patients were randomized to immediate open necrosectomy, and 43 patients were randomized to the step-up approach. Baseline patient characteristics were similar in both groups. Outcomes were significantly better in the step-up group compared to the open surgery group. Death or major morbidity occurred in 40% of the step-up group compared with 69% of the open necrosectomy group; mortality was similar in both groups (19% vs 16%). Twelve percent of patients in the step-up group experienced new-onset multiorgan failure compared to 42% in the open necrosectomy group. Long-term morbidity including incisional hernia (7% vs 24%), new-onset diabetes mellitus (16% vs 38%), pancreatic enzyme use (7% vs 33%), and cost of care were all significantly lower in the step-up group. Notably, 35% of patients in the step-up group did not require necrosectomy.

One confounder when comparing open vs minimally invasive surgery is the issue of timing. The literature supports delayed surgery leads to better outcomes. The step-up protocol is based on delaying surgery utilizing drains and observation. When comparing series of minimally invasive surgery with open surgery, it may be that the delay explains the improved outcomes rather than the route of surgical intervention. While there are case series showing early laparoscopic surgical interventions can be done safely, none compare laparoscopic-assisted pancreatic debridement to open intervention. Given what we know about the disease process and the dismal outcomes associated with open necrosectomy, it is unlikely that a large-scale randomized trial is feasible.

The potential learning curve associated with this procedure must also be recognized. While the Dutch papers show impressive improvements in outcomes, they are small and have not been widely reproduced in other populations. While acute care surgeons have significant experience in managing ill patients with distorted anatomy, they may not have extensive experience with this disease process and approaching it from a retroperitoneal point of view. With the introduction of all new surgical techniques, one must acknowledge that outcomes may improve over time as the surgeons develop their skill set. No published literature on the subject addresses the outcomes as the beginning of the series when compared to the end of the series.

SUMMARY

Acute care surgeons are uniquely trained to care for patients with pancreatic necrosis due their training in critical care and complex surgery with ongoing shock. During the first 30 days of symptoms with infected necrotic collections, patients should only undergo surgical debridement if the patients fail to improve after radiologic or endoscopic drainage. The preferred route of surgical intervention is the step-up approach.

Traditionally, the most widely used approach to infected necrosis has been open surgical necrosectomy. Most cases can now be managed using minimally invasive techniques in specialized centers with the appropriate expertise. Percutaneous catheter drainage, endoscopic and laparoscopic methods are all feasible approaches for treating infected necrosis. Combination approaches may be useful in selected patients with extensive peripancreatic necrosis. Current evidence favors endoscopic necrosectomy or percutaneous catheter drainage early in an effort to delay surgery followed by a step-up approach necrosectomy if needed.

The overriding principle of interventions for necrosis is that no single approach is optimal for all patients. The best approach is multimodal and adaptable to the individual patient to achieve the best outcomes.

SUGGESTED READINGS

Aboelsoud MM, Siddique O, Morales A, Seol Y, Al-Qadi MO. Fluid choice matters in critically-ill patients with acute pancreatitis: lactated Ringer's vs. isotonic saline. *R I Med J*. 2016;99(10):39.

Acute Respiratory Distress Syndrome Network; Brower RG, Matthay MA, Morris A, Schoenfeld D, Thompson BT, Wheeler A. Ventilation with lower tidal volumes as compared with traditional tidal volumes for acute lung injury and the acute respiratory distress syndrome. *N Engl J Med*. 2000;342(18):1301-1308.

Adams DB, Harvey TS, Anderson MC. Percutaneous catheter drainage of infected pancreatic and peripancreatic fluid collections. *Arch Surg*. 1990;125(12):1554-1557.

Agarwal AK, Kumar KR, Agarwal S, Singh S. Significance of splenic vein thrombosis in chronic pancreatitis. *Am J Surg*. 2008;196(2):149-154.

Aultman DF, Bilton BD, Zibari GB, McMillan RW, McDonald JC. Nonoperative therapy for acute necrotizing pancreatitis. *Am Surg*. 1997;63(12):1114-1117; discussion 1117-1118.

Babu BI, Sheen AJ, Lee SH, O'Shea S, Eddleston JM, Siriwardena AK. Open pancreatic necrosectomy in the multidisciplinary management of postinflammatory necrosis. *Ann Surg*. 2010;251(5):783-786.

Badalov N, Baradarian R, Iswara K, Li J, Steinberg W, Tenner S. Drug-induced acute pancreatitis: an evidence-based review. *Clin Gastroenterol Hepatol*. 2007;5(6):648-661.

Bakker OJ, van Brunschot S, van Santvoort HC, et al. Early versus on-demand nasoenteric tube feeding in acute pancreatitis. *N Engl J Med*. 2014;371(21):1983-1993.

Bakker OJ, van Santvoort HC, van Brunschot S, et al. Endoscopic transgastric vs surgical necrosectomy for infected necrotizing pancreatitis: a randomized trial. *JAMA*. 2012;307(10):1053-1061.

Balthazar EJ, Fisher LA. Hemorrhagic complications of pancreatitis: radiologic evaluation with emphasis on CT imaging. *Pancreatology*. 2001;1(4):306-313.

Banks PA, Bollen TL, Dervenis C, et al. Classification of acute pancreatitis—2012: revision of the Atlanta classification and definitions by international consensus. *Gut*. 2013;62(1):102-111.

Basit H, Ruan GJ, Mukherjee S. Ranson criteria. In: *StatPearls*. StatPearls Publishing Copyright © 2020, StatPearls Publishing LLC; 2020.

Beger HG, Buchler M, Bittner R, Oettinger W, Block S, Nevalainen T. Necrosectomy and postoperative local lavage in patients with necrotizing pancreatitis: results of a prospective clinical trial. *World J Surg*. 1988;12(2):255-262.

Bergert H, Hinterseher I, Kersting S, Leonhardt J, Bloomenthal A, Saeger HD. Management and outcome of hemorrhage due to arterial pseudoaneurysms in pancreatitis. *Surgery*. 2005;137(3):323-328.

Besselink M, van Santvoort H, Freeman M, et al. IAP/APA evidence-based guidelines for the management of acute pancreatitis. *Pancreatology*. 2013;13(4 suppl 2):E1-E15.

Besselink MG, Verwer TJ, Schoenmaeckers EJ, et al. Timing of surgical intervention in necrotizing pancreatitis. *Arch Surg*. 2007;142(12):1194-1201.

Bhansali SK, Shah SC, Desai SB, Sunawala JD. Infected necrosis complicating acute pancreatitis: experience with 131 cases. *Indian J Gastroenterol*. 2003;22(1):7-10.

Bryner BS, Smith C, Cooley E, Bartlett RH, Mychaliska GB. Extracorporeal life support for pancreatitis-induced acute respiratory distress syndrome. *Ann Surg*. 2012;256(6):1073-1077.

Buchler MW, Gloor B, Muller CA, Friess H, Seiler CA, Uhl W. Acute necrotizing pancreatitis: treatment strategy according to the status of infection. *Ann Surg*. 2000;232(5):619-626.

Carr RA, Rejowski BJ, Cote GA, Pitt HA, Zyromski NJ. Systematic review of hypertriglyceridemia-induced acute pancreatitis: a more virulent etiology? *Pancreatology*. 2016;16(4):469-476.

Carter CR, McKay CJ, Imrie CW. Percutaneous necrosectomy and sinus tract endoscopy in the management of infected pancreatic necrosis: an initial experience. *Ann Surg*. 2000;232(2):175-180.

Chang Y-s, Fu H-q, Xiao Y-m, Liu J-c. Nasogastric or nasojejunal feeding in predicted severe acute pancreatitis: a meta-analysis. *Crit Care*. 2013;17(3):R118.

Connor S, Alexakis N, Raraty MG, et al. Early and late complications after pancreatic necrosectomy. *Surgery*. 2005;137(5):499-505.

Crockett SD, Wani S, Gardner TB, et al. American Gastroenterological Association Institute guideline on initial management of acute pancreatitis. *Gastroenterology*. 2018;154(4):1096-1101.

Cutts S, Talboys R, Paspula C, Prempeh EM, Fanous R, Ail D. Adult respiratory distress syndrome. *Ann R Coll Surg Engl*. 2017;99(1):12-16.

Cuschieri A. Pancreatic necrosis: pathogenesis and endoscopic management. *Semin Laparosc Surg*. 2002;9(1): 54-63.

da Costa DW, Bouwense SA, Schepers NJ, et al. Same-admission versus interval cholecystectomy for mild gallstone pancreatitis (PONCHO): a multicentre randomized controlled trial. *Lancet*. 2015;386(10000): 1261-1268.

Dasgupta R, Davies N, Williamson R, Jackson J. Haemosuccus pancreaticus: treatment by arterial embolization. *Clin Radiol*. 2002;57(11):1021-1027.

De Waele JJ, Hoste E, Blot SI, Decruyenaere J, Colardyn F. Intra-abdominal hypertension in patients with severe acute pancreatitis. *Crit Care*. 2005;9(4): R452-R457.

de-Madaria E, Herrera-Marante I, González-Camacho V, et al. Fluid resuscitation with lactated Ringer's solution vs normal saline in acute pancreatitis: a triple-blind, randomized, controlled trial. *United European Gastroenterol J*. 2018;6(1):63-72.

Eatock FC, Chong P, Menezes N, et al. A randomized study of early nasogastric versus nasojejunal feeding in severe acute pancreatitis. *Am J Gastroenterol*. 2005;100(2):432-439.

Feller JH, Brown RA, Toussaint GPM, Thompson AG. Changing methods in the treatment of severe pancreatitis. *Am J Surg*. 1974;127(2):196-201.

Fernandez-del Castillo C, Rattner DW, Makary MA, Mostafavi A, McGrath D, Warshaw AL. Debridement and closed packing for the treatment of necrotizing pancreatitis. *Ann Surg*. 1998;228(5):676-684.

Fortenberry JD, Bhardwaj V, Niemer P, Cornish JD, Wright JA, Bland L. Neutrophil and cytokine activation with neonatal extracorporeal membrane oxygenation. *J Pediatr*. 1996;128(5 Pt 1):670-678.

Foster BR, Jensen KK, Bakis G, Shaaban AM, Coakley FV. Revised Atlanta classification for acute pancreatitis: a pictorial essay. *Radiographics* 2016;36:675-687.

Fotoohi M, D'Agostino HB, Wollman B, Chon K, Shahrokni S, vanSonnenberg E. Persistent pancreatocutaneous fistula after percutaneous drainage of pancreatic fluid collections: role of cause and severity of pancreatitis. *Radiology*. 1999;213(2):573-578.

Freeny PC, Hauptmann E, Althaus SJ, Traverso LW, Sinanan M. Percutaneous CT-guided catheter drainage of infected acute necrotizing pancreatitis: techniques and results. *AJR Am J Roentgenol*. 1998;170(4): 969-975.

Frey CF. Hemorrhagic pancreatitis. *Am J Surg*. 1979;137(5): 616-623.

Friedman G, Flávia Couto CL, Becker M. Randomized study to compare nasojejunal with nasogastric nutrition in critically ill patients without prior evidence of altered gastric emptying. *Indian J Crit Care Med*. 2015;19(2):71-75.

Gagner M. Laparoscopic treatment of acute necrotizing pancreatitis. *Semin Laparosc Surg*. 1996;3(1):21-28.

Gan SI, Edwards AL, Symonds CJ, Beck PL. Hypertriglyceridemia-induced pancreatitis: a case-based review. *World J Gastroenterol*. 2006;12(44): 7197-7202.

Gardner TB, Vege SS, Chari ST, et al. Faster rate of initial fluid resuscitation in severe acute pancreatitis diminishes in-hospital mortality. *Pancreatology*. 2009;9(6):770-776.

Garg R, Rustagi T. Management of hypertriglyceridemia induced acute pancreatitis. *Biomed Res Int* 2018;2018:4721357.

Gluck M, Ross A, Irani S, et al. Dual modality drainage for symptomatic walled-off pancreatic necrosis reduces length of hospitalization, radiological procedures, and number of endoscopies compared to standard percutaneous drainage. *J Gastrointest Surg*. 2012;16(2):248-256; discussion 256-257.

Goyal H, Smith B, Bayer C, Rutherford C, Shelnut D. Differences in severity and outcomes between hypertriglyceridemia and alcohol-induced pancreatitis. *N Am J Med Sci*. 2016;8(2):82-87.

Guay J, Ochroch EA, Kopp S. Intraoperative use of low volume ventilation to decrease postoperative mortality, mechanical ventilation, lengths of stay and lung injury in adults without acute lung injury. *Cochrane Database Syst Rev*. 2018;7(7):CD011151.

Guda NM, Muddana V, Whitcomb DC, et al. Recurrent acute pancreatitis: international state-of-the-science conference with recommendations. *Pancreas*. 2018;47(6):653-666.

Hartwig W, Maksan SM, Foitzik T, Schmidt J, Herfarth C, Klar E. Reduction in mortality with delayed surgical therapy of severe pancreatitis. *J Gastrointest Surg.* 2002;6(3):481-487.

Haydock MD, Mittal A, Wilms HR, Phillips A, Petrov MS, Windsor JA. Fluid therapy in acute pancreatitis: anybody's guess. *Ann Surg.* 2013;257(2):182-188.

Hernandez V, Pascual I, Almela P, et al. Recurrence of acute gallstone pancreatitis and relationship with cholecystectomy or endoscopic sphincterotomy. *Am J Gastroenterol.* 2004;99(12):2417-2423.

Holodinsky JK, Roberts DJ, Ball CG, et al. Risk factors for intra-abdominal hypertension and abdominal compartment syndrome among adult intensive care unit patients: a systematic review and meta-analysis. *Crit Care.* 2013;17(5):R249.

Horvath K, Brody F, Davis B, et al. Minimally invasive management of pancreatic disease: SAGES and SSAT pancreas symposium, Ft. Lauderdale, Florida, April 2005. *Surg Endosc.* 2007;21(3):367-372.

Horvath K, Freeny P, Escallon J, et al. Safety and efficacy of video-assisted retroperitoneal debridement for infected pancreatic collections: a multicenter, prospective, single-arm phase 2 study. *Arch Surg.* 2010;145(9):817-825.

Howard TJ, Patel JB, Zyromski N, et al. Declining morbidity and mortality rates in the surgical management of pancreatic necrosis. *J Gastrointest Surg.* 2007;11(1):43-49.

Hu Y, Xiong W, Li C, Cui Y. Continuous blood purification for severe acute pancreatitis: a systematic review and meta-analysis. *Medicine (Baltimore).* 2019;98(12):e14873.

Huber W, Malbrain ML. Goal-directed fluid resuscitation in acute pancreatitis: shedding light on the penumbra by dynamic markers of preload? *Intensive Care Med.* 2013;39(4):784-786.

Iqbal U, Anwar H, Scribani M. Ringer's lactate versus normal saline in acute pancreatitis: a systematic review and meta-analysis. *J Dig Dis.* 2018;19(6):335-341.

Jain P, Rai R-R, Udawat H, Nijhawan S, Mathur A. Insulin and heparin in treatment of hypertriglyceridemia-induced pancreatitis. *World J Gastroenterol.* 2007;13(18):2642-2643.

Jiang HL, Xue WJ, Li DQ, et al. Influence of continuous veno-venous hemofiltration on the course of acute pancreatitis. *World J Gastroenterol.* 2005;11(31):4815-4821.

Jordan GL Jr, Spjut HJ. Hemorrhagic pancreatitis. *Arch Surg.* 1972;104(4):489-493.

Kelm DJ, Perrin JT, Cartin-Ceba R, Gajic O, Schenck L, Kennedy CC. Fluid overload in patients with severe sepsis and septic shock treated with early goal-directed therapy is associated with increased acute need for fluid-related medical interventions and hospital death. *Shock.* 2015;43(1):68-73.

Kirby JM, Vora P, Midia M, Rawlinson J. Vascular complications of pancreatitis: imaging and intervention. *Cardiovasc Intervent Radiol.* 2008;31(5):957-970.

Knoch M, Köllen B, Dietrich G, Müller E, Mottaghy K, Lennartz H. Progress in veno-venous long-term bypass techniques for the treatment of ARDS. Controlled clinical trial with the heparin-coated bypass circuit. *Int J Artif Organs.* 1992;15(2):103-108.

Lee A, Thompson CC. Direct endoscopic necrosectomy in retroflexion when using a lumen-apposing transmural covered metal stent. *Gastrointest Endosc.* 2016;83:255.

Lee MJ, Rattner DW, Legemate DA, et al. Acute complicated pancreatitis: redefining the role of interventional radiology. *Radiology.* 1992;183(1):171-174.

Leppäniemi A, Tolonen M, Tarasconi A, et al. 2019 WSES guidelines for the management of severe acute pancreatitis. *World J Emerg Surg.* 2019;14(1):27.

Lin Y, He S, Gong J, et al. Continuous veno-venous hemofiltration for severe acute pancreatitis. *Cochrane Database Syst Rev.* 2019;10(10):CD012959.

Lu Y, Zhang H, Teng F, Xia WJ, Sun GX, Wen AQ. Early goal-directed therapy in severe sepsis and septic shock: a meta-analysis and trial sequential analysis of randomized controlled trials. *J Intensive Care Med.* 2018;33(5):296-309.

Machicado JD, Papachristou GI. Intravenous fluid resuscitation in the management of acute pancreatitis. *Curr Opin Gastroenterol.* 2020;36(5):409-416.

Marik PE, Monnet X, Teboul J-L. Hemodynamic parameters to guide fluid therapy. *Ann Intensive Care.* 2011;1(1):1.

Marik PE. Fluid responsiveness and the six guiding principles of fluid resuscitation. *Crit Care Med.* 2016;44(10):1920-1922.

Marshall JC, Cook DJ, Christou NV, Bernard GR, Sprung CL, Sibbald WJ. Multiple organ dysfunction score: a reliable descriptor of a complex clinical outcome. *Crit Care Med.* 1995;23(10):1638-1652.

McClave SA, Chang WK, Dhaliwal R, Heyland DK. Nutrition support in acute pancreatitis: a systematic review of the literature. *J Parenter Enteral Nutr.* 2006;30(2):143-156.

McKay C, Imrie C. The continuing challenge of early mortality in acute pancreatitis. *Br J Surg.* 2004;91(10):1243-1244.

Medich DS, Lee TK, Melhem MF, Rowe MI, Schraut WH, Lee KKW. Pathogenesis of pancreatic sepsis. *Am J Surg.* 1993;165(1):46-52.

Mentula P, Hienonen P, Kemppainen E, Puolakkainen P, Leppäniemi A. Surgical decompression for abdominal compartment syndrome in severe acute pancreatitis. *Arch Surg.* 2010;145(8):764-769.

Mier J, Leon EL, Castillo A, Robledo F, Blanco R. Early versus late necrosectomy in severe necrotizing pancreatitis. *Am J Surg.* 1997;173(2):71-75.

Mirtallo JM, Forbes A, McClave SA, et al. International consensus guidelines for nutrition therapy in pancreatitis. *J Parenter Enteral Nutr.* 2012;36(3):284-291.

Mounzer R, Langmead CJ, Wu BU, et al. Comparison of existing clinical scoring systems to predict persistent organ failure in patients with acute pancreatitis. *Gastroenterology*. 2012;142(7):1476-1482.

Mowery NT, Bruns BR, MacNew HG, et al. Surgical management of pancreatic necrosis: a practice management guideline from the Eastern Association for the Surgery of Trauma. *J Trauma Acute Care Surg*. 2017;83(2):316-327.

Muckart DJ, Bhagwanjee S. American College of Chest Physicians/Society of Critical Care Medicine Consensus Conference definitions of the systemic inflammatory response syndrome and allied disorders in relation to critically injured patients. *Crit Care Med*. 1997;25(11):1789-1795.

Oda S, Hirasawa H, Shiga H, Nakanishi K, Matsuda K-I, Nakamura M. Continuous hemofiltration/hemodiafiltration in critical care. *Ther Apher*. 2002;6(3): 193-198.

Olah A, Belagyi T, Bartek P, Poharnok L, Romics L Jr. Alternative treatment modalities of infected pancreatic necrosis. *Hepatogastroenterology*. 2006;53(70): 603-607.

Osborn TM. Severe sepsis and septic shock trials (ProCESS, ARISE, ProMISe): what is optimal resuscitation? *Crit Care Clin*. 2017;33(2):323-344.

Papachristou GI, Takahashi N, Chahal P, Sarr MG, Baron TH. Peroral endoscopic drainage/debridement of walled-off pancreatic necrosis. *Ann Surg*. 2007;245(6):943-951.

Parekh D. Laparoscopic-assisted pancreatic necrosectomy: a new surgical option for treatment of severe necrotizing pancreatitis. *Arch Surg*. 2006;141(9):895-902; discussion 902-903.

Parikh PY, Pitt HA, Kilbane M, et al. Pancreatic necrosectomy: North American mortality is much lower than expected. *J Am Coll Surg*. 2009;209(6):712-719.

Park SK, Shin SR, Hur M, Kim WH, Oh EA, Lee SH. The effect of early goal-directed therapy for treatment of severe sepsis or septic shock: a systemic review and meta-analysis. *J Crit Care*. 2017;38:115-122.

Peek GJ, White S, Scott AD, et al. Severe acute respiratory distress syndrome secondary to acute pancreatitis successfully treated with extracorporeal membrane oxygenation in three patients. *Ann Surg*. 1998;227(4):572-574.

Petrov MS, Correia M, Windsor JA. Nasogastric tube feeding in predicted severe acute pancreatitis. A systematic review of the literature to determine safety and tolerance. *JOP*. 2008;9(4):440-448.

Petrov MS, Yadav D. Global epidemiology and holistic prevention of pancreatitis. *Nat Rev Gastroenterol Hepatol*. 2019;16(3):175-184.

Pupelis G, Austrums E, Snippe K, Berzins M. Clinical significance of increased intra-abdominal pressure in severe acute pancreatitis. *Acta Chir Belg*. 2002;102(2):71-74.

Pupelis G, Plaudis H, Zeiza K, Drozdova N, Mukans M, Kazaka I. Early continuous veno-venous haemofiltration in the management of severe acute pancreatitis complicated with intra-abdominal hypertension: retrospective review of 10 year" experience. *Ann Intensive Care*. 2012;2(1):S21.

Raraty MG, Halloran CM, Dodd S, et al. Minimal access retroperitoneal pancreatic necrosectomy: improvement in morbidity and mortality with a less invasive approach. *Ann Surg*. 2010;251(5):787-793.

Räty S, Pulkkinen J, Nordback I, et al. Can laparoscopic cholecystectomy prevent recurrent idiopathic acute pancreatitis?: A prospective randomized multicenter trial. *Ann Surg*. 2015;262(5):736-741.

Reddy M, Jindal R, Gupta R, Yadav TD, Wig JD. Outcome after pancreatic necrosectomy: trends over 12 years at an Indian centre. *ANZ J Surg*. 2006;76(8): 704-709.

Regli A, De Keulenaer B, De Laet I, Roberts D, Dabrowski W, Malbrain ML. Fluid therapy and perfusional considerations during resuscitation in critically ill patients with intra-abdominal hypertension. *Anaesthesiol Intensive Ther*. 2015;47(1):45-53.

Rivers EP, Coba V, Whitmill M. Early goal-directed therapy in severe sepsis and septic shock: a contemporary review of the literature. *Curr Opin Anaesthesiol*. 2008;21(2):128-140.

Rocha FG, Benoit E, Zinner MJ, et al. Impact of radiologic intervention on mortality in necrotizing pancreatitis: the role of organ failure. *Arch Surg*. 2009;144(3):261-265.

Rosas JMH, Soto SN, Aracil JS, et al. Intra-abdominal pressure as a marker of severity in acute pancreatitis. *Surgery*. 2007;141(2):173-178.

Ross A, Gluck M, Irani S, et al. Combined endoscopic and percutaneous drainage of organized pancreatic necrosis. *Gastrointest Endosc*. 2010;71(1):79-84.

Rotman N, Mathieu D, Anglade MC, Fagniez PL. Failure of percutaneous drainage of pancreatic abscesses complicating severe acute pancreatitis. *Surg Gynecol Obstet*. 1992;174(2):141-144.

Samaraee AA, McCallum IJD, Coyne PE, Seymour K. Nutritional strategies in severe acute pancreatitis: a systematic review of the evidence. *Surgeon*. 2010;8(2):105-110.

Sarr MG. Early fluid "resuscitation/therapy" in acute pancreatitis: which fluid? What rate? What parameters to gauge effectiveness? *Ann Surg*. 2013;257(2): 189-190.

Segal D, Mortele KJ, Banks PA, Silverman SG. Acute necrotizing pancreatitis: role of CT-guided percutaneous catheter drainage. *Abdom Imaging*. 2007;32(3):351-361.

Stevens CL, Abbas SM, Watters DAK. How does cholecystectomy influence recurrence of idiopathic acute pancreatitis? *J Gastrointest Surg*. 2016;20(12): 1997-2001.

Sunday ML, Schuricht AL, Barbot DJ, Rosato FE. Management of infected pancreatic fluid collections. *Am Surg*. 1994;60(1):63-67.

Targarona Modena J, Barreda Cevasco L, Arroyo Basto C, Orellana Vicuna A, Portanova Ramirez M. Total enteral nutrition as prophylactic therapy for pancreatic necrosis infection in severe acute pancreatitis. *Pancreatology*. 2006;6(1):58-64.

Tenner S, Baillie J, DeWitt J, Vege SS. American College of Gastroenterology guideline: management of acute pancreatitis. *Am J Gastroenterol*. 2013;108(9):1400-1415.

Tenner S, Dubner H, Steinberg W. Predicting gallstone pancreatitis with laboratory parameters: a meta-analysis. *Am J Gastroenterol*. 1994;89(10):1863-1866.

Trikudanathan G, Navaneethan U, Vege SS. Current controversies in fluid resuscitation in acute pancreatitis: a systematic review. *Pancreas*. 2012;41(6):827-834.

Tsiotos GG, Luque-de Leon E, Sarr MG. Long-term outcome of necrotizing pancreatitis treated by necrosectomy. *Br J Surg*. 1998;85(12):1650-1653.

Uhl W, Warshaw A, Imrie C, et al. IAP guidelines for the surgical management of acute pancreatitis. *Pancreatology*. 2002;2(6):565-573.

Underwood MJ, Pearson JA, Waggoner J, Lunec J, Firmin RK, Elliot MJ. Changes in "inflammator" mediators and total body water during extra-corporeal membrane oxygenation (ECMO). A preliminary study. *Int J Artif Organs*. 1995;18(10):627-632.

van Baal MC, van Santvoort HC, Bollen TL, et al. Systematic review of percutaneous catheter drainage as primary treatment for necrotizing pancreatitis. *Br J Surg*. 2011;98(1):18-27.

van Brunschot S, Schut AJ, Bouwense SA, et al. Abdominal compartment syndrome in acute pancreatitis: a systematic review. *Pancreas*. 2014;43(5):665-674.

van Brunschot S, van Grinsven J, van Santvoort HC, et al. Endoscopic or surgical step-up approach for infected necrotising pancreatitis: a multicentre randomised trial. *Lancet*. 2018;391(10115):51-58.

van Santvoort HC, Bakker OJ, Bollen TL, et al. A conservative and minimally invasive approach to necrotizing pancreatitis improves outcome. *Gastroenterology*. 2011;141(4):1254-1263.

van Santvoort HC, Besselink MG, Bakker OJ, et al. A step-up approach or open necrosectomy for necrotizing pancreatitis. *N Engl J Med*. 2010;362(16):1491-1502.

van Santvoort HC, Besselink MG, Bakker OJ, et al. A step-up approach or open necrosectomy for necrotizing pancreatitis. *N Engl J Med*. 2010;362(16):1491-1502.

Warndorf MG, Kurtzman JT, Bartel MJ, et al. Early fluid resuscitation reduces morbidity among patients with acute pancreatitis. *Clin Gastroenterol Hepatol*. 2011;9(8):705-709.

Werner J, Feuerbach S, Uhl W, Buchler MW. Management of acute pancreatitis: from surgery to interventional intensive care. *Gut*. 2005;54(3):426-436.

Whitcomb DC. Acute pancreatitis. *N Engl J Med*. 2006;354(20):2142-2150.

Windsor A, Kanwar S, Li A, et al. Compared with parenteral nutrition, enteral feeding attenuates the acute phase response and improves disease severity in acute pancreatitis. *Gut*. 1998;42(3):431-435.

Wittau M, Scheele J, Golz I, Henne-Bruns D, Isenmann R. Changing role of surgery in necrotizing pancreatitis: a single-center experience. *Hepatogastroenterology*. 2010;57(102-103):1300-1304.

Working Party of the British Society of Gastroenterology; Association of Surgeons of Great Britain and Ireland; Pancreatic Society of Great Britain and Ireland; Association of Upper GI Surgeons of Great Britain and Ireland. UK guidelines for the management of acute pancreatitis. *Gut*. 2005;54(Suppl 3):iii1-iii9.

Wu BU, Hwang JQ, Gardner TH, et al. Lactated Ringer's solution reduces systemic inflammation compared with saline in patients with acute pancreatitis. *Clin Gastroenterol Hepatol*. 2011;9(8):710-717.e711.

Xu JY, Chen QH, Liu SQ, et al. The effect of early goal-directed therapy on outcome in adult severe sepsis and septic shock patients: a meta-analysis of randomized clinical trials. *Anesth Analg*. 2016;123(2):371-381.

Yan X-W, Li W-Q, Wang H, Zhang Z-H, Li N, Li J-S. Effects of high-volume continuous hemofiltration on experimental pancreatitis associated lung injury in pigs. *Int J Artif Organs*. 2006;29(3):293-302.

Yokoe M, Takada T, Mayumi T, et al. Japanese guidelines for the management of acute pancreatitis: Japanese Guidelines 2015. *J Hepatobiliary Pancreat Sci*. 2015;22(6):405-432.

Yu H, Chi D, Wang S, Liu B. Effect of early goal-directed therapy on mortality in patients with severe sepsis or septic shock: a meta-analysis of randomized controlled trials. *BMJ Open*. 2016;6(3):e008330.

Zhao G, Wang C-Y, Wang F, Xiong J-X. Clinical study on nutrition support in patients with severe acute pancreatitis. *World J Gastroenterol*. 2003;9(9):2105-2108.

Zhou ZG, Zheng YC, Shu Y, et al. Laparoscopic management of severe acute pancreatitis. *Pancreas*. 2003;27(3):e46-e50.

Zhu JF, Fan XH, Zhang XH. Laparoscopic treatment of severe acute pancreatitis. *Surg Endosc*. 2001;15(2):146-148.

Zyromski NJ, Vieira C, Stecker M, et al. Improved outcomes in postoperative and pancreatitis-related visceral pseudoaneurysms. *J Gastrointest Surg*. 2007;11(1):50-55.

CHAPTER

15 Biliary Tree Disease

Tanya Egodage, Laura N. Godat, and Lillian S. Kao

CLINICAL PRESENTATION

A 43-year-old female presents with epigastric and right upper quadrant (RUQ) abdominal pain. She endorses nausea, vomiting, and a subjective fever that has been episodic over several days. Her bowel function has been normal. She has a medical history of hypertension and surgical history of a Roux-en-Y gastric bypass 7 years ago. Examination reveals mild scleral icterus and RUQ tenderness. Her vital signs are blood pressure of 131/98 mm Hg, heart rate of 113 beats/min, respirations of 14 per minute, and temperature of 102 °F. She also had elevated total bilirubin to 3 mg/dL, indicating possible biliary obstruction. Because of her fever and concern for cholangitis, she was started on empiric antibiotics.

Question: *What would be the next test of choice in confirming the patient's diagnosis and how would you treat her?"*

Answer: *Transabdominal ultrasound to evaluate the presence of gallstones and the caliber of the biliary ducts. This patient was found to have dilated extrahepatic common bile duct. Percutaneous transhepatic drainage of her biliary tract was performed; a cholangiogram through the tube demonstrated choledocholithiasis. Due to a lack of gastrointestinal expertise at her hospital, she was transferred to a tertiary care center. Given her prior Roux-en-Y gastric bypass, she had a laparoscopic-assisted ERCP with sphincterotomy and stone retrieval followed by an uncomplicated laparoscopic cholecystectomy.*

INTRODUCTION

Differential Diagnosis

The differential diagnosis of patients presenting with epigastric and RUQ abdominal pain is extensive. Gastrointestinal etiologies include biliary colic, acute cholecystitis, choledocholithiasis, peptic ulcer disease, gastritis, acute pancreatitis, and hepatitis. Cardiac and pulmonary etiologies should also be considered. Cardiac dysfunction such as acute myocardial infarction or congestive heart failure should be ruled out. Additionally, pulmonary disease such as pneumonia or pulmonary infarction may present with RUQ pain. Other infectious processes such as acute pyelonephritis, acute appendicitis, or infectious mononucleosis causing hepatomegaly should also be considered. In the above scenario, biliary tree diseases such as acute calculous cholecystitis or cholangitis are high in the differential diagnosis.

Etiology and Epidemiology

Cholelithiasis or gallstones may be classified as cholesterol stones, pigment stones, or mixed. Cholesterol stones are most common, with pigment stones (either brown or black) occurring with lesser frequency, and mixed stones in the minority. Black pigment stones result from hemolytic disorders or cirrhosis, whereas brown pigment stones predominantly occur with biliary infections in those residing in East Asia. Several risk factors including female gender, older age, obesity, Native American ancestry, and rapid weight loss predispose to cholelithiasis formation.

The spectrum of biliary disease ranges from asymptomatic cholelithiasis to more severe manifestations such as cholangitis or severe gallstone pancreatitis. Cholelithiasis is a fairly common condition, occurring in ~10%-20% of the population in developed nations. Approximately 80% of patients with cholelithiasis remain asymptomatic. Symptoms can arise from transient or persistent obstruction of the cystic duct or gallbladder neck/infundibulum, from obstruction of the common bile or pancreatic duct, or erosion into an adjacent structure such as the duodenum or stomach. Complications occur at an approximate rate of 4% per year in those who have cholelithiasis.

Diagnosis

A complete history and physical exam should be performed in patients suspected to have cholelithiasis or a related complication. Patients may report RUQ and/or epigastric pain, both of which occur frequently. Characteristics and duration of the pain should be noted. Patients with symptomatic gallstones often present with biliary colic, defined as episodic RUQ or epigastric pain lasting 30 minutes in duration or greater. The pain can occur with or without radiation. In acute cholecystitis, pain may radiate to the right shoulder, whereas pain may radiate to the back in gallstone pancreatitis. Other biliary-related symptoms can include nausea, vomiting, and bloating. These biliary symptoms may be provoked by meals, especially those high in fat. Attention should be paid to the presence of fever or evidence of shock, such as altered mental status. Jaundice, as manifested by acholic stools or dark-colored urine, may indicate biliary tract obstruction.

Physical examination should begin with a review of vital signs to ensure that the patient is hemodynamically stable. Given the differential diagnosis, a complete pulmonary and cardiac examination should be performed. An abdominal examination should note the presence or absence of abdominal tenderness, guarding, or rebound. Evaluation for Murphy sign or cessation of breathing with deep RUQ palpation should be performed. The presence of scleral icterus or yellowish skin should be noted.

Laboratory evaluation may include a basic metabolic panel to evaluate electrolyte abnormalities from emesis or renal dysfunction related to dehydration. Leukocytosis may be present in acute cholecystitis or cholangitis. However, leukocytosis alone is neither specific nor sensitive for acute cholecystitis; its specificity increases when present with associated fever. C-reactive peptide (CRP) may be helpful when elevated, although it may be normal in the very early phases of acute cholecystitis (the initial 6-12 hours of the disease process). Even so, CRP has generally not been proven useful in the diagnosis of biliary disease. Similarly, procalcitonin has not been demonstrated as useful in the diagnosis of biliary tract disease.

Acute cholecystitis can be associated with an elevation in liver function tests, but no single abnormality in the liver function examination is sensitive or specific for the diagnosis of cholecystitis. Elevated liver function tests may be seen in patients with suspected choledocholithiasis or gallstone pancreatitis. Amylase and lipase should be measured when pancreatitis is suspected; serum lipase offers better sensitivity than serum amylase in defining pancreatitis. Serial measurement of laboratory tests may be useful, such as in the prognostication of acute pancreatitis.

Several imaging modalities are useful in the evaluation of biliary tract disease. Transabdominal ultrasound is the gold standard for the diagnosis of gallstones and can also be used to evaluate acute cholecystitis and choledocholithiasis. Cholescintigraphy (hepatobiliary iminodiacetic acid, HIDA) can be used to diagnose acute cholecystitis, biliary dyskinesia, and biliary leaks. Computed tomography (CT) scan can be used to evaluate for both biliary and other intra-abdominal pathology. In addition, it is used in the evaluation for complications of biliary tract disease, such as necrotizing pancreatitis. Magnetic resonance imaging (MRI) can also be used to evaluate the gallbladder, biliary tract, and pancreas.

Acute Calculous Cholecystitis

Patients with acute calculous cholecystitis often present with RUQ and/or epigastric pain. They may also report nausea, emesis, anorexia, bloating, and fever. On examination, patients may have RUQ tenderness and/or guarding. The presence of Murphy sign increases the likelihood of acute calculous cholecystitis. As noted above, leukocytosis or an elevated CRP may be present, but neither is diagnostic. A mild elevation in liver function tests may be seen due to adjacent liver inflammation. Additional laboratory tests may help classify patients based on the severity of the disease as described below.

Abdominal ultrasound is the recommended initial imaging test. Although the sensitivity and specificity of abdominal ultrasound vary in the literature, ultrasound is easily accessible, low cost, and noninvasive. Ultrasound evidence of acute cholecystitis includes gallbladder wall thickening, gallbladder distension, and pericholecystic fluid.

HIDA scan can also be performed; nonvisualization of the gallbladder is diagnostic for acute cholecystitis. Although the sensitivity and specificity of a HIDA scan are greater than that of an abdominal ultrasound, limited availability, prolonged duration of the procedure, and radiation dose prevent its widespread use over ultrasound. MRI has comparable accuracy to that of abdominal ultrasound, but resource restrictions make it prohibitive as a first-line diagnostic tool. CT may be utilized in patients with equivocal ultrasound results or with unclear history of biliary disease. CT findings of acute cholecystitis include gallbladder distension or wall thickening, pericholecystic fluid and fat enhancement, edema, and bile attenuation within the gallbladder. Oral cholecystography is no longer commonly utilized.

The 2018 Tokyo Guidelines (TG18) and the World Society for Emergency Surgery (WSES)

TABLE 15.1 ■ Tokyo Guidelines 18 Grades of Acute Cholecystiti

Grade	Description
I (mild)	Acute cholecystitis without organ dysfunction
II (moderate)	Associated with any single following conditions: WBC > 18 000/mm^3 Symptoms >72 h Marked local inflammation (gangrenous cholecystitis, pericholecystic abscess, hepatic abscess, biliary peritonitis, emphysematous cholecystitis)
III (severe)	Associated with any organ dysfunction of the following: Cardiovascular: Hypotension requiring vasopressors Neurologic: Decreased level of consciousness Respiratory $PaO_2/FiO_2 < 300$ Renal: Oliguria, creatinine >2.0 mg/dL Hepatic: PT-INR > 1.5 Hematologic: Platelets <100 000/mm^3

Yokoe M, Hata J, Takada T, et al. Tokyo Guidelines 2018: diagnostic criteria and severity grading of acute cholecystitis (with videos). *J Hepatobiliary Pancreat Sci*. 2018;25(1):41-54.

guidelines have both recommended combining patient history, clinical examination, and diagnostic criteria in determining whether a patient has acute cholecystitis. Per TG18, a definitive diagnosis of cholecystitis includes local signs of inflammation (either Murphy sign or RUQ pain/tenderness/or mass) with systemic signs of inflammation (fever, elevated CRP, or leukocytosis) and imaging evidence of cholecystitis. While the WSES guidelines also state that a combination of history, clinical examination, laboratory evaluation, and imaging studies is recommended, the guidelines note that the best combination remains unknown.

Acute cholecystitis includes a spectrum of disease. For example, more severe and less common pathologies include suppurative cholecystitis or gallbladder empyema, gangrenous cholecystitis, emphysematous cholecystitis, and perforation of acute cholecystitis with either pericholecystic abscess or generalized peritonitis. Grading of cholecystitis has aided in delineating the severity of disease and identifying surgical risk. In addition to the TG18 grades (**Table 15.1**), the American Association for the Surgery of Trauma (AAST) has also developed an anatomically based severity grading system for cholecystitis (**Table 15.2 and Figure 15.1**). Although the AAST grading system

TABLE 15.2 ■ AAST Grades of Acute Cholecystitis

Grade	Description	Imaging	Operative
I	Localized gallbladder inflammation	Wall thickening, pericholecystic fluid, nonvisualization of the gallbladder	Localized inflammatory changes
II	Distended gallbladder with purulence or hydrops, necrosis/gangrene of wall noted without iatrogenic perforation	Above plus air in the gallbladder lumen, wall, or biliary tree	Distended gallbladder with pus/hydrops, nonperforated wall necrosis/gangrene
III	Noniatrogenic perforation with bile located to RUQ	Extraluminal fluid collection limited to RUQ	Noniatrogenic gallbladder wall perforation with bile limited to RUQ
IV	Pericholecystic abscess, bilioenteric fistula, gallstone ileus	RUQ abscess, bilioenteric fistula, gallstone ileus	Pericholecystic abscess, bilioenteric fistula, gallstone ileus
V	Grade IV disease with generalized peritonitis	Free intraperitoneal fluid	Above with generalized peritonitis

Staudenmayer KL, Shafi S, et al. The American Association for the Surgery of Trauma grading scale for 16 emergency general surgery conditions: disease-specific criteria characterizing anatomic severity grading. *J Trauma Acute Care Surg*. 2016;81(3):593-602.

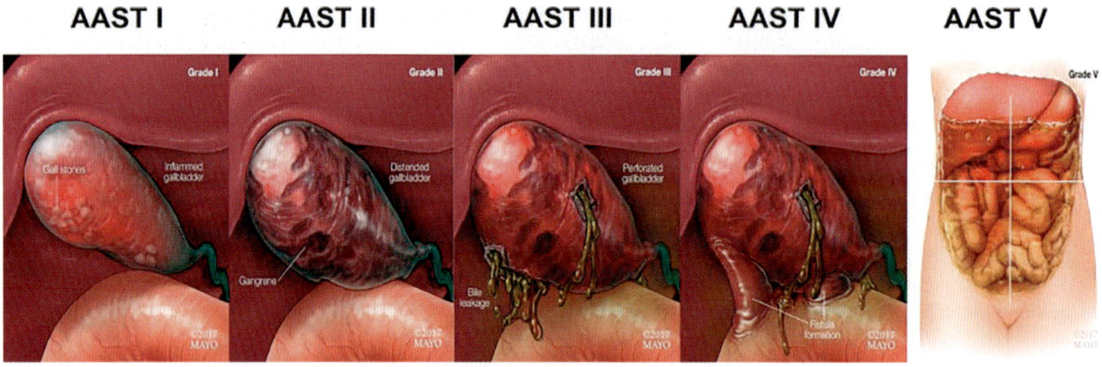

Figure 15.1 AAST grades of acute cholecystitis. (Reprinted from Hernandez M, Murphy B, Aho JM, et al. Validation of the AAST EGS acute cholecystitis grade and comparison with the Tokyo guidelines. *Surgery.* 2018;163(4):739-746, with permission from Elsevier.)

requires further prospective validation, at least one study suggested that it outperformed the TG18 grades for key clinical outcomes.

Chronic Cholecystitis

Although acute calculous cholecystitis remains the most common biliary tract disorder, other pathologies must be considered. Chronic cholecystitis results from ongoing inflammation of the gallbladder that is largely due to calculous disease. Symptoms are congruent with acute cholecystitis, although they can also be more vague, especially in the elderly population. In chronic cholecystitis, the gallbladder may appear contracted on imaging or may be associated with a decreased ejection fraction on HIDA.

Functional Disorders of the Gallbladder

Other gallbladder pathology includes functional disorders of the gallbladder. Biliary dyskinesia can manifest as episodic pain with decreased ejection of bile from the gallbladder. Ultrasound assessment of the gallbladder before and following a meal can lend to the diagnosis, as can HIDA scan. A decreased ejection fraction of approximately <40% supports but does not confirm the diagnosis of biliary dyskinesia. Other functional disorders include sphincter of Oddi dysfunction or stenosis and cystic duct dysmotility. Specifics regarding diagnosis and management of these functional gallbladder disorders are delineated in the Rome IV consensus criteria.

Choledocholithiasis

Choledocholithiasis is the mechanical obstruction of the biliary tract by gallstones. This can lead to further pathology including cholangitis and acute pancreatitis, which confer significant morbidity and mortality to patients. Clinically, patients can present with RUQ pain and signs of jaundice such as scleral icterus, clay-colored stools, and dark-colored urine. Laboratory examinations may reveal elevated bilirubin and alkaline phosphatase. Workup for the etiology of suspected obstructive jaundice includes several imaging modalities including transabdominal ultrasound, endoscopic ultrasound (EUS), magnetic resonance cholangiopancreatography (MRCP), and endoscopic retrograde cholangiopancreatography (ERCP). The sensitivity and specificity of EUS and MRCP are both high and comparable to each other. MRCP is less invasive than EUS but has lower resolution.

The American Society for Gastrointestinal Endoscopy (ASGE) classifies the risk of choledocholithiasis as low, intermediate, or high (**Table 15.3**). The ASGE risk stratification schema can help guide diagnostic strategy, which depends on the pretest probability of choledocholithiasis and patient factors and resource availability (**Figure 15.2**). For example, patients with a low risk for choledocholithiasis may need no additional workup. In patients with intermediate risk, a preoperative EUS or MRCP may be performed. Alternatively, intraoperative cholangiography or ultrasound may be performed during laparoscopic cholecystectomy. In patients with a high-risk, preoperative ERCP or intraoperative laparoscopic common bile duct (CBD), exploration may be performed.

Acute Cholangitis

Biliary infection as a result of any obstructing biliary etiology can be classified as acute cholangitis. Traditionally, Charcot triad of RUQ pain, fever, and jaundice has been used to diagnose acute cholangitis. However, the sensitivity of this clinical tool ranges from 50% to 70%. Other schema for the diagnosis and grading of severity of acute cholangitis has been developed, such as the TG18

TABLE 15.3 ■ ASGE Risk Stratification for Choledocholithiasis

Strength	**Predictors**
Moderate	Abnormal liver biochemical test other than bilirubin Age older than 55 y Clinical gallstone pancreatitis
Strong	Dilated CBD on ultrasound >6 mm (with gallbladder *in situ*) Bilirubin level 1.8-4 mg/dL
Very strong	CBD stone on transabdominal ultrasound Clinical ascending cholangitis Bilirubin >4 mg/dL
Risk strata	
Low	No predictors present
Intermediate	All patients who are not in the low- or high-risk strata
High	Presence of any very strong predictor Presence of both strong predictors

Based on Committee ASoP, Buxbaum JL, Abbas Fehmi SM, Sultan S, et al. ASGE guideline on the role of endoscopy in the evaluation and management of choledocholithiasis. *Gastrointest Endosc.* 2019;89(6):1075-1105 e15.

criteria (**Table 15.4**). The sensitivity of the TG18 criteria is higher than that of Charcot triad. Whereas the sensitivity of ultrasound in this scenario is somewhat low, the specificity is higher. CT scan provides information on concomitant complications, including adjacent abscesses or thrombosis. Both dynamic CT and MRI may be useful in this diagnosis, although further literature is required.

Gallstone Pancreatitis

As an etiology of pancreatitis, gallstones occur in up to 55% of patients presenting with pancreatitis. Diagnosis involves meeting two of three criteria: upper abdominal pain, levels of serum amylase or lipase or both three or more times above normal, and imaging consistent with acute pancreatitis. In identifying a biliary etiology, transabdominal ultrasound is recommended to determine the presence or absence of gallstones or sludge. Additionally, liver function tests can also be used to assist in diagnosis. CT and MRI may be useful in the early phase (first week) if the diagnosis is uncertain or after initial presentation (after 48-72 hours) to detect complications such as hemorrhage or development of peripancreatic fluid collections.

Acute pancreatitis is classified as either interstitial edematous or necrotizing (see Chapter 14: Acute Pancreatitis). Interstitial edematous pancreatitis tends to be more common and is often self-limiting, while necrotizing pancreatitis is more severe and can result in complications such as infection and hemorrhage. Multiple classification systems have been used to classify the severity of pancreatitis; one of the more commonly used is the revised Atlanta classification (**Table 15.5**). The AAST also has developed acute pancreatitis grades based on clinical, imaging, operative, and pathologic criteria.

Management

Biliary Colic

Immediate management of an episode of biliary colic includes pain control if needed. Subsequent alternatives for management include medical vs surgical strategies. Medical management

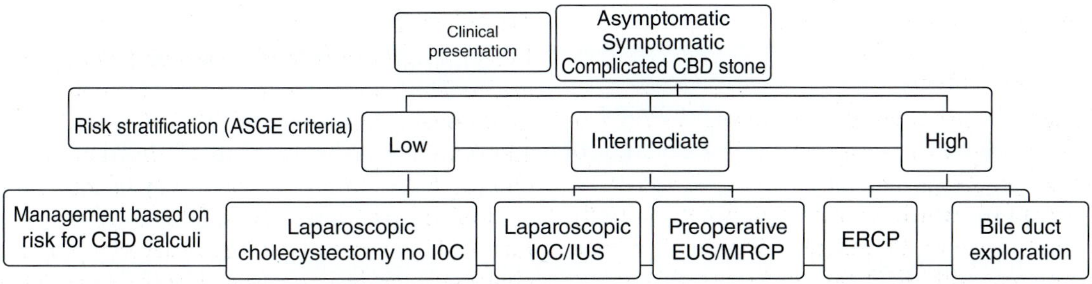

Figure 15.2 Algorithm for management of common bile duct stones.

TABLE 15.4 ■ Tokyo Guidelines 18 Severity Grading for Acute Cholangitis

Grade	Conditions
I (mild)	Does not meet criteria of grades II or III acute cholangitis at initial diagnosis
II (moderate)	Any 2 of the following: Abnormal WBC count (>12 000/mm^3, <4000/mm^3) High fever (≥39 °C) Age (≥75 y) Hyperbilirubinemia (total bilirubin ≥5 mg/dL) Hypoalbuminemia (less than lower limit of normal value × 0.7)
III (severe)	Associated with any organ dysfunction of the following: Cardiovascular: Hypotension requiring vasopressors Neurologic: Decreased level of consciousness Respiratory PaO_2/FiO_2 < 300 Renal: Oliguria, creatinine >2.0 mg/dL Hepatic: PT-INR > 1.5 1. Hematologic: Platelets <100 000/mm^3

Based on Kiriyama S, Kozaka K, Takada T, et al. Tokyo Guidelines 2018: diagnostic criteria and severity grading of acute cholangitis (with videos). *J Hepatobiliary Pancreat Sci.* 2018;25(1):41-54.

consists primarily of watchful waiting or expectant management. Dietary modification and avoidance of foods that may exacerbate symptoms (ie, fatty foods) are often recommended. Oral dissolution therapy such as ursodeoxycholic acid has been prescribed but has not proven to reduce the risk of biliary complications or improve symptoms. Extracorporeal shock wave lithotripsy has also been utilized but is not considered a first-line treatment option. In suitable patients who seek operative intervention or fail expectant management, laparoscopic cholecystectomy is typically the procedure of choice.

Acute Calculous Cholecystitis

Laparoscopic cholecystectomy is the preferred treatment for acute calculous cholecystitis in patients who are surgical candidates. Although a diagnosis of cholecystitis and nonelective operation increase the operative difficulty of laparoscopic cholecystectomy, guidelines are consistent that whenever possible, laparoscopic cholecystectomy should be performed during index admission for acute cholecystitis, ideally within 48 hours of admission. Other predictors of a difficult cholecystectomy include age, American Society of Anesthesiologists classification, male gender, thick-walled gallbladders, CBD dilation, and preoperative ERCP. Operative strategies for the difficult gallbladder are discussed later in this chapter and include conversion to open, a fundus-down approach, subtotal cholecystectomy, and placement of an open cholecystostomy tube as a bailout procedure. Although laparoscopic cholecystectomy is still the preferred initial treatment in high-risk patients when feasible, percutaneous cholecystostomy tube drainage is an option in patients in whom the surgical risks outweigh the benefits. Endoscopic transpapillary gallbladder drainage is a newer technique that has been reported to be an option for poor-risk candidates. Antibiotics are not indicated for uncomplicated acute cholecystitis but should be administered for complicated acute cholecystitis.

Choledocholithiasis

There are several therapeutic options for the management of choledocholithiasis. Choice of management strategy should consider the probability of the

TABLE 15.5 ■ Revised Atlanta Classification of Pancreatitis Severity

	Mild	Moderate	Severe
Organ failure	No	Resolving <48 h (transient organ failure)	Persistent >48 h
Local or systemic complications	No	Without persistent organ failure	Single or multiple organ failure

Based on Banks PA, Bollen TL, Dervenis C, et al. Classification of acute pancreatitis—2012: revision of the Atlanta classification and definitions by international consensus. *Gut.* 2013;62(1):102-111.

diagnosis along with local expertise and resources. Options for management include ERCP with sphincterotomy and stone retrieval; timing can be pre-, intra-, or postoperatively. Alternatively, patients may undergo laparoscopic cholecystectomy with CBD exploration. If unsuccessful, a transcystic bile duct stent can be placed to ensure biliary drainage. In patients with large biliary ductal stones (>1 cm), endoscopic sphincterotomy with large balloon dilation is conditionally recommended over sphincterotomy alone. Mechanical lithotripsy, cholangioscopy-guided intraductal laser, and electrohydraulic lithotripsy can also be considered for these patients. When all else fails, open CBD exploration with or without transduodenal sphincterotomy or sphincteroplasty remain options.

Cholangitis

Mortality rates of cholangitis can be as high as 8%-10%, depending on severity. Thus, prompt resuscitation and treatment are required upon diagnosis. TG18 provides management recommendations based on severity. All grades of acute cholangitis should be treated with antibiotic coverage. Empiric antibiotic coverage should include treatment for *Escherichia coli* and *Klebsiella* species, given that they are the two predominant pathogens in acute cholangitis. Antibiotics are aimed at preventing the systemic spread of infection and assisting with the control of primary infection. Blood cultures should be obtained for grades II and III cholangitis and any hospital-associated cholangitis. Analgesics have not been demonstrated to mask the pain associated with cholangitis and should be administered. Of note, however, opioid analgesics result in the contraction of the sphincter of Oddi, potentially exacerbating the cholangitis.

In patients with grade III or severe cholangitis (as indicated by end-organ dysfunction), urgent biliary drainage with supportive care remains the mainstay of treatment. Biliary drainage may be accomplished via an endoscopic approach with sphincterotomy or via a percutaneous transhepatic approach. Single-stage ERCP with sphincterotomy and laparoscopic choledocholithotomy may also be considered, although further data are still pending on these outcomes. If biliary drainage is not available, patients with grades II and III cholangitis should be transferred to centers with these capabilities.

Gallstone Pancreatitis

Several scoring systems have been proposed to classify the severity of pancreatitis and to predict outcome. Historically, Ranson criteria, consisting of five criteria evaluated on admission and six criteria assessed after 48 hours into admission, were used. Recently, the International Association of Pancreatology and American Pancreatic Association have conferred that systemic inflammatory response syndrome criteria are better aligned with the classification of acute pancreatitis. The revised Atlanta classification has also been utilized as a severity classification system. In cases of acute pancreatitis without evidence of infection, antibiotic prophylaxis is not indicated. Enteral nutrition is encouraged, via oral, nasogastric, or nasojejunal routes, if tolerated by the patient. Early ERCP and endoscopic sphincterotomy should be considered in the setting of cholangitis or ongoing biliary obstruction; however, routine ERCP is not indicated. Multiple randomized trials and meta-analyses have demonstrated that laparoscopic cholecystectomy should be performed during the index admission for mild gallstone pancreatitis when possible. Although a few studies have suggested that cholecystectomy within the first 72 hours of admission is safe for mild gallstone pancreatitis, even in the absence of resolution of pain and improvement in laboratory values, further trials are needed.

Interventions may be indicated for complications of severe or necrotizing gallstone pancreatitis. Hemorrhage secondary to pseudoaneurysm formation may require angioembolization. Infected peripancreatic fluid collections may require percutaneous, endoscopic, videoscopic, or open drainage. Additionally, operative intervention is indicated for infected pancreatic necrosis with a decline in the patient's clinical status. If possible, it is ideal for giving an interim of 4 weeks from onset of pathology to operative intervention to allow for walling off of necrosis and ease of operative success.

Surgical Techniques

Once cholecystectomy is indicated, then an operative approach to the patient should be decided. In 1987, Phillipe Mouret performed the first laparoscopic cholecystectomy in France. Within 5 years, this became the primary method of cholecystectomy in the United States. The available options are open cholecystectomy, laparoscopic cholecystectomy, and robotic cholecystectomy. Bailout procedures such as subtotal cholecystectomy and cholecystostomy tube should also be in the surgeon's armamentarium.

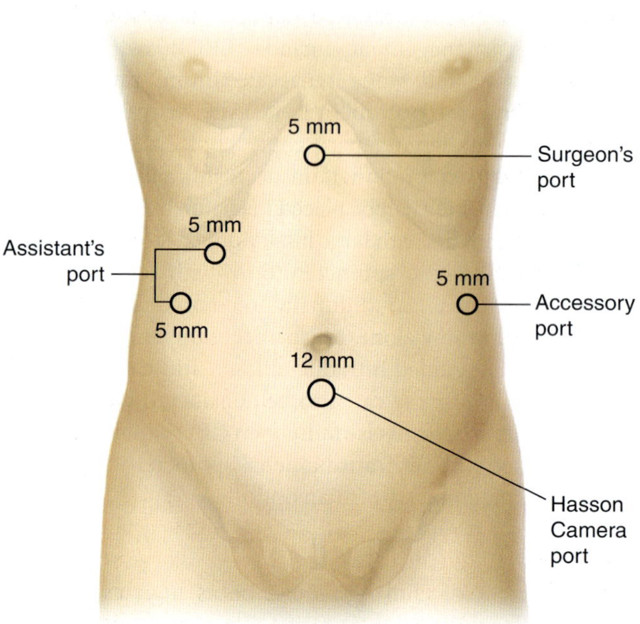

Figure 15.3 Example of port placement for laparoscopic cholecystectomy. Typically, ports *A*, *B*, and *C* are working ports with *D* serving as the camera port. Depending on surgeon preference, port *C* or *D* is a larger 10- to 12-mm port for eventual retrieval of the gallbladder, with the remaining ports being 5 mm. (Modified from Lillemoe Master *Techniques in Surgery: Hepatobiliary and Pancreatic Surgery*. 2nd ed. Wolters Kluwer; 2020.)

Laparoscopic Cholecystectomy

The laparoscopic approach, which became standard by the mid-1990s, is the procedure of choice for many surgeons. However, in preparation for any laparoscopic procedure, surgeons should also prepare the patient for the possibility of an open operation in the event this is deemed necessary intraoperatively. The open approach will be addressed later.

The patient should be prepared from the nipples to the lower mid abdomen. Initial access can be obtained in any manner the surgeon feels is most appropriate; options include an open Hasson technique at the umbilicus, Veress needle insufflation, or optical trocar insertion under direct visualization. The resultant port placement is classically described as three additional ports in the RUQ—one epigastric, one midaxillary, and the other along the anterior axillary line (**Figure 15.3**). Surgeons will often have some preferred variation on these port placements to adjust for personal ergonomics.

The most lateral RUQ port is typically used to grasp and retract the fundus of the gallbladder in the anterior and cephalad direction to expose the cystic structures. The midaxillary port is used to retract the infundibulum inferiorly and laterally. This retraction aims to elongate the cystic structures away from the CBD to create the optimal retraction for the "critical view" (**Figure 15.4**). This retraction can be thought of as a line running up the cystic structures and making a right angle at the infundibulum straight up the body and fundus of the gallbladder. This up and out retraction is one of the keys to success. Dissection typically begins with opening the peritoneum over the infundibulum and extending this up onto the

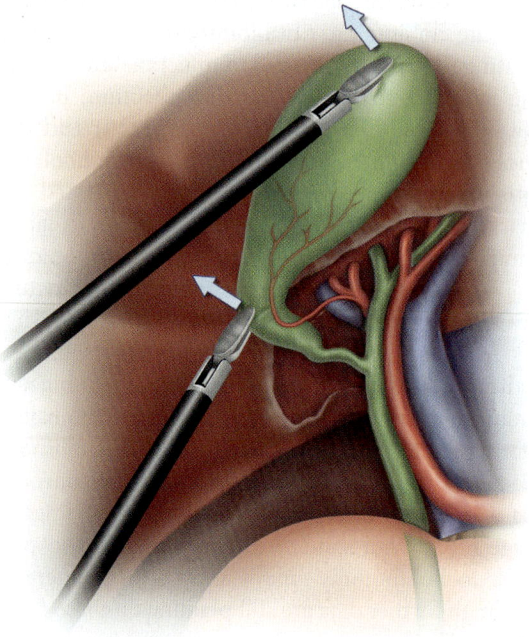

Figure 15.4 Retraction of the gallbladder during laparoscopic cholecystectomy. Retraction of the gallbladder away from the common bile duct during dissection and creating the critical view of safety is key to the operation. This can be achieved by retracting the gall bladder away from the common bile duct and creating a right angle.

gallbladder fossa, working to expose the cystic structures.

Use of the "critical view of safety" is recommended to minimize the risk of bile duct injury.

The critical view of safety:

1. Clear the hepatocystic triangle.
2. Expose at least the lower one-third of the cystic plate.
3. Leave only two structures entering the gallbladder.

The critical view of safety is obtained by clearing the hepatocystic triangle (inferior liver edge, cystic duct, and common hepatic duct) of fat and fibrous tissue and then dissecting the lower one-third of the gallbladder from the liver bed to expose the cystic plate. The resulting dissection should reveal the cystic duct and cystic artery as the only two structures that should be seen entering the gallbladder; if this is not the case, additional dissection is needed to assess aberrant anatomy before transection of any structures. Depending on the degree and chronicity of inflammation, this dissection can be very challenging. A top-down or fundus-first approach may be employed if there is extensive scaring, similar to how an open cholecystectomy is done. However, caution should be used as the top-down approach can lead to devastating injuries if the anatomy is misinterpreted. Thus, it is important to note that if there is a question regarding the dissection, exposure, or uncontrolled bleeding, converting to an open operation may be the safest approach.

To reduce complications such as bile duct injuries associated with laparoscopic cholecystectomy, the Society of American Gastrointestinal Endoscopic Surgeons (SAGES) has published "The SAGES Safe Cholecystectomy Program." The program outlines six strategies surgeons can employ to "adopt a universal culture of safety for cholecystectomy and minimize the risk of bile duct injury." These include the following:

1. Use the critical view of safety.
2. Understanding aberrant anatomy.
3. Liberal use of biliary tree imaging intraoperatively.
4. Use of an intraoperative "pause" before transection of any ductal structure.
5. Recognize when your dissection is approaching the "zone of significant risk" and convert to another method, ie, perform a subtotal cholecystectomy, place a cholecystostomy tube, or convert to an open operation.
6. Ask for help from another surgeon in challenging cases with difficult dissections or unclear anatomy.

The listed strategies should be employed to minimize the risk of bile duct injury, which is a highly morbid and potentially life-altering complication for patients. Nonetheless, even when using these strategies, surgeons need to be aware of potential errors to avoid injury.

Although the critical view of safety is described as essential for every cholecystectomy to minimize the risk of CBD injuries, it is only achieved about 60% of the time. It is important to keep in mind that misinterpretation of normal anatomy, especially in an inflamed and infected field, can lead to injury and misadventures during cholecystectomy. Strasberg error traps describe circumstances in which techniques employed to ensure safety can contribute to misinterpretations of anatomy. The first of these is the "infundibular view," in which 360° dissection facilitates a three-dimensional funnel shape of the lower end of the gallbladder going into the cystic duct. Injuries occur most frequently in a field of chronic inflammation when a false view is obtained, meaning the CBD, being mistaken for the cystic duct, is followed up to the gallbladder. In these types of conditions, the gallbladder and cystic duct may be adherent to the CBD in the inflammatory mass, scarring down and obliterating the triangle of Calot. In addition, the potential to misinterpret anatomy is further increased with the presence of a large stone impacted in the gallbladder neck, and a thickened, distended, or contracted gallbladder due to scarring and difficulty with retraction.

Another dissection error trap is associated with the fundus-down or "top-down" method for cholecystectomy. Injuries related to this technique tend to be the most severe, especially after conversion from laparoscopic to open cholecystectomy. In the inflamed and scarred-in field, the gallbladder can be adherent to the hepatic bile ducts, arteries, and portal venous structures, contributing to the inadvertent transection of these structures. Concomitant vascular injuries can cause infarction of all or part of the liver and can ultimately require resection.

In challenging cases, a landmark of note is the Rouviere sulcus, defined initially as the groove of the caudate lobe. It can be found between the right lobe of the liver and the caudate process. Occurring in ~80% of patients, this anatomic landmark may range from a small but visible slit to a deep sulcus. During laparoscopic cholecystectomies, the required pneumoperitoneum results in increased visibility of this landmark. The dorsum, or floor, of this sulcus houses the right portal vein, right hepatic artery, and right hepatic bile duct. The base confers the direction of the CBD. Therefore, dissection should be maintained ventral to this landmark.

Open Cholecystectomy

Conversion from laparoscopic to open cholecystectomy is indicated when the procedure cannot be completed safely, such as in the setting of hemorrhage, perforation, or pregnancy. Risk factors for conversion include increased gallbladder wall thickness, contracted gallbladder, older age, male sex, and acute cholecystitis. Other reasons for open cholecystectomy may include the inability of the patient to tolerate pneumoperitoneum, anticipated difficulties with laparoscopic cholecystectomy such as due to coagulopathy or adhesions, or plan to perform a concomitant open procedure. Open cholecystectomy can be done either through a subcostal or an upper midline incision. In a "top-down" fashion, the peritoneum is opened at the gallbladder fundus and liver edge interface, taking the gallbladder down off the fossa to the pedicle of the cystic duct and artery. When the cystic structures cannot be positively identified or the scarring is too extensive, consider a subtotal cholecystectomy, which has been shown to have comparable morbidity rates to total cholecystectomy and is considered safe in the setting of a difficult gallbladder.

Subtotal Cholecystectomy

When there is too much inflammation in the hepatocystic triangle to safely identify the anatomy, an option is to perform a subtotal cholecystectomy. Although partial and subtotal have been used synonymously in the past, the term subtotal cholecystectomy is preferred as it implies near-total removal of the gallbladder. Subtotal cholecystectomy can be performed either via a laparoscopic or an open approach. If the gallbladder wall is adherent to the liver, it may be left in place and the mucosa fulgurated. There is no consensus on how best to manage the remnant in a subtotal cholecystectomy. Options include an attempt to close the gallbladder (reconstituting) or to leave it open (fenestrated) (**Figure 15.5**). At least one closed suction drain is placed. No randomized trials exist comparing reconstituting to fenestrate subtotal cholecystectomies. However, retrospective data suggest that there is no significant difference in the rates of complications. There may be more long-term recurrent biliary events despite a higher need for completion cholecystectomy with fenestration.

Robotic Cholecystectomy

As the popularity of robotics has entered the surgical world, robotic cholecystectomy has been employed. Studies suggest that robotic cholecystectomy is not safer and only adds time to the procedure, especially in the preparatory phase. There

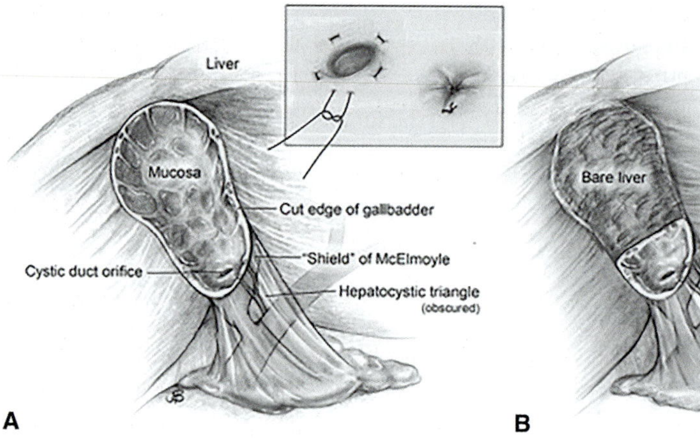

Figure 15.5 Fenestrated subtotal cholecystectomy. **A.** Demonstrates excision of the peritonealized portion of the gallbladder, except for the area near the cystic duct to avoid entering the hepatocystic triangle. **B.** Shows excision of all of the gallbladder except for the portion adherent to the liver near the cystic duct. The inset illustrates the option of closing the cystic duct with a purse-string suture. (From Strasberg SM, Pucci MJ, Brunt LM, Deziel DJ. Subtotal Cholecystectomy-"Fenestrating" vs "Reconstituting" Subtypes and the Prevention of Bile Duct Injury: Definition of the Optimal Procedure in Difficult Operative Conditions. *J Am Coll Surg*. 2016 Jan;222(1):89-96.)

is also evidence that robotic cholecystectomy may be associated with increased cost.

Cholangiography

It is important to ensure that patients with elevated bilirubin do not have obstructing stones left unmanaged. Though there are multiple options for assessing the biliary ducts, including preoperative MRCP or ERCP, intraoperative cholangiography can also be used. There is controversy regarding the use of routine vs selective fluoroscopic intraoperative cholangiography; regardless, this should be a skill that surgeons have available, especially if biliary anatomy is unclear or there is a question of injury to the common duct. This requires cannulation of the cystic duct for injection of contrast into the duct during live fluoroscopy.

A newer option for anatomic identification of the bile ducts intraoperatively is near-infrared fluoroscopy. This method has the benefit of not needing to incise and cannulate the cystic duct. The water-soluble fluorescent dye, indocyanine green, is given to the patient intravenously in the preoperative area, giving it time to be taken up by the liver and start to be excreted into the biliary tree. This method has been shown to reduce operative times when compared to traditional fluoroscopic cholangiography. The downsides to this method are that it does not detect retained stones and may be less effective in bloody fields or in patients with increased body mass index. In addition, the laparoscope has to be equipped with near-infrared technology.

The other option that has been described but is not often used is laparoscopic ultrasonography. This has the benefit of being noninvasive, does not require contrast injection, and its overall low cost. It can also identify stones in addition to ductal anatomy, especially in situations where anatomy is obscured. However, the learning curve for this can be steep, and thus, the technique has not been widely adopted.

Although cholangiography can help define anatomy, it is important to recognize that it does not prevent injuries. Misidentification of anatomy is still possible. One trap to be aware of is the aberrant right hepatic duct. This duct can join with the cystic duct prior to it joining the common duct.

Common Bile Duct Exploration

Common bile duct (CBD) exploration has become less common with the technical advancements in ERCP for the management of choledocholithiasis. Overall, randomized controlled trials comparing a single-stage laparoscopic cholecystectomy and CBD exploration to a two-staged laparoscopic cholecystectomy followed by ERCP show no significant differences in effectiveness in clearing the duct or complications between the two approaches. With this in mind, the choice of approach may be operator dependent. The surgical approach to CBD exploration is described below.

Open CBD exploration is performed through a choledochotomy in the CBD. This is performed after an extensive Kocher maneuver and clearance of the CBD for 3-5 cm in the region of the cystic duct, stay sutures are placed, and a longitudinal incision is made in the CBD for ~1 cm distal to the cystic duct. It is important that the opening is large enough to minimize trauma from instrument insertion. Multiple instruments exist to clear stones, including balloon catheters, irrigating catheters, scoops, and graspers. In addition, a choledochoscope can be used to facilitate exploration and stone extraction with balloons and baskets. Once the duct is cleared, the choledochotomy is closed over a T-tube using an absorbable suture. A closing cholangiogram should be performed to confirm the clearance of stones.

Laparoscopic CBD exploration can be performed via a transcystic approach, whereby a cystic ductotomy is made, a cholangiogram balloon catheter is inserted, and a cholangiogram can be performed at this time to confirm position and anatomy. The duct can be flushed using 20-30 mL saline, which may flush small stones out. To facilitate the ability to flush out gallstones, glucagon may be administered to assist with the relaxation of the sphincter of Oddi. The next option is to pass a Fogarty balloon to pull stones out through the cystic duct. If this is not successful, then the use of the choledochoscope may be needed. To perform this, a transcystic guidewire is placed into the CBD. The cystic duct orifice must then be dilated to accommodate the scope with an 8-Fr angioplasty balloon. A 12-Fr introducer catheter is then placed as a conduit for entry into the biliary tree and facilitates multiple reentries. Similar to the open procedure, balloons, graspers, and baskets can be used to retrieve stones via the choledochoscope. *If the transcystic approach is not possible, a choledochotomy can be made in the CBD and a choledochoscope used as described for the open approach; the CBD should be closed over a T-tube.* The T-tube should be left in place for drainage for 4 weeks. A cholangiogram can then be performed to confirm patency of the ducts and stone clearance, followed by removal of the tube.

In patients with previous Roux-en-Y gastric bypass, a laparoscopic-assisted ERCP can be performed. Indications include choledocholithiasis requiring stone retrieval and sphincterotomy and cystic duct stump leaks with stent placement and later stent retrieval. This technique involves the performance of a laparoscopic gastrotomy in the gastric remnant to introduce the endoscope into the stomach. This can be facilitated by tacking the stomach to the anterior abdominal wall with stay sutures and introducing a 15-mm trocar to insert the scope through. If needed, a gastrostomy tube may be placed for later access if a stent needs to be retrieved or another therapeutic intervention needs to be performed.

Cholecystostomy

In patients considered high risk for cholecystectomy, percutaneous or open cholecystostomy tube drainage can be considered. Per TG18, patients to be considered for cholecystostomy are those with grade II disease and >96 hours of symptoms and grade II disease and high risk for surgery. Cholecystostomy may also be a temporizing measure for those with grade III disease.

In 2018, Loozen et al. published the results of their multicenter randomized controlled trial (CHOCOLATE) comparing laparoscopic cholecystectomy to percutaneous cholecystostomy tube in high-risk patients. High-risk patients in this trial were primarily identified as those with an Acute Physiology and Chronic Health Evaluation (APACHE) II of 7-15. In this population, percutaneous cholecystostomy tube as compared to laparoscopic cholecystectomy was associated with higher mortality (9% vs 3%, $p = .27$) and more major complications (65% vs 12%, $p < .001$). Complications included infectious and cardiopulmonary complications within 1 month and any type of reintervention or recurrent biliary disease within 1 year. These results may not be generalizable to all patients since the trial excluded patients with a prohibitive surgical risk as demonstrated by an APACHE II score of ≥15, symptoms for >7 days on presentation, pregnancy, decompensated liver cirrhosis, or ICU admission at the time of diagnosis of cholecystitis.

The use of percutaneous or surgical cholecystostomy should be considered in patients who are truly critically ill with acute cholecystitis as a temporizing measure with significant consideration for interval cholecystectomy. However, the timing of laparoscopic cholecystectomy after percutaneous cholecystostomy tube drainage is controversial. The other indication may be in those with significant comorbidities in whom the surgical risk outweighs the benefit. Although age is often considered a risk factor for poor outcomes, age alone should not be an indication for avoiding cholecystectomy.

Complications

The overall complication rate for cholecystectomy is ~10%. The most feared complication is bile leak or common bile duct injury; the rates of these complications are 0.1%-1.5%. However, they can carry significant morbidity and mortality.

Bile leak after cholecystectomy is an important complication to diagnose and treat early, with a reported incidence of 1%-4% after laparoscopic cholecystectomy. Postoperatively, patients may present with fever, right upper quadrant pain, sepsis, and even septic shock from bile peritonitis. Serum bilirubin may be elevated in laboratory studies. Imaging may include ultrasound, CT scan, or MRI to assist in this diagnosis by finding a fluid collection in the previous surgical bed. A HIDA scan may demonstrate an active bile leak. The priority for management should be control of contamination. Percutaneous drainage may be performed if there is a localized fluid collection. In contrast, surgical washout and drainage may be required if there is bile peritonitis or the patient is critically ill. Then the bile leak needs to be managed. For a cystic duct stump leak, duct of Luschka, or even a small CBD injury, this often is done via ERCP with sphincterotomy and stent placement to divert bile. For more significant CBD injuries, delayed reconstruction may be required after resolution of intra-abdominal sepsis, improvement of inflammation, and optimization of nutritional status.

Intraoperatively, *common bile duct injury*, if small and identified at the time of surgery, may be managed by repair over a T-tube. However, if noted at the time of surgery, the most important step, especially for the young surgeon, is to stop and call for help. It is critical that if you injure a duct, first do no further harm and do not persist with the operation as this is likely to worsen the injury. Early referral to a specialty center and delayed repair for complex bile duct injuries such as a complete transection confer favorable outcomes. Surgical repair, if needed, may include either end-to-end ductal anastomosis or hepaticojejunostomy.

Other complications of surgery for biliary disease may include postoperative bleeding. Potential sources include the cystic plate, cystic artery, hepatic vessels, or port sites. For the unstable patient, immediate return to the operating room is required. The other complication to be aware of is bowel injury. It is important to remember the proximity of the surgical field to the duodenum and the potential for inadvertent injury, especially during challenging dissections. A high index of suspicion must be maintained to detect and treat these complications.

Additional Pathology

Acute Acalculous Cholecystitis

Acute acalculous cholecystitis is an uncommon variant of acute cholecystitis that should be suspected in critically ill patients as a potential source of sepsis, particularly in those patients with unexplained fever, leukocytosis, and/or upper abdominal pain. Risk factors include cholestasis due to total parental nutrition and/or prolonged bowel rest, shock, and prolonged narcotic use. Timing is typically weeks after the initial insult.

For diagnosis, an abdominal ultrasound should be performed. Suggestive findings include a thickened wall, gallbladder distension, and absence of stones or sludge. Second, a HIDA scan should be obtained. Nonvisualization of the gallbladder after morphine challenge is consistent with acute acalculous cholecystitis. The combination of positive findings on ultrasound and HIDA scan are highly sensitive and specific.

Given that most patients with acute acalculous cholecystitis are critically ill, the initial treatment is typically percutaneous cholecystostomy tube; this serves to decompress the gallbladder and generally provides source control. After resolution of the critical illness, drains can be used to obtain a cholecystogram to assess the patency of the biliary tree. If the gallbladder empties and the patient is asymptomatic with the tube clamped, the patient will likely tolerate tube removal. Otherwise, cholecystectomy should be considered when the patient has recovered from their critical illness if they are an operative candidate. In poor-risk patients, a cholecystostomy tube may be the definitive treatment.

Mirizzi Syndrome

In certain patients presenting with signs and symptoms of cholecystitis or choledocholithiasis, workup may demonstrate extrinsic compression onto the CBD; this is Mirizzi syndrome. A common etiology is an impacted stone in the infundibulum of the gallbladder or the cystic duct. Patients often present with obstructive jaundice. ERCP is the gold standard for diagnosis, although MRCP is also useful. Five Csendes types have been described, ranging from simple external compression to cholecystobiliary or cholecystoenteric fistulae. The complication rate of laparoscopic surgery is high in these cases, especially without a preoperative diagnosis. Therefore, open surgery is sometimes considered safer.

Gallstone Ileus

Gallstone ileus is an infrequent complication, occurring in up to 4% of patients with cholelithiasis. Chronic mucosal inflammation from an impacted gallstone results in fistulization, commonly presenting as a cholecystoduodenal fistula (85%). Less frequent fistulae include cholecystocolonic, cholecystogastric (Bouveret syndrome), and others. Despite the misnomer, gallstone ileus is a mechanical bowel obstruction, present in up to 0.5% of patients with bowel obstruction, with a stone most commonly impacted at the ileocecal valve. The frequency increases in elderly patients and has a greater prevalence among elderly women rather than men.

Patients generally present with signs and symptoms of bowel obstruction, including nausea, vomiting, and abdominal distension, occurring intermittently. Infrequently, hematemesis may be present due to the presence of fistula formation. Laboratory values may demonstrate a leukocytosis; however, the presence of laboratory anomalies is relatively nonspecific. Abdominal films may demonstrate the classic signs of bowel obstruction, including dilated loops of bowel and air-fluid levels. Additionally, pneumobilia or air in the biliary tree may be present. CT scan has remarkable sensitivity and specificity for this process, demonstrating findings of cholecystitis, bowel obstruction, and the presence of an obstructing gallstone. Ultrasound examination may reveal cholecystitis, pneumobilia, and an obstructing stone, although sensitivity is low. HIDA scan is similarly of low sensitivity, although it may identify a fistula tract. MRCP may be used to demonstrate a fistula tract and the additional findings of gallstone ileus; however, a CT scan is the preferred method for diagnosis. Stones generally range in size from 2 to 5 cm.

Given that gallstone ileus may be a subacute or even chronic condition in elderly patients, treatment includes resuscitation and optimization of patient comorbidities. Surgical treatment is primarily directed at relieving the obstruction by performing an enterolithotomy to remove the obstructing stone. This has been described generally via a laparotomy, although laparoscopy is also an option, depending on surgeon ability and patient tolerance. After milking the stone proximally, an enterotomy should be created on the antimesenteric portion of the bowel longitudinally and closed transversely. Occasionally, a bowel resection is required if the stone is immobile, if there is bowel perforation or ischemia. The rest of the gastrointestinal tract should be examined for additional stones. The decision regarding whether or not to perform a concomitant cholecystectomy and fistula closure at the time of enterolithotomy depends on the patient's risk for complications due to physiologic status and comorbidities. Cholecystectomy in this setting may be very difficult and is generally not indicated. In high-risk patients in whom cholecystectomy is deferred, delayed cholecystectomy is recommended if there are residual or recurrent biliary symptoms and if the patient can be medically optimized.

A variant of gallstone ileus is Bouveret syndrome, where a stone that has passed through a cholecystoduodenal fistula results in gastric outlet obstruction. Whereas enterolithotomy alone is not optimal for patients with cholecystoduodenal fistulas, literature is still evolving on the use of enterolithotomy alone for patients with Bouveret syndrome.

Special Considerations

Pregnancy

Surgical management of biliary disease, including symptomatic cholelithiasis, acute cholecystitis, and choledocholithiasis, should be considered in pregnancy. Nonoperative management is associated with high rates of recurrent symptoms, especially for those presenting in the 1st trimester. For patients with uncomplicated disease, the risk of preterm labor and fetal demise are similar for operative and nonoperative management. However, the rate of developing complicated disease is 1:4 to 1:5 patients, which is associated with preterm labor and fetal loss. Available evidence and SAGES support early surgical management in the 1st or 2nd trimester with laparoscopic cholecystectomy preferred to open cholecystectomy. Controversy exists regarding the safety of laparoscopic cholecystectomy in the 3rd trimester vs deferral until after delivery. CBD stones should be attended to when present. These can be managed with standard techniques with attention to minimizing ionizing radiation to the fetus.

Cirrhosis

Patients with cirrhosis who develop cholecystitis present a significant clinical decision-making challenge. Morbidity following surgical intervention has been reported around 20%-30%, with 2%-4% mortality. As may be expected with the increased severity of cirrhosis, the risk of poor outcomes increases in this patient population. The rate of conversion to open from laparoscopy and bleeding complications can also be higher. Operative management of acute cholecystitis in cirrhotic patients is possible; however, careful consideration and patient selection are important.

Elderly

Elderly patients may present with atypical signs and symptoms of biliary disease, so a high index of suspicion is required. Furthermore, operative management should be strongly considered in elderly patients with an acceptable risk profile. In particular, the risk of recurrent symptoms and gallstone-related complications must be weighed against their comorbidities. Retrospective studies of cholecystectomy in elderly patients with acute cholecystitis and acute gallstone pancreatitis have reported low mortality rates. Thus, age alone should not be used as a contraindication to operative management in the elderly.

Prophylactic Cholecystectomy

Prophylactic cholecystectomy has been considered for various special patient populations but has dwindled in popularity over time. For example, although there is a paucity of data, prophylactic cholecystectomy has been considered in patients with asymptomatic gallstones undergoing heart transplantation. Another subset of patients in whom prophylactic cholecystectomy has been suggested is patients undergoing bariatric surgery who are expected to have rapid weight loss. However, the literature supports a low incidence of biliary complications and that prophylactic cholecystectomy increases operative morbidity during bariatric surgery. Prophylactic cholecystectomy has also been suggested in patients undergoing gastrectomy for gastric cancer. These patients may have an increased incidence of cholelithiasis due to vagal branch damage and the gastrointestinal reconstruction. A multicenter randomized trial by Bencini et al. demonstrated that concomitant prophylactic cholecystectomy was associated with a decreased number of biliary abnormalities but did not reduce cholelithiasis-free survival.

SUMMARY

Acute care surgeons commonly encounter biliary tract disease. Knowledge of the spectrum of disease and the management strategies is necessary to provide safe and effective care. A multidisciplinary approach to management is often required given the advancements in techniques, particularly regarding endoscopic and radiologic-assisted adjuncts to the management of complicated biliary disease.

SUGGESTED READINGS

ASGE Standards of Practice Committee; Buxbaum JL, Abbas Fehmi SM, Sultan S, et al. ASGE guideline on the role of endoscopy in the evaluation and management of choledocholithiasis. *Gastrointest Endosc.* 2019;89(6):1075-1105 e15.

Banks PA, Bollen TL, Dervenis C, et al. Classification of acute pancreatitis—2012: revision of the Atlanta classification and definitions by international consensus. *Gut.* 2013;62(1):102-111.

Bencini L, Marchet A, Alfieri S, et al. The Cholegas trial: long-term results of prophylactic cholecystectomy during gastrectomy for cancer—a randomized-controlled trial. *Gastric Cancer.* 2019;22(3):632-639.

Brunt LM, Deziel DJ, Telem DA, et al. Safe cholecystectomy multi-society practice guideline and state-of-the-art consensus conference on prevention of bile duct injury during cholecystectomy. *Surg Endosc.* 2020;34: 2827-2855.

Cotton PB, Elta GH, Carter CR, Pasricha PJ, Corazziari ES. Rome IV. Gallbladder and Sphincter of Oddi disorders. *Gastroenterology.* 2016;150(6):1420-1429.

Expert Panel on Gastrointestinal Imaging; Porter KK, Zaheer A, Kamel IR, et al. ACR Appropriateness Criteria(R) acute pancreatitis. *J Am Coll Radiol.* 2019; 16(11S):S316-S330.

Han C, Shan X, Yao L, et al. Robotic-assisted versus laparoscopic cholecystectomy for benign gallbladder diseases: a systematic review and meta-analysis. *Surg Endosc.* 2018;32(11):4377-4392.

Hernandez M, Murphy B, Aho JM, et al. Validation of the AAST EGS acute cholecystitis grade and comparison with the Tokyo guidelines. *Surgery.* 2018;163(4):739-746.

Kilic A, Sheer A, Shah AS, Russell SD, Gourin CG, Lidor AO. Outcomes of cholecystectomy in US heart transplant recipients. *Ann Surg.* 2013;258(2):312-317.

Loozen CS, van Santvoort HC, van Duijvendijk P, et al. Laparoscopic cholecystectomy versus percutaneous catheter drainage for acute cholecystitis in high risk patients (CHOCOLATE): multicentre randomised clinical trial. *BMJ.* 2018;363:k3965.

Mayumi T, Okamoto K, Takada T, et al. Tokyo Guidelines 2018: management bundles for acute cholangitis and cholecystitis. *J Hepatobiliary Pancreat Sci.* 2018;25(1):96-100.

Pisano M, Allievi N, Gurusamy K, et al. 2020 World Society of Emergency Surgery updated guidelines for the diagnosis and treatment of acute calculus cholecystitis. *World J Emerg Surg.* 2020;15(1):61.

Sedaghat N, Cao AM, Eslick GD, Cox MR. Laparoscopic versus open cholecystectomy in pregnancy: a systematic review and meta-analysis. *Surg Endosc.* 2017;31(2):673-679.

Singh M, Prasad N. The anatomy of Rouviere's sulcus as seen during laparoscopic cholecystectomy: a proposed classification. *J Minim Access Surg.* 2017;13(2):89-95. doi:10.4103/0972-9941.201731

Society of American Gastrointestinal and Endoscopic Surgeons (SAGES). Guidelines for diagnosis, treatment and use of laparoscopy for surgical problems during pregnancy. 2016. http://www.sages.org/publications/guidelines/guidelines-for-diagnosis-treatment-and-use-of-laparoscopy-for-surgical-problems-during-pregnancy/

Society of American Gastrointestinal and Endoscopic Surgeons (SAGES). The SAGES Safe Cholecystectomy Program. https://www.sages.org/safe-cholecystectomy-program/

Staudenmayer KL, Shafi S, et al. The American Association for the Surgery of Trauma grading scale for 16 emergency general surgery conditions: disease-specific criteria characterizing anatomic severity grading. *J Trauma Acute Care Surg.* 2016;81(3): 593-602.

Strasberg SM. Error traps and vasculo-biliary injury in laparoscopic and open cholecystectomy. *J Hepatobiliary Pancreat Surg* 2008;15:284-292.

Strasberg SM, Pucci MJ, Brunt LM, Deziel DJ. Subtotal cholecystectomy-"fenestrating" vs "reconstituting" subtypes and the prevention of bile duct injury: definition of the optimal procedure in difficult operative conditions. *J Am Coll Surg.* 2016;222(1): 89-96.

Tsuda S. Laparoscopic Common Bile Duct Exploration. www.sages.org. https://www.sages.org/wiki/laparoscopic-common-bile-duct-exploration/

Tustumi F, Bernardo WM, Santo MA, Cecconello I. Cholecystectomy in patients submitted to bariatric procedure: a systematic review and meta-analysis. *Obes Surg.* 2018;28(10):3312-3320.

Vlek SL, van Dam DA, Rubinstein SM, et al. Biliary tract visualization using near-infrared imaging with indocyanine green during laparoscopic cholecystectomy: results of a systematic review. *Surg Endosc.* 2017;31(7): 2731-2742.

Wang X, Yu WL, Fu XH, Zhu B, Zhao T, Zhang YJ. Early versus delayed surgical repair and referral for patients with bile duct injury: a systematic review and meta-analysis. *Ann Surg.* 2020;271(3):449-459.

Yokoe M, Hata J, Takada T, et al. Tokyo Guidelines 2018: diagnostic criteria and severity grading of acute cholecystitis (with videos). *J Hepatobiliary Pancreat Sci.* 2018;25(1):41-54.

CHAPTER

16 Peptic Ulcer Disease

Kimberly A. Davis, Jamie J. Coleman, and Nicole Goulet

CASE PRESENTATION

A 73-year-old female without significant past medical or surgical history presented with a 2-day history of abdominal pain associated with nausea and vomiting. Her pain initially began in the epigastrium but spread diffusely across her abdomen prior to presentation. On exam, she was afebrile with normal hemodynamics but was markedly tender with generalized peritonitis. A chest x-ray revealed free intraperitoneal air (**Figure 16.1**). A CT demonstrated marked thickening of the wall of the gastric antrum with free air and free fluid (**Figures 16.2 and 16.3**). She was taken for exploration. Findings included free gastric contents in the abdomen with a 2 × 3 cm prepyloric gastric perforation. Multiple biopsies were taken which were negative for malignancy on frozen section. The perforation was closed in layers given its size and reinforced with an omental patch. She required ICU admission and resuscitation for septic shock with slow improvement. A contrast study on postoperative day 4 did not demonstrate a leak, and her nasogastric tube was removed and her diet advanced. She was discharged home on postoperative day 8. Final pathology was negative for malignancy, positive for *H pylori* and she was treated with a course of triple therapy.

Question: *Which different clinical presentation my prompt nonoperative management of a perforated peptic ulcer?*

Answer: *Had the CT demonstrated a contained perforation without free fluid the patient could have been considered for nonoperative management.*

INTRODUCTION

Peptic ulcer disease was once very common and a significant cause of hospitalizations and mortality worldwide. Over the past 30 years, however, multiple countries have shown a decrease in hospitalization rates by 40%-50% along with a sharp decrease in mortality associated with the disease. Duodenal ulcers are more common than gastric ulcers, although the greatest decrease in incidence has occurred with duodenal ulcers. These changes correspond with the identification, treatment, and now decreasing incidence of *H pylori* infections as well as the widespread use of histamine 2 receptor antagonists and proton pump inhibitors (PPIs). Despite the decreasing rate of hospitalization and mortality, peptic ulcer disease remains relatively common, with a lifetime prevalence of 5%-10% in the United States, and an incidence of 0.1%-0.3% per year. Additionally, the complication rate for peptic ulcer disease remains high at 10%-20%. Peptic ulcer disease is associated with the male sex, smoking, and increasing age. Males represent ~1.5 times the number of peptic ulcer disease as females, with complications of peptic ulcer disease occurring most frequently in individuals over 60 years of age. Other risk factors for the development of peptic ulcer disease are infection with *H pylori* and chronic use of nonsteroidal anti-inflammatory drugs. Complications of peptic ulcer disease include bleeding, perforation, and obstruction, with bleeding as the most common complication. Overall, despite the decreased hospitalization and mortality rates associated with peptic ulcer disease, it remains a complex medical problem with which today's surgeon ought to be well versed. Importantly, operations for peptic ulcer disease currently are to treat the complication (bleeding or perforation), not to eradicate the ulcer disease.

HEMORRHAGE

Diagnosis

Clinical symptoms and the severity of those symptoms for patients with peptic ulcer disease can vary widely, and peptic ulcer disease is the most common cause of upper gastrointestinal (GI) bleeding. Bleeding from a gastric or duodenal ulcer typically

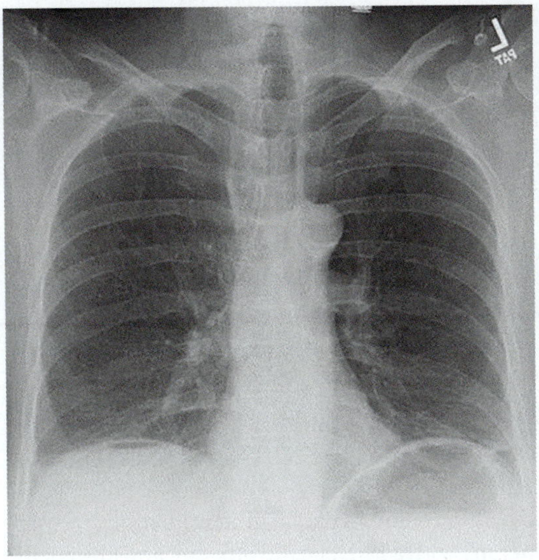

Figure 16.1 Chest x-ray shows pneumoperitoneum.

presents with melena or hematemesis, yet if the bleeding is particularly brisk, it can also present as hematochezia. (See Chapter 13: Gastrointestinal Hemorrhage in Emergency Surgery.) Up to 50% of patients who present with GI bleeding do so without prior symptoms of peptic ulcer disease. The hospitalization rate for patients with GI bleeding has been declining due to available medical management; yet, this complication still carries a mortality rate of 5%-10%.

The first step in evaluation of a patient with bleeding from a presumed upper gastrointestinal source is to assess the circulation of the patient with monitoring of hemodynamics, establishing vascular access, and restoring blood volume if needed. Laboratory tests should be sent for hemoglobin/hematocrit, blood typing, and assessment of coagulation. Next, localize the source of the bleed. A nasogastric tube may be placed but is not required, nor is it highly accurate in determining the location of the hemorrhage. The gold standard for this is an upper endoscopy, or esophagogastroduodenoscopy (EGD), performed early after presentation to the hospital. Several scoring systems both pre- and postendoscopy have been developed and described to predict need for intervention, rebleeding, need for operation, and death. One of the most commonly used and studied is the Glasgow Blatchford score (**Table 16.1**), which is calculated pre-endoscopy and has been shown to be highly accurate in predicting need for treatment and mortality. (See Chapter 13: Gastrointestinal Hemorrhage in Emergency Surgery.)

Nonoperative Management

Most bleeding from peptic ulcer disease resolves without endoscopic or operative intervention (**Table 16.2**). Early, empiric intravenous administration of PPIs is recommended at the time of the patient's presentation, as this decreases the need for intervention at the time of endoscopy. Prokinetic medications can be used prior to endoscopy to aid in emptying of the stomach and improving visualization. Upper endoscopy serves as both a diagnostic and therapeutic tool. Endoscopic intervention is required ~25%. Endoscopic treatment is recommended when active bleeding, high-risk stigmata such as a visible vessel or adherent clot are present. Endoscopic treatment techniques include epinephrine injection, thermal therapy, and application of clips. A combination of modalities is often performed as this reduces recurrence of bleeding and need for operative intervention. Gastric ulcers should be biopsied at the time of endoscopy given the 4%-6% incidence of malignancy. Intravenous PPI administration should continue for 72 hours after endoscopic interven-

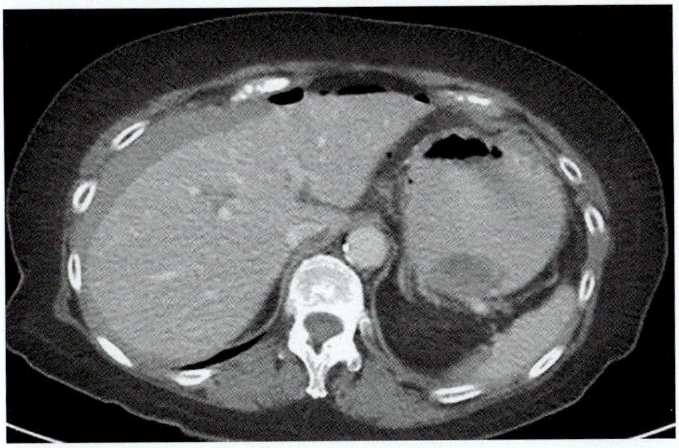

Figure 16.2 CT demonstrates free intraperitoneal fluid and air.

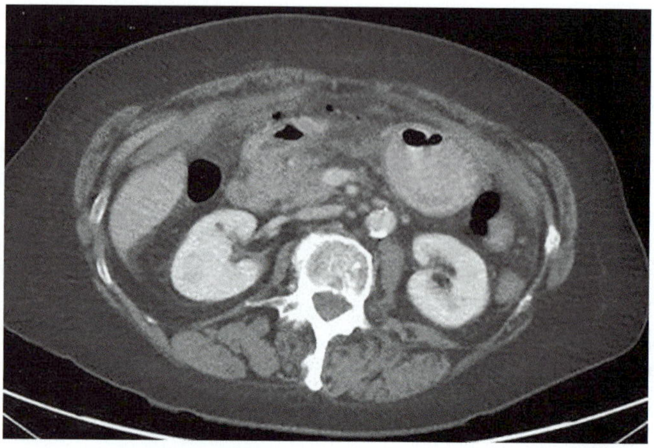

Figure 16.3 CT shows marked thickening of the gastric antrum.

tion to reduce risk of rebleeding followed by twice oral administration for 6-8 weeks. Continuation of PPI treatment is dependent upon etiology of the ulcer and the presence of continued risk factors such as continued use of nonsteroidal anti-inflammatory drugs (NSAIDs) and the presence of *H pylori*. *H pylori* should be tested for and if positive, undergo 14 days of clarithromycin triple therapy with a PPI, clarithromycin, and amoxicillin or metronidazole. In areas with increased (>15%) clarithromycin resistance, a bismuth-containing quadruple therapy (PPI, bismuth subcitrate, tetracycline, and metronidazole) or a nonbismuth-based quadruple therapy (PPI, clarithromycin, amoxicillin, and metronidazole) should be used instead. Repeat EGD is typically performed 4-6 weeks after treatment to evaluate healing.

TABLE 16.1 ■ Glasgow Blatchford Score

Risk Factor on Admission	Score
Blood urea (mmol/L)	2
≥6.5 to <8	3
≥8 to <10	4
≥10 to <25	6
≥25	
Hemoglobin (g/L) (male)	1
≥12 to <13	3
≥10 to <12	6
<10	
Hemoglobin (g/L) (female)	1
≥10 to <12	6
<10	
Systolic blood pressure (mm Hg)	1
≥100 to <109	2
≥90 to <100	3
<90	
Pulse ≥100/min	1
Melena	1
Syncope	2
Hepatic disease	2
Cardiac failure	2

Modified from: Blatchford O, Murray WR, Blatchford M. A risk score to predict need for treatment for upper-gastrointestinal haemorrhage. *Lancet*. 2000;356(9238):1318-1321.

Recurrent bleeding occurs in 5%-15% of patients, who should be treated with a second attempt at EGD with endoscopic treatment modalities given the lower complication rate as compared to emergent surgical treatment. Factors associated with failure of endoscopic management include ulcers >2 cm in diameter and hemorrhagic shock during the rebleed event. If repeat endoscopic treatment fails, referral to interventional radiology for embolization of the gastroduodenal artery should occur if this resource is available. Angiography with embolization has also shown to have lower mortality rates than emergent surgery and is successful in 90%-95% of patients.

Operative Management

Emergent operative management is required in 2%-8% of patients who present with upper GI bleeding from peptic ulcer disease and carries a mortality of 25%-30%. Consider operation for patients who have failed repeat endoscopic treatment and/or angiographic embolization or in health care delivery systems in which these resources are not available. Consider urgent operative intervention in patients without repeat endoscopy if the patient is hemodynamically unstable or if rebleeding occurs in a patient in whom the ulcer was >2 cm on initial endoscopy or has failed endovascular embolization.

TABLE 16.2 ■ Medical Management of Hemorrhage From Peptic Ulcer Disease

Management of Peptic Ulcer Disease		
Before Endoscopy →	**During Endoscopy →**	**After Endoscopy**
• Resuscitate if hemodynamically unstable • Assess for coagulopathy and reverse if present • Cessation of and consider reversal of anticoagulants or antiplatelet agents • Transfuse for hemoglobin <7 g/dL • Calculate Glasgow-Blatchford score • Initiate proton pump inhibitor (PPI) • Consider prokinetic agents	• Endoscopy within 24 hours of presentation after resuscitation and optimization • Assess for high-risk stigmata (visible vessel, clot) or active bleeding • Perform indicated therapy • Add second line of treatment when able (thermal, clipping, epinephrine injection)	• High-dose IV PPI for 72 hours (if high-risk stigmata seen) • Repeat scope only if recurrent bleeding • If continued bleeding after second endoscopy→surgery and interventional radiology consults • Treat for *H pylori* • Consideration for long-term PI

Perform a midline laparotomy. Bleeding gastric ulcers should be treated with resection if technically feasible. Intraoperative endoscopy can help identify and localize the bleeding ulcer(s). If the location of the ulcer is not amenable for resection, a gastrotomy is most often performed followed by biopsies to excluded malignancy and oversew of the ulcer for hemostasis. Biopsies should be taken from all four quadrants of the ulcer edge for maximum diagnostic yield. If the ulcer is present along the lesser curvature at the incisura and the ulcer requires resection, an antrectomy with a Billroth I or Billroth II reconstruction should be considered. For duodenal ulcers, persistent bleeding is typically caused by an ulcer in the posterior wall, which has eroded into the gastroduodenal artery. The duodenum is mobilized with a Kocher maneuver, and a duodenotomy made with a longitudinal incision along the anterior wall of the stomach, starting ~2 cm proximal to the pylorus, extending through the pylorus and onto the anterior wall of the duodenum for ~3-4 cm in length. The gastroduodenal artery is then ligated by placing three sutures in a figure of eight fashion at the site of the bleeding vessel within the ulcer, in the superior, inferior, and medial positions (**Figure 16.4**). This three-point ligation (visualizing the face of a clock: 12, 3, and 6) is imperative given the collateral blood supply from the transverse pancreatic arteries with permanent suture. When performing the three-point ligation, it is important to be

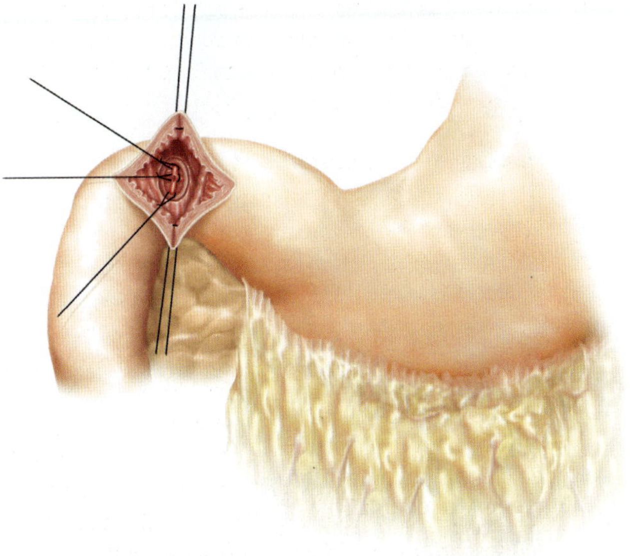

Figure 16.4 Three-point suture ligation of bleeding duodenal ulcer. The culprit is usually the gastroduodenal artery. The ligation can be done with individual stitches or a single "u-stitch" but must be sure to include the side branch. (From Fischer JE. *Fischer's Mastery of Surgery*. 7th ed. Wolters Kluwer; 2019. Figure 86.1.)

cognizant of the location of the ampulla of Vater. A probe or small catheter may be used in the ampulla to help identify its location and prevent injury to the common bile duct. After hemorrhage control is obtained, the longitudinal duodenotomy is then closed in a transverse fashion, thereby constructing a Heineke-Mikulicz pyloroplasty. Although this surgery was classically described in conjunction with a truncal vagotomy, a vagotomy is no longer routinely performed given the success of *H pylori* treatment.

STRESS GASTRITIS

Stress gastritis most commonly occurs in patients who undergo a traumatic event that is associated with shock, sepsis, respiratory failure requiring mechanical ventilation, hemorrhage, or multisystem organ failure. Traumatic brain injury patients and burn victims are at an especially increased risk. In this stressed state, there is disruption of the mucosal barrier (due to decreased blood flow) along with elevated levels of acetylcholine and histamine that lead to increased acid production in the stomach resulting in gastritis. It often presents 3-10 days from the initial injury and most commonly occurs in the fundus. Diagnosis can start with NGT lavage and fecal occult blood test but definitive diagnosis consists of endoscopic examination of acute mucosal ulcerations that are multiple, diffuse shallow areas of erythema and friability. The primary treatment focuses on resolution of the underlying injury and shock, and management of gastric pH with H_2 blockers or PPI. A major complication of stress gastritis is bleeding which is associated with increased mortality. The greatest risk factors for bleeding are respiratory failure (mechanical ventilation) and coagulopathy. Bleeding can be treated with selective angiography or endoscopically with cautery and injection. In critically ill patients, focus should be placed on stress ulcer prophylaxis. Early enteral feeding has been shown to be very effective in stress ulcer prophylaxis and should be employed when able. In addition, H_2-receptor antagonists or PPIs should also be used in patients at high risk of stress gastritis, which many studies suggest are equivalent in clinically important bleeding prevention from stress gastritis.

PERFORATION

The main risk factors for gastric ulceration are NSAID use, tobacco smoking, and *H pylori* colonization (**Figure 16.5**). Around 85%-90% of patients with a gastric ulcer are colonized with *H pylori* and if left untreated, fewer than 30% will recur within a year. Ten to thirty-five percent of people diagnosed with a gastric ulcer will have a serious complication that includes bleeding, perforation, or obstruction/stricture. As opposed to duodenal ulcers, malignancy needs to be considered in all gastric ulcers as it is present in 10%-13% of gastric ulcers. Therefore, biopsies should always be taken.

The main risk factors for duodenal ulcers are similar to that of gastric and include *H pylori* (90%), NSAID use, and tobacco smoking (see **Figure 16.5**).

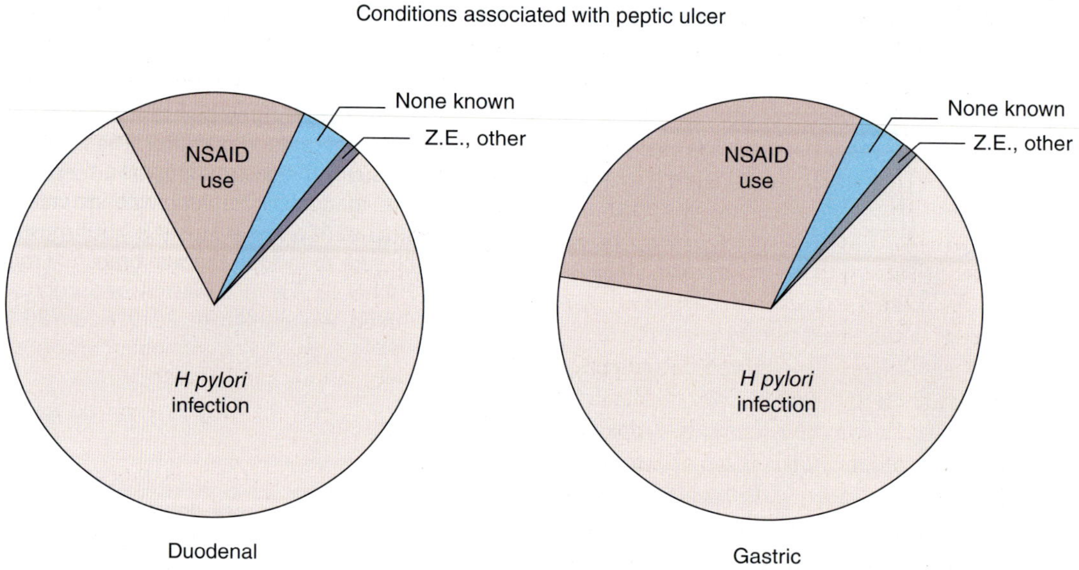

Figure 16.5 Causes of peptic ulcer disease. Z.E., Zollinger-Ellison syndrome. (Derived from Brunicardi FC, Andersent DK, Billiar TR, et al. *Schwartz's Principles of Surgery*. 11th ed. McGraw-Hill; 2019. Data from Graham DY, Lew GM, Klein PD, et al. Effect of treatment of Helicobacter pylori infection on the long-term recurrence of gastric or duodenal ulcer. A randomized, controlled study. *Ann Intern Med*. 1992;116(9):705–708.)

The majority of ulcers occur in the first portion of the duodenum (90%) and patients have a 10% lifetime risk of perforation. Although rare (1%-2%), Zollinger-Ellison syndrome (gastrinoma) must be considered in the differential of patients who have no other risk factors are refractory to medical management and especially if an ulcer is located distal to the first portion of the duodenum.

Diagnosis

When evaluating a patient with possible gastric or duodenal ulcer perforation, perform a thorough history and physical. Obtaining a patient's history of ulcer disease, prior treatments, time onset of acute symptoms, and risk factors including NSAID use, tobacco use, alcohol, chronic steroids, and cocaine are important in the management of these patients. Both types of ulcer perforation have similar presentations and diagnostic work-up. Symptoms include acute epigastric pain, tenderness, peritoneal signs, and possible radiation to the back (if ulcer has eroded into the pancreas). Patients may present with either a contained perforation or free perforation, which is often associated with sepsis or septic shock. Patients who present with hemodynamic lability or instability will require aggressive resuscitation.

There are five types of ulcers (see Chapter 13, Figure 13.1) and management of each varies. Type I is the most common (60%) and occurs along lesser curvature proximal to the incisura; type II has two ulcers: one in body of stomach near incisura and second in duodenum; type III is prepyloric (20%), found within 2-3 cm from the pylorus and can be multiple; type IV is located on the lesser curve near the GE junction (<10%); and type V is located anywhere in stomach and is associated with NSAIDs. Only types II and III are associated with acid hypersecretion.

The diagnosis of perforation related to NSAID use may be challenging, as these are often on the posterior wall of the stomach and may perforate in the retrogastric position, resulting in a contained perforation that may not manifest as free air on plain radiography. Liberal CT scanning should be employed, depending on the index of suspicion for perforation.

Work-up includes imaging that most commonly consists of an upright CXR that often will demonstrate air under the diaphragm (pneumoperitoneum). In perforated duodenal ulcers, 20% of patients will not have pneumoperitoneum on the CXR so if the patient is hemodynamically stable, obtain a CT scan of the abdomen. Prompt diagnosis and treatment is important as treatment beyond 12 hours is associated with increased morbidity and mortality.

Nonoperative Management

In patients who are hemodynamically stable and do not have peritoneal signs, obtain a CT scan of the abdomen. Nonoperative management may be considered in patients with a contained or sealed duodenal perforation as documented by imaging. The medical management of contained perforations includes the administration of broad-spectrum antibiotics and PPIs, DVT prophylaxis, nasogastric decompression, and IV fluids. All patients should be tested for *H pylori*. If positive or if unable to test patients, empirically treat, given the high rate of prevalence and recurrence if left untreated. Careful selection of the patient for nonoperative management must be thoughtful, as mortality increases with failure of nonoperative management, especially with delay >12-24 hours to operation. Patients should also be instructed to abstain from NSAIDs, steroids, drugs, and tobacco. Patients with significant comorbidities, hemodynamic instability, free perforation on imaging, or peritonitis should be managed operatively.

Operative Management

Operative management can be performed in an open technique or minimally invasively (**Figure 16.6**). If the patient is hemodynamically unstable, laparotomy is preferred, as insufflation can exacerbate hypotension. Patients with sepsis and septic shock need prompt resuscitation with intravenous fluids, IV PPI, broad-spectrum antibiotics, and nasogastric decompression in preparation for the operating room. Increased operative mortality has been shown in patients with preoperative shock, coexisting medical illness, location of the ulcer, and perforation for >48 hours. When planning the operation for a perforated duodenal ulcer, the surgeon must answer 6 questions (Feliciano, 1992; Lagoo, 2002):

1. Is the operation indicated?
2. Is an omental plication sufficient or is a definitive ulcer operation indicated?
3. Is the patient stable enough to undergo a definitive ulcer operation?
4. Which definitive operation is indicated?
5. Should the availability of newer medical treatments influence the choice of operation?
6. Should the procedure be approached via laparoscopy or laparotomy?

When considering a minimally invasive approach, patient selection and surgeon expe-

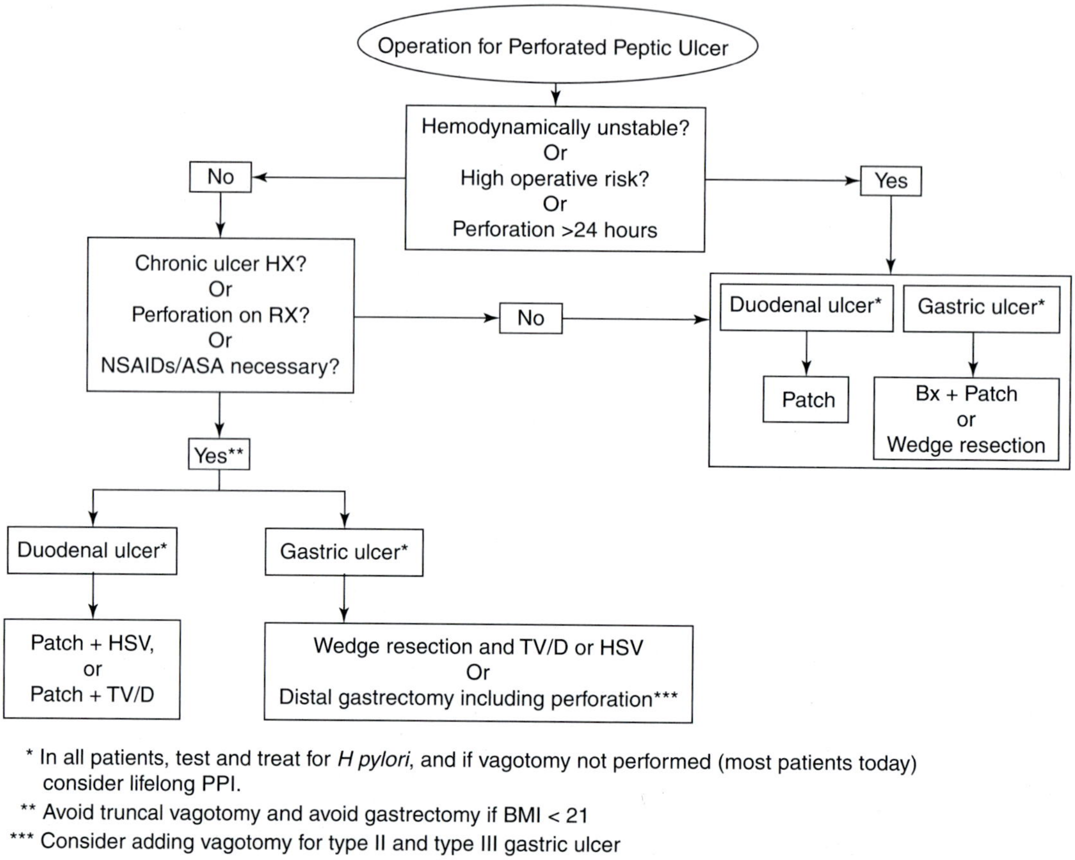

Figure 16.6 Algorithm for operation for perforated peptic ulcer. ASA, acetylsalicylic acid; BMI, body mass index; Bx, biopsy; HSV, highly selective vagotomy; Hx, history; PPI, proton pump inhibitor; Rx, treatment; TV/D, truncal vagotomy and drainage. (Derived from Brunicardi FC, Andersen DK, Billiar TR, et al. *Schwartz's Principles of Surgery*. 11th ed. McGraw-Hill; 2019.)

rience should be considered. Laparoscopic approaches have improved rates of wound infection and pain control, but there is no difference in length of stay or rates of postoperative complications, and mortality. Operative treatment of both gastric and duodenal ulcers will depend on patient factors, hemodynamic stability, and the location and type of ulcer. A critical principle in the management of perforated peptic ulcer disease: **the simplest operative solution is generally the best approach.**

Gastric ulcer perforation has a 10%-13% risk of malignancy, so resection is recommended. The location and type of ulcer will dictate where and how the resection is performed and could include wedge resection (if amenable and if patient is unstable) or antrectomy. If an antrectomy is performed, this will be followed by Billroth I (preferential), Billroth II or Roux-en-Y reconstruction. Given that type II and III ulcers are associated with acid hypersecretion, vagotomy may also be considered. This is especially prudent if patient is noncompliant or has already failed medical management of prior ulcer disease with PPI/*H pylori* eradication. If the patient has never trialed a PPI or *H pylori* eradication prior to perforation, it is reasonable to try these measures prior to vagotomy given the potential debilitating side effects of the operation. Although truncal vagotomy can have a 60%-70% acid reduction (85% if antrectomy is also performed), treatment with PPIs has clinical equipoise. Type IV ulcers can be challenging, and resection could include Pauchet or Csendes procedures (**Figures 16.7 and 16.8**). For patients who are hemodynamically unstable, have a low suspicion for malignancy, or have prepyloric ulcers, an omental patch can be considered (**Figure 16.9**). In the type II or III ulcer in which scarring prevents adequate dissection of the pylorus, the Bancroft procedure can be used. After completed removal of all antral mucosa, a muscular cuff of the antrum is utilized to close the duodenal stump. The right gastric and right gastroepiploic arteries must be preserved to maintain blood supply (**Figure 16.10**).

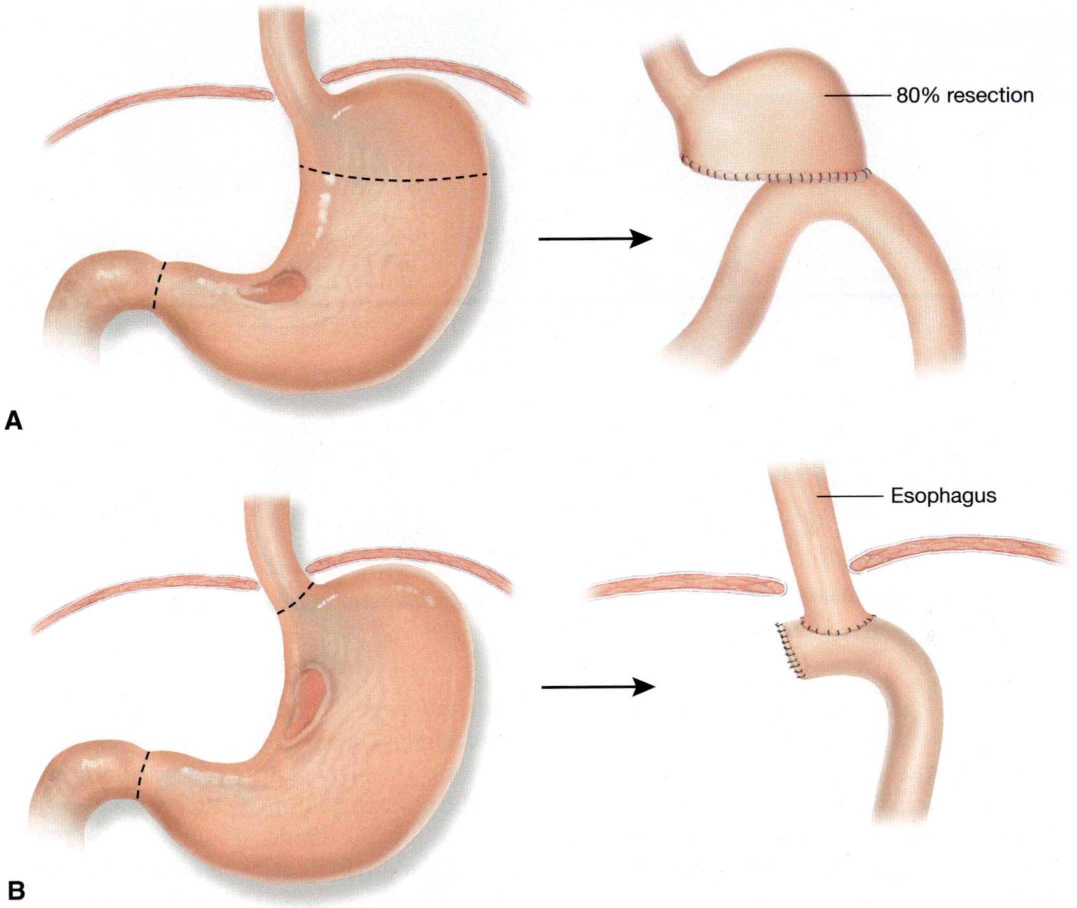

Figure 16.7 Resection lines for partial gastrectomy.

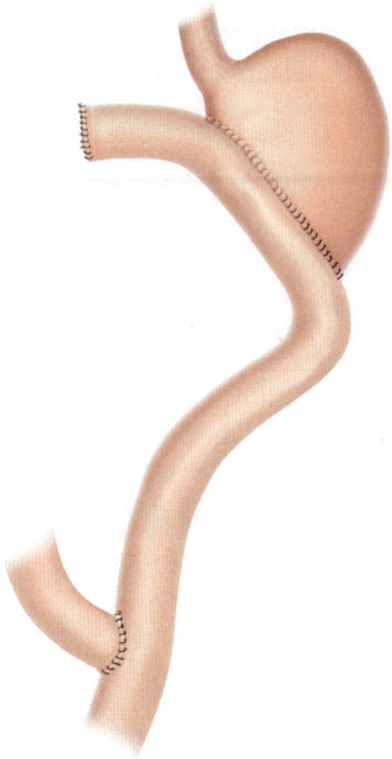

Figure 16.8 Csendes procedure for type IV gastric ulcers.

If able, intraoperative biopsies should still be taken to evaluate for malignancy or a future endoscopic evaluation and biopsies should be performed. In addition, *H pylori* should be tested and treated.

Duodenal ulcer perforation is mostly associated with *H pylori* and acid hypersecretion and does not have as high a risk of malignancy as gastric ulcers. Therefore, the hallmark of operative management for small prepyloric ulcers is closure or patch as opposed to resection. In patients who are healthy, have <24 hours of symptoms and who have a perforation that is prepyloric and <5 mm, a simple suture closure can be performed.

If the perforation is >5 mm, the patient is unstable, has delayed presentation, or significant comorbidities or risk factors, an omental patch should be performed.

The giant duodenal ulcer, defined as >2 or 3 cm depending on the reference, creates an operative dilemma and there is currently no consensus on management. In a hemodynamically unstable patient, a closure and patch should be performed.

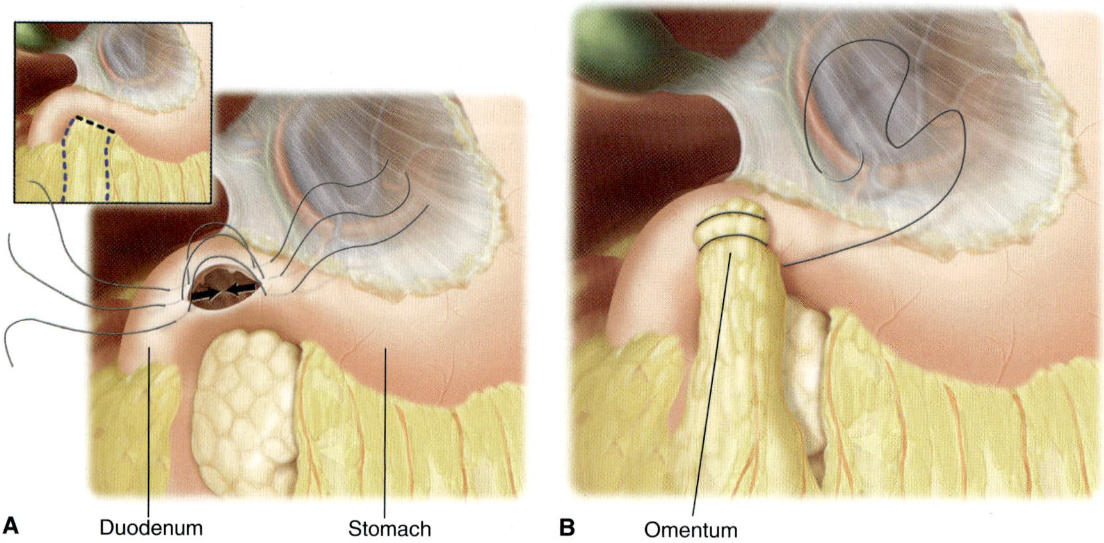

Figure 16.9 Omental patch of a perforated ulcer. (Reprinted with permission from Khan S, Schuchert V, Zuckerbraun BS. Inflammatory conditions of the small and large intestine. In: Britt LD, Peitzman AB, Barie PS, Jurkovich GJ, eds. *Acute Care Surgery*. 2nd ed. Wolters Kluwer; 2019. Figure 60.4.)

Other surgical considerations include (1) duodenostomy tube into the duodenal ulcer; (2) pyloric exclusion +/− gastrojejunostomy (**Figure 16.11**); (3) a retrograde jejunostomy tube, feeding jejunostomy tube, and pyloric exclusion +/− gastrojejunostomy; or (4) resection and reconstruction. No single technique is superior as far as morbidity or mortality. The choice of operative technique depends on the size of the ulcer, loss of duodenal tissue, the degree of inflammation of the duodenum, the proximity to the ampulla, and stability of the patient. The **posterior duodenal ulcer** with penetration of the ulcer into the pancreas often results in loss of a portion of the posterior duodenal wall. This may require gastric resection, leaving the ulcer bed *in situ*, with a Nissen procedure used to close the duodenal stump (**Figure 16.12**).

Similar to gastric ulcer perforations, in patients who will be noncompliant with *H pylori* eradication, who have failed medical management, or who will continue to smoke tobacco or take NSAIDs, consider acid reduction surgery in addition to the omental patch (see above types). If possible, a highly selective vagotomy or a vagotomy

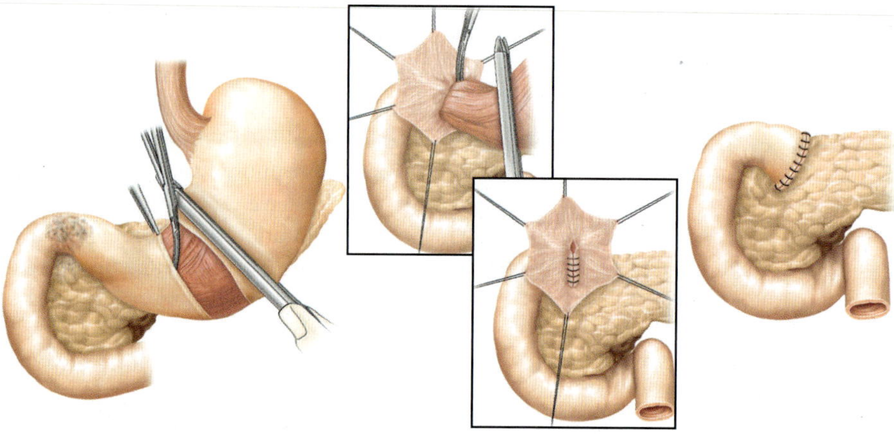

Figure 16.10 Bancroft procedure/closure. In this method of duodenal stump closure, the stomach is transected 3 to 4 cm proximal to the pylorus, where tissue is less fibrotic. The antral mucosa in the duodenal stump is then dissected away from the submucosa beyond the pylorus and into the duodenum. This is secured with a purse-string suture, and the seromuscular layer is closed over the stump. (From Nussbaum M. *Master Techniques in Surgery: Gastric Surgery*. Wolters Kluwer; 2013. Figure 60.4).

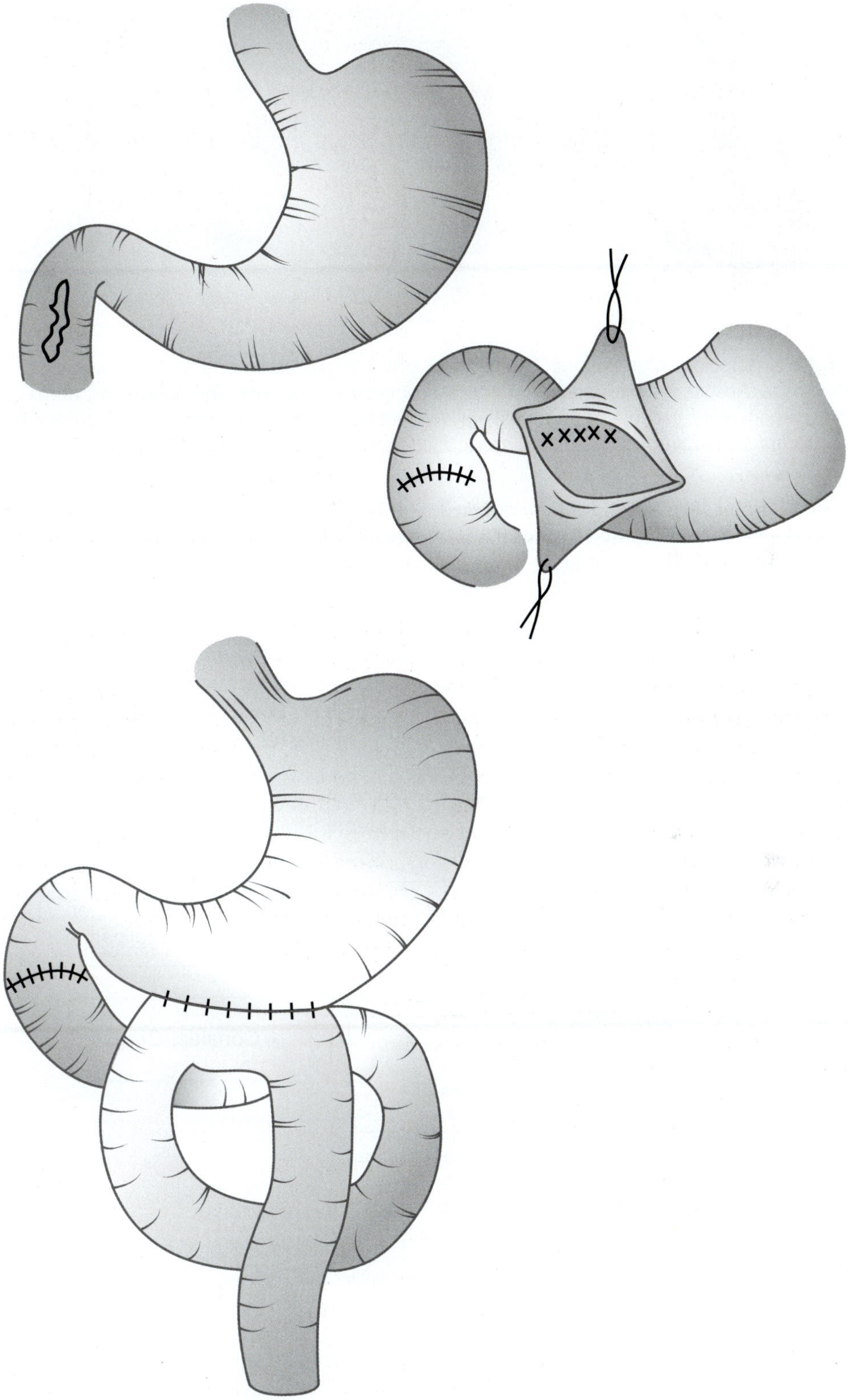

Figure 16.11 Pyloric exclusion. (From Peitzman AB, et al. *The Trauma Manual*. 5th ed. Wolters Kluwer; 2020. Figure 37.11.)

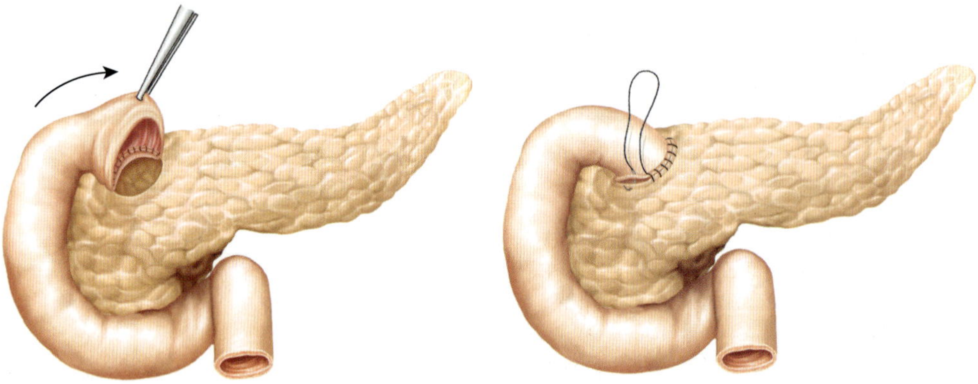

Figure 16.12 Nissen closure/procedure. This method, often employed when the duodenum is scarred to the pancreatic capsule, is performed by first transecting the duodenum. The duodenal stump is then sutured to the pancreatic capsule or duodenal wall left in place on the pancreatic capsule. (From Nussbaum M. *Master Techniques in Surgery: Gastric Surgery*. Wolters Kluwer; 2013. Figure 14.1A.)

with drainage procedure should be performed over a vagotomy and antrectomy, because the latter is associated with higher morbidity.

DUODENAL STUMP LEAK

A duodenal stump leak generally presents 5-10 days postoperatively. The common symptoms are abdominal pain, fever, and tachycardia. Delay to diagnosis and treatment of the duodenal stump leak increases morbidity and mortality. A contrast-enhanced CT (including oral contrast) is the diagnostic test of choice. Management of a duodenal stump leak depends on the clinical status of the patient (**Figure 16.13**). Start broad-spectrum antibiotics, fluid resuscitation, and initiate NPO. In the hemodynamically stable, nonseptic patient, conservative management is generally successful. This approach continues NPO,

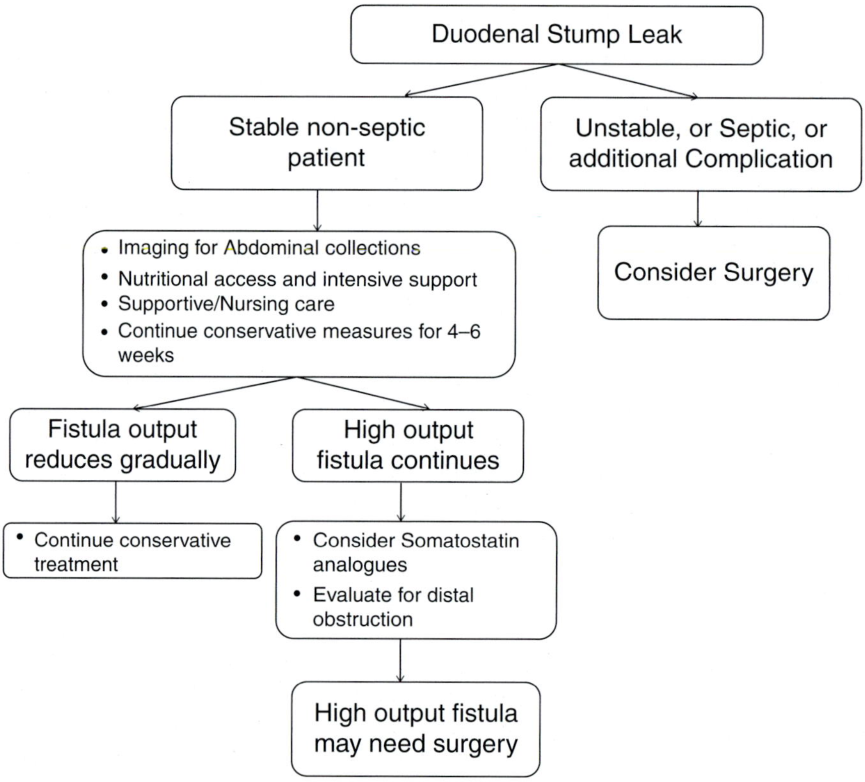

Figure 16.13 Flowchart for the management of a duodenal stump leak.

possibly a nasogastric tube, IV antibiotics, enteral or parental nutrition (if enteral is not tolerated or feasible), percutaneous drainage, and consideration of somatostatin analogues. Be certain to exclude a distal obstruction as an etiology in the duodenal leak. The unstable or septic patient requires emergent operative intervention. The goal of this operation is to convert the leak into a controlled duodenal fistula. If the duodenal stump seems reasonable, suture closure and an omental patch can be attempted. If not, a soft tube is placed into the duodenal stump defect as a tube duodenostomy (**Figure 16.14**). The area is widely drained with closed suction catheters. Some authors advocate biliary diversion as well.

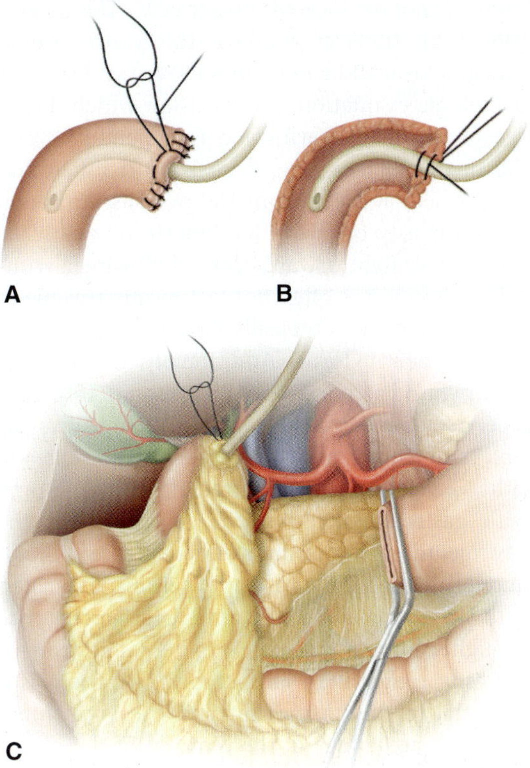

A B

C

Figure 16.14 A-C. Tube duodenostomy for aduodenal stump. **A.** First purse string suture. **B.** Second purse string suture.

OBSTRUCTION

Diagnosis

Peptic ulcer disease is rarely the etiology of obstruction given the widespread use of *H pylori* and acid suppression treatment strategies. Most gastric outlet obstruction (GOO) is caused by malignancy, often of pancreatic origin. Of benign causes of GOO, peptic ulcer disease is the most common cause, accounting for ~90% of cases. Computed tomography with oral contrast is commonly the initial test performed for evaluation and can easily identify a complete obstruction or stricture. An EGD is then performed to assess the rest of the gastric mucosa and obtain biopsies to rule out a malignant cause of the obstruction or stricture. It is important to note patients with GOO are frequently malnourished. Before an operation is performed, correct any electrolyte abnormalities and nutritional deficiencies.

Medical Management

Once a patient has been diagnosed with GOO due to peptic ulcer disease, the first step is nasogastric decompression in association with treatment of the underlying condition. *H pylori* testing and eradication with a triple therapy regimen is indicated. Chronic NSAID use should be discontinued, and an acid suppression medication initiated. If medical management fails to resolve the obstruction, the next step is endoscopic intervention with balloon dilation, if a balloon can be passed through the stricture. Repeated and stepwise dilation may be needed in very tight or narrow strictures, and overall, repeated dilations may be needed dependent upon clinical response. The frequency of repeated dilatation sessions remains variable and is highly patient dependent. Once adequate dilation has been achieved, the success rate for a lasting clinical response has been reported in 70%-80% of patients. Stents have also been used in patients who did not clinically respond to dilation with a reported long-term success rate of 67.5%, although further study is needed to fully assess the effectiveness of stents as compared to balloon dilation.

Operative Management

Surgical intervention is uncommonly required for benign GOO secondary to peptic ulcer disease due to the relatively high success rates of medical treatment and endoscopic management. In patients who have either failed multiple endoscopic dilations or in whom endoscopic dilation cannot be performed, surgery is indicated. Once the patient's nutritional status has been optimized, perform a truncal vagotomy in conjunction with a drainage procedure—either a pyloroplasty, gastroduodenostomy, antrectomy, or gastrojejunostomy. To adequately perform a truncal vagotomy, the distal segment of the esophagus must be exposed well. The left vagus nerve runs along the anterior aspect of the esophagus, and the right vagus nerve is located posteriorly. The nerves should be transected above the gastroesophageal junction, and a portion removed and sent for pathologic evaluation. The decision which drainage procedure is performed is dependent upon the degree of scarring, fibrosis, and inflammation present at the antrum and pylorus. Although a pyloroplasty or gastroduodenostomy would be the most straightforward option following a truncal vagotomy, it is often not technically feasible in these patients who typically have significant scarring of their pylorus. Additionally, a vagotomy with pyloroplasty is associated with an 10%-15% ulcer recurrence rate. The more technically feasible and commonly performed operations are either a vagotomy with antrectomy or vagotomy with gastrojejunostomy. The advantage of the gastrojejunostomy is the avoidance of a difficult duodenal resection and complications associated with a scarred duodenal stump. Ulcer recurrence is higher in patients who undergo gastrojejunostomy rather than antrectomy, and there is a potential to miss a malignancy. The antrectomy offers the advantage of the removal of the physical obstruction and a complete pathologic review of the ulcer yet is associated with a higher mortality and complication rate. The choice of operation should depend upon the surgeon's experience with these operations and the feasibility of resection.

POSTGASTRECTOMY SYNDROMES

While postgastrectomy syndromes are rare (1%-3%), they can be disabling, difficult to diagnosis, and, in rare cases, difficult to treat. The two most common syndromes are dumping and alkaline reflux gastritis.

Mechanical Disorders

Afferent Limb Syndrome

This disorder can occur from a Billroth II, Roux-en-Y reconstruction, and less commonly with a loop gastrojejunostomy. It occurs when there is an obstruction due to stricture, adhesions, internal hernia, or recurrent cancer at the gastroenterostomy or enteroenterostomy leading to the inability of the biliopancreatic limb (afferent limb) to deliver pancreatic secretions and bile into the distal segments of intestine. It can also occur when the afferent limb is too long. Symptoms may occur early after surgery or several years later. They consist of signs of a mechanical obstruction and pain (mostly right upper quadrant) after eating which is often relieved with bilious emesis (will not vomit undigested food). Work-up should include a CT scan of the abdomen, which may show dilation of the biliopancreatic limb (but not always). In addition, an endoscopy can be performed to better visualize the anastomosis and assess for the cause such as marginal ulcer or recurrent cancer. Treatment will depend on the acuity of symptoms and the etiology and will mostly consist of operative intervention. Takedown of the anastomosis may be required, and re-anastomosis should be performed with a shorter afferent limb. Bowel resection may be required depending on the viability of the bowel. If a patient has a gastrojejunostomy, conversion to a Roux-en-Y anastomosis is recommended.

Efferent Limb Syndrome

This disorder occurs when there is obstruction of the efferent limb (or Roux limb) that normally receives ingested food from the stomach and transports it distally. The obstruction is most commonly due to an ulcer at the gastrojejunal anastomosis or from an internal hernia but can result also from adhesions or recurrent cancer. Patients experience early satiety but mainly have obstructive symptoms that are relieved with emesis but unlike afferent limb syndrome, the vomitus will consist of ingested food as opposed to just liquid and bile. Treatment mainly consists of operative management. Revision of the gastrojejunostomy is normally required with possible further gastric resection if the etiology is ulceration. Endoscopic management with stents or dilation can also be performed, especially for palliation in the setting of recurrent cancer.

Internal Hernias

The most common internal hernia after gastrectomy with Roux-en-Y reconstruction is a Petersen hernia (**Figure 16.15**). This occurs when a loop of small bowel herniates through the space posterior to the gastrojejunal anastomosis. In the case of a retrocolic anastomosis, the bowel herniates between the mesentery of the Roux limb and the retroperitoneum. In an antecolic anastomosis, the bowel herniates between the Roux limb and the colon. Other potential sites of internal hernia include the mesocolonic defect and the entero-enterostomy defect. Symptoms may be acute or vague in nature. A high index of suspicion is needed given that imaging in the form of CT scan or small bowel follow-through is only diagnostic in 65% of patients. A diagnostic laparoscopy should

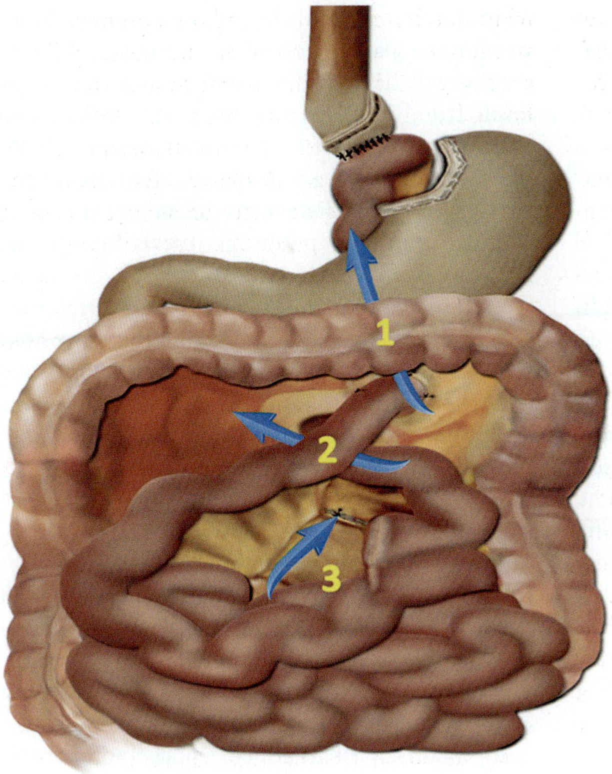

Figure 16.15 Mesenteric defects in Roux-en-Y gastric bypass: *1*, transverse colon-mesenteric defect/window; *2*, Petersen defect; *3*, biliopancreatic defect. (From Peitzman AB, Yealy DM, Fabian TC, Schwab CW, Guyette FX, Seamon MJ,. *Zuckerbraun BS. The Trauma Manual*. 5th ed. Wolters Kluwer; 2020. Figure 74.4.)

be performed if there is suspicion and treatment involves reduction of the hernia, possible bowel resection, and closure of the defect.

Functional Disorders

(Early) Dumping Syndrome

This syndrome can occur following gastric resection or after vagotomy in 5%-10% of patients. It is due to the rapid emptying of contents into the small intestine and the symptoms are related to the neurohormonal response to this rapid emptying. Dumping syndrome predominately occurs after liquid consumption and carbohydrate-rich meals. It occurs secondary to resection or disruption of the pylorus that leads to loss of regulation of gastric emptying. The addition of a vagotomy worsens dumping syndrome by interrupting the receptive relaxation of the stomach which is vagally mediated. In addition, the duodenum contains mucosal receptors that provide feedback to slow gastric emptying and by bypassing this, that mechanism is lost, and early dumping syndrome is exacerbated. Symptoms of dumping syndrome are nausea, bloating, crampy abdominal pain that is associated with tachycardia, flushing, and palpitations. They occur early after ingestion of food (10-20 minutes) and can be followed by diarrhea 2-3 hours later. These symptoms subside in most patients over time especially with diet modification. Avoiding liquids at meals and avoiding meals high in carbohydrates improves symptoms. It is rare that symptoms continue for a prolonged period (1%-2%) but occur more frequently in patients who have had a vagotomy, and symptoms can continue for months to years. If symptoms persist despite diet modification, a trial of octreotide (50-100 mg) before each meal can help. In the rare instance where symptoms are still persistent despite these measures, operative management can be pursued. In the case of Billroth I or II, these can be converted to Roux-en-Y, which will help slow gastric emptying. In the case of pyloroplasty, the pylorus should be reconstructed. Other operations such as a jejunal pouch or reversed jejunal segment are mostly historic and are rarely performed as they have been shown to provide minimal benefit and are associated with complications.

Gastroparesis

Gastroparesis can occur after gastrectomy and is very common during the first 2-6 weeks postoperatively but generally resolves. The chronic form is mostly associated with vagotomy, is more common in women than men, and develops months to years after surgery. While a vagotomy prevents proximal receptive gastric relaxation, which leads to rapid emptying of liquids, it also prevents the pylorus from fully relaxing and thereby prevents gastric emptying of solids. A pyloroplasty or pyloromyotomy can attenuate this but gastroparesis can still occur. Symptoms include early satiety and emesis of undigested foods more than 6 hours after eating. When diagnosing postgastrectomy/postvagotomy gastroparesis, first exclude mechanical obstruction, usually by CT scan. An EGD can then assist with the diagnosis by visualizing undigested food remaining in the stomach, along with lack of gastric distension or wall thickening. In addition, gastric emptying studies can also be obtained. Treatment starts with medical management through diet modification consisting of soft foods that are easily broken down. In addition, there is utility in the use of the prokinetic agent, erythromycin (low dose before meals), and, to a lesser degree, metoclopramide. If symptoms persist, consider operative treatment. The only useful operation for this, however, is a near-total gastrectomy with Roux-en-Y reconstruction given that the culprit is the proximal stomach where there is a lack of tonic contractions or coordinated distal phasic, peristaltic gastric contractile activity. Even with a near-total gastrectomy, only 50% of patients have complete relief and can maintain adequate nutrition. Therefore, consider a jejunostomy for supplemental enteral nutrition.

Noninsulinoma Pancreatogenous Hypoglycemia Syndrome

Sometimes referred to as the *"late dumping syndrome,"* this reactive hypoglycemia entails a true hypoglycemia that occurs 90-150 minutes postprandially. It is caused by a rapid entry of carbohydrates into the small intestine, leading to a rapid increase in glucose 30-60 minutes postprandially, which can be associated with dumping syndrome frequently, but not always. Bypass of the duodenum also increases the risk of late dumping syndrome. The rapid increase of blood glucose subsequently leads to an uncontrolled release of insulin, thereby causing hypoglycemia. This occurs months to years following surgery. Patients experience symptoms of hypoglycemia including tachycardia, palpitations, diaphoresis, and in severe cases, seizure, syncope, and altered mentation. Patients suspected to have this disorder should undergo a work-up first to exclude other causes of hypoglycemia including insulinoma and medications. They should then have serial serum glucose measurements performed starting 30 minutes postprandially every 15 minutes. Noninsulinoma pancreatogenous hypoglycemia syndrome will have a characteristic rise in glucose levels from 30 to 60 minutes postprandially and then a drastic fall 60-90 minutes postprandially, down to levels below 40 mg/dL. Treatment consists primarily of dietary modifications similar to those in dumping syndrome: meals low in carbohydrates and avoidance of liquids with meals. Octreotide can also occasionally be helpful. Surgical options consist of redirecting the Roux limb into the duodenum to restore the flow of ingested contents into the duodenum. Improvement of symptoms after such an operation can take 6-12 months.

Postvagotomy Diarrhea

This disorder occurs in up to 20% of patients after truncal vagotomy with only 4% being severe. It consists of watery diarrhea 15-30 minutes postprandially. The pathophysiology of postvagotomy diarrhea is still not well understood, and it is a diagnosis of exclusion. Dietary modification is the mainstay of treatment consisting of small, frequent, low-fat meals. The addition of bulking agents such as fiber can help. Treatments that have been suggested but do not have strong evidence to support them are octreotide, cholestyramine, and a reversed segment of jejunum.

Roux Stasis Syndrome

Roux stasis is rare and can sometimes be misdiagnosed as gastroparesis. It occurs when disruption of the myenteric plexus occurs during transection of the bowel. The normal intestinal pacemaker center in the duodenum that controls the myenteric plexus and leads to antegrade propagation of ingested contents can be relocated with this disruption of the bowel. If the new ectopic pacemaker center is located very distal to the transection, it can lead to retrograde contractions which in turn cause a functional obstruction of the Roux limb. Patients experience early satiety and emesis, as in gastroparesis. Most patients who have experienced this have undergone vagotomy with gastrectomy. A true mechanical obstruction must be ruled out and the diagnosis is one of exclusion. Gastric motility tests and EGD can be helpful in the diagnosis. If patients have any remnant of stomach remaining, the diagnosis is most likely gastroparesis as opposed to Roux stasis. Treatment is similar to gastroparesis and consists of dietary modification (soft or liquid foods); distal enteric supplemental feeds may be required through a jejunostomy. Erythromycin and metoclopramide occasionally improve symptoms. Operative interventions have little data to support their success, most suggesting shortening the Roux limb to move the pacemaker center more proximally.

Alkaline (Bile) Reflux Gastritis

Bile reflux occurs after functional disruption of the pylorus along with gastroparesis that can occur after vagotomy. Esophagitis can also occur when there is an incompetent lower esophageal sphincter (LES). Interruption of the pylorus leads to the free reflux of bile into the stomach. Symptoms consist of bilious emesis that can have associated epigastric pain and are most common between meals when there are few food particles to mix with the bile. It occurs transiently in 10%-20% of patients, persists in only 1%-2% of patients and mostly commonly presents months to years after operation. Diagnosis can be made based on symptoms as well as EGD and histologic findings of gastritis/esophagitis combined with pooling of bile in the stomach. If solid gastric contents are also present with a large amount of bile pooling, gastroparesis should also be suspected. Other causes of gastritis such as Zollinger-Ellison syndrome or retained gastric antrum (checking gastrin level) should be ruled out. Treatment focuses on conversion to a Roux-en-Y reconstruction with the Roux limb at least 50-60 cm.

Metabolic Disorders

Vitamin B_{12} deficiency is the most common deficiency after gastrectomy. Absorption requires intrinsic factor (IF), which is produced by the proximal stomach and R-factor, which binds to B_{12} in the stomach and requires an acidic environment. Absence of these factors and the binding process in the stomach, along with bypassing the duodenum where IF binds to B_{12}, leads to this deficiency. It most commonly presents with symptoms relating to anemia that include fatigue. Neurologic symptoms are unusual and are usually late findings. In its most severe form, the B_{12} deficiency can present as Wernicke encephalopathy. Even with gastrectomy, the intestine can absorb up to 1% of free B_{12}, so daily oral supplementation can prevent deficiency. Replacement can also be achieved through monthly injections, which is generally preferred.

Iron-deficiency anemia is also common following gastrectomy as iron is primarily absorbed in the duodenum. In addition, an acidic environment is also required to oxidize iron to the preferred absorptive ferric ion (Fe^{3+}). Acute blood loss should first be ruled out by fecal occult blood test and work-up should then include iron studies. Calcium deficiency and osteopenia can also occur following gastrectomy, as early as 2-3 years postoperatively. It is caused by decreased dissolution and ionization of calcium salts in the acid-free environment. Lastly, copper deficiency has also been seen following gastrectomy and presents as ataxia, myelopathy, and peripheral neuropathy. In addition to oral or injectable B_{12}, daily multivitamin, iron and micronutrient supplementation is pertinent early in the postoperative course to prevent these deficiencies.

SUMMARY

Most gastrointestinal hemorrhage due to peptic ulcer disease can be managed medically with pharmaceuticals and endoscopy. Only in rare cases is surgical intervention required. However, it is important that the surgeon understand all potential interventions and have the ability to address related complications to optimize outcomes for their patients. Peptic ulcer disease may also be complicated by GOO or perforation. Gastric and duodenal ulcer perforation is managed based on location and whether caused by high acid production. In general, the simplest operative solution is the best. Treatment of *H pylori* is an important facet of peptic ulcer management.

SUGGESTED READINGS

Abdel-Misih RZ, Larson JD, et al. The stomach. In: Cameron JL, Cameron AM, eds. *Current Surgical Therapy*. 11th ed. Elsevier Saunders; 2014:69-107.

Aurello P, Sirimarco D, Magistri P, et al. Management of duodenal stump fistula after gastrectomy for gastric cancer. *World J Gastroenterol*. 2015;21:7571-7576.

Becker HD, Caspary WF. *Postgastrectomy and Postvagotomy Syndromes*. Springer-Verlag; 1980.

Bertleff MJOE, Halm JA, Bemelman WA, et al. Randomized clinical trial of laparoscopic versus open repair of the perforated peptic ulcer: the LAMA trial. *World J Surg*. 2009;33:1368-1373.

Blatchford O, Murray WR, Blatchford M. A risk score to predict need for treatment for upper-gastrointestinal haemorrhage. *Lancet*. 2000;356(9238):1318-1321.

Bolton JS, Conway C II. Postgastrectomy syndromes. *Surg Clin North Am*. 2011;91:1105-1122.

Britt LD, Blake DP. Gastroduodenal operations for upper gastrointestinal bleeding and perforation. In: Cioffi WG, Asensio JA, eds. *Atlas of Trauma/Emergency General Surgery Techniques.* Chapter 20. Elsevier/Saunders; 2014:219-226.

Chey WD, Leontiadis GI, Howden CW, Moss SF. ACG clinical guideline: treatment of helicobacter pylori infection. *Am J Gastroenterol.* 2017;112(2):212-239.

Chung KT, Shelat VG. Perforated peptic ulcer: an update. *World J Gastroinest Surg.* 2017;9:1-12.

Clinch D, Damskos D, diMarzo F, et al. Duodenal ulcer perforation: a systematic literature review and narrative description of surgical techniques to treat large duodenal defects. *J Trauma Acute Care Surg.* 2021;91:748-758.

Feliciano DV. Do perforated duodenal ulcers need an acid reducing procedure now that omeprazole is available? *Surg Clin North Am.* 1992;72:369-380.

Kavitt RT, Lipowska AM, Anyane-Yeboa A, et al. Diagnosis and treatment of peptic ulcer disease. *Am J Med.* 2019;132(4):447-456.

Kempenich JW, Sirinek KR. Acid peptic disease. *Surg Clin North Am.* 2018;98(5):933-944.

Kurdia K, Singh RK. Post total gastrectomy complications: duodenal stump leak. In: Baretta SG, Shrikhande SV, eds. *Dilemmas in Abdominal Surgery.* CRC; 2020:63-68.

Lagoo S, McMahon RL, Kakihara M, et al. The sixth decision regarding perforated duodenal ulcer. *JSLS.* 2002;6:359-368.

Lanas A, Chan FK. Peptic ulcer disease. *Lancet.* 2017;390:613-624.

Lee CW, Sarosi GA. Emergency ulcer surgery. *Surg Clin North Am.* 2011;91(5):1001-1013.

Mulholland MW. Gastroduodenal ulceration. In: Mulholland MW, Lillemoe KD, Doherty GM, et al., eds. *Greenfield's Surgery: Scientific Principles and Practice.* 6th ed. Lippincott Williams & Wilkins; 2017:725-735.

Nelms DW, Pelaez CA. The acute upper gastrointestinal bleed. *Surg Clin North Am.* 2018;98:1047-1057.

Quah GS, Eslick GD, Cox MR. Laparoscopic repair for perforated peptic ulcer disease has better outcomes than open repair. *J Gastrointest Surg.* 2019;23:618-625.

Reid KM, Sarr MG. Postgastrectomy syndromes in the current era. In: Fischer JE, et al., eds. *Fischer's Mastery of Surgery.* 7th ed. Lippincott Williams & Wilkins; 2018:1148-1165.

Roses RE, Dempsey DT. Stomach. In: Brunicardi FC, Andersen DK, Billiar TR, et al., eds. *Schwartz's Principles of Surgery.* 11th ed. McGraw-Hill; 2019:69-87.

Soreide K, Thorsen K, Harrison EM, et al. Perforated peptic ulcer. *Lancet.* 2015;386:1288-1298.

Stanley AJ, Laine L, Dalton HR, et al. Comparison of risk scoring systems for patients presenting with upper gastrointestinal bleeding: international, multicenter prospective study. *BMJ.* 2017;356:i6432.

Tarasconi A, Coccolini F, Biffl WL, et al. Perforated and bleeding peptic ulcer: WSES guidelines. *World J Emerg Surg.* 2020;15:3.

Teitelbaum EN, Hungness ES, Mahvi DM. Stomach. In: Townsend C, ed. *Sabiston Textbook of Surgery.* Chapter 48. Elsevier; 2017:1188-1236.

Tringali A, Giannetti A, Adler DG. Endoscopic management of gastric outlet obstruction disease. *Ann Gastroenterol.* 2019;32(4):330-337.

Vakayil V, Bauman B, Joppru K, et al. Surgical repair of perforated peptic ulcers: laparoscopic versus open approach. *Surg Endosc.* 2019;33:281-292.

Zittel TT, Jehle EC, Becker HD. Surgical management of peptic ulcer disease today—indication, technique and outcome. *Langenbecks Arch Surg.* 2000;385(2):84-96.

Zizzo M, Ugoletti L, Ruiz CC, et al. Management of duodenal stump fistula after gastrectomy for malignant disease. *BMC Surg.* 2019;19:55. doi:10.1186/s12893-019-0520-x

CHAPTER

17 Acute Appendicitis

Shahin Mohseni and Dennis Y. Kim

CASE PRESENTATION 1

A previously healthy 3-year-old boy presents to the emergency department with anorexia, high fever, vomiting (past 4 days), diarrhea (past 2 days), and abdominal pain (last day). He has generalized abdominal pain, hyponatremia, a significant increase in his white blood count (WBC), and C-reactive protein (CRP), with a normal urinalysis and glucose level. His heart rate (HR) is 120 bpm and blood pressure (BP) is 100/70 mm Hg. He is lethargic on exam with guarding in all quadrants.

Question: *What is the optimal management of this patient's presumed intra-abdominal sepsis?*

CASE PRESENTATION 2

A 79-year-old male presents with 2 days of lower abdominal pain, nausea, and fever. He has a history of hypertension and myocardial infarction 8 years ago. He is currently on beta-blocker therapy. Surgical history is significant for an open cholecystectomy (Kocher incision) 35 years ago. On presentation, he is febrile, HR is 60 bpm, and BP is 140/90 mm Hg. Laboratory investigations reveal an increased WBC with right shift and elevated CRP. His abdominal exam reveals focal peritonitis in the right lower quadrant with a positive Rovsing sign.

Question: *What is the optimal management of this patient's abdominal pain?*

Suspicion for intra-abdominal sepsis should be high in both of these patients. Recognition and risk assessment for sepsis should be carried out as part of the initial evaluation and patient triage. Risk assessment for frailty, delirium, and deep vein thrombosis should be part of initial assessment in all elderly patients. Aggressive fluid resuscitation and early initiation of antibiotics is of paramount importance when intra-abdominal sepsis is suspected. Early involvement of surgical critical care or intensivists for correction of electrolyte imbalance, especially hyponatremia in children, is warranted. Definitive diagnosis is often accomplished with the use of ultrasonography (US) or computed tomography (CT). Initiate ongoing resuscitative efforts prior to and concurrent with these investigations should not delay definitive source control (ie, appendectomy). Undertake surgery as soon as possible provided that there are no absolute medical contraindications for general anesthesia. In both cases, if laparoscopic equipment and expertise are available, and the patient is hemodynamically stable without contraindications, a laparoscopic approach may be attempted first.

INTRODUCTION

Despite being one of the most common diagnoses in general surgery, occurring with an overall incidence of 8% in the Western general population, acute appendicitis (AA) remains a challenge in clinical practice. One reason is that not all patients fit the classic description found in most medical textbooks, which includes symptoms and signs of anorexia, migratory pain to the right lower abdominal quadrant, fever, and leukocytosis. The differential diagnoses, depending on sex and age, can range from gynecological conditions to Meckel diverticulitis or colon cancer. For the purpose of this chapter, we will concentrate on three special populations, namely children, pregnant, and elderly patients. Further, we will focus primarily on complicated appendicitis (gangrenous or perforated), thus highlighting the challenges in diagnosing and treating appendicitis. Finally, we will also discuss some controversies in the diagnosis of appendicitis and existing treatment options.

APPENDICITIS IN CHILDREN

Clinical Presentation

Young children presenting with abdominal pain pose a diagnostic challenge due to communication barriers, which may result in an unreliable history or inability to perform a reliable physical exam. In children, especially those of younger age (<6 years), abdominal pain can be caused by other inflammatory and infectious conditions remote from the abdominal cavity, such as pneumonia or acute otitis media. Furthermore, the typical findings of abdominal rigidity or rebound tenderness on physical examination are not usually present in the youngest children (<4 years). This means that serious intra-abdominal pathology, such as gangrenous or perforated appendicitis, can go unrecognized, which makes the diagnosis of AA more challenging. Existing risk assessment tools yield low sensitivity and specificity in diagnosing AA. However, low scores without an increase in inflammatory laboratory values (WBC, CRP) can exclude AA in children with a high probability. Take caution when considering CT investigations for the diagnosis of AA in children; attempt to minimize radiation exposure. For this reason, US is currently recommended as first-line imaging for the diagnosis of AA in children. However, it has been reported that US exhibits low specificity and sensitivity, which may be due to patient-specific factors such as high body mass index (BMI) or operator dependent. In cases where suspicion is high, a negative US should not delay surgery or result in additional radiologic investigations.

Surgical Approach

Laparoscopic appendectomy is safe and recommended in children of all ages where equipment and surgical expertise is available. Many centers do not have laparoscopic equipment for the smallest children, and in these cases, a right lower quadrant incision (McBurney incision) is an acceptable surgical approach. If other causes of abdominal pain need to be ruled out, such as perforated Meckel diverticulitis, a lower midline approach is recommended to achieve better extensile access to the intra-abdominal structures. Data suggest an increased risk of surgical site and wound infections in children when endoloops are used instead of endostaplers for managing stump closure in uncomplicated appendicitis. In complicated AA, using an endostapler may have the advantage of more precise closure of the base of the appendix, and in cases of proximal perforations, a wedge cecal resection can be performed. There are no advantages to inverting the appendiceal stump.

What to Do When Encountering the Unexpected

As mentioned, children may have several different causes of abdominal pain that can be mistaken for appendicitis. It is not uncommon that with a high clinical suspicion of AA, many surgeons perform a diagnostic laparoscopy in children. In cases where the appendix is macroscopically found to be uninflamed, it is important to rule out other intra-abdominal sources of pain. If no surgically treatable intra-abdominal source is detected, the authors recommend an appendectomy be carried out due to a lifetime risk of AA vs the low incidence of postoperative complications.

It is not uncommon that both clinically, and on ultrasound, a Meckel diverticulum is mistaken for the appendix (**Figure 17.1**). If Meckel diverticulum is present at the time of surgery in children, we recommend its removal either laparoscopically or by conversion to open surgery, depending on the surgical expertise available.

APPENDICITIS DURING PREGNANCY

Clinical Presentation

Appendicitis during pregnancy is a rare, and often delayed, diagnosis. Perforated appendicitis is a potentially life-threatening condition for both the mother and the fetus. There are no validated risk assessment tools for diagnosing AA during pregnancy and physical exam can be highly unreliable in the later stages of pregnancy due to the displacement of the abdominal viscera. High suspicion of AA in pregnant women with abdominal pain on the right side, fever, and increased inflammatory markers is warranted and mandates an aggressive approach for the diagnosis and subsequent treatment. Depending on body habitus, trimester, and size of the uterus, different imaging investigations can be pursued. In the early stages of gestation, US is recommended, and if inconclusive, MRI is the next radiological tool of choice. CT, if more readily available or deemed necessary in addition to US and MRI, should not be withheld from a pregnant patient. Diagnostic laparoscopy is also a viable option if suspicion of AA remains, and the patient is in the early stages of pregnancy.

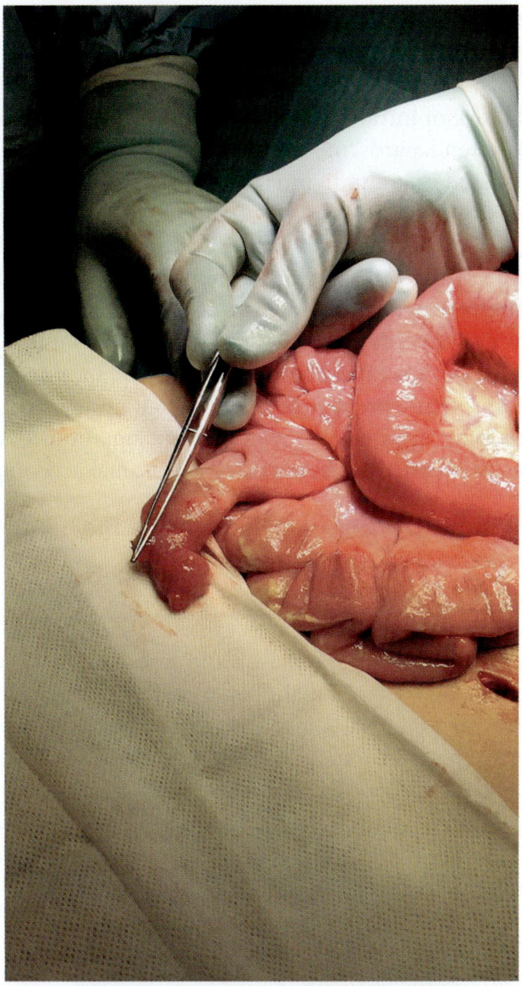

Figure 17.1 A 6-year-old boy (22 kg, 110 cm) seeking health care for low abdominal pain twice, 3 days apart. Initial presentation with no fever, normal appetite, and normal laboratory tests (electrolytes, WBC, CRP). Abdominal examination revealed mild subumbilical tenderness, no guarding or peritonitis. No radiology investigation was performed. The second presentation with high fever, vomiting, markedly increased WBC and CRP. On examination, there was a generalized peritonitis. Resuscitation and intravenous antibiotics were started from the ED and he was taken to OR within 3 hours of admission for diagnostic laparoscopy. Laparoscopically, the intra-abdominal space contained large amounts of pus and small bowel content, which lead to a decision to convert to open approach by lower midline incision. A perforated Meckel diverticulum was detected, which was removed by wedge resection at the base and a primary anastomosis was completed.

Surgical Approach

Pregnancy is not a contraindication to laparoscopic surgery. However, depending on the gestational age and the patient's body habitus, laparoscopic surgery might be challenging and associated with a high risk of iatrogenic injury. In the first and second trimesters, laparoscopic appendectomy should be attempted. Modify the trocar placement accordingly (**Figure 17.2**). We discourage laparoscopic appendectomy in the third trimester due to the distorted intraperitoneal anatomy and the limited space provided. In the case where an open approach is planned from the onset, gather as much information from preoperative radiological investigations as possible to localize the exact position of the inflamed appendix. This information will help plan the incision, which should preferably be a "modified" McBurney's (**Figure 17.3**). The surgical team should have contacted an obstetrician well in advance in case an emergency cesarian section is necessary.

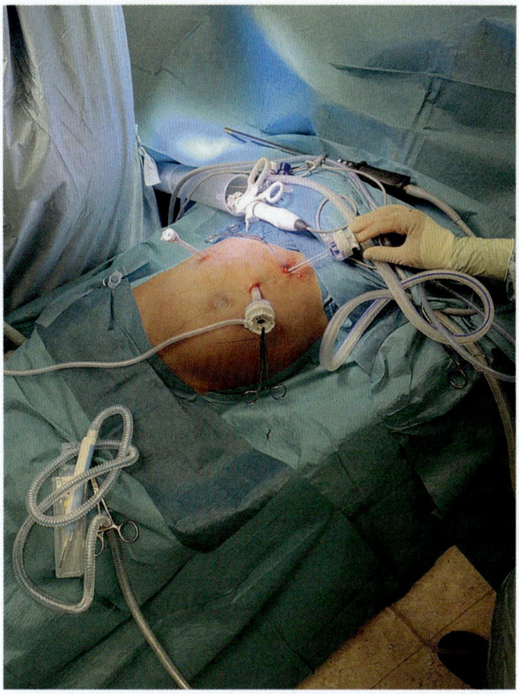

Figure 17.2 Trocars placement modification in case of acute appendicitis in pregnancy.

What to Do when Encountering the Unexpected

If an uninflamed appendix is encountered intraoperatively, and no alternative source for the clinical presentation is detected, proceed with an appendectomy.

If other surgical conditions are encountered that might lead to more extensive or complex surgical procedures, a multidisciplinary decision-making process should take place between

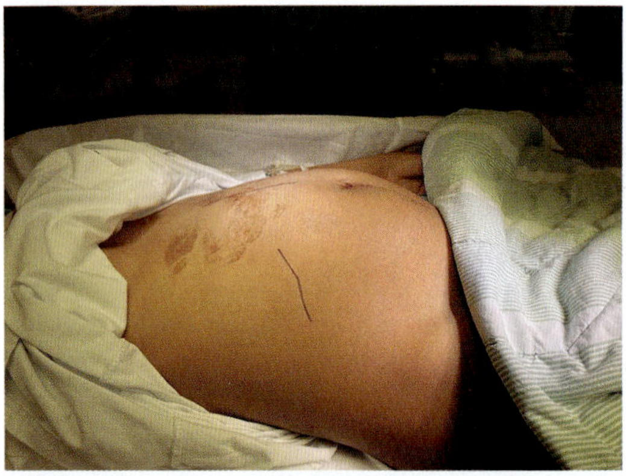

Figure 17.3 Modified McBurney incision in pregnancy.

members of the health care team (surgery, anesthesiology, obstetrics, and neonatology) intraoperatively. Also, when possible, preoperatively discuss with the patient and their loved ones how to proceed. The authors also strongly suggest, due to the rarity of these conditions, that a senior surgeon is present throughout the surgery in all pregnant patients undergoing an appendectomy.

APPENDICITIS IN THE ELDERLY

Clinical Presentation

With an increase in life expectancy, the size of the geriatric population (>65 years) will increase substantially in the coming years, which will lead to a rise in the incidence of appendicitis in this potentially vulnerable population. Compared to younger patients, clinical signs, physical exam, and laboratory values may be misleading due to higher rate of multipharmacy, different pain perception, and at times communication barriers, leading to a low specificity and sensitivity of current risk assessment tools for AA diagnosis when used in the elderly. Also, physicians must always take into account more life-threatening conditions due to the higher prevalence of comorbidities in geriatric patients with acute abdominal pain. For these reasons, several medical societies and guidelines recommend liberal and early use of CT in this patient population for diagnosing AA and to detect or rule out other conditions that may cause acute abdominal pain. It is also of outmost importance to complete preoperative risk assessment for delirium, frailty, and deep venous thrombosis, all strongly associated with worse postoperative outcome in geriatric surgical patients, and to individualize factors such as pre- and postoperative level of care, pain, and anesthesiology medications. This will optimize postoperative outcome.

Surgical Approach

There is a higher prevalence of previous abdominal surgery in geriatric patients, which increases the risk of intraperitoneal adhesions. The decision between laparoscopic and open surgery should be assessed on an individual basis where a history of previous major abdominal surgery exists. Based on the risk assessment and the surgeon's level of experience with laparoscopic surgery, an attempt with a laparoscopic approach is recommended, even if patients have had prior abdominal surgery. If the peritoneal environment is hostile or a decision is made preoperatively not to attempt a laparoscopic approach, a lower midline laparotomy is recommended for better intra-abdominal access.

What to Do When encountering the Unexpected

In the elderly patient, there is always a risk of underlying malignancy as cause of the abdominal pain. Intraoperatively, if the suspicion is high for a diagnosis of malignancy, a judicious decision on whether to, and how to, proceed with the surgery is warranted (**Figure 17.4**). In cases where a malignancy of the appendix or cecum (colon)

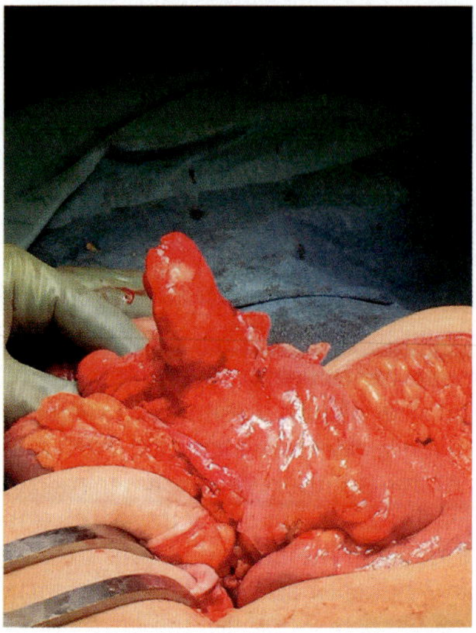

Figure 17.4 A 70-year-old female with right lower abdominal pain for last 4 days, normal appetite, fever, and mildly elevated WBC and CRP admitted to surgical service. No cancer diagnosis in immediate relatives. CT was interpreted as perforated appendicitis and suspicion of abscess formation. Intraoperatively, high suspicion for malignancy leads to conversion from laparoscopy to midline laparotomy, and subsequent right-sided hemicolectomy. Pathological examination of the specimen revealed adenocarcinoma.

is suspected, and a decision is made to proceed with surgery, perform a right-sided hemicolectomy. The authors suggest that, in these instances, if the surgeon does not perform cancer resection surgery on regular basis, that a colorectal cancer surgeon is consulted for assistance to achieve the best oncological results.

AMYAND HERNIA

Amyand hernia, a rare condition where an inguinal hernia contains an appendix, may be encountered. The surgical approach and intervention in these cases are individualized based on patient-specific risk factors and whether the appendix is inflamed or perforated. In setting where the appendix is incarcerated within the hernia sac with acute inflammation without perforation, an appendectomy and herniorrhaphy with (or without) mesh can be performed. In cases with perforated appendicitis, the authors suggest herniorrhaphy be performed without mesh placement due to the increased risk of foreign body infection. Laparoscopy is recommended in both non- and perforated appendicitis for both herniorrhaphy and appendectomy; however, the threshold for conversion to open surgery should be low.

COMPLICATED APPENDICITIS

Although a common surgical procedure with a low rate of complication, an appendectomy can be challenging if the appendix is perforated. Perforated appendicitis is almost twice as common in children and the elderly compared to the rest of the general population. It is commonly associated with a delayed diagnosis due to atypical presentation, communication difficulties, unreliable physical examination and laboratory values, and in-hospital delays to surgery. On the other hand, it has been suggested that ruptured appendicitis is a different disease than nonruptured appendicitis from the onset.

The combination of an increased burden of comorbidities and frailty in elderly patients leads to worse outcomes across emergency medical conditions. In addition, the physiologic stress induced by an operation may augment this response, potentially resulting in even worse outcomes. Children, on the other hand, are more resilient with increased physiological capacity, which may mislead acute care physicians regarding physiological stability despite serious conditions such as ongoing sepsis. For the aforementioned reasons, it is of paramount importance that perforated appendicitis be suspected, diagnosed, and treated expeditiously. Start fluid and intravenous antibiotic therapy immediately when intra-abdominal sepsis is suspected, with a sense of urgency to investigate and determine the correct diagnosis, and subsequent intervention for source control. There is a body of evidence that laparoscopic appendectomy for perforated appendicitis is both safe and associated with fewer postoperative complications than appendectomy with open surgical approach. In the elderly, the minimally invasive approach is preferred as the resulting reduction in surgical stress leads to less postoperative pain, earlier rehabilitation/mobilization, and earlier discharge from hospital. There is no evidence supporting the use of intra-abdominal drainage after an appendectomy in the context of complicated appendicitis. Its use has been associated with longer hospital stay and, in some instances, an increased risk of adverse outcomes. The authors do not recommend aggressive high-volume intra-abdominal irrigation in these instances either, since current data have shown no benefit for such practice. In contrast, there is some evidence for abscess formation at other intra-abdominal locations, remote from the perforation site, suggesting dissemination of bacteria via the irrigation fluid.

An ongoing debate on how to best manage appendiceal abscesses still remains, with opinions divided between initial nonoperative management (antibiotics with or without percutaneous drainage) and early surgical intervention. The data support early laparoscopic appendectomy in experienced hands, and this approach has been associated with fewer complications, re-interventions, less antibiotic use, decreased postoperative hospital length of stay, and fewer readmissions. However, many experts including the authors still recommend the nonoperative approach as the first step when laparoscopic expertise is not available and among patients with prior abdominal surgery. Interval appendectomy after nonoperative management of appendiceal abscess is another area of controversy. In children, there is no need for interval appendectomy. However, recent data demonstrate an increased risk for malignancy with increasing age in elderly patients with complicated appendicitis. These data suggest the risk of malignancy may be as high as 20% in patients ≥40 years. However, based on the evidence available today and the recommendation from several surgical societies, the decision for interval appendectomy in this patient population should be individualized. The data are scarce on the management in pregnant patients with appendiceal perforations and abscesses. At present, therefore, we recommend the same treatment algorithms in these instances. In cases where a caesarean section is performed for other reasons such as contractions and labor in a pregnant patient with complicated appendicitis, simultaneous appendectomy should be undertaken.

ANTIBIOTICS ONLY VS APPENDECTOMY

In the last decade, more attention has been given to a nonoperative, antibiotics only management strategy for uncomplicated appendicitis, for example, no fecalith, perforation, or abscess on the admission CT. This issue remains controversial. The presence of a fecalith or a dilated appendix (>10-12 mm) significantly increases the risk of failure for antibiotics only approach and should be considered as an contraindication when present. A nonoperative approach is not recommended in the immunosuppressed or pregnant patient. Several studies have shown that uncomplicated appendicitis in children can be managed with antibiotics alone at index admission. However, some follow-up data have shown that up to 50% of these cases underwent an appendectomy within the first year after nonoperative management. Since the risk of perforation in children is higher than in the general population, appendectomy at index admission in this patient population is recommended. In elderly patients, who to a larger extent are frail with several comorbidities, there would be a rationale to undertake a nonoperative approach avoiding the risk of anesthesia and surgery. However, there is always a risk of treatment failure, which would undoubtedly lead to more physiological strain and an inevitable surgical intervention. A recent study demonstrated that one in six elderly patients failed within 6 months of antibiotic treatment, requiring operation, with higher morbidity and mortality. Knowing that there is a higher risk of perforation in this group, the authors strongly recommend against nonoperative management with antibiotics if there are no absolute contraindications to surgery. Finally, another concern with antibiotic only treatment in clinical practice at this time is the lack of agreement on the type, mode of administration, and length of antibiotic treatment for uncomplicated appendicitis (most recommend 10 days) as the studies in the field have all used different protocols. Despite these caveats, recent recommendations from the American Association for the Surgery of Trauma, World Society of Emergency Surgery, and the American College of Surgeons support antibiotic only initial treatment for uncomplicated appendicitis excluding the contraindications discussed above. Surgery or antibiotics alone are now considered reasonable approaches in selected patients. Nonetheless, 30%-40% of patients initially treated with antibiotics alone will undergo appendectomy within 5 years.

TIMING OF APPENDECTOMY: THE SOONER THE BETTER

Several studies have demonstrated that out-of-hours appendectomy is safe even when performed during the late night/early morning hours, while other studies have shown increased complications with delayed surgery. Consequently, if there is no medical reason for postponing the procedure, it should be undertaken as soon as possible. Furthermore, a delay may result in perforation of the appendix and suboptimal outcome, especially in the special patient groups discussed in the current chapter.

POSTOPERATIVE CARE

Early postoperative enteral nutrition and mobilization should be the rule after any appendectomy, even in cases where open appendectomy has been performed. Treat uncomplicated, nonperforated appendicitis with a preoperative dose of IV antibiotics; extended postoperatively antibiotic therapy is neither needed nor recommended. To date, there are no solid data on the length or mode (intravenous or oral administration) for postoperative antibiotic treatment after surgery for complicated appendicitis, thus such therapy should be tailored based on preoperative risk factors, clinical course, and by following infection parameters such as laboratory values. Thromboembolic prophylaxis should be given to all patients with preoperative risk factors for deep venous thrombosis, pregnant patients, and those patients with a long operation time (>2 hours) or when conversion to open surgery was performed; at least until there are no signs of ongoing severe infection or sepsis and the patient is fully mobilized. Maintain a low threshold for postoperative CT in all cases of suspected postoperative complications or surgical site infection/abscess after complicated appendicitis. If intra-abdominal abscess is detected on CT, percutaneous drainage with extended antibiotic coverage should be undertaken.

SUMMARY

Acute appendicitis continues to pose diagnostic and treatment challenges, especially in the pediatric, pregnant, and elderly populations, where early clinical suspicion and diagnosis are key factors for successful treatment and favorable outcomes. Early radiological imaging is highly recommended for establishing diagnosis but should not delay surgical intervention if deemed necessary. When abdominal sepsis is suspected, it is of paramount importance that simultaneous resuscitation according to sepsis guidelines is started as soon as possible along with diagnostic measures. Laparoscopic surgery is recommended as surgical approach for complicated appendicitis in children, elderly, during pregnancy, and even in those with previous abdominal surgery, whenever equipment and surgical expertise exists.

SUGGESTED READINGS

Camron JL, Cameron AM. *Current Surgical Therapy*. 13th ed. Elsevier; 2020.

Chehab M, Ditillo M, Khurrum M, et al. Managing acute uncomplicated appendicitis in frail geriatric patients: a second hit may be too much. *J Trauma Acute Care Surg*. 2021;90:501-506.

de Virgilio C, Frank PN, Grigorian A. *Surgery: A Case Based Clinical Review*. 2nd ed. Springer International Publishing; 2020.

Di Saverio S, Podda M, De Simone B, et al. Diagnosis and treatment of acute appendicitis: 2020 update of the WSES Jerusalem guidelines. *World J Emerg Surg*. 2020;15(1):27.

Helling TS, Soltys DF, Seals S. Operative vs nonoperative management in the care of patients with complicated appendicitis. *Am J Surg*. 2017;214:1195-1200.

Mallinen J, Rautio T, Gronroos J, et al. Risk of appendiceal neoplasm in periappendicular abscess on patients treated with interval appendectomy vs followup with MRI. 1-year outcomes of the periappendicitis Acuta randomized clinical trial. *JAMA Surg*. 2019;154:200-207.

Moris D, Paulson EK, Pappas TN. Diagnosis and management of acute appendicitis in adults: a review. *JAMA*. 2021;326:2299-2311.

Nimmagadda N, Matsushima K, Piccinini A, et al. Complicated appendicitis: immediate operation or trial of nonoperative management. *Am J Surg*. 2019;217:713-717.

O'Leary DP. Walsh SM, Bolger J, et al. A randomized clinical trial evaluating the efficacy and quality of life of antibiotic-only treatment of acute uncomplicated appendicitis: results of the COMMA trial. *Ann Surg*. 2021;274:240-247.

Podda M, Gerardi C, Cillara N, et al. Antibiotic treatment and appendectomy for uncomplicated acute appendicitis in adults and children: a systematic review and meta-analysis. *Ann Surg*. 2019;270:1028-1040.

Rushing A, Bugaev N, Jones C, et al. Management of acute appendicitis in adults: a practice management guideline from the Eastern Association for the Surgery of Trauma. *J Trauma Acute Care Surg*. 2019;87(1):214-224.

Saar S, Mihnovitš V, Lustenberger T, et al. Twenty-four hour versus extended antibiotic administration after surgery in complicated appendicitis: a randomized controlled trial. *J Trauma Acute Care Surg*. 2019;86(1):36-42.

Symer MM, Abelson JS, Sedrakyan A, et al. Early operative management of complicated appendicitis is associated with improved surgical outcomes in adults. *Am J Surg*. 2018;216:431-437.

Talan DA, DiSaverio S. Treatment of acute uncomplicated appendicitis. *N Engl J Med*. 2021;385:1116-1123.

CHAPTER

18 Inflammatory Disease of the Small Bowel and Colon

Brian S. Zuckerbraun, Sean F. Monaghan, and Samuel Wade Ross

CASE PRESENTATION

A 71-year old female with a history of diabetes, asthma, lupus, and hypertension presents to the emergency department with a 2-day history of right lower quadrant pain and associated nausea and vomiting. The pain has been increasing in severity and she had a new fever to 39.2 °C today. She has been passing liquid stool and admits to several year history of diarrhea and tenesmus. Her only prior surgery is a hysterectomy 20 years ago. On exam, she is alert, oriented, heart rate is 125/min, blood pressure 95/54 mm Hg, and is mildly diaphoretic and toxic appearing. Abdominal exam reveals diffuse tenderness to palpation with focal rebound and guarding in the right lower quadrant. Laboratory studies: creatinine of 1.9 mg/dL, WBC is 21 000 mm^3, and lactate of 3.5 mmol/L. A representative cut of a noncontrasted CT of the abdomen and pelvis shows (**Figure 18.1**) free fluid, diffuse terminal ileal thickening, and stranding in the mesentery. She is taken emergently to the operating room, is started on vasopressors intraoperatively, and 20 cm of ischemic terminal ileum is found with associated creeping fat and perforation. She undergoes terminal ileal resection, is left in discontinuity, and a temporary abdominal dressing is placed for damage control laparotomy due to hemodynamic instability and lactic acidosis. She improves in her hemodynamics and acid-base status and returns to the operating room within 24 hours for ileocecectomy, primary isoperistaltic anastomosis, and abdominal closure. Gastroenterology is consulted and she is started on biologic suppression therapy 6 weeks postoperatively.

Questions: *What is the underlying disease process in this patient? What indications does she have for emergent surgery? What nonoperative modalities are available to nonemergent cases of this disease? When adjuncts should be considered in addition to surgical resection and what additional considerations should be kept in mind for this disease process?*

Answers: *Crohn's disease with ileal perforation, peritonitis, and sepsis. Free air, peritonitis, septic shock. Medical therapy, steroids, and biologic therapy. In patients without signs of free perforation and/or sepsis, minimally invasive strategies should be employed with percutaneous drainage, IV antibiotics, and bowel rest. The minimal amount of bowel resection should be performed when required given the recurrent nature of the disease. Bowel anastomoses should be performed in isoperistoltic fashion given the need for frequent endoscopy in these patients.*

INTRODUCTION

This chapter reviews diseases of the small bowel and colon. The focus of this chapter is on inflammatory processes that require prompt recognition of the patient who requires immediate surgical intervention. Common presentations include obstruction, ischemia, perforation, abscess, bleeding, and fistula. Gastrointestinal bleeding, bowel obstruction, and mesenteric ischemia are covered in Chapters 11, 12, and 13.

INFLAMMATORY BOWEL DISEASE

Inflammatory bowel disease (IBD) is a spectrum of autoimmune diseases that can target anywhere in the gastrointestinal (GI) tract, but most commonly in the small and large intestine, as well as anorectal disease. IBD is comprised of ulcerative colitis (UC), which exists only in the colon and rectum while Crohn disease (CD) can occur anywhere along the gastrointestinal tract. We will review the epidemiology, presentation, diagnosis, medical and surgical

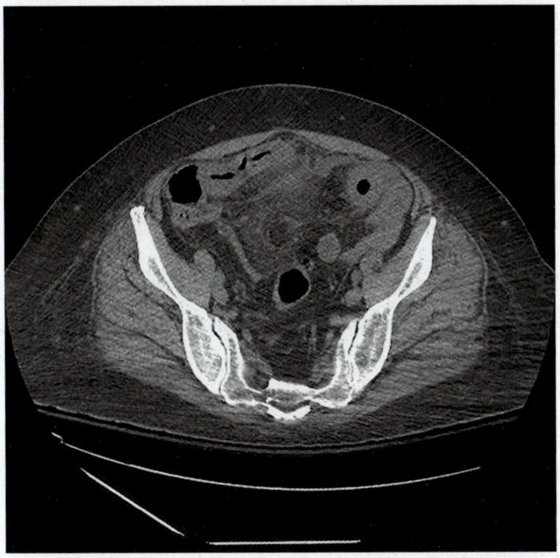

Figure 18.1 A 71 year-old female presenting with RLQ pain, obstructive symptoms, sepsis, and new terminal ileal thickening on CT abdomen/pelvis.

treatment, and emergent surgical indications for CD and UC separately and based on anatomic presentation to the small intestine, colon, or anorectal. Special considerations to surgical evaluation and management, surgical technique, and postoperative care will be discussed.

TABLE 18.1 ■ Risk Factors for Crohn Disease

Genetic	Ashkenazi Jew
	Caucasian
	Family history of IBD
History/ environment	Smoking
	Appendectomy
	Lack of exercise
	High stress/anxiety
Diet	High fat
	Low vitamin D3
	Low fiber
	High refined carbohydrates
Microbiome	*E coli* predominant
	Bacteroides enterotype
	No pet/farm animal exposure
	Not breast-feed
	Cleanliness
Medications	NSAIDs
	Aspirin
	Oral Contraceptive pills

CROHN DISEASE

Epidemiology

Crohn disease is a chronic autoimmune inflammatory disease of the gastrointestinal tract with symptoms that occur in a relapsing and recurring manner, with a varied spectrum of severity and penetrance of disease. The incidence of CD has been increasing since the end of World War II, but particularly in urban and developed nations with lower rates of prevalence in rural areas and developing nations. Prevalence of the disease is highest in Europe, Canada, and the United States with cases of roughly 200-300 per 100 000 in these countries. Typically, there is a bimodal distribution of age of onset with a first peak in the teens to 30s and then again in the 50-70 age range.

Risk factors for Crohn disease are summarized in **Table 18.1** and are associated with genetics, race, nutrition, microbiome, immune, and environmental factors. Typically, those of Asian and African descent have the lowest associated risk while descendants of Ashkenazi Jewish ancestry have 3-4× the risk of non-Jewish cohorts. Certain genes have been found to predispose to CD, especially those related to bacterial activation and Th17 lymphocyte function. This cell produces Il-17, which has been implicated in the pathogenesis of CD. However, clinical variations in these genes do not completely account for CD phenotype and, therefore, tests for them are not used in the clinical practice of CD. Tobacco use has been well linked to risk of developing CD and at a younger age, likely due to oxidative stress, transient ischemia, nitric oxide production, and changes to the GI microbiome.

Like many realms of clinical science today, scientists are finding that the interplay between host physiology and cell function and the bacterial microbiota are vital to understanding the pathophysiology of CD. The prevailing thought is that without a large reservoir of bacteria or even parasites for the immune system to learn self from foreign, the body erroneously attacks self-antigens leading to chronic inflammation. Many studies have demonstrated that a decreased diversity in GI microbiome bacteria is associated with higher rates of IBD; specifically increased rates of *E coli* and fungal dysbiosis and decrease in *Bacteroides* and *Clostridium* species. A myriad host of factors can affect this balance of life in the GI tract, some of which have been shown to decrease risk of CD: large family size, exposure to pets and farm animals, breast-feeding, poor hygiene, decreased stress, and eastern diet.

Similarly, medications that can eradicate microbiome biodiversity such as antibiotics within the first year of life have been associated with CD. Other medications that have been associated are nonsteroidal anti-inflammatory medications, oral contraceptives, and aspirin use. One extreme example of this is the fact that appendectomy is associated with higher rates of CD, perhaps due to the appendix acting as a reservoir for the microbiome to repopulate the GI tract after illness.

Nutrition has been widely implicated as having a key role in the development of CD, specifically western high in fat and protein diets. In contrast, eastern diets high in grains, vegetables, and fiber foster different bacterial phenotypes, such as *Prevotella* and Firmicutes, based on the dietary intake. Additionally, lack of vitamins and micronutrients (zinc, iron, vitamin D3) play key roles in the development of CD and can be important in the treatment. Vitamin D3 <20 ng/mL has been associated with increased CD rates, need for hospitalization, and surgery within CD, and supplementation can decrease the risk of these for patients with CD.

Pathophysiology

The pathophysiologic genesis of Crohn disease is multifactorial and based on the above risk factors and increasingly understood, the microbiome present, but generally can be summarized into three categories: mucosal barrier dysfunction, innate immune activation, and adaptive immune propagation. In CD, changes in the microbiome, diet, and innate genetic risk factors result in dysregulation of the buffer zone created by the GI columnar epithelium. Lack of the buffer, through damage, mutation, or emulsifiers present in the diet promote bacterial translocation. Dysfunction of lysosomal degradation and/or exportation of bacteria can lead to bacterial translocation and immune activation. Invasion of bacteria due to damage or dysfunction of the tight junctions between cells can similarly lead to bacterial invasion beyond the mucosa.

Innate immunity is nonspecific and is triggered by activation of toll-like receptors (TLR) on immune cells from bacteria or erroneously on self-antigens and NOD-like receptors in the cytoplasm. Both receptors have been found to be dysregulated in IBD and will trigger activation of dendritic cells, neutrophils, monocytes, natural killer cells, and macrophages. Importantly, mucosal innate lymphoid cells respond to similar cues and excrete several cytokines, most notably TNF-α. Additionally, deficits in IL-23 and genes associated with autophagy have been associated with development of CD as directed cell death is impaired. Adaptive immune response is specific to antigens and in CD is related to increased IL-2 and interferon gamma on mucosal Th1 cells. More recent research also implicates Th17 and IL-23 in the initiation of CD. These mechanisms lead to increased dendritic cell activation in Peyer patches and systemic recruitment of T and B cells.

Presentation

Crohn disease can be an insidious and misdiagnosed disease process that can affect anywhere in the GI tract from the mouth to the perineum with emergent, acute, and chronic presentations. Its hallmark characteristic is transmural inflammation, but initial presentation and subsequent recurrence can occur in a myriad of ways. Typical disease types are described later in this chapter, but signs and symptoms can be indolent to fulminant on first diagnosis. In general, symptoms follow disease location and severity and can include nonspecific symptoms such as fatigue, anorexia, weight loss, or diarrhea. Classic presentation of right lower quadrant pain, diarrhea, and weight loss should raise suspicions if present on history; especially if presenting later with complicated disease such as abscess, obstruction, or fistula. Presence of fever and/or hemodynamic instability on evaluation should raise concern for developing sepsis from complicated CD. Distribution of intestinal disease is the terminal ileum and cecum roughly 50% of the time, 25% with ileitis only, and 25% with colitis only. Perianal disease can be present in up to 1/3 of CD. The presence of a noncentrally located fissure and/or multiple anal strictures or fistulae should raise suspicion for CD. Upper GI location is only present in around 5%-10% of CD. Extra-GI manifestations include erythema nodosum, pyoderma gangrenosum, large joint arthritis, uveitis, iritis, and episcleritis being present usually only if active intestinal disease is present.

Crohn disease is classified according to its age, location, and symptoms at patient presentation in a system that was first codified in 1998, the Vienna Classification. This was further modified in 2005 for the Montreal Classification, which is summarized in **Table 18.2**. While these are helpful to classify the disease phenotype, the activity and progression of the patient's CD are also important to consider when deciding on medical and surgical management. The 3rd European Congress on the Diagnosis and Management of Crohn Disease in 2016 helped define a common vernacular for evaluating CD. These definitions uniformly rely on the Crohn Disease Activity Index (CDAI), which is a validated symptom-based scoring elements summarized in **Table 18.3**. Defini-

TABLE 18.2 ■ Montreal Crohn Disease Classification

	Designation	Criteria
Age	A1	<16
	A2	17-40
	A3	>40
Location	L1	Ileal
	L2	Colonic
	L3	Ileocolonic
	L4	Upper GI
Behavior	B1	Nonstricturing, nonpenetrating
	B2	Structuring
	B3	Penetrating
	P	Perianal disease modifier

tions based on the above guidelines and with reference CDAI are summarized in **Table 18.4**.

Disease Types

Crohn disease can present in a variety of ways as the above symptoms indicate, and complicated disease has various definitions. However, nonpenetrating nonstricturing intraluminal disease has the least severe symptoms and presentation in general. This is characterized in the classic presentation of weight loss, right lower quadrant pain, and diarrhea. Transmural persistent inflammation that is usually present in the terminal ileum is the hallmark of active disease. A closeup of transmural inflammation is shown in **Figure 18.2**. Longitudinal studies have demonstrated that the patient with uncomplicated intraluminal CD who is in remission for 1 year has an 80% likelihood to continue remission for the next year. For those with active CD, there is a 70% chance they will have active disease in the next year. Only 13% of patients will be relapse free once in remission.

Persistent subclinical disease, while patients are in remission, is thought to lead to complicated CD processes such as strictures, phlegmon, abscesses, and fistulae, which are due to progressive bowel inflammation and damage. About 20% of patients will have complicated disease at initial presentation and risk of bowel damage increases overtime. Of patients with a history or presence of complicated CD, 20% will require admission per year and 14% will undergo a permanent ostomy. Complicated CD usually presents as one of two phenotypic types: *stricturing* or *penetrating*, with possibility of perianal involvement in both. *Stricturing* disease can lead to proximal dilation and obstruction, with nausea and vomiting as the initial presentation. Ileal stricture with proximal

TABLE 18.3 ■ Crohn Disease Activity Index (CDAI)

Variable	Qualification	Weight
Liquid stool count	Per week	×2
Abdominal pain (0-3)	Sum of score per day for week	×5
General wellbeing (0-4)	Sum of score per day for week	×7
Antidiarrheal use	Any in a week	×30
Extraintestinal complications	Per complication	×20
Arthralgias		
Skin lesion		
Iritis/uveitis		
Perianal disease		
Fistula		
Abscess		
Fever >37.8 °C		
Abdominal mass (0-5)	0 = none, 2 = equivocal, 5 = present	×10
Hematocrit		
Male	47-hematocrit = x	×6
Female	42-hematocrit = x	
Underweight	100 × (1-[ideal body weight/actual weight])	×1

TABLE 18.4 ■ Crohn Disease Activity and Progression Definitions

Term	Definition	CDIA
Active disease	High CDAI and/or CRP>10 mg/L	>220
Mild	No complicating features, mild symptoms and weight loss <10%	150-220
Moderate	Intermittent vomiting, >10% weight loss, abdominal mass or tenderness, no obstruction	220-450
Severe	Persistent symptoms despite treatment, complicated features such as obstruction, abscess, fistulizing disease, cachectic, low BMI	>450
Response	Decrease in CDIA from baseline	Baseline −70 points
Remission	Decrease to less than mild disease for 12 months or more	<150
Relapse	Flare of disease confirmed by imaging, laboratory, and endoscopic findings	>150 and +70 from baseline
Infrequent	<1 episode per year	
Frequent	>2 episodes per year	
Continuous	active CD without remission	
Recurrence	Return of mucosal lesions after resection, usually at the neo-terminal ileum or at a prior anastomosis	
Local disease	<30 cm of bowel involved	
Extensive disease	>100 cm of bowel involved	
Steroid dependent	Unable to reduce steroids <10 mg/day within 3 months of starting without suffering recurrent active disease	
Steroid refractory	Active disease despite at least 0.75 mg/kg/d prednisolone over 4 weeks	

small bowel dilation requiring resection is seen in **Figure 18.3**. **Penetrating** disease refers to fistulizing processes with overt enterocutaneous, enteroenteric, and enterocolic fistulae; however, it can also present as more of a phlegmon or interloop abscesses. Around 15% of patients will present with penetrating disease at the time of diagnosis. An example of a resected enteroenteric fistula with abscess is displayed in **Figure 18.4**.

Perianal disease can present as both stricturing and/or fistulizing disease and is present in 20%-30% of CD patients over their lifetime. Exam under anesthesia is usually required for suspected CD given the extent of disease and evaluation of painful anal fissures or fistulae. Any noncentrally located fissure should lead to suspicion for CD if not already confirmed. Multiple fistulas can present

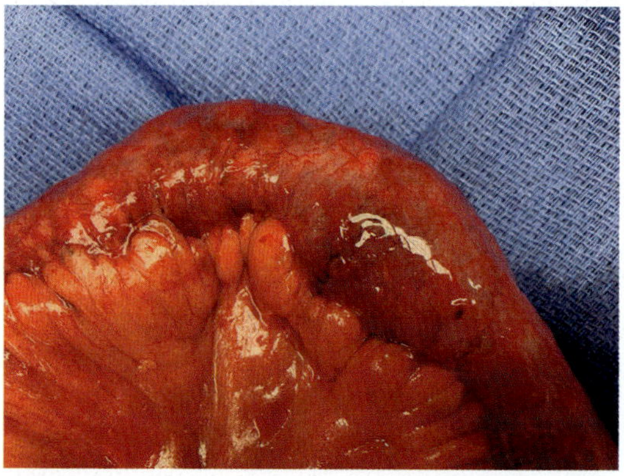

Figure 18.2 Transmural inflammation from nonstricturing nonpenetrating Crohn disease.

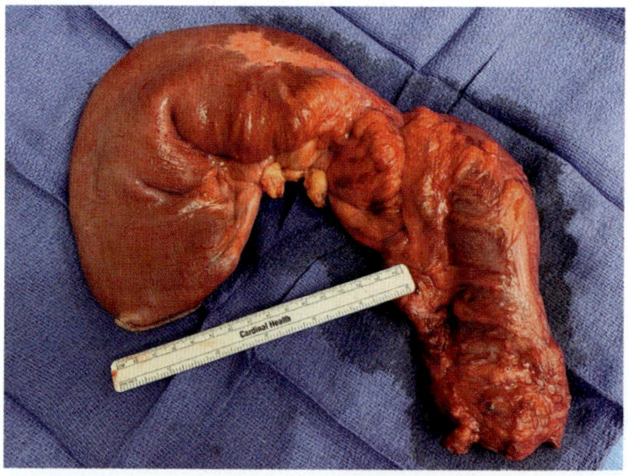

Figure 18.3 Ileocecectomy specimen: terminal ileal stricture with creeping fat with chronic massive small bowel dilatation proximally.

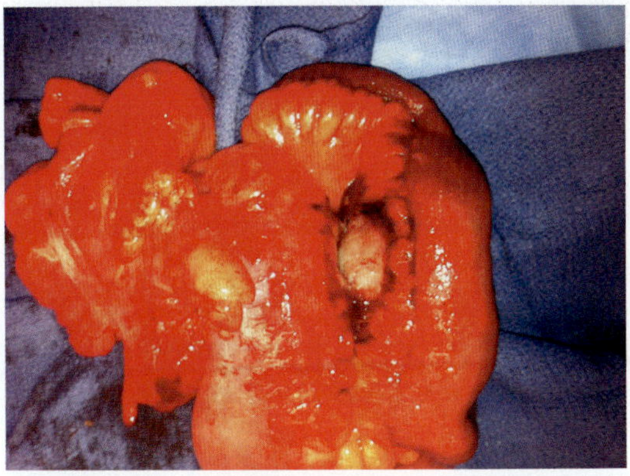

Figure 18.4 Enteroenteric fistula with interloop abscess in Crohn disease.

with a so-called "watering can" appearance and can require fecal diversion for the fistula to heal.

Evaluation, Diagnosis, and Management

Diagnosis of suspected CD should proceed first with evaluation of the patient's hemodynamic status, fluid balance, and evidence of infectious process. Determine first if sepsis is present, which requires emergent intervention. Placement of two intravenous lines and fluid resuscitation should begin in the likely setting of dehydration, weight loss, and malnutrition with emergency room presentation of CD. Patients with suspected or confirmed CD with a sepsis presentation should receive broad-spectrum antibiotics, IV fluid bolus of 40 mL/kg, with goal-directed therapy, early surgical consultation, evaluation for peritonitis, ICU admission, and cross-sectional imaging to evaluate for an intra-abdominal source of infection.

Next, laboratory evaluation should proceed with a complete blood count, basic metabolic panel, erythrocyte sedimentation rate (ESR), C-reactive protein (CRP), liver function tests, iron studies, vitamin B12, and vitamin D-3 levels. Complete blood count is likely to show an elevated white blood count in active disease and especially if sepsis is present, as well as an anemia of chronic disease. ESR and CRP are nonspecific but sensitive markers for IBD and CRP is usually >10 mg/dL in active CD. Hypoalbuminemia is also common, especially if recent weight loss is present. Fetal calprotectin has gained recent use for screening symptomatic patients with levels <40 μg/g suggestive of irritable bowel syndrome and levels between 50 and 250 μg/g diagnostic for CD. High postoperative levels are also indicative of early recurrence.

Radiologic evaluation with cross-sectional imaging is usually the next line of inquiry given the nonspecific constellation of findings that can exist with CD. Differential diagnosis can be broad including common processes such as acute appendicitis, adhesive small bowel disease, lymphadenitis, infectious or ischemic colitis, intra-abdominal abscess, typhlitis, intestinal neoplasm, to more rare occurrences including microscopic colitis, Behçet disease, intestinal angioedema, recurrent appendicitis, and other autoimmune intestinal syndromes. Initial evaluation with plain radiographs may have no specific findings in most CD cases but can show small bowel dilatation and air fluid levels in cases of stricture and obstruction. High-resolution computed tomography (CT) of the abdomen and pelvis, preferably with IV and oral contrast, is the most common radiologic modality for differentiating these processes on presentation. CT has a sensitivity of 95.2% in diagnosis of CD and can demonstrate transmural thickening and inflammation (**Figure 18.5**). Other signs that can be seen on CT are enlarged mesenteric lymph nodes, ulcerations, associated masses, abscesses, fistulae, and perforation with free air.

After diagnosis of CD is confirmed in the nonseptic patient, CT enterography or MRI enterography should be performed to evaluate the extent of disease and for complicating features such as fistulae and stenosis. When nonemergent and available, MRI enterography is preferred to limit the cumulative ionizing radiation exposure to the patient given the high burden of lifetime imaging required for patients with CD. Sensitivity and specificity of MRI enterography for CD diagnosis is 78% and 83%, respectively. Ultrasound can also

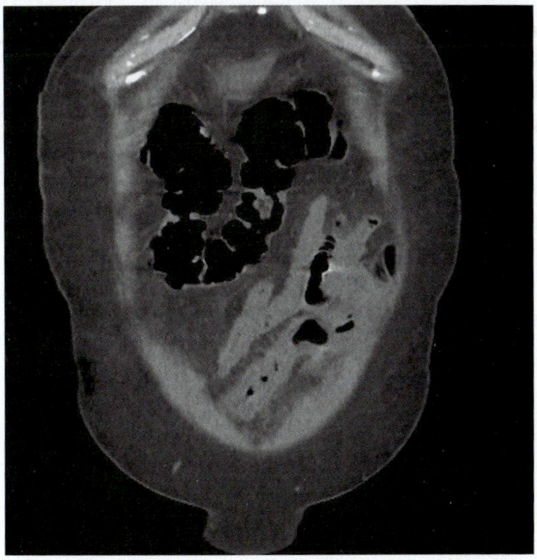

Figure 18.5 Diffuse transmural thickening of small bowel in active Crohn disease.

be a useful modality to evaluate CD complications and perform radiographic guided interventions. In some studies, the sensitivity of ultrasound for diagnosing small bowel CD was around 85%; however, this modality is user dependent and can be severely limited by obese body habitus.

The gold standard for CD diagnosis still relies on endoscopic evaluation and tissue biopsy with pathologic examination. Endoscopic evaluation typically includes a mechanical bowel preparation and colonoscopy with terminal ileoscopy and biopsy. The colon should be examined for any signs of fistula invasion and/or intrinsic ulceration to suggest colonic CD and to differentiate from UC. Typical patterns in the terminal ileum are segmental aphthoid ulceration and inflammation (**Figure 18.6**). With severe chronic inflammation, serpiginous ulcerations and nodular edematous mucosa give a "cobble-stoning" appearance to the mucosa, which is pathognomonic for CD (**Figure 18.7**). Biopsy results in CD typically show transmural chronic inflammation with lymphocyte and plasma cell invasion, with focal crypt irregularities, granulomas, and irregular villous architecture. At least two of these features are required for endoscopic biopsy confirmation of CD and typically three of these findings are used to evaluate surgical specimens for CD.

Upper endoscopic evaluation should be used to assess upper endoscopic manifestations of CD once diagnosed, especially if symptomatic with reflux, heartburn, dyspepsia, bloating, brash, regurgitation, or other upper GI symptoms. Capsule endoscopy can be a valuable adjunct to evaluate jejunal Crohn disease without evidence of terminal ileitis on imaging or endoscopy. However, the capsule itself is 11 × 26 mm and should not be used if there is any concern for stricturing

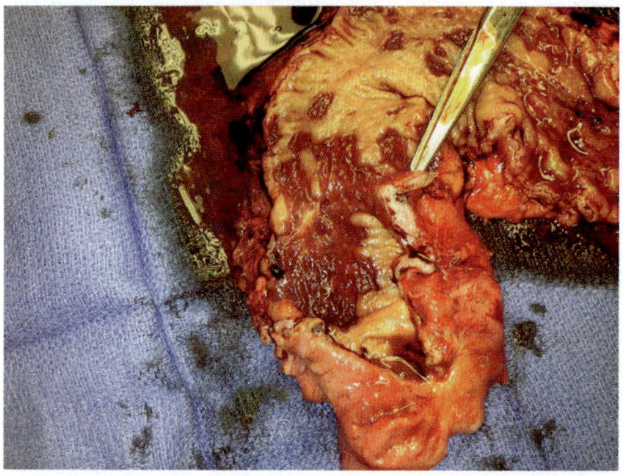

Figure 18.6 Terminal ileal specimen with severe segmental apthoid ulcers.

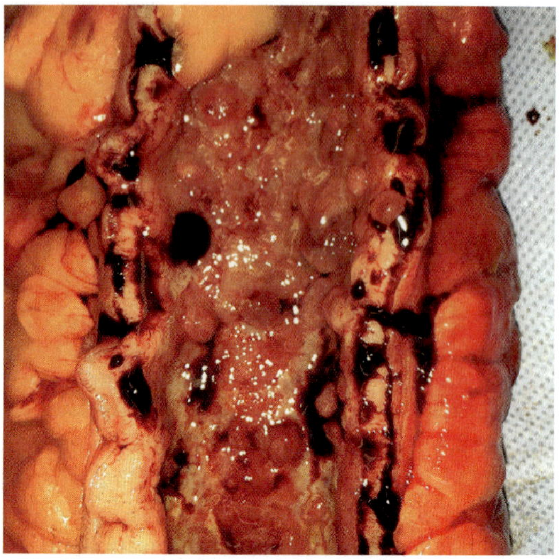

Figure 18.7 Terminal ileal specimen with "cobblestone" mucosa which is pathognomonic for Crohn disease.

disease on imaging or history as this can precipitate a complete small bowel obstruction and accelerate the need for emergent surgery and bowel resection. In addition to diagnosis, endoscopy is used to follow progression of disease and a typical goal after medical or surgical treatment is remission on endoscopic evaluation, not only by imaging or symptoms. Several indices have been created to score endoscopic severity on follow-up endoscopy and to guide medical management, such as the Crohn Disease Index of Severity, Simple Endoscopic Score for CD and Rutgeert Score; however, these are beyond the scope of this chapter.

Medical Management

After diagnosis of CD is confirmed, in nonemergent scenarios, medical therapy begins with an induction phase to achieve remission, followed by maintenance therapy to prevent recurrence. It is important as emergency surgeons to understand the medical regimen a patient has had previously to identify where in the natural history and spectrum of CD the patient currently is living prior to their emergency presentation. The classic treatment strategy was to "step-up" modalities in ever increasing tiers of medication complications and surgical invasiveness based on the patient's disease and tolerance of medications. However, a newer strategy is a "top-down" or "step-down" approach with more aggressive therapy up front designed to induce remission quickly and then titrate off medications based on side effects and patient tolerance. This second approach has improved remission rates and now a treat-to-target strategy of achieving endoscopic and histologic remission, in addition to symptom resolution, has become the goal therapy in CD. The process of eliminating CD that is symptom free but endoscopically active and, therefore, likely still creating chronic bowel damage has now become protocolized into more frequent endoscopic evaluation, biopsy, and radiologic monitoring. This approach results in slower progression to surgery and fewer hospital admissions.

Induction for mild to moderate disease first utilizes oral steroids to decrease intraluminal inflammation. Typically, budesonide is used for milder cases as it has a more localized mucosal effect and less systemic symptoms that the alternative, prednisone. However, budesonide has decreased response. Systemic steroids with methylprednisolone should be utilized for nonileal and severe disease. Around 30% of patients will become steroid dependent, which can predispose to long-term effects of oral steroids such as diabetes, osteopenia, avascular necrosis, hypertension, and infectious risk.

Many centers are now using biologics as induction therapy and several studies are examining their efficacy compared to steroids. In widespread practice, after steroid induction, typical maintenance regimens now generally utilize biologic agents such as monoclonal antibodies to TNF-α. These include infliximab, adalimumab, and certolizumab pegol. Infliximab also has the benefit of resulting in perianal fistula disease regression in a randomized control trial and is first-line therapy for severe perianal Crohn disease. However, long-term use of these medications can result in immunogenicity, where response to disease is lost over time. Side effects include decreased postsurgical healing, increased infection rates, and the possible risk of increased skin cancer risk. Given the increased use and tolerance of patients to these agents, surgery is no longer considered a contraindication when patients are on these regimens.

The mainstay of therapy for decades in Crohn disease has been oral immunosuppressants. Azathioprine and mercaptopurine are in the thiopurine class and have been used for CD, other immune disorders, and posttransplant immune suppression for decades but can cause increased rates of lymphoma, skin cancer, and other malignancies. Methotrexate is a similar folate-metabolism analog but is a teratogen and contraindicated in child-bearing age women. 5-Aminosalicylate has been found to be ineffective compared to other modern therapy, and in general is no longer used to treat CD.

Other Considerations

Unfortunately, in addition to malignancies associated with IBD treatment, the chronic inflammation associated with CD predisposes to several malignancies. CD patients with extensive colitis have 1.7 times the odds of colorectal cancer. Anal cancer is also increased when perianal CD is present at 0.2 per 1000 patient years. Intestinal lymphoma is similarly at absolute low rates at 0.5 per 1000 patient years but increased compared to the general population. Small bowel adenocarcinoma, however, is 20-30× more prevalence in CD patients with an incidence of 0.5 per 1000 patient years. Extraintestinal manifestations of malignancy are also more common in immune organs with higher rates of systemic lymphoma, splenic lymphoma, melanoma and other skin cancers, urinary tract cancer, and cervical cancer.

Given the increased need for operative intervention in these patients and need for repeated multiple bowel resections with refractory and recurrent disease, CD patients are at risk for developing short bowel syndrome (SBS). Patients with <180 cm are at risk of developing SBS, but the presence of an intact ileocecal valve can significantly decrease symptoms of malabsorption and fluid loss. Additionally, the more colon remaining after resection can help contribute to fluid resorption and decrease dehydration symptoms. Patients with high output ileostomy with SBS are at high risk for mortality and morbidity, require parental nutrition, and should be referred to a small bowel failure and intestinal transplant center.

While nutrition is vital to healing, CD patients usually present initially with malnutrition, possible weight loss, and protein loss. Ninety-two percent of CD patients have been found to malnourished and chronic GI inflammation leads to the loss of specific vitamins and micronutrients both due to increased consumption and malabsorption. B12, calcium, iron, vitamin D3, zinc, and folate have been reported at low levels in CD patients. Additionally, the fat-soluble ADEK vitamins are absorbed in the terminal ileum and with inflammation or resection can have decreased absorption of these, which can in turn affect liver synthetic function. Every effort should be taken to continue enteral nutrition and to replace these vitamins and minerals in CD patients unless perforation, obstruction, or abscess is present. Parental nutrition should be restricted to patients the above contraindications, short gut syndrome, and high output fistulas and ostomies.

Women of child-bearing age with CD should discuss with the physicians before attempting to become pregnant and stop methotrexate therapy 3-6 months beforehand. Most other IBD medications are considered safe for pregnancy. There is a small increased risk of preterm birth, stillbirth, and small gestational age with CD; however, fertility rates are not affected. There is some thought but little evidence that anti-TNF biologic medications should be stopped in the second trimester in patients in remission. Babies born to mothers on anti-TNF medications should not have live vaccines for 6 months following delivery.

Surgical Indications

In general, surgery is reserved for cases of CD that have failed medical therapy and the ongoing disease burden and symptoms are not amendable or refractory to further medical intervention. This can include problems that are chronic, subacute, acute, and emergent, all of which the General and Acute Care Surgeon can encounter in practice. Surgical resection is not usually a cure for patients and symptom recurrence occurs in 20%-40% of patients within a year of surgery. However, surgery is directed at relieving structural and anatomic disease burden that is the result of ongoing inflammation and bowel damage. Some principles of surgical management are to minimize bowel resection in the small intestine when possible and perform segmental resection of colonic disease when required. This is due to CD patients requiring a subsequent surgery within 5 years in 25% of patients and 35% in 10 years. Therefore, strict surveillance colonoscopies should be performed 6 months following surgery and continue every 1-3 years based on findings and patient symptoms. Additionally, high-risk patients should be started on postoperative anti-TNF medications to prevent early recurrence of disease. When resection and anastomosis is performed, do so in an isoperistaltic fashion as this is easier to traverse with an endoscope rather than the 180° turn of an antiperistaltic anastomosis. This is important due to the close endoscopic follow-up and surveillance required in CD.

Stricture

Obstruction is one of the classic and most common reasons for operative intervention in CD patients. Stricturing disease can cause an indolent small bowel obstruction with chronic dilatation of the proximal small bowel with small bowel fecalization and obstructive symptoms. Eventually this will convert to a complete obstruction and require surgical intervention. Obstruction due to stricture accounts for 25% of CD surgical indications. Patients first should be managed with nasogastric tube decompression, IV access, and rehydration with isotonic IV fluids. If no systemic signs of sepsis are present, obtain cross-sectional imaging to further characterize the location of the obstruction. Adhesive small bowel disease is equally as likely in patients with multiple prior abdominal surgeries. MRI enterography can be useful in these settings to determine if a stricture is present and additionally if the stricture appears to be fibrotic or inflammatory in nature. Fibrotic strictures will not respond to further medical therapy and induction and will require surgery, while a purely inflammatory obstruction may resolve with induction dose steroids and biologic agents.

Balloon endoscopic dilation is also a temporary option for fibrotic strictures with 90% reporting technical success and ~75% of patients experiencing relief. However, almost 75% require repeat dilation within 2 years and nearly 50% require surgery in that same time frame. Surgical management includes either bowel resection or stricturoplasty. An example of ileocecectomy for terminal ileum stricture with proximal dilation is shown in **Figure 18.8**. When short segments of stricture are present with no or little prior small bowel resection, segmental resection is appropriate. However, when there is extensive stricturing disease or multiple prior resections, stricturoplasty in a Heineke-Mikulicz fashion with longitudinal

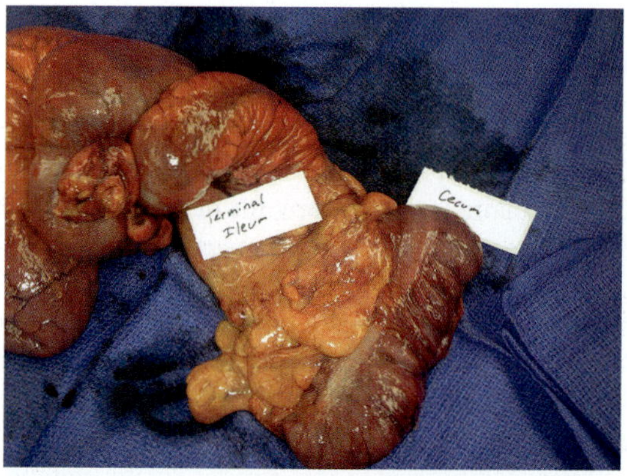

Figure 18.8 Terminal ileum and cecum segmental resection for stricture (screen left) and proximal small bowel obstruction.

opening and transverse closure is warranted. Strictures in the colon in the presence of known CD should raise suspicion for underlying malignancy, and oncologic resection should be performed in the emergency setting. If able to temporize the patient with colonic stenting and biopsies, this could lead to a segmental resection if no malignancy is confirmed by endoscopic biopsy.

Hemorrhage

Gastrointestinal hemorrhage can occur in UC and CD but is more common in UC due to pancolitis. In CD, GI hemorrhage is usually due to ulceration into the intestinal wall and erosion into an associated mesenteric vessel. The approach to management should proceed similar to other lower gastrointestinal bleeding with IV fluid resuscitation, type and cross, ICU admission, and endoscopic evaluation, followed by angiography if warranted. If upper GI bleeding is present, proceed with nasogastric tube placement and upper endoscopy. In one series up to 30% of patients with GI bleeding in CD was due to a bleeding duodenal ulcer. Total abdominal colectomy is an immediate viable option for hemorrhage control in UC. However, in CD, localizing the bleed is very important as it could occur anywhere along the GI tract. If angiography is not diagnostic, a tagged red blood cell scan may also be used. Additionally, capsule endoscopy can be utilized to localize slow persistent bleeds. The final option to localize the bleeding location is on table push endoscopy with hand-assisted telescoping of the small bowel over the upper endoscope from duodenum to terminal ileum to discover the source of bleeding. Once the bleeding is localized, surgical resection is recommended. Provocative angiography is not recommended for CD as the likely small bowel source will be difficult to identify surgically due to large amount of luminal bleeding and nonspecific location on angiography in the small bowel. If the location is in the colon, this may be a viable option in CD to localize to the right or left colon to preserve the contralateral colon for anastomosis. However, if unable to localize to any source, and patient is unstable, an end ileostomy and total abdominal colectomy can be performed if no ileal blood is found.

Perforation

Overt free perforation for CD is rare but classically accounted for 2%-3% of all surgical indications for CD. This is usually secondary to stricturing disease with proximal dilation of the small bowel and perforation of the proximal segment. A CT scan showing perforation with free air in a CD patient with distal ileal inflammatory stricture is shown in **Figure 18.9.** Surgical management should include initiation of broad-spectrum antibiotic coverage, IV fluid resuscitation, and prompt surgical exploration. Typically, resection of the perforation site and any distal stricture is indicated, with or without ileocecectomy if in the terminal ileum and cecum. If in the distal ileum, end ileostomy with or without mucus fistula should be considered for certain patient populations. Large amount of contamination, abscess, complex fistulae, malnourished or cachectic patients, multiple prior resections, or who are critically ill should be considered for ileostomy and possibly for damage control surgery. These are relative indications, and if not present or the patient is otherwise healthy, then primary anastomosis should be considered with or without fecal diversion with loop ileostomy.

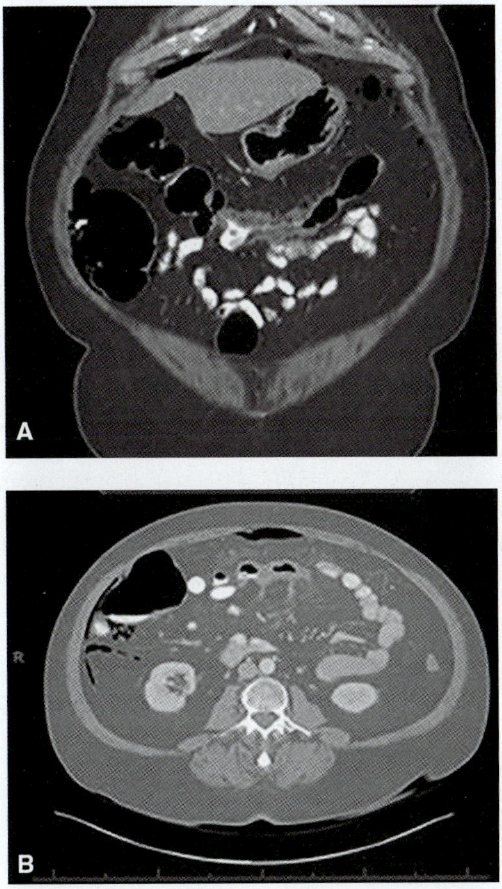

Figure 18.9 Terminal ileal inflammatory stricture with proximal small bowel dilation (**A**) and perforation with free air (**B**).

Abscess and Phlegmon

Intra-abdominal abscess accounts for 10%-25% of indications for CD surgical management and characterized by acute on chronic transmural inflammation and microperforation. This develops into an abscess or phlegmon over time and is usually located in the right lower quadrant given the predominance of terminal ileal disease. Similar to other emergent indications, evaluation and initial management should be early broad-spectrum antibiotics, IV fluid resuscitation, cross-sectional imaging, and evaluation for signs and symptoms of sepsis. However, if the patient is stable, nonsurgical management can be appropriate and should be attempted, as radiologic intervention can temporarily be successful in more than 90% of cases. Up to 75% of patients will go on to require bowel resection for the source of the abscess. If there is an abscess located at the base of the mesentery or covered by multiple loops of small bowel, such as **Figure 18.10**, laparoscopic or open washout and drain placement can be required to address the infectious source. Small bowel resection of the source of the abscess and anastomosis can be performed if inflammatory adhesions are not too dense and would not require long length of bowel resection at that time. If this is not safe to perform, planned second operation with bowel resection can be performed once the inflammation has subsided.

Phlegmon associated with CD can be associated with abscess and/or fistula of the small bowel and present with overt signs of sepsis and/or obstruction. An example of a heterogenous phlegmon with forming abscess is shown in **Figure 18.11**. Multiple enteroenteric fistulas and intervening abscess can create a "spider web" of inflammation and adhesions between the small bowel loops that unfortunately may require a long segment of bowel resection in the acute setting if presenting with obstruction, abscess, or sepsis. If the patient presents subacutely and is able to start induction therapy and biologic anti-TNF therapy, this should be pursued to limit the amount of bowel needed to be resected. An intraoperative example of a subacute phlegmon is seen in **Figure 18.12**.

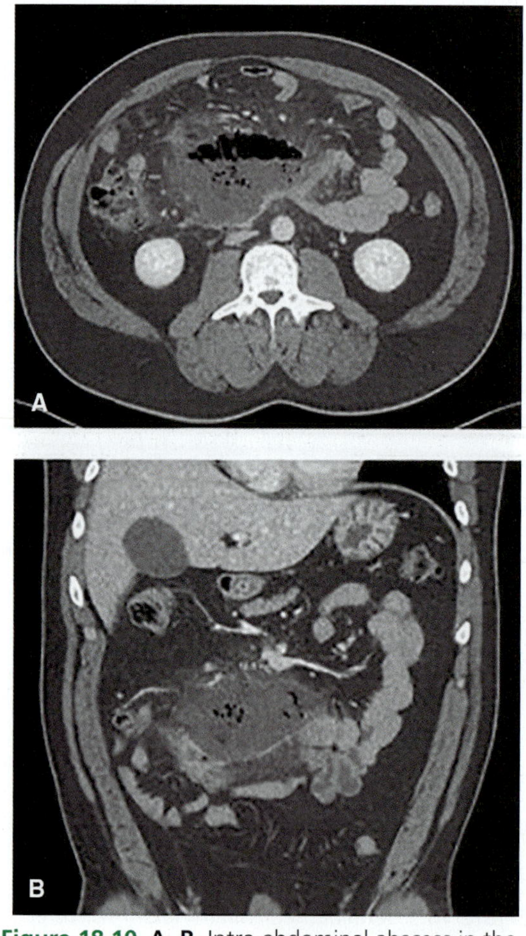

Figure 18.10 A, B. Intra-abdominal abscess in the mid-abdomen not amendable to percutaneous drainage.

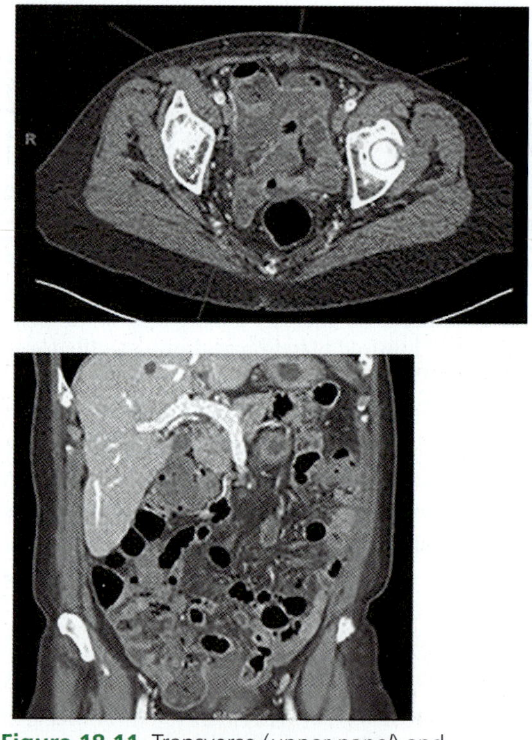

Figure 18.11 Transverse (*upper panel*) and coronal (*lower panel*) CT abdomen view of pelvic phlegmon.

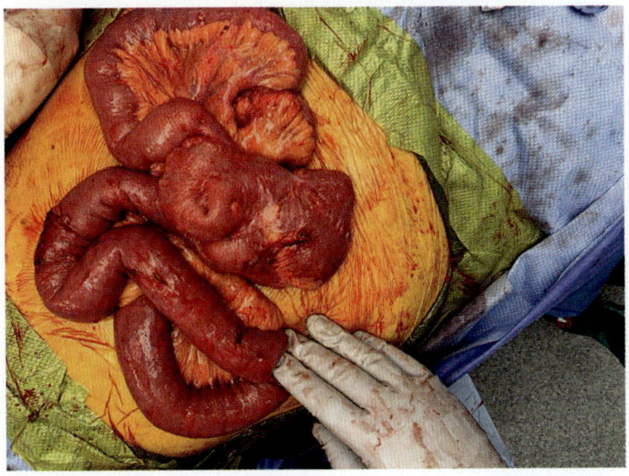

Figure 18.12 Small bowel phlegmon at time of surgical resection with multiple interloop adhesions, woody inflammation, and purulence.

Enteric Fistula

Penetrating disease in CD refers to the creation of fistula that can occur into any other organ, the skin, the gyneco-urologic system, peritoneum (abscess), and in CD also has a predilection for forming connections to other sites in the GI tract such as distal small bowel, colon, and even stomach. A fistula to the skin or another hollow organ itself usually presents subacutely without signs of significant sepsis unless an cystoenteric fistula causes a urinary tract infection. However, these can bring create distress and symptoms to the patient, which can lead to emergency room presentation. High volume stool can be an indicator of a coloenteric fistula. Enterocutaneous fistulas can begin as erythema, cellulitis, and small draining sinuses before overt feculent output. In general, medical induction therapy should begin along with nutritional therapy and daily output evaluation of the fistula. In small studies, 28%-67% of patients with EC fistulas had a decrease in output with anti-TNF therapy, but many progress to require resection. Imaging with a fistologram to evaluate the location of the fistula in the GI tract and any other associated organs should be performed. High output fistulas (more than 300 mL/day) and proximal fistulas are less likely to heal on their own. Low output fistulas and distal fistulas are more likely to heal spontaneously (30%) and the addition of octreotide and bowel rest with parental nutrition can increase this up to 57%. If medical management fails, planned resection with nutritional optimization and prehabilitation of the patient should be performed, followed by resection of the site of CD fistula origination and closure of site at the affected organ.

ULCERATIVE COLITIS

CASE PRESENTATION

A 20-year-old male presents with bloody diarrhea occurring over the last 2 weeks. He denies any fevers or chills but reports feeling weak and fatigued. He has stopped eating because of the large amount of diarrhea as a way to control the number of bowel movements. He came into the ER because the diarrhea did not improve despite attempts to use multiple over the counter medications. He has no sick contacts and has not changed his diet. He reports a family history of colitis in many uncles and his father died early from colon cancer. He also reports he remembers his father always having diarrhea. He has recently stopped smoking and started NSAID for knee injury while playing soccer. He takes no other medications and has no allergies. On exam, he appears diaphoretic and pale. His heart rate is 110/min, respiratory rate 16/min, and blood pressure is 90/40 mm Hg. He is alert and orientated to person place and time. His heart and lung exam are normal. He has some abdominal pain but is not peritoneal. Rectal exam shows bloody stool and no hemorrhoids. He has an elevated white blood cell count to 14 000/mm^3 and his hemoglobin is 8 g/dL (last check for a physical 10 months ago it was 14 g/dL). A thromboelastogram revealed normal coagulation. A CT scan with IV contrast reveals diffuse inflammation of the colon with no active extravasation.

Question: *What is the next step in treatment?*

Answer: *Twenty percent of patients with ulcerative colitis will experience a similar severe flare. This flare requires hospitalization to first stabilize his hemodynamics. Defined by his heart rate and blood pressure, the patient is between class 2 and 3 hemorrhagic shock from bloody diarrhea. Start with IV fluid resuscitation and correction of electrolytes. Blood transfusion could be indicated if his hemodynamics do not improve with fluid resuscitation. His thromboelastogram was normal but hemoglobin should be followed serially. Due to his lack of oral intake, nutritional support with TPN may be needed. Despite the history* *(family with colitis, age, recent smoking cessation, and increased NSAID use), a bacterial or viral infection must be ruled out. It is especially important to rule out Clostridium difficile or CMV infection. If a bacterial or viral infection is found, treatment must be started, but ulcerative colitis remains the most likely diagnosis. Once the bleeding has subsided and blood work is stable, thromboprophylaxis can be started. If the symptoms persist, intravenous corticosteroids are the first-line treatment for ulcerative colitis in patients in this age range. Due to his age, it is hoped that bleeding will be self-limited and not require an emergency colectomy. If the IV steroids are not effective within 3-5 days of hospital admission, treatment may need to progress to more aggressive immune therapies (infliximab). If all medical therapies (to be described later) fail, the patient may need a colectomy as a lifesaving intervention. If the patient does respond to treatment, a colonoscopy with biopsies is needed to confirm diagnosis (full workup described later in the chapter).*

Pathophysiology

Immune

The exact mechanism of ulcerative colitis is not known. However, inflammation of the intestinal mucosa is the hallmark. This inflammation is present in the rectum and usually proceeds contiguously toward the cecum (although there are cases of involvement of the rectum with extension proximally, with some cecal inflammation). The impact of the immune system on ulcerative colitis can be characterized as an initial antigen presentation that results in a dysregulated immune response and subsequent recruitment of additional immune cells resulting in a hyperinflammatory environment. Patients with ulcerative colitis appear to have increased dendritic cells in the intestinal epithelium, and it is through these cells that antigens are presented to the cells of the adaptive arm and lead to the above described dysregulated immune response. Dendritic cells are also responsible for homeostasis with the intestinal microbial populations through TLR. Again, in ulcerative colitis, the type of TLR is altered (more TLR4 in ulcerative colitis). The signals from the dendritic cells in ulcerative colitis to the cells of the adaptive immune system (B and T cells) are more a Th2 response with an emphasis on natural killer T cells. This altered cellular response leads to many changes in cytokines. TNF-alpha is elevated in patients with ulcerative colitis and is the target of treatment. Genome wide association studies have also identified immune system genes as targets in ulcerative colitis; notably HLA and interleukin 23 and 10. As will be described later, the immune system is the target of the majority of medical intervention for ulcerative colitis. Despite extensive immune evidence, it also appears that the microbial population of the colon influences the development of ulcerative colitis.

Microbial

Two interventions impact the intestinal microbial populations: probiotics and fecal microbiota transplantation (FMT). Both treatments attempt to promote a population of symbiotic bacteria (*Bacteroides*, *Bifidobacterium*, and *Peptococcus*). With these bacteria as the dominant population, other bacteria such as *Enterococcus* and *Enterobacter* remain in a steady state. The interplay between these five species and the epithelial and dendritic cells promotes a healthy intestinal barrier. In some patients with ulcerative colitis, common bacteria such as *Akkermansia muciniphila* are reduced or the overall diversity of the population is decreased. In many studies, the bacteria are treated as passive bystanders, changing in population when an opportunity arises. However, bacteria are complex organisms that can sense the environment may be changing due to signals from the immune system or dietary factors. Although the impact of the microbial populations is important, the diet of the patient can influence that population as well as the immune response.

Diet

A patient's diet has been associated with ulcerative colitis, as evidenced by the increased incidence in North American and European countries, and the increase in incidence when someone moves from an area of low prevalence to an area of higher prevalence. Despite the epidemiological evidence that diet is important, studies to identify trigger foods to avoid or diets that promote remission have mixed results. Dairy, particularly milk, has been studied as a food to eliminate to prevent relapses; however, there are not clear statistical differences in randomized trials. Elimination of carrageenan (extract from seaweed used as a thickener) has shown success in some small trials. Elimination of sugars and sugared beverages and the FODMAP diet also has some modest results. A novel personalized medicine technique is to eliminate foods that the patient has IgG antibodies to in the blood. Despite much research on diet, there does not appear to be a single food that can be eliminated, but rather the focus must remain on the interplay of the host immune system, the microbial environment, and the nutrients that interact with both.

The combination of these factors, immune, microbial, and dietary, result in reduced mucin production and the destruction of the epithelial barrier. This then results in continued inflammation and more subsequent damage and eventual clinical presentation.

Presentation

Ulcerative colitis is typically identified in patients in North America and Europe, although its incidence in other areas in increasing. Ulcerative colitis is also more common than Crohn disease. Most patients have their first symptoms in their 20s, but some patients do not have symptoms until their 50s. Many factors put patients at risk for ulcerative colitis. A family history of ulcerative colitis, particularly among first-degree relatives, increases risk and numerous genes are associated with ulcerative colitis (many related to the immune system). Taking antibiotics and nonsteroidal anti-inflammatory drugs are associated with development of ulcerative colitis. In addition, infection with some bacteria (*Campylobacter* and *Salmonella*) is noted around the development of ulcerative colitis. These associations are all dependent upon self-report, but many of these observations are repeated. Interestingly, cigarette smoking appears protective against ulcerative colitis. As in the clinical case, smoking cessation can sometimes lead to ulcerative colitis symptoms; however, cigarette smoking is never suggested as a treatment of ulcerative colitis.

Bloody diarrhea is the classic presenting symptom reported by the patient early in the course of ulcerative colitis. Other symptoms include abdominal pain and urgency to stool. Manifestations of ulcerative colitis outside the colon are well known. Skin lesions associated with the immune response, erythema nodosum, and pyoderma gangrenosum are present in some patients. Arthritis is also seen. Primary sclerosing cholangitis can be seen with ulcerative colitis and this portends increased hepatobiliary cancer risk.

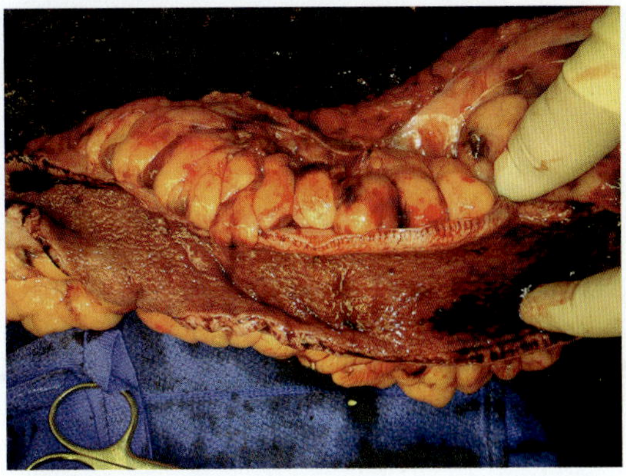

Figure 18.13 Ulcerative colitis with burned out mucosa.

Diagnosis

The definitive diagnosis of ulcerative colitis is only confirmed by histological evaluation of colonic samples from endoscopic biopsies. Classic findings on endoscopy are ascending areas of mucosal ulcerations with burned out mucosa in terminal UC (**Figure 18.13**). Other causes of diarrhea (infectious and noninfectious) must be excluded by microbial testing or metabolic assessment prior to endoscopic evaluation. In ulcerative colitis, the extent of inflammation should be assessed, and it typically starts at the rectum. The extent of inflammation is directly correlated to degree of illness. In addition, local disease can be treated with topical medications (via enema) rather than systemic formulations. Once a diagnosis is made, the severity of the disease is based upon the number of stools and systemic inflammation (ie, systemic inflammatory response syndrome criteria: fever, tachypnea, tachycardia, leukocytosis).

Medical Treatment

Treatment is best defined by the severity of the disease when treatment is started and can be categorized by the target of the intervention (see **Table 18.5**). In the clinical case, the patient had severe disease on presentation. However, medical treatment is the primary option for mild and moderate disease. In addition, treatments are designed to treat active disease or maintain remission (see **Table 18.5**).

Mesalamine (a 5-aminosalicylate) is the typical treatment for mild and moderate ulcerative colitis. There is an oral formulation, which is standard, but topical (via suppository) is the best option for inflammation in the rectum alone. More diffuse disease should be treated with oral formulations

TABLE 18.5 ■ Target of Therapeutic Intervention

Immune System	Colon Microbial Population	Diet
5-Aminosalicylate corticosteroids Thiopurines Anti-TNF Calcineurin Inhibitors Adhesion molecule inhibitor	Stool transplant Probiotics	Carrageenan free diet

and the combination of both (oral and topical) has the best effectiveness for remission.

Corticosteroids are typically given during an acute episode requiring hospitalization due to severe colitis. Steroids can also be given in an outpatient setting to induce remission. Steroids can be given systemically or locally via enema if disease is limited (per endoscopic evaluation). Steroids are not typically given as maintenance treatment. If steroids do not control symptoms (30% of cases), further immune targeting medications are given.

If steroids are successful, treatment shifts to thiopurine as a medication for continued remission. If this medication is used, testing is required to understand the patient's metabolism of the drug and must be avoided in some patients. Sometimes infliximab, adalimumab, or golimumab (all anti-TNF medications) are used in combination with thiopurine. Anti-TNF medications are also sometimes used when steroids fail to induce remission. Anti-TNF may lead to increased risk of lymphoma, complicating medication selection. Cyclosporine (a calcineurin inhibitor) is no longer commonly used for ulcerative colitis, except in hospitalized patients who fail steroids. However, recent data suggest that anti-TNF treatment is equivocal, with the benefit of continuing the anti-TNF treatment as a maintenance therapy. Vedolizumab is an adhesion molecule inhibitor that blocks white blood cell migration in the gut. This drug has been used in patients unresponsive to anti-TNF treatment. It is also important to remember the impact of biosimilars as it relates to these immune modulating medications and the long-term impact of treatment.

Stool transplant is a recent treatment strategy for many colonic disease processes. The goal is to normalize the intestinal microbiota and return the immune interactions to a steadier state. Donors typically come from friends/relatives in the same home or healthy controls. Clinical response rate to transplant is around 30% and there are suggestions that multiple transplants are more effective than a single one. More success from this modality may come from transplants from healthy donors rather than friends/relatives as it may change the flora, but more research is needed to prove this.

Probiotics attempt to restore balance to the microbial environment of the colon. This is done by first maintaining the delicate balance of microbes at the epithelial border. With steady state of bacteria, there is enhanced mucosal barrier function and the interplay of the immune system and the microbes is constant. Probiotics have been shown to increase remission in patients with ulcerative colitis.

Dietary management of ulcerative colitis has been extensively studied. Although numerous diets (cow milk/dairy elimination, high fiber, and specific anti-inflammatory diets) have been attempted, only a carrageenan-free diet has reported significant benefits in well-designed and controlled trials. Carrageenan is derived from red seaweed and is a common thickener in processed foods.

Patients with ulcerative colitis (and Crohn disease) are at increased risk for colorectal cancers. Patients should be screened with a colonoscopy 8-10 years after initial diagnosis and then every 1-2 years. If cancer or dysplasia is identified, surgical management is necessary. A daily inpatient assessment and medical management plan for UC is presented in **Table 18.6.**

Surgical Management

Urgent surgery is indicated in patients with ulcerative colitis for reasons similar to other GI processes: perforation, bleeding that is not controlled, and systemic illness such as that due to toxic megacolon. These three emergency presentations are described in further detail later in this chapter. In the emergency setting, a total colectomy with blind-ended sigmoid loop and an end ileostomy is the operation of choice. Reconstruction of the GI tract should be performed when the patient recovers from the initial surgery and the overall inflammatory burden is reduced.

Patients may also progress to operation if there is failure of medical therapy or dysplasia/cancer

TABLE 18.6 ■ UC Management Protocol

Day	Tests/Goals	Treatments
Daily assessment and consideration for patients with acute ulcerative colitis		
Day 1	• Complete set of labs (chem7, CBC, prealbumin, ESR, CRP, cholesterol) • PPD • *C diff* testing • Stool culture • CMV PCR • Abdominal film • Begin diary of stool/blood/urgency • GI medicine consult • Surgery consult if signs of megacolon or patient has been on steroid therapy	• IV steroids • Pharmacological DVT prophylaxis • IV fluids • NPO
Day 2	• Labs (chem7, CBC, CRP) • Flexible sigmoidoscopy • Diary of stool/blood/urgency	• IV steroids • Pharmacological DVT prophylaxis • IV fluids • NPO
Day 3	• Labs (chem7, CBC, ESR, CRP) • Flexible sigmoidoscopy • Diary of stool/blood/urgency • Biopsy results • PPD results • Calculate predictive scores • Abdominal film • Consult surgery	• IV steroids • Pharmacological DVT prophylaxis • IV fluids • Clear diet if hungry
Day 4	• Labs • Continue diary	• IV steroids • Pharmacological DVT prophylaxis • IV fluids • Soft diet if hungry
Day 5	• Labs • Calculate predictive scores • Abdominal film if not improving	• IV steroids • Not improving or not eating, then NPO • If not improving then decide on medical salvage versus surgery • If improving then advance diet and consider oral steroid taper

of the colon. The patients who fail medical therapy may need an urgent operation if they no longer respond to steroids. In the setting of an urgent operation, the procedure should be similar to that of an emergency (colectomy with end ileostomy) and allow for reconstruction at a later time. In a patient where elective surgery is planned (failure of medical management or cancer/dysplasia), the standard operation is proctocolectomy with ileal pouch and anal anastomosis with diverting loop ileostomy to prevent pelvic sepsis. Once the initial reconstruction is healed, a second operation reverses the loop ileostomy. After this procedure, the patient can expect to have 4-6 bowel movements a day and 1-2 each night. Medications and dietary habits can control this number.

Emergency Presentation

Toxic colitis occurs when the inflammatory burden in the colon leads to systemic illness. This can be due to a bacterial infection (*C difficile*) or a combination of host and bacterial inflammation interplay as seen in ulcerative colitis. In ulcerative colitis, the uncontrolled inflammation leads to barrier dysfunction and toxins from the colon lumen (from pathogens) can enter the blood stream. In addition, cytokine signals from the host immune cells in the colon (dendritic cells and others attracted to the site) promote further inflammation and impact the clinical status. The patient reports a week's long history of worsening condition. On presentation, the patient exhibits multiple signs of systemic inflammation (tachycardia, tachypnea, blood pressure changes). The patient will also have derangements in laboratory values such as elevated white blood count, hemoconcentration, and electrolyte abnormalities. If the inflammation is severe, it can lead to toxic megacolon. The diameter of the colon enlarges, and blood flow is reduced. In addition, the risk of perforation increases. An upright chest x-ray or abdominal film could show the classic thumb printing signifying edema of the bowel wall due to inflammation. A CT scan would also show inflammation and edema. If the patient is hemodynamically unstable due to the colitis, then an emergency damage control operation is warranted. In the emergency setting, perform a total colectomy with end ileostomy. The goal of the operation is to remove the colon that is causing the uncontrolled inflammation. An image of megacolon with resection is seen in **Figure 18.14**. Reconstruction can be accomplished at a later time. If the patient responds to fluid resuscitation, steroids can be attempted. Failure of steroids would result in a similar urgent operation.

Hemorrhage as seen by bloody diarrhea occurs in almost all patients with ulcerative colitis. Despite ubiquitous bloody diarrhea in this population, continued bleeding accounts for only a small portion of emergent colectomies for ulcerative colitis. If the patient presents in hemorrhagic shock (as in the case presentation), initial resuscitation is imperative. An urgent operation is needed if this treatment fails. In the urgent setting, perform a subtotal colectomy and monitor the rectal stump for continued bleeding. If possible, prior to operation, sigmoidoscopy can identify significant rectal bleeding and push the operation to a colectomy with proctectomy. A bleeding colon and associated mucosa requiring total colectomy are shown in **Figure 18.15**.

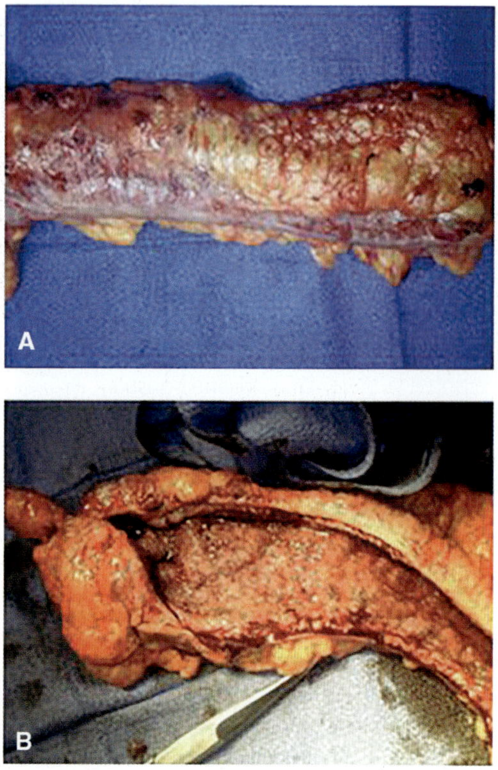

Figure 18.15 A, B. Ulcerative colitis requiring resection for bleeding, with characteristic mucosal ulcerations.

Perforation is a complication of ulcerative colitis as the inflammatory state results in weakened barrier defenses of the colonic epithelium. In addition, toxic megacolon can result in perforation as the colon enlarges and the blood supply is compromised. Perforated cancer can also occur in ulcerative colitis. It is paramount to note that the mortality from perforation in a patient with ulcerative colitis is significantly higher than patients who do not have a perforation. For this reason,

Figure 18.14 Toxic megacolon causing sepsis on laparotomy (*left panel*) and resection (*right panel*).

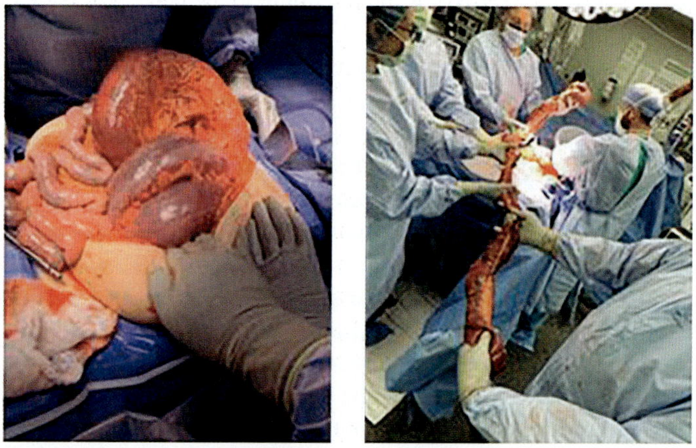

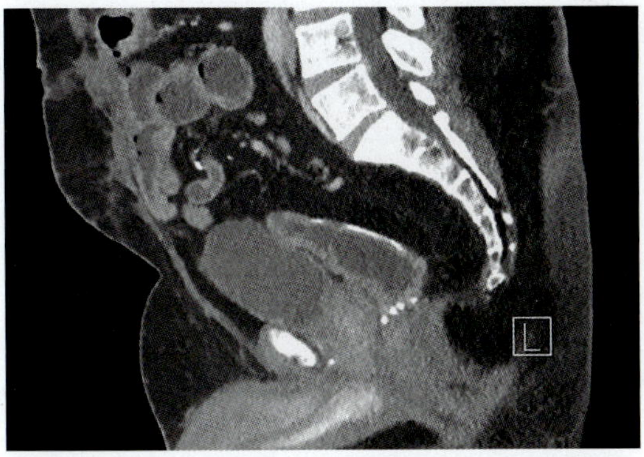

Figure 18.16 Ulcerative colitis patient status post total abdominal colectomy and J-pouch ileal anal anastomosis returns with pouchitis seen on CT.

any sign of perforation (free air on x-ray, peritonitis) should initiate emergency colectomy. In addition, since patients are sometimes on steroids or immune modulating therapies, peritoneal findings may not be present and free air on imaging may be the only definitive finding. With perforation, proceed with colectomy with end ileostomy. After an emergency colectomy, reconstruction with an ileal pouch and anal anastomosis is delayed until the inflammation in the abdomen is resolved. After ileal pouch and anal anastomosis, evaluation for recurrence at the anal cuff is important as this can cause recurrent rectal bleeding if UC tissue is left at the anal margin. More commonly bacterial, overgrowth and pouchitis can present with abdominal pain, urgency, and signs of systemic illness, as is seen in **Figure 18.16**.

DIVERTICULAR DISEASE

Diverticula can occur anywhere in the gastrointestinal tract. Diverticula are either acquired as in the small bowel or colon or congenital as in Meckel diverticulum. Congenital diverticula are true diverticula, incorporating all layers of the intestine. Acquired diverticula are "false" diverticula, containing only mucosa and submucosa.

Small Bowel Diverticuli

Diverticula of the small bowel are relatively rare; <4% of small bowel diverticula will cause clinically significant symptoms in a patient's lifetime.

Duodenal diverticula account for the vast majority of diverticula in the small bowel (50%-75%) but <1% require treatment. These usually occur on the mesenteric side of the duodenum and within 2 cm of the ampulla. Duodenal diverticula are generally asymptomatic and should not be treated. However, if causing hemorrhage, perforation, biliary or pancreatic obstruction, operative intervention with diverticulectomy is indicated.

GI bleeding from a duodenal diverticulum should be evaluated endoscopically whenever possible. Upper endoscopy can both diagnose and often treat bleeding from the diverticulum. Angiography/embolization may also treat the bleeding. Massive hemorrhage unable to be controlled by endoscopy or angioembolization will require operation. Hemorrhage may be controlled by performing a lateral duodenotomy and oversewing the vessel.

Consider CT or an upper GI study to diagnose a duodenal diverticulum (when diverticulitis or perforation is not suspected). Endoscopic retrograde cholangiopancreatography (ERCP) can be both diagnostic and therapeutic in evaluation of the biliopancreatic tree.

Perforation is most often limited with focal abscess formation. This can often be treated by resuscitation, intravenous antibiotics, and bowel rest. Exploration with resection and closure is reserved patients with uncontrolled abdominal sepsis. The operation for a duodenal diverticulum can be an open, laparoscopic, or robotic procedure. The key steps include kocherization of the duodenum, opening the antimesenteric border, cannulation of the ampulla to prevent stenosis, inversion and diverticulectomy, and primary closure with or without buttress from omentum, falciform ligament, or jejunal serosal patch. Roux-en-Y hepaticojejunostomy can be required if the ampulla is involved or injured. If perforation is present with significant retroperitoneal inflammation and contamination, external drainage with efferent and afferent duodenostomy tubes, peritoneal drains, and distal feeding access is indicated. Duodenal pyloric exclusion with gastrostomy tube or diversion with gastrojejunostomy can also facilitate healing of this area in combination with triple tube therapy. Gastrojejunostomy should also be performed if after diverticulectomy and closure there is significant duodenal stenosis operatively or on endoscopy.

Jejunal/ileal diverticula are less common, present in only 2% of the population but more likely to be symptomatic. Up to 5% present with diverticula throughout the small bowel, with 80% isolated to the jejunum, and 15% in the ileum alone. Most of these diverticula are diagnosed incidentally at the time of surgery for other indications. However, symptoms can include abdominal pain, steatorrhea, chronic anemia, and rarely pneumatosis and free air with microperforation. These processes are related to bacterial overgrowth. After diagnosis with small bowel contrasted study (fluoroscopy or CT enterography), the mainstay of therapy is antibiotic suppression with metronidazole and a beta-lactam antibiotic (Augmentin, cefpodoxime). If medical therapy fails or perforation is present, surgical intervention with segmental resection is indicated.

Meckel Diverticulum

An isolated true diverticulum of the small bowel on the antimesenteric border can be an incidental or pathologic finding in an adult. Meckel diverticulum accounts for 25% of all small bowel diverticula and can contain embryonic heterotopic mucosa for pancreas or stomach. Meckel diverticula occur in 2% of the population, are usually 2 in. long, and are found within 2 ft of the ileocecal valve. The heterotopic mucosa can lead to downstream ulceration and lower gastrointestinal bleeding. A Meckel scan with tagged radionucleotides for heterotopic mucosa can identify the diverticulum in cases of occult GI hemorrhage. Most presentations of symptomatic Meckel diverticula are abdominal pain related to acute diverticulitis or obstruction and can be confused with other etiologies. Obstruction may occur from intussusception with the diverticulum acting as a lead point, volvulus around the fibrous band attaching the diverticulum to the umbilicus, stricture secondary to chronic diverticulitis, or entrapment of intestine by a mesodiverticular band.

A Meckel diverticulum may be found at the time of surgery for other indications and is classically confused for appendicitis. Therefore, incidental appendectomy is recommended when diverticulectomy is performed or in cases of incidentally found Meckel diverticulum to avoid future appendicitis. If found at the time of surgery and there is evidence of obstruction or diverticulitis, diverticulectomy or segmental resection is warranted. Resection may be preferred if there is a wide base or significant inflammation of the adjacent bowel or the cause of a GI bleed. In the later case, resection should occur just distal enough on the small bowel segment to resect the downstream ulceration. An image of a wide mouthed Meckel diverticulum prior to segmental resection is shown in **Figure 18.17**. Incidental diverticulectomy is not indicated in adults if found at the time of surgery for other nonemergent indications.

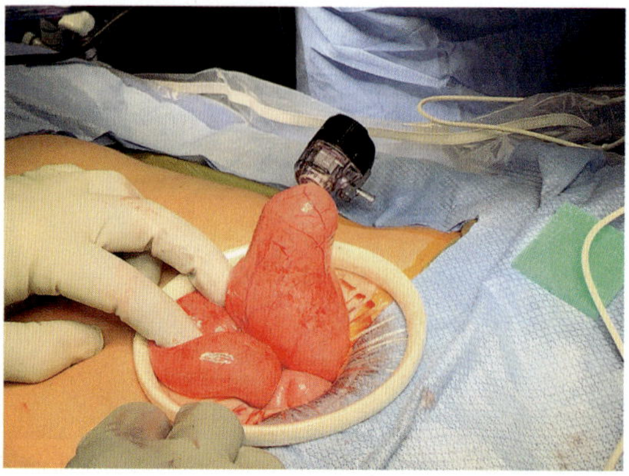

Figure 18.17 A wide mouthed Meckel diverticulum causing small bowel obstruction in patient with no prior surgery due to anchor like effect of intraluminal contents into the pelvis.

Colonic Diverticular Disease

Colonic diverticula are acquired false diverticula that tend to occur at areas of weakness where the vasa recta enter the muscularis. In western countries, colonic diverticula most commonly occur in the sigmoid colon (~75%); in Asian countries, more commonly in the right colon. The incidence of diverticulosis increases with age, with two-thirds of adults over 85 with diverticulosis. Only 4%-20% of patients with diverticulosis ever become symptomatic. Furthermore, the vast majority of patients with acute diverticulitis can be managed nonoperatively.

Clinical Manifestations

Patients who have acute uncomplicated diverticulitis typically present with a triad of left lower quadrant pain, fever, and leukocytosis. They may also have symptoms of nausea, vomiting, dysuria, or constipation.

Complicated diverticulitis may present with the previously mentioned triad as well as diffuse abdominal tenderness and rebound tenderness. Progression of this process may present with septic shock secondary to gross contamination of the abdomen. Complicated diverticulitis may also present with symptoms of large bowel obstruction (due to stricture or abscess), pneumaturia or urinary tract infection (colovesicular fistula), fecal drainage from the vagina (colovaginal fistula), retroperitoneal abscess, or as a necrotizing soft tissue infection.

Diagnostic Evaluation

Clinical exam alone in diagnosis of acute diverticulitis is incorrect in >50%. This is especially

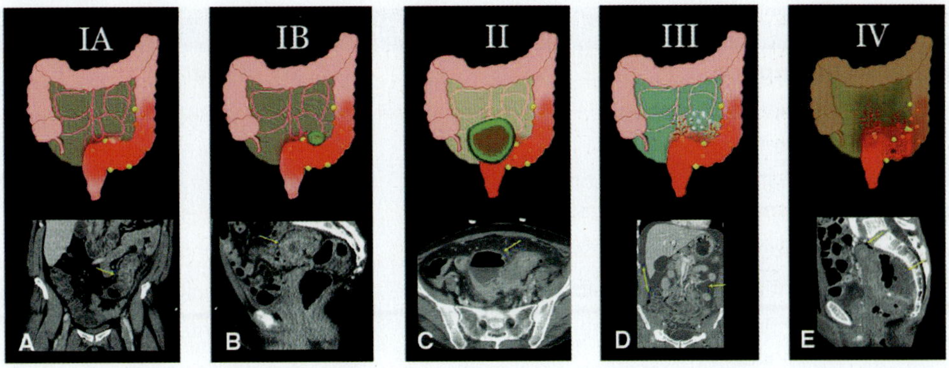

Figure 18.18 CT images of Hinchey grades of acute diverticulitis. Arrows point to the area of complicated diverticulitis. **A. Hinchey Ia** diverticulitis is characterized by a pericolonic phlegmon with associated inflammation; no fluid is present. **B. Hinchey Ib** diverticulitis is characterized by the additional finding of a pericolonic abscess <4 cm, adjacent to the area of diverticulitis. **C. Hinchey II** diverticulitis is characterized by the presence of a pelvic or interloop abscess, or an abscess >4 cm. **D. Hinchey III** diverticulitis is feculent peritonitis. **E. Hinchey IV** diverticulitis is feculent peritonitis. (Reprinted by permission from Springer Nature: From Bates DD, Fernandez MB, Ponchiardi C, et al. Surgical management in acute diverticulitis and its association with multidetector CT, modified Hinchey classification, and clinical parameters. *Abdom Radiol*. 2018;43:2060-2065.)

true in the patient without a previous diagnosis of diverticular disease. CT with IV contrast is the diagnostic test of choice. This will detect localized abscess formation, determine the degree of inflammation, or detect other pathology as the source of the symptoms (**Figure 18.18**; **Tables 18.7** to **18.9**). Any quantity of extraluminal air on CT does not mandate operative intervention in the stable, immunocompetent patient without peritonitis. If the air is pericolonic and small volume (few locules), the patient may be observed closely. The presence of an associated abscess or distant free air predicts the need for operation. Measurement of CRP has been recommended by some to help diagnose and differentiate complicated from uncomplicated diverticulitis.

Barium enema or lower endoscopy should not be performed in patients with acute diverticulitis for risk of perforation and extravasation of barium. The risk of a colorectal cancer concomitant with complicated diverticulitis is 8%-11%. These tests may be performed >6 weeks later if indicated to exclude obstruction/stricture and malignancy.

Acute Uncomplicated Diverticulitis

More than 70% of cases of acute diverticulitis are uncomplicated. The classical initial treatment for mild diverticulitis has been broad-spectrum oral antibiotics and a liquid diet, managed as an outpatient. More recent data suggest that acute uncomplicated diverticulitis can be managed without antibiotics, although this should only be employed in healthy, low-risk patients without comorbidities. Immunosuppressed patients should routinely receive antibiotics for acute diverticulitis.

If symptoms do not resolve after 48 hours, CT should be performed and patients should be

TABLE 18.7 ■ WSES Classification for Complicated Diverticulitis

1A	Pericolic air bubbles or little pericolic fluid without abscess
1B	Abscess ≤4 cm
2A	Abscess >4 cm
2B	Distant air (>5 cm from inflamed bowel segment)
3	Diffuse fluid without distant free air (no hole in colon)
4	Diffuse fluid with distant free air (persistent hole in colon)

TABLE 18.8 ■ Modified Hinchey Classification for Acute Diverticulitis

0	Mild clinical diverticulitis
IA	Pericolic phlegmon and inflammation
IB	Pericolonic inflammation and abscess <4 cm, adjacent to the area of diverticulitis
II	Pelvic, intra-abdominal, retroperitoneal abscess, or an abscess >4 cm
III	Purulent peritonitis
IV	Feculent peritonitis

TABLE 18.9 ■ AAST Classification for Acute Diverticulitis

AAST Grade	Description	Clinical Criteria
I	Colonic inflammation	Pain; leukocytosis; minimal or no tenderness
II	Colon microperforation or pericolic phlegmon without abscess	Localized tenderness (single or multiple areas) without peritonitis
III	Localized pericolic abscess	Localized peritonitis
IV	Distant and/or multiple abscesses	Localized peritonitis at multiple locations
V	Free colonic perforation with generalized peritonitis	Generalized peritonitis

admitted for IV antibiotics and bowel rest. Continue antibiotic treatment for 7-10 days with a broad-spectrum antibiotic as long as the patient continues to improve. If the patient is failing to progress after 72 hours or worsens, reimaging or operation may be needed. Free intra-abdominal fluid and the length of the segment with acute diverticulitis are associated with risk of disease progression. If the patient's pain improves and oral intake is tolerated, finish a 7-10 days course of oral antibiotics as an outpatient.

The management of acute diverticulitis has significantly evolved as medical therapy is shown to be successful in 75%-91% of uncomplicated diverticulitis. Elective resection after uncomplicated diverticulitis is on "a case by case basis"; not mandated by age or number of recurrences. Resection is performed for complicated diverticulitis or repeat episodes of uncomplicated diverticulitis with a negative effect on the patient's quality of life, often smoldering diverticulitis.

Complicated Diverticulitis

Diverticulitis of the colon may be complicated by abscess, fistula, obstruction, or free perforation.

Abscess. Abscess may be due to a microperforation causing pericolonic inflammation. These usually become small well-contained abscesses (**Tables 18.7** to **18.9**). These patients may be treated nonoperatively with IV antibiotics. Larger contained abscesses (>3-4 cm) should be treated by percutaneous drainage and antibiotics to control sepsis. Patients who are unable to be drained percutaneously can be treated by antibiotics alone or laparoscopic-assisted drainage. Repeat CT if the patient fails to improve. Patients who fail nonoperative therapy will require an operation. After treatment of a diverticular abscess with drainage, the risk of recurrent diverticulitis or later operation is 40%-70%, especially with a pelvic or distant abscess. Thus, an elective resection following a complicated episode with abscess drainage must be considered; although some surgeons only offer elective resection if symptoms persist or the patient continues to have multiple episodes.

Fistula. Formation of a fistula with diverticular disease most commonly involves the bladder. These fistulas occur twice as commonly in men compared to women (protective effect of the uterus). Colovesicular fistulas account for 50% of all diverticular-related fistulas. They may present with pneumaturia, fecaluria, or recurrent urinary tract infections. Colovaginal fistulas comprise 25% of diverticular-related fistulas. These fistulas are treated by colonic segmental resection generally as delayed procedure after the acute episode has resolved. Repair of the bladder or vaginal wall is often not necessary but should be interrogated thoroughly (cystoscopy, full pelvic examination).

Obstruction. Patients may present with obstruction from either narrowing of the colonic lumen during an attack or by a loop of small bowel incorporated into the inflammatory phlegmon causing obstruction. This may resolve with nonoperative management but should be closely monitored for potential need for operation. Cancer must always be excluded in this evaluation.

Free perforation. Free perforation of colonic diverticula with peritonitis is a morbid complication associated with up to a 35% mortality rate. This is the first manifestation of diverticular disease in 70% of patients with free perforation. Institute intravenous broad-spectrum antibiotics and prompt fluid resuscitation immediately. Then proceed directly to the operative suite.

Operative Indications/Management

Indications include the following:

- Diffuse peritoneal signs on initial examination, due to free, nonlocalized perforation.
- Clinical deterioration 48-72 hours after medical management is instituted.
- Obstruction with failure of nonoperative management.
- Complex abscess unable to be drained percutaneously.

Acute operation is rarely indicated for a diverticular fistula to the bladder, vagina. or another segment of intestine. Acute treatment is IV antibiotics to help resolve inflammation, followed by a delayed, elective operation.

The goal of the operation for acute perforated diverticulitis should be resection of the diseased bowel under most circumstances. If there is little pericolonic inflammation and minimal contamination of the peritoneal cavity without peritonitis, in the appropriate patient, perform a primary anastomosis with or without proximal diversion. The acute physiologic status of the patient, the degree of contamination, and the chronic medical condition of the patient should be considered (**Table 18.10**). If the patient has peritonitis, or has significant pericolonic inflammation or large amounts of gross contamination, a Hartmann procedure is generally performed with resection of the perforated segment, end colostomy and stapled blind rectal pouch. (In the unstable patient, this may invoke a damage control approach.)

If a Hartmann procedure is selected, the index resection should be limited to the involved segment of sigmoid colon, essentially a "perforectomy." When completing the definitive resection for diverticulitis at either the index operation or as a takedown of the colostomy after the Hartmann procedure: (1) all colon with diverticuli need not be resected; (2) the proximal resection margin must be to healthy colonic wall, avoiding diverticuli within the anastomosis; and (3) distally to upper rectum. Failure to resect to true rectum results in higher recurrence of diverticulitis.

For many reasons, 35%-40% of patients never have their colostomy reversed after a Hartmann procedure. This results in poor quality of life. Furthermore, the morbidity of the second operation for colostomy reversal is well documented. Thus, based on both randomized prospective studies and meta-analyses, several societies and reviews have advocated for definitive resection and primary anastomosis at the index operation. This recommendation is for Hinchey III and possibly Hinchey IV diverticulitis. The majority of authors recommend a diverting loop ileostomy. Factors that mitigate against a resection and primary anastomosis are listed in 18.10. Despite such data, recent series of acute perforated sigmoid diverticulitis report that a Hartmann procedure was done in >90% of cases with primary anastomosis in only 4%-7%

Another area of controversy has been the role of laparoscopic lavage and drainage without resection in the operative management of Hinchey III diverticulitis. Several prospective studies with somewhat conflicting results have investigated this approach. One study was stopped early because of high incidence of patient harm. Very selected patients with Hinchey III peritonitis may avoid a stoma, colon resection, or prolonged hospital stay. However, laparoscopic lavage has a high risk of failure, abscess formation, fistula, need for further intervention—and cancers are missed. In summary of the data, resection is still the safest treatment for acute perforated diverticulitis.

TABLE 18.10 ■ Mannheim Peritonitis Index (MPI)

Risk Factor	Scores
Age >50 years	5
Female	5
Organ failure	7
Malignancy	4
Preoperative duration of peritonitis >24 hours	4
Origin of sepsis not colonic	4
Diffuse generalized peritonitis	6
Exudate	
Clear	0
Cloudy, purulent	6
Fecal	12

Reprinted with permission from Biondo S, Borao JL, Millan M, et al. Current status of the treatment of acute colonic diverticulitis: a systematic review. *Colorectal Dis*. 2011;14:e1–e11.

COLITIS

Colonic inflammation or colitis may be of etiologies ranging from IBD, as discussed, to infectious, neutropenic, and ischemic colitis (see Chapter 12: Mesenteric Ischemia). Here, we will further discuss the management and definitive treatments of these other colidities.

Infectious Colitis

Infectious colitis may be secondary to overgrowth of a pathogenic bacteria, virus, fungi, or parasite. These tend to occur more commonly in immunocompromised individuals who cannot defend against these pathogens, with transplant patients having some of the highest risk.

Clostridium difficile Colitis

Introduction

The incidence and severity of *Clostridium difficile* infection (CDI) has markedly increased in the last 30 years. Currently, CDI is the most common cause of diarrhea in hospitalized patients and a common cause of hospital acquired infections, leading to 30 000 deaths annually in the United States.

The development of CDI is affected by several factors including age, comorbidities, immunosuppressive diseases and drugs, malnutrition, IBD, and particularly important, a previous use of antibiotics in the hospital setting. Surgical interventions can either predispose patients to CDI or are part of the multiple management strategies used to care for patients with severe forms of CDI.

Etiology and Pathophysiology

Clostridium difficile infection is cause by *Clostridioides difficile*, formerly known as *Clostridium difficile*, a gram-positive, obligate anaerobe spore producing organism. The spores survive in aerobic conditions and are the main contributing factor to transmission in the health care setting. Colonization in adults occurs in 5%-15% of individuals via the fecal-oral route.

The spores, shed by both symptomatic and asymptomatic patients, remain viable on surfaces for up to 5 months and are not easily eradicated with alcohol-based and other traditional surface cleaners. It becomes obvious that contact with the health care environment or health care workers' hands increases the risk of acquiring the infection. Several infection control measures including, but not limited to, patient isolation and contact precautions, the use of personal protective equipment, hand washing with soap and water, and use of sporicidal agents for cleaning surfaces, are used to prevent hospital-acquired infections caused by *C difficile*.

Spores acquired via the fecal-oral route are not susceptible to the acidic environment of the stomach and reach the small intestine where they are transformed into the vegetative form and produce toxins causing clinical disease.

Two toxins, Toxin A (TcdA) and Toxin B (TcdB), are responsible for the recruitment of inflammatory cells to the colon wall, which leads to watery diarrhea. In addition to copious diarrhea, more severe forms of the disease include pseudomembranous colitis and toxic megacolon, leading to multiorgan failure and eventually death, depending on the virulence of the strain of *C difficile* infecting the host.

Due to the increased use of fluoroquinolones, hypervirulent strains such as the BI/NAP1/027 produce the toxin *C difficile* transferase, which causes more toxin production, higher recurrence rates, and increased mortality rates compared to other strains. Therefore, antimicrobial stewardship strategies are critically important to control CDI in hospitalized patients.

Clinical Presentation and Diagnosis

Clinical manifestations usually occur within the first 5-10 days after exposure to antibiotics but can vary from 1 day to several weeks. Diarrhea is the most common symptom of CDI, although it may not be present initially due to colonic dysmotility from previous colonic diseases or because of CDI in patients with postoperative ileus.

Diarrhea without any systemic symptoms, such as fever, renal failure, or hemodynamic instability, characterizes mild disease, which is usually associated with mild abdominal pain and cramps. Electrolyte imbalance and volume depletion are common and should be diagnosed and treated aggressively in the postoperative period to minimize systemic complications.

Moderate disease is characterized by profuse diarrhea accompanied by abdominal pain and distension, fever, tachycardia, leukocytosis, and, commonly, oliguria.

Severe or fulminant disease results in occult bleeding, renal failure, hemodynamic instability requiring vasopressor support, and respiratory failure requiring mechanical ventilation. This severe form of the disease is relatively infrequent, developing in 1%-3% of cases. However, when present, it may lead to toxic megacolon, intestinal necrosis with perforation, multisystem organ failure, and death.

The astute surgeon must be attentive to patients with recent or current antibiotic use who appear systemically sick with a sudden decrease in the volume and frequency of diarrhea, fever (temperature >38.5 °C) without obvious cause, abdominal distension with or without tenderness, altered mental status, severe leukocytosis (WBC > 15 × 10^3 cells/mL), increased serum lactate (>4 mmol/L), and vasopressor requirements. In those circumstances, a high level of suspicion for CDI is necessary to provide timely care and prompt intervention. Other important laboratory findings include an increase in serum creatinine level >1.5 times the baseline level and albumin <2.5 g/dL.

Clostridium difficile infection recurrence after the initial treatment occurs in 10%-30% of patients, which is associated with an impaired immune response to the *C difficile* toxins and/or alterations of the colonic flora. Recurrent episodes are usually less severe than the first episode and multiple recurrences may occur either due to reinfection or the presence of remaining spores from the initial infection resistant to treatment with antibiotics. Toxins produced by *C difficile* bacteria can be usually detected in a sample of stool.

Patients with known risk factors for CDI (recent antibiotic use, history of recent hospitalization, or advanced age) who have >3 loose stools in a 24-hour period without alternative reason for signs and symptoms, such as use of stool softener or enteral nutrition, should undergo stool testing.

Patients with formed stool should not be tested due to the potential of over diagnosing CDI in potential carriers. Patients with ileus who are unable to produce a stool specimen, performing polymerase chain reaction testing of perirectal swabs, provide an acceptable alternative.

The diagnosis of CDI is established via either a positive nucleic acid amplification test (NAAT) for *C difficile* toxin B gene or a positive stool test for *C difficile* toxin(s).

Other tests are also acceptable with different degrees of sensitivity and specificity and include a) enzyme immunoassay for *C difficile* glutamate dehydrogenase, b) enzyme immunoassay for *C difficile* toxins A and B, c) cell culture cytotoxicity assay, and d) selective anaerobic culture.

CT imaging is recommended for patients with clinical manifestations of severe CDI (severe abdominal pain, abdominal distention with apparent ileus, fever, hypovolemia, lactic acidosis, hypoalbuminemia, and/or marked leukocytosis) or fulminant colitis (hypotension or ileus) to evaluate for presence of bowel perforation or toxic megacolon. Significant colon dilatation >7 cm in diameter in patients with signs and symptoms of CDI confirms the diagnosis of toxic megacolon.

CT findings of CDI include colonic wall thickening (pancolitis), dilation of the colon, peri colonic stranding, "accordion sign" (high-attenuation oral contrast in the colonic lumen alternating with low-attenuation inflamed mucosa), "target sign" (IV contrast displaying varying degrees of attenuation caused by submucosal inflammation), "thumb printing" (scalloping of the bowel wall) due to submucosal edema, and ascites. CT diagnosis of CDI has a sensitivity of 52%, specificity of 93%, positive and negative predictive values of 88% and 67%, respectively.

Endoscopically, CDI is characterized by the presence of ulcers, plaques, and pseudomembranes, which are present in 90% of fulminant colitis cases. Due to the risk of perforation, endoscopy is rarely used to diagnose CDI.

Medical Management of the Initial Episode of CDI

Either oral vancomycin 125 mg four times daily or fidaxomicin 200 mg oral twice daily is recommended over metronidazole for an initial episode of CDI in adults, regardless of severity, for a period of 10-14 days. If vancomycin or fidaxomicin are unavailable or contraindicated, oral metronidazole is indicated.

The IDSA/SHEA guidelines recommend using leukocyte count of >15 000 cells/mL or a serum creatinine level >1.5 mg/dL as indicators of severe disease. The clinical cure rate with fidaxomicin is noninferior to vancomycin, but the rate of recurrence is significantly lower, thus fidaxomicin may be reserved for patients at increased risk of CDI recurrence.

Fulminant CDI

Fulminant CDI may be characterized by hypotension or shock, ileus, or megacolon. Treatment is higher dose vancomycin, 500 mg orally four times daily for 10 days. If ileus is present, rectal instillation of vancomycin 500 mg in 100 mL normal saline every 6 hours as a retention enema should be considered (**Table 18.1**). Intravenous metronidazole 500 mg every 8 hours is recommended as an addition to oral or rectal vancomycin if ileus is suspected. If the response to vancomycin and metronidazole is inadequate, tigecycline or intravenous immunoglobulins may be used, but studies have provided limited evidence of their effectiveness. Studies have shown that a rising WBC count (>25 000 cells/mL) or rising lactate level (>5 mmol/L) is associated with higher mortality and early surgical intervention is key for survival; hence, expert surgical consultation must be sought earlier in the course of fulminant CDI with ileus.

Treatment of Recurrent CDI

Recurrent CDI occurs in ~25% of patients. Risk factors for recurrence include administration of antibiotics during or after treatment of previous CDI, increased severity of underlying disease, advanced age, and immunosuppression. Recurrent CDI can result from the same strain (relapse) or a different *C difficile* strain (new infection), but the management is the same regardless of etiology.

Treatment of the first recurrent episode varies based on the agent used to treat the initial episode of CDI. Patients who received metronidazole in the initial episode must be treated with a standard 10-day course of oral vancomycin 125 mg four times daily. Patients who received a standard course of oral vancomycin as initial treatment must be treated with a tapered, pulse-dose regimen of vancomycin, or a 10-day course of fidaxomicin. Metronidazole is not recommended for recurrent CDI. Patients with multiple recurrent CDIs may receive an extended course of oral vancomycin (tapered or pulse regimen), or oral vancomycin followed by rifaximin, or fidaxomicin.

Fecal microbiota transplantation has been used successfully to correct the antibiotic-related dysbiosis in the gut microbiome, which contributes to the development of CDIs. Reported success rates of FMT are high regardless of route of installation of feces and range from 77% to 94% with the highest success rates with colonic instillation. There is no consensus on the number of antibiotic treatment courses for recurrent CDI before using FMT, but IDSA/SHEA recommends appropriate antibiotic treatment of at least 2 recurrences, or a total of 3 CDI episodes, before initiating FMT. Complications of FMT include infectious complications and physical complications from the instillation of the fecal solution, while long-term consequences are unknown at this time.

Bezlotoxumab, a toxin-B binding monoclonal antibody, was approved in 2016 and demonstrated significant promise to reduce the risk of recurrence in adult patients who were concomitantly receiving antibiotics for CDI.

Surgical Management

Patients with fulminant colitis progressing to systemic toxicity require surgical intervention. Age (>70 years), prior CDI, leukocytosis (>18 000/mm^3), hemodynamic instability, use of antiperistaltic medications, increasing abdominal pain, distension, diarrhea, and mental status change are predictive signs and symptoms of fulminant colitis. Delays in surgical intervention increase the likelihood of poor outcomes. Therefore, in cases of severe CDI with systemic toxicity and/or organ failure, emergency colectomy provides a survival benefit compared to medical management with antibiotics. Early surgery before the onset of cardio/pulmonary failure or vasopressor requirements, especially in patients <65 years of age, leads to lower mortality rates. Although the ideal timing for surgery in patients with CDI has not been well defined, most surgeons agree that patients who are worsening or not improving clinically 3-5 days after the initial diagnosis should be considered for operative intervention.

Total abdominal colectomy with end ileostomy should be considered when treating patients with fulminant colitis, and it is the most common operation performed for cases presenting with fulminant colitis. Segmental colon resection is inadequate for fulminant CDI.

The surgeon should not be dissuaded in the operating room by the external appearance of the colon, as it may appear relatively benign. However, more often the colon is markedly dilated, filled with large amounts of fluid, the colonic wall is edematous, and pericolic inflammation and sterile ascites are also commonly found in nonperforated cases. When surgery is delayed, the colonic wall may be necrotic with or without perforation.

Surgical intervention must be performed expeditiously, open, and the rectum should be divided at or near the peritoneal reflection. To facilitate a quick resection, the mesenteric vessels should be ligated before they branch out.

A laparoscopic diverting loop ileostomy with antegrade colonic lavage with warmed polyethylene glycol 3350/electrolyte solution is a colon preserving alternative to total colectomy in patients with hemodynamic stability, complemented with postoperative antegrade instillation of vancomycin flushes via the ileostomy. Using this operation relatively early (any signs of progressive organ failure) has made the need for total abdominal colectomy uncommon in our hands. Exceptions are the patient who presents late in the course of disease or the patient with abdominal compartment syndrome. Preprocedure predictors of mortality for colonic lavage include age, elevated serum lactate levels, timing of operation, vasopressor use, and presence of acute renal failure.

NEUTROPENIC ENTEROCOLITIS

Neutropenic enterocolitis is also referred to as typhlitis. It is an acute life-threatening condition characterized by transmural inflammation of the cecum, commonly with involvement of the ascending colon and ileum.

Risk factors include chemotherapy, malignancy, and systemic antibiotics changing the bowel flora. It is more common in children than adults. With more patients undergoing chemotherapy and novel immune modulating treatments, colitis has become a common complication of these treatments. Neutropenic colitis is the classic chemotherapy-induced colitis, typical in patients with leukemia and is associated with low neutrophil counts. The cause of the colitis is secondary to the toxic effects of chemotherapeutic agents on the mucosa of the colon secondary to its rapidly dividing nature. Enterocolitis is believed to occur when the injured bowel mucosa develops microbial invasion in the face of immunosuppression.

Diagnosis is by history, physical, and CT findings of acute inflammation. Neutropenic enterocolitis varies in presentation based on severity of disease. Most commonly, it presents as abdominal distension, with abdominal tenderness focused in the right lower quadrant, and shock.

Diagnostic evaluation includes *CBC with differential* (anemia, neutropenia, and thrombocytopenia may be present); *stool studies* (to exclude *C difficile* and other infectious etiologies); and CT of the abdomen is the diagnostic imaging of choice. It may demonstrate cecal and ascending colonic wall thickening, pericecal inflammation, as well as more ominous signs such as portal venous gas or free air.

Treatment of neutropenic colitis includes bowel rest and antibiotics, steroids in more severe cases. Medical management with antibiotics and fluid resuscitation can be successful if neither necrosis nor ischemia is present. Operative indications include peritonitis, perforation, pneumoperitoneum, or unrelenting intra-abdominal sepsis, or abscess formation. Resect all areas of transmural necrosis. Second-look operation may be necessary.

CYTOMEGALOVIRUS (CMV) ENTEROCOLITIS

Cytomegalovirus enterocolitis is a rare entity in immunocompetent patients but more common in those who are immunocompromised; 2%-16% risk in patients after solid organ transplant and 3%-5% risk of those with HIV. Primary infection occurs in patients who are seronegative, then exposed to CMV. Reactivation of latent CMV occurs in patients who become immunocompromised and is associated with significant morbidity and mortality. Risk factors include immunosuppressive medications, IBD in immunocompetent hosts, HIV, transplant patients (especially those receiving CMV + organs), hemodialysis, malnutrition, and collagen vascular disease.

Cytomegalovirus targets multiple organs, with the esophagus and colon as the most common sites of infection. Thus, the clinical presentation may include fever, anorexia, malaise, abdominal pain, ulceration in GI mucosa, mucosal hemorrhage, and chronic watery or bloody diarrhea.

Diagnostic evaluation includes CT, which may demonstrate bowel wall thickening, mucosal ulceration, and luminal narrowing. In addition to standard laboratory studies, perform an immunoassay for CMV. Diagnosis may be further confirmed by sigmoidoscopy or colonoscopy, allowing direct visualization of ulceration and nodular plaque or polypoid lesions. This also allows biopsy of tissue to aid in diagnosis.

Treatment of CMV colitis begins immediately with aggressive fluid resuscitation and antiviral therapy. Indications for operation are peritonitis, pneumoperitoneum, and perforation. Patients who require colectomy have a 30% mortality.

SUMMARY

- Crohn disease presents with inflammatory, stricturing, and penetrating disease with or without perianal involvement. Medical management of Crohn disease with induction therapy with steroids and anti-TNF agents is preferred if no signs of sepsis are present. Perforation, abscess, fistula, and obstruction can be emergent presentations of Crohn disease that require emergent surgical intervention. Ulcerative colitis can present as an outpatient problem or an emergency situation due to toxic megacolon, hemorrhage, or perforation. Treatment is typically multimodal focusing on the immune system, colonic microbiota, and dietary changes. Surgery is typically the last resort after multiple medical treatments have failed, except in the emergency presentations.
- Small bowel diverticula are relatively uncommon. Most remain asymptomatic, requiring no treatment. They may present with bleeding, contained diverticulitis, or free perforation.

- Colonic diverticulosis increases in frequency with older age. In western cultures, left-sided diverticula are more common. In eastern cultures, right-sided diverticula are more common. Most remain asymptomatic and require no treatment. Most cases of acute diverticulitis can be managed without operation. Management of Hinchey III and IV diverticulitis should generally involve sigmoid resection. Several randomized studies recommend primary anastomosis rather than a Hartmann procedure after resection. However, over 90% of patients still are managed with a colostomy after resection for acute perforated colonic diverticulitis.
- Infectious colidities for which surgeons may be consulted include CMV, neutropenic colidities, and *Clostridioides difficile*, formerly known as *Clostridium difficile* (CDI). Fulminant cases of CDI may require operation. Effective surgical management depends upon operative intervention prior to progressive organ failure. The two operative options are total abdominal colectomy or laparoscopic diverting loop ileostomy with antegrade colonic lavage with warmed polyethylene glycol 3350/electrolyte solution, complemented with postoperative antegrade instillation of vancomycin flushes via the ileostomy. The latter approach is effective in the hemodynamically stable patient with early signs of organ dysfunction.

SUGGESTED READINGS

Abt MC, McKenney PT, Pamer EG. Clostridium difficile colitis: pathogenesis and host defence. *Nat Rev Microbiol.* 2016;14(10):609-620. doi:10.1038/nrmicro.2016.108

Bagdasarian N, Rao K, Malani PN. Diagnosis and treatment of Clostridium difficile in adults: a systematic review. *JAMA*. 2015;313:398-408.

Bates DD, Fernandez MB, Ponchiardi C, et al. Surgical management in acute diverticulitis and its association with multi-detector CT, modified Hinchey classification, and clinical parameters. *Abdom Radiol (NY)*. 2018;43:2060-2065.

Berg DF, Bahadursingh AM, Kaminski DL, Longo WE. Acute surgical emergencies in inflammatory bowel disease. *Am J Surg*. 2002;184(1):45-51.

Biondo S, Ramos E, Fraccalvieri D, et al. Comparative study of left colonic Peritonitis Severity Score and Mannheim Peritonitis Index. *Br J Surg* 2006;93:616-622.

Bitton A, Peppercorn MA. Emergencies in inflammatory bowel disease. *Crit Care Clin*. 1995;11(2):513-529.

Boland GW, Lee MJ, Cats AM, Gaa JA, Saini S, Mueller PR. Antibiotic-induced diarrhea: specificity of abdominal CT for the diagnosis of Clostridium difficile disease. *Radiology*. 1994;191:103-106.

Brandt LJ, Aroniadis OC, Mellow M, et al. Long-term follow-up of colonoscopic fecal microbiota transplant for recurrent Clostridium difficile infection. *Am J Gastroenterol.* 2012;107:1079-1087.

Carchman EH, Peitzman AB, Simmons RL, Zuckerbraun BS. The role of acute care surgery in the treatment of severe, complicated Clostridium difficile-associated disease. *J Trauma Acute Care Surg*. 2012;73:789-800.

Cauley CE, Patel R, Bordeianou L. Use of primary anastomosis with diverting ileostomy in patients with acute diverticulitis requiring urgent operative intervention. *Dis Colon Rectum*. 2018;61:586-592.

Chan S, Kelly M, Helme S, Gossage J, Modarai B, Forshaw M. Outcomes following colectomy for Clostridium difficile colitis. *Int J Surg*. 2009;7:78-81.

Chen H, Li H, Liu Z. Interplay of intestinal microbiota and mucosal immunity in inflammatory bowel disease: a relationship of frenemies. *Therap Adv Gastroenterol.* 2020;13:1756284820935188.

Chen P, Zhou G, Lin J, et al. Serum biomarkers for inflammatory bowel disease. *Front Med (Lausanne)*. 2020;7:123.

Choi J, Bessoff K, Bromley-Dulfano R, et al. Prospectively assigned AAST grade versus modified Hinchey class and acute diverticulitis outcomes. *J Surg Res.* 2021;259:555-561.

Clanton J, Fawley R, Haller N, et al. Patience is a virtue: an argument for delayed surgical intervention in fulminant Clostridium difficile colitis. *Am Surg*. 2014;80:614-619.

Dahmus J, Rosario M, Clarke K. Risk of lymphoma associated with Anti-TNF therapy in patients with inflammatory bowel disease: implications for therapy. *Clin Exp Gastroenterol.* 2020;13:339-350.

De Simone B, Alberici L, Ansaloni L, Sartelli M, Coccolini F, Catena F. Not all diverticulites are colonic: small bowel diverticulitis: a systematic review. *Minerva Chir*. 2019;74(2):137-145.

Fekety R, Kim KH, Brown D, Batts DH, Cudmore M, Silva J Jr. Epidemiology of antibiotic-associated colitis; isolation of Clostridium difficile from the hospital environment. *Am J Med*. 1981;70(4):906-908.

Ferrada P, Callcut R, Zielinski MD, et al.; EAST Multi-Institutional Trials Committee. Loop ileostomy versus total colectomy as surgical treatment for Clostridium difficile-associated disease: an Eastern Association for the Surgery of Trauma multicenter trial. *J Trauma Acute Care Surg*. 2017;83:36-40.

Feuerstein JD, Cheifetz AS. Ulcerative colitis: epidemiology, diagnosis, and management. *Mayo Clin Proc.* 2014;89(11):1553-1563.

Gajendran M, Loganathan P, Catinella AP, Hashash JG. A comprehensive review and update on Crohn's disease. *Dis Mon*. 2018;64(2):20-57.

Gionchetti P, Dignass A, Danese S, et al. 3rd European evidence-based consensus on the diagnosis and management of Crohn's disease 2016: part 2: surgical management and special situations. *J Crohns Colitis.* 2017;11(2):135-149.

Girotra M, Kumar V, Khan JM, et al. Clinical predictors of fulminant colitis in patients with Clostridium difficile infection. *Saudi J Gastroenterol.* 2012;18:133-139.

Gkikas K, Gerasimidis K, Milling S, Ijaz UZ, Hansen R, Russell RK. Dietary strategies for maintenance of clinical remission in inflammatory bowel diseases: are we there yet? *Nutrients.* 2020;12(7).

Goldstone RN, Steinhagen RM. Abdominal emergencies in inflammatory bowel disease. *Surg Clin North Am.* 2019;99(6):1141-1150.

Gomollon F, Dignass A, Annese V, et al. 3rd European evidence-based consensus on the diagnosis and management of Crohn's disease 2016: part 1: diagnosis and medical management. *J Crohns Colitis.* 2017;11(1):3-25.

Gough E, Shaikh H, Manges AR. Systematic review of intestinal microbiota transplantation (fecal bacteriotherapy) for recurrent Clostridium difficile infection. *Clin Infect Dis.* 2011;53:994-1002.

Gourarzi M, Seyedjacadi SS, Goudarzi H, Mehdizadeh Aghdam E, Nazeri S. Clostridium difficile infection: epidemiology, pathogenesis risk factors and therapeutic options. *Scientifica (Cairo).* 2014;2014:916826.

Hall J, Hardiman K, Lee S, et al. The American Society of Colon and Rectal Surgeons Clinical Practice Guidelines for the treatment of left-sided colonic diverticulitis. *Dis Colon Rect* 2020;m63:728-747.

Hamilton MJ, Weingarden AR, Sadowsky MJ, Khoruts A. Standardized frozen preparation for transplantation of fecal microbiota for recurrent Clostridium difficile infection. *Am J Gastroenterol.* 2012;107:761-767.

Hanna MH, Kaiser AM. Update on management of sigmoid diverticulitis. *World J Gastroenterol.* 2021;27:760-781.

Hansen CC, Soreide K. Systematic review of epidemiology, presentation, and management of Meckel's diverticulum in the 21st century. *Medicine (Baltimore).* 2018;97(35):e12154.

Haut ER, Johnson E, Praba-Egge A, et al. Timing and type of surgical treatment of Clostridium difficile-associated disease: a practice management guideline from the Eastern Association for the Surgery of Trauma. *J Trauma Acute Care Surg.* 2014;76:1484-1493.

Hindryckx P, Jairath V, D'Haens G. Acute severe ulcerative colitis: from pathophysiology to clinical management. *Nat Rev Gastroenterol Hepatol.* 2016;13(11):654-664.

Jorup-Rönström C, Håkanson A, Sandell S, et al. Fecal transplant against relapsing Clostridium difficile-associated diarrhea in 32 patients. *Scand J Gastroenterol* 2012;47:548-552.

Kaiser AM, Hogen R, Bordeianou L, Alavi K, Wise PE, Sudan R; CME Committee of the SSAT. Clostridium Difficile Infection from a Surgical Perspective. *J Gastrointest Surg.* 2015;19:1363-1377.

Keshteli AH, Madsen KL, Dieleman LA. Diet in the pathogenesis and management of ulcerative colitis; a review of randomized controlled dietary interventions. *Nutrients.* 2019;11(7).

Khan A, Hawkins AT. Challenging surgical dogma. Controversies in diverticulitis. *Surg Clin North Am.* 2021;101:967-980.

Kim MJ, Kim BS, Kwon JW, et al. Risk factors for the development of Clostridium difficile colitis in a surgical ward. *J Korean Surg Soc.* 2012;83:14-20.

Kim PK, Zhao P, Teperman S. Evolving treatment strategies for severe clostridium difficile colitis: defining the therapeutic window. In: Sartelli M, Bassetti M, Martin-Loeches I, eds. *Abdominal Sepsis. Hot Topics in Acute Care Surgery and Trauma.* Springer; 2018.

Lamontagne F, Labb AC, Haeck O, et al. Impact of emergency colectomy on survival of patients with fulminant Clostridium difficile colitis during an epidemic caused by a hypervirulent strain. *Ann Surg.* 2007;245:267-272.

Lee JH, Ahn BK, Lee KH. Conservative treatment of uncomplicated right sided diverticulitis: a systematic review and meta-analysis. *Int J Colorect Dis.* 2021;36:1791-1799.

Lee DY, Chung EL, Guend H, Whelan RL, Wedderburn RV, Rose KM. Predictors of mortality after emergency colectomy for Clostridium difficile colitis: an analysis of ACS-NSQIP. *Ann Surg.* 2014;259:148-156.

Lessa FC, Gould CV, McDonald LC. Current status of Clostridium difficile infection epidemiology. *Clin Infect Dis.* 2012;55:65-70.

Lessa FC, Mu Y, Bamberg WM, et al. Burden of Clostridium difficile infection in the United States. *N Engl J Med.* 2015;372:825-834.

Lins Neto MÁ F, Verdi GMX, Veras AO, Veras MO, Caetano LC, Ursulino JS. Use of metabolomics to the diagnosis of inflammatory bowel disease. *Arq Gastroenterol.* 2020;57:311-315.

MacConnachie AA, Fox R, Kennedy DR, Seaton RA. Faecal transplant for recurrent Clostridium difficile-associated diarrhoea: a UK case series. *QJM.* 2009;102:781-784.

Mahadevan U, Silverberg MS. Inflammatory bowel disease-gastroenterology diamond jubilee review. *Gastroenterology.* 2018;154(6):1555-1558.

Mattila E, Uusitalo-Seppälä R, Wuorela M, et al. Fecal transplantation, through colonoscopy, is effective therapy for recurrent Clostridium difficile infection. *Gastroenterology.* 2012;142:490-496.

McDonald LC, Gerding DN, Johnson S, et al. Clinical practice guidelines for Clostridium difficile infection in adults and children: 2017 update by the Infectious Diseases Society of America (IDSA) and Society for Healthcare Epidemiology of America (SHEA). *Clin Infect Dis.* 2018;66:e1-e48.

Mona-Lopez L, Ruiz-Edo N, Estrada-Ferrer O, et al. Efficacy and safety of nonantibiotic outpatient treatment in mild acute diverticulitis (DINAMO-study). *Ann Surg*. 2021;274:e435-e442.

Moriichi K, Fujiya M, Okumura T. The endoscopic diagnosis of mucosal healing and deep remission in inflammatory bowel disease. *Dig Endosc*. 2021;33:1008-1023.

Neal MD, Alverdy JC, Hall DE, Simmons RL, Zuckerbraun BS. Diverting loop ileostomy and colonic lavage: an alternative to total abdominal colectomy for the treatment of severe, complicated Clostridium difficile associated disease. *Ann Surg*. 2011;254:423-437.

Nebbia M, Yassin NA, Spinelli A. Colorectal cancer in inflammatory bowel disease. *Clin Colon Rectal Surg*. 2020;33(5):305-317.

Nicolaides S, Vasudevan A, Long T, van Langenberg D. The impact of tobacco smoking on treatment choice and efficacy in inflammatory bowel disease. *Intest Res*. 2021;19:158-170.

Ordás I, Eckmann L, Talamini M, Baumgart DC, Sandborn WJ. Ulcerative colitis. *Lancet*. 2012;380(9853):1606-1619.

Peery AF, Shaukat A, Strate LL. AGA Clinical practice update in medical management of colonic diverticulitis: expert review. *Gastroenterology*. 2021;160:906-911.

Portugal R, Nucci M. Typhlitis (neutropenic enterocolitis) in patients with acute leukemia: a review. *Expert Rev Hematol*. 2017;10(2):169-174.

Poxton IR, McCoubrey J, Blair G. The pathogenicity of Clostridium difficile. *Clin Microbiol Infect*. 2001;7(8):421-424.

Rangan V, Lamont JT. Small bowel diverticulosis: pathogenesis, clinical management, and new concepts. *Curr Gastroenterol Rep*. 2020;22:4.

Rodrigues MA, Brady RR, Rodrigues J, Graham C, Gibb AP. Clostridium difficile infection in general surgery patients; identification of high-risk populations. *Int J Surg*. 2010;8:368-372.

Sartelli M, Di Bella S, McFarland LV, et al. 2019 update of the WSES Guidelines for Management of Clostridium difficile infection in Surgical Patients. *World J Emerg Surg*. 2019;14:8. doi:10.1186/s13017-019-0228-3

Sartelli M, Moore FA, Ansaloni L, et al. A proposal for a CT driven classification of Left colon acute diverticulitis. *World J Emerg Surg*. 2015;10:3. https://doi.org/10.1186/1749-7922-10-3

Sartelli M, Weber DG, Kluger Y, et al. 2020 update of the WSES guidelines for the management of acute colonic diverticulitis in the emergency setting. *World J Emerg Surg*. 2020;15:32. https://doi.org/10.1186/s13017-020-00313-4

Satsangi J, Silverberg MS, Vermeire S, Colombel JF. The Montreal classification of inflammatory bowel disease: controversies, consensus, and implications. *Gut*. 2006;55(6):749-753.

Schultz JK, Azhar N, Binda GA, et al. European Society of Coloproctology: guidelines for the management of diverticular disease of the colon. *Colorectal Dis*. 2020;22:5-28.

Seder CW, Villalba MR Jr, Robbins J, et al. Early colectomy may be associated with improved survival in fulminant Clostridium difficile colitis: an 8-year experience. *Am J Surg*. 2009;197:302-307.

Shafi S, Priest EL, Crandall ML, et al. Multicenter validation of AASR grading system for acute colonic diverticulitis and its use for emergency general surgery quality improvement program. *J Trauma Acute Care Surg*. 2016;80:405-411.

Shen ZH, Zhu CX, Quan YS, et al. Relationship between intestinal microbiota and ulcerative colitis: mechanisms and clinical application of probiotics and fecal microbiota transplantation. *World J Gastroenterol*. 2018;24(1):5-14.

Stewart DB, Hollenbeak CS, Wilson MZ. Is colectomy for fulminant Clostridium difficile colitis life saving? A systematic review. *Colorectal Dis*. 2013;15:798-804.

Talathi S, Baig KKK. Biosimilars in inflammatory bowel disease. *J Dig Dis*. 2020;21:610-620.

Tan P, Li X, Shen J, Feng Q. Fecal microbiota transplantation for the treatment of inflammatory bowel disease: an update. *Front Pharmacol*. 2020;11:574533.

Tatiya-Aphiradee N, Chatuphonprasert W, Jarukamjorn K. Immune response and inflammatory pathway of ulcerative colitis. *J Basic Clin Physiol Pharmacol*. 2018;30(1):1-10.

Tian Y, Abu-Sbeih H, Wang Y. Immune checkpoint inhibitors-induced colitis. *Adv Exp Med Biol*. 2018;995:151-157.

To KB, Napolitano LM. Clostridium difficile infection: update on diagnosis, epidemiology, and treatment strategies. *Surg Infect*. 2014;15:490-502.

Toh JW, Stewart P, Rickard MJ, Leong R, Wang N, Young CJ. Indications and surgical options for small bowel, large bowel and perianal Crohn's disease. *World J Gastroenterol*. 2016;22(40):8892-8904.

Torres J, Mehandru S, Colombel JF, Peyrin-Biroulet L. Crohn's disease. *Lancet*. 2017;389(10080):1741-1755.

Young-Fadok TM. Diverticulitis. *N Engl J Med*. 2018;379:1635-1642.

Zangenberg MS, Horesh N, Kopylov U, El-Hussuna A. Preoperative optimization of patients with inflammatory bowel disease undergoing gastrointestinal surgery: a systematic review. *Int J Colorectal Dis*. 2017;32(12):1663-1676.

Zhang YZ, Li YY. Inflammatory bowel disease: pathogenesis. *World J Gastroenterol*. 2014;20(1):91-99.

CHAPTER

19 Anorectal Emergencies

Bogdan Diaconescu and Tudor Marinescu

CASE PRESENTATION

Overnight, a 62-year-old patient with poorly controlled diabetes mellitus presented to the emergency department with perianal pain. A tender perianal region with increasing inflammatory signs made standing and walking more difficult for the patient. Pain assessment was 7/10 at rest, localized in perianal region, without radiation, worsened during walking or standing. The patient had a fever and anal pain for the past 12 hours. Upon examination, cellulitis was observed.

The patient's clinical status deteriorated rapidly. Within the next 3 hours, crepitus, skin necrosis, and hemorrhagic bullae developed. Sensory loss of the overlying skin was also noted. Abnormal labs included WBC 15.500/mm^3 with neutrophilic predominance, Hgb 11.5 g/dL, normal platelets, sodium 130 mmol/L, creatinine 1.7 mg/dL (baseline 1.2 mg/dL), glucose 265 mg/dL, and CRP 180 ng/L. The Laboratory Risk Indicator for Necrotizing Fasciitis (LRINEC) score was 9, so we had a high index of suspicion for fasciitis. The patient's condition deteriorated rapidly, and he was soon in septic shock.

The patient was taken to the operating room for excision of all devitalized tissue (**Figure 19.1**): the wound was left open. At the time of surgery, pus and samples of necrotic tissue were collected and sent for microbiological examination (culture and antibiogram).

Initially, the patient received broad-spectrum antibiotics and was transferred to the intensive care unit. Culture revealed *Staphylococcus aureus* and *Escherichia coli* sensitive to cephalosporins, leading to antibiotic adjustment. Fluid resuscitation and close monitoring were essential to avoid further deterioration.

A second surgical debridement was required 48 hours after the initial debridement. Forty-eight hours later, a diverting colostomy was performed, and secondary closure was performed 5 weeks later (**Figure 19.2**). Colostomy reversal was performed 3 months after the initial surgery.

Question: *What is the patient diagnosis? What are the priorities in the management for this patient and the steps for treatment?*

Answer: *NSTI are severe conditions that may alter patients within hours. The priority is to proceed a radical surgical debridement. Early recognition and treatment by extensive debridement can avoid a fatal outcome due to its fulminant progression. Rapid deterioration of patient's clinical status rushed us to a rapid resuscitation followed by early and aggressive surgical exploration and debridement of necrotic tissue. A staged debridement was planned to minimize damage to healthy tissue. Extensive incisions that extend outside the area of superficial involvement was necessary. Decision for diverting colostomy was made after few stages debridement due to huge contamination of surgical wound.*

INTRODUCTION

Acute swelling in the anorectal region, associated with pain, bleeding, fever, or intestinal obstruction, represents a condition that may require urgent surgical management. These anorectal emergencies include infectious emergencies (anorectal abscesses, perineal necrotizing fasciitis—also known as Fournier gangrene), hemorrhoidal emergencies (bleeding, thrombosed, or strangulated), traumatic emergencies (anorectal trauma or retained foreign bodies), and obstructive emergencies (obstructing anorectal tumors, anorectal prolapse, or intussusception). Careful clinical evaluation and assessment of the situation should guide the surgeon to successful treatment (operative or nonoperative). Any delay in decision-making may lead to complications or inappropriate treatment with poor outcomes.

INFECTIOUS EMERGENCIES

Anorectal abscesses and fistulas are among the most frequent anorectal lesions. Abscesses and

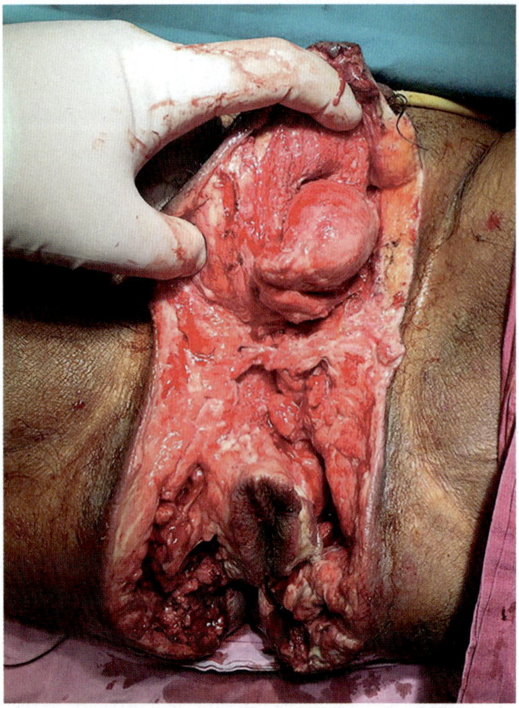

Figure 19.1 A case of Fournier gangrene after extensive debridement.

fistulas are two phases of the same disease, fistulous abscess. However, for practical and therapeutic reasons, they will be considered separately. An abscess represents acute inflammation in the anorectal region, and the anal fistula represents the chronic complication of an anal abscess.

Anal Abscess

The crypts and anal glands above the dentate line in the anal canal can become infected by feces; penetration into the anal wall can lead to an anal abscess. Infection can spread to surrounding tissues and develop into an intrasphincteric or intersphincteric abscess. Infection usually spreads along the pathway of minimum resistance: caudally into the intersphincteric space resulting in a perianal abscess; cephalad inside the longitudinal muscle layer within the gut wall, causing an intermuscular abscess; or cephalad outside the gut wall resulting in a supralevator abscess. The infection may spread across the external sphincter at any level, resulting in an ischiorectal abscess, which may also extend cephalad or caudad.

Classification

Anorectal abscess is classified by its relations with the anal sphincter: perianal, intersphincteric, ischiorectal, or supralevator (**Figure 19.3A-E**).

Perianal abscess is located superficially in the subcutaneous fat tissue and does not pass deep to the external sphincter (**Figure 19.4**). Intersphincteric abscesses develop between the two anal

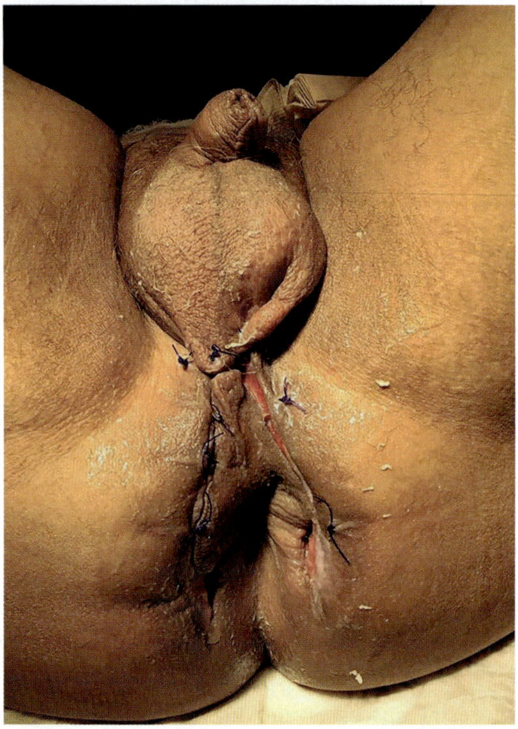

Figure 19.2 Final aspect with secondary suture post perineal fasciitis.

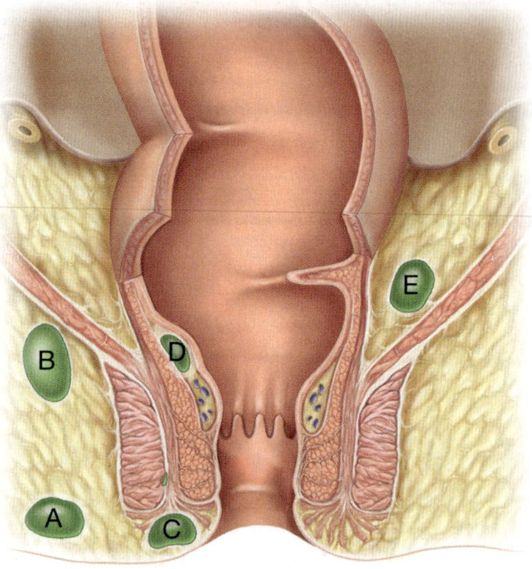

A. Perianal abscess
B. Perineal abscess
C. Ischiorectal abscess
D. Submucosal abscess
E. Perirectal/ supralevator abscess

Figure 19.3 Perianal abscess (*A*), perineal abscess (*B*), ischiorectal abscess (*C*), submucosal abscess (*D*), and perirectal/supralevator abscess (*E*).

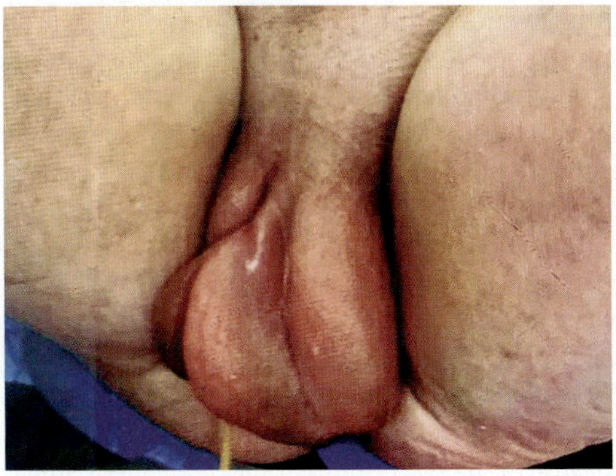

Figure 19.4 A perineal abscess.

sphincters (internal and external) and are contained at that level. This results in severe pain. In many case, only a digital rectal examination may identify the abscess in the anal canal. Anoscopy is useful in such cases.

An ischiorectal fossa abscess may extend to the opposite side as a "horseshoe abscess" (**Figure 19.5**). It develops in such a way by passing through the deep postanal space.

Supralevator abscess develops above the levator ani muscle. It occurs due to cranial extension of an intersphincteric abscess or caudal extension of rectal or colonic inflammatory disease.

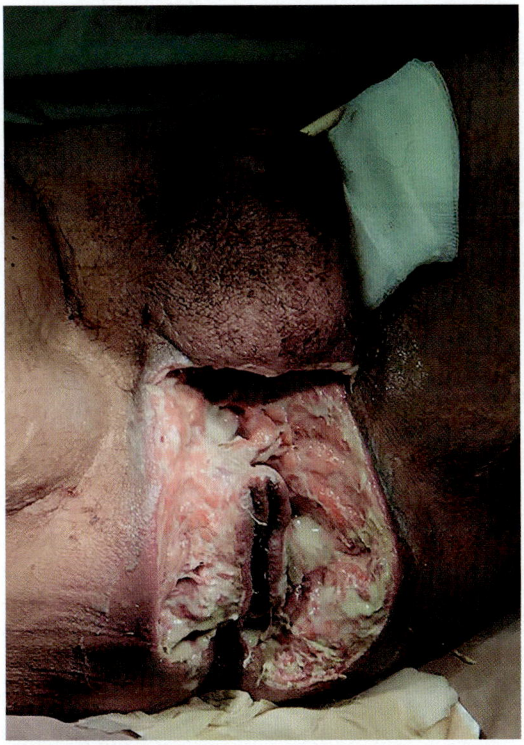

Figure 19.5 An ischiorectal abscess.

Assessment and Diagnosis

Collections of pus may lead to perianal pain, swelling, and discomfort. The symptoms develop within hours or days. They are aggravated by sitting, walking, coughing, or defecation. Intersphincteric or supralevator abscesses may be accompanied by severe rectal pain, dysuria, or acute urinary retention. Associated rectal bleeding has been reported (rarely). It is essential to note the anal incontinence score before and after any fistula surgery. Perianal abscesses are common and can vary from a small perianal abscess to large horseshoe perianal collections. Superficial cellulitis or even gangrenous skin lesions can be observed.

Inspection reveals erythema with a tender, fluctuant swelling. Due to an increased amount of fat in the perianal area, a fluctuant anorectal abscess may be more challenging to identify and assess. At times, a central orifice can be seen; pus can exit either spontaneously or with finger expression. Patients may complain of severe pain without the evident findings of an abscess; this may reflect a deeper infectious process. In this case, a careful rectal examination can reveal a protuberance or tenderness of the rectal wall, or pus may be found within the anal canal. A small intersphincteric abscess may be very painful and is sometimes confused with an acute anal fissure. A digital rectal examination should be performed to identify the infected anal crypt that led to an abscess, rectal inflammation, infection, or a perforated anorectal tumor. Examination under general anesthesia can help palpation of a small abscess within the intersphincteric space.

A fluctuant mass palpated during a digital rectal examination suggests an intersphincteric abscess. They develop between the internal and external anal sphincters; thus, no changes are observed outside the anal canal.

A perforated colonic tumor or diverticulum, or complicated Crohn disease may lead to a caudal migration of the infection, creating a supralevator abscess. This condition is rare. The main symptoms are severe perianal pain, fever, and often acute urinary retention. Clinical examination reveals no signs in the perianal area, but a digital rectal examination will identify a fluctuant area with inflammation, usually above the anal sphincter. Blood samples usually demonstrate leukocytosis.

In some instances, a CT scan may be helpful. Endoanal ultrasound is not well tolerated and therefore is not recommended. MRI is the method of choice in assessing an anal abscess and its relations with the sphincters and surrounding fat tissue. It can also assess a chronic evolution of an anal abscess toward a fistula, evaluation of a perforated Crohn disease or complex and recurrent fistula.

Treatment

The key to a successful surgery is immediate and adequate drainage of the abscess. Antibiotics alone may allow development of more complex lesions and delay the needed surgery. Complete resolution of an anal abscess without surgical treatment is highly unlikely. Patients should be informed about this situation. Extremely uncommon, a neglected anal abscess may lead to septic shock and, if untreated correctly, even death.

Perform an adequate incision under local, spinal, or general anesthesia in case of a perianal abscess. The goal is to obtain adequate drainage of pus and prevent early closure of the incision. Subsequent fistula development is prevented by an anal verge incision (as close as possible to the verge). Packing to control the bleeding and curettage should be avoided. If an internal fistula is noticed during surgical drainage of the anal abscess, it should be treated similar to a chronic abscess—incision and/or excision and local repair.

For intersphincteric abscesses, locoregional or general anesthesia is required to achieve adequate exposure. While palpating the intersphincteric abscess, utilize needle aspiration to confirm pus. Then, a longitudinal incision is performed by transecting the internal sphincter fibers along the abscess cavity. The incision should run between the lower end of the internal sphincter, dentate line, and the most superior part of the abscess cavity. Curettage is performed in the intersphincteric space to remove any trace of the infected anal gland.

A diffuse, ill-defined tender or fluctuant area within the buttocks may suggest an ischiorectal abscess or perirectal abscess and requires surgical treatment under spinal or general anesthesia. If the fistulous tract can be identified and catheterized easily, a drainage seton should be placed.

Establishing the origin of a supralevator abscess is the main goal as both the cause and resultant abscess must be treated. Supralevator abscess can occur as a cranial extension of an intersphincteric abscess or as a caudal extension of a pelvic abscess. If preoperative or intraoperative evaluation confirms extension into the perirectal supralevator space, the most cephalad septic cavities should be drained by dividing the levator muscle. A silicon tube is inserted and fixed to the skin with a stitch. After gentle curettage, the wounds are packed with a mesh dressing for 24-48 hours. A second stage will be required to treat the transsphincteric fistulous tract.

A perianal fistula with a pelvic abscess extending from the anal canal should not be drained into the rectum because it will result in an extrasphincteric fistula, which is a significantly more complex problem to solve. A pelvic abscess may originate from a perforated hollow viscus, such as acute perforated appendicitis, perforated diverticulitis, perforated fallopian abscess, or perforated Crohn disease. In this case, drain the abscess transabdominally.

For a posterior abscess, the primary opening is usually located in a crypt in the posterior midline. It is easy to identify when the pus can be seen draining from it. A probe should be passed into the tract of the deep postanal space to allow free drainage of pus. Immediate fistulotomy should not be undertaken because of the risk of unnecessary sphincter damage. Seton (vessel loop) drainage is placed to permit better drainage and allow easy identification of the tract at a later stage. In more complex abscesses with lateral and anterior extension, the abscess is drained by one or more separate round incisions on each side. Curettage is performed in the lateral extensions of the abscess, which are then drained and packed separately.

Some technical details are important: the incision should be performed close to the anal verge, thereby reducing the amount of tissue that might need to be transected in case of a fistula. The size of the catheter should match that of the abscess.

The wounds are dressed with dry gauze. The patient should bathe after each defecation and clean the wound initially at least once daily, and after a short hospital stay, the wound must be evaluated weekly until complete restoration.

Antibiotic therapy is essential for patients with comorbidities such as prosthetic cardiac valves, concomitant systemic illness, immunosuppression, or extensive local cellulitis. Incision and drainage of an anal abscess results in a fistula in 30% of cases; patients should be informed of this possibility. Anal sphincter continence can be affected due to an inappropriate transection of the external sphincter during incision and drainage. Prolonged packing of a drained abscess may damage continence by inhibiting the development of granulation tissue.

Perineal Necrotizing Fasciitis—Fournier Gangrene

Fournier gangrene is a severe life-threatening condition that develops as an acute severe infection of the skin and soft tissue in the anal and perianal areas (see Chapter 21: Necrotizing Soft Tissue Infections). An untreated infection such as anorectal abscess, genital infections, or skin infections may lead to this condition. The infection contains multiple pathogens and is likely to occur in immunosuppressed patients, morbid obesity, or patients with diabetes mellitus.

Despite advances in antibiotic therapy, surgical management, and supportive care, necrotizing fasciitis remains an aggressive infection, with multiple organisms, due to the synergistic action of anaerobes and aerobes. Fournier gangrene is associated with significant morbidity, organ failure, and high mortality. The high mortality is due in part to the aggressive nature of the infection and to the underlying comorbid disease present in these patients. The rapid progression makes expeditious diagnosis and treatment critical. The two most common pitfalls in management are failure of early diagnosis and inadequate surgical debridement.

These infections are often mistaken for cellulitis or innocent wound infections, and this leads to diagnostic delay. The many predisposing factors include diabetes mellitus, alcoholism, immunosuppression, renal and hepatic disease, vascular disease, and obesity. The main goals of successful treatment include early diagnosis, aggressive surgical debridement, antibiotics, and supportive intensive care unit treatment. Incision and drainage alone are inadequate treatment for necrotizing soft tissue infections (NSTIs); excisional debridement is mandatory. Hyperbaric oxygen therapy may be useful, but it has limited indications.

Survival is higher among patients who receive early aggressive surgical treatment. Although there are clinical practice guidelines, debate persists as to which antibiotics should be used and for how long, the timing of initial surgical therapy, and adjuvant therapies. Many factors can influence the outcome, such as age, the extent of necrosis, and comorbidities.

Assessment and Diagnosis

The main symptoms of Fournier gangrene are high fever and severe perineal pain. The perineal infection can involve skin, adipose tissue, muscles, and fascia. Gas-producing germs can be present; therefore, underlying crepitance can be palpated, while skin erythema, tenderness, or even gangrene may also be obvious initially. Necrotizing infections may be suggested by dark areas. This severe condition may be associated with septic shock and renal failure.

Clinical examination is the most important element in diagnosis—tenderness of abdominal wall or perineum, swelling at the buttocks or perineum, or skin necrosis. Often, inflammation begins with the appearance of a black spot, called Brodie sign (**Figure 19.6**). From this moment, the necrotic inflammation spreads briskly, moving along the fascial planes and extending into the surrounding areas (perineum, scrotum, hypogastrium, and at times affecting the region from the thigh up to the diaphragm), causing rapid deterioration of the patient.

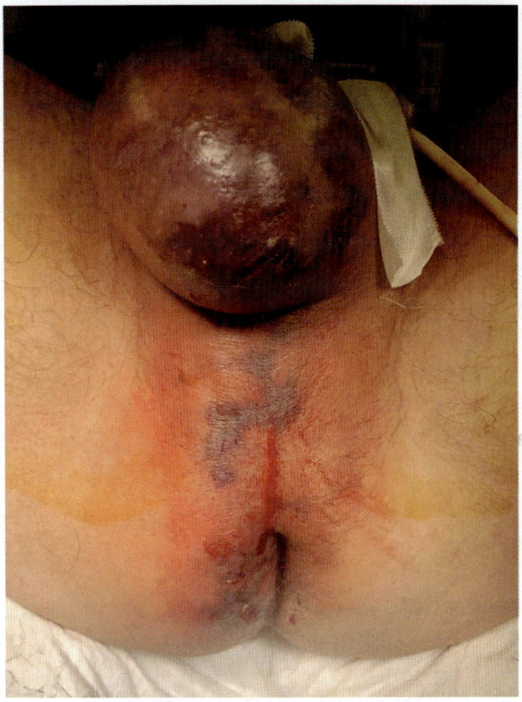

Figure 19.6 The black spot in Fournier gangrene—Brodie sign.

A diagnostic scoring system, the Laboratory Risk Indicator for Necrotizing Fasciitis (LRINEC), has been applied in the diagnosis of necrotizing fasciitis (**Table 19.1**). However, recent studies reported that an LRINEC score ≥6 was insensitive for diagnosis and only moderately specific. A score ≥8 increased the specificity but at reduced sensitivity. In addition, a low LRINEC score was insufficient to rule out the diagnosis. They cautioned that the score itself had poor diagnostic accuracy for NSTI.

Necrotizing soft tissue infections can involve the epidermis, dermis, subcutaneous tissue, fascia, and muscle and thus define the clinical forms of

TABLE 19.1 ■ Risk Groups According to LRINEC Criteria (NSTI: Necrotizing Soft Tissue Infection)

Risk Category	LRINEC Score, Points	Probability of NSTI, %
Low	<5	<50
Intermediate	6-7	50-75
High	>8	>75

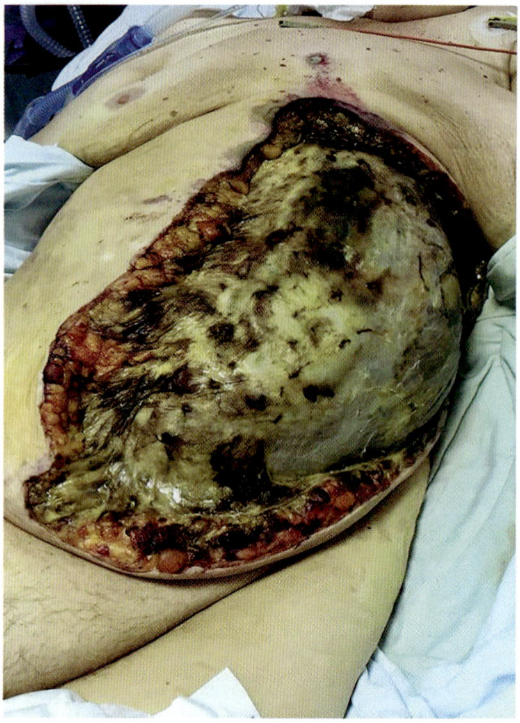

Figure 19.7 Severe necrotizing fasciitis.

fasciitis, myositis, and cellulitis (**Figure 19.7**). These infections are characterized clinically by systemic signs of toxicity and high mortality. Necrotizing infection may be categorized based on microbiology and presence or absence of gas in the tissues.

Rapid assessment may be done using CT scan of abdominal wall—which identifies the extent of the infection. However, imaging should not delay the initial debridement. NSTI is a diagnosis that is confirmed surgically, in the operating room, not by imaging.

Treatment

Necrotizing soft tissue infection is a surgical emergency, and surgical debridement of necrotic tissue is the treatment of choice. A planned reintervention is generally needed, with the aim of controlling the infection. Return to the operating room usually should be within 24 hours; earlier if concerns about adequacy of source control.

Early diagnosis followed by fluid resuscitation, aggressive surgery along with broad-spectrum IV antibiotics may decrease morbidity and mortality. A multiantibiotic regimen including a carbapenem or beta-lactam/beta-lactamase inhibitor (eg, piperacillin-tazobactam), clindamycin, and an anti-MRSA antibiotic (eg, vancomycin) should be used until cultures dictate otherwise. Accompanying coagulopathy, respiratory insufficiency, and renal failure must be aggressively treated. The best surgical treatment is sequential aggressive surgical debridement of necrotic tissue to stop the infection. Surgical treatment must be expeditious and aggressive consisting of extensive radical debridement until healthy tissue is encountered.

It is essential to realize that the preoperative skin changes can be minimal compared to the operative findings, which may demonstrate edema and necrosis of subcutaneous tissues, pus formation, and extensive necrosis of underlying fascia. Programmed reinterventions are necessary for complete debridement of necrotic tissue and also provides examination of tissue, wound, and dressing. A diverting colostomy to avoid wound contamination and facilitate perineal closure has been recommended by some authors. While still under debate, recent studies recommend colostomy in case of bowel perforation, sphincter incontinence, or in immunosuppressed patients.

Perineal reconstruction may be facilitated by vacuum-assisted closure, skin grafts, or (muscular, cutaneous, or myocutaneous) flaps.

Anal Fistula

A fistula is an abnormal connection between two epithelial-lined surfaces: anal fistula is an abnormal communication between rectum and anal canal with surrounding perianal skin, containing granulation connective tissue. The majority of fistulae are cryptoglandular in origin and are preceded by anorectal abscesses. Fistulae are often recurrent.

Assessment and Diagnosis

Anorectal fistula causes intermittent swelling, chronic purulent evacuation with skin irritation, pain, and even fever. Spontaneous rupture and drainage may lead to subjective clinical improvement, but this still requires surgical attention. More frequently, a fistula is seen as an orifice draining in the perineal area without acute discharge. Some patients have a long history resulting in the formation of several lateral secondary openings. In the absence of inflammation, palpation is painless. Digital examination is useful to identify the fibrous tract crossing the external sphincter and to palpate the anal crypt with fibrosis and retraction at the level of anal crypt.

Injection of air into the superficial lumen followed by the passage of air into the anal lumen is confirmed by digital perception of air bubbles or visualization by anoscopy. This technique identifies the anorectal opening and may dilate the fistula. Fistulography may be useful to identify the multiple tracts in selected cases of complicated fistulas. Endoanal ultrasonography is helpful to allow precise identification of any fistulous tracts and septic diverticula that may not be detected by palpation. Injection of hydrogen peroxide may be useful because as it enhances the contrast.

CT and especially magnetic resonance imaging have been used to establish the location of fistulous tracts. They provide precise information on high tracts with or about the extension to adjacent organs. The use of the contrast enhancement is recommended.

Goodsall rule predicts the fistula course by assessing the position of the perianal orifice: an imaginary horizontal line is drawn to divide the anus in two parts: anterior and posterior. An anterior orifice is suggestive of a short fistula that opens directly into anus. A posterior orifice suggests a longer and curved course that opens posteriorly, along the midline. There is also a correlation between the complexity of the fistula course and the distance in between anal orifice and fistula orifice: the longer the distance, the more complex the fistula.

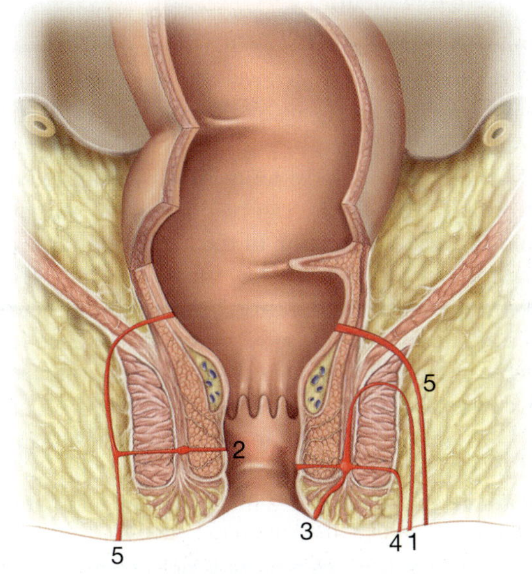

Figure 19.8 Types of fistulae: (*1*) suprasphincteric fistula, (*2*) transsphincteric fistula, (*3*) submucosal fistula, (*4*) intersphincteric fistula, and (*5*) extrasphincteric fistula.

Various classifications of anal fistulae have been described, but the most useful is that of Parks (**Figure 19.8**):

1. Intersphincteric:
   a. Simple low tract
   b. High blind tract
   c. High tract (with a rectal opening)
   d. Rectal opening (with no a perineal opening)
   e. Extrarectal extension
   f. Following pelvic disease
2. Transsphincteric:
   a. Uncomplicated
   b. High blind tract
3. Suprasphincteric:
   a. Uncomplicated
   b. High blind tract
4. Extrasphincteric are secondary to:
   a. Anal fistula
   b. Trauma
   c. Anorectal disease
   d. Pelvic inflammation

Treatment

Surgery is the main treatment for anal fistula. Surgery must achieve two goals: treat the fistula with preservation of continence and promote as little scar tissue formation as possible. Many surgical techniques have been described. The choice must be adapted to the course of the tract in relation to the sphincter. Even if continence is normal at the time of fistula operation, it can result in incontinence. Preoperative assessment of anal continence is essential.

Fistulotomy involves an incision of the fistulous tract along a probe and leaving it open. Fistulectomy consists of excision of the fistulous tract and granulation fibrous tissues that creates a larger wound, increasing the separation of the ends of the sphincter with a longer healing time and a higher risk of incontinence.

In case of perineal fistula, intersphincteric fistula or low transsphincteric fistula, fistula excision, or fistula transection can be easily performed. If the fistulous tract traverses the external sphincter, a lay-open technique or fistulotomy may result in some sphincter damage, depending on the amount of sphincter that is divided. After surgery for a fistulous tract, the wound is left open for healing by second intention. Wounds are irrigated or cleaned several times a day by a nurse during the hospital stay or by the patients themselves. Seton drainage allows restoration of the external wound with fibrous tissue connecting the external sphincter to the external fistulous tract.

Anal Fissure

Represents the most common cause of acute anal pain, also one of the most common benign anorectal conditions. It is a longitudinal rupture of anal mucosa or skin, below dentate line, overlying distal half of internal anal sphincter. Most anal fissures are solitary and occur in the posterior midline; only 10% occur in the anterior midline or atypical places. Atypical position or multiple sites should suggest a particular condition: inflammatory bowel disease, HIV, anal intercourse, malignancy, or tuberculosis. Multiple mechanisms has implicated in the development of anal fistula anal fistula development: trauma of the anal canal due to hard fecal mass leads to anal sphincter spasm; sometimes severe, ischemia of anal mucosa has been demonstrated in cadaveric specimens (leads to delayed healing); trauma during vaginal childbirth (due to indirect internal sphincter shearing); rare conditions like anal trauma, malignancy, anal finger dilatation, Crohn disease; infectious conditions like HIV, syphilis, or tuberculosis. Anal fissure can associate with a sentinel pile or a fissure-fistula complex can occur.

Assessment and Diagnosis

History of the disease is often suggestive for the diagnosis—excruciating anal pain after stool passage with or without minimal bleeding. Proper positioning of patient, followed by gentle retraction of buttocks and effacement of anal verge offers visual identification of the fissure. Rectal examination should be done with extreme gentleness due to the extremely painful condition. It can reveal the fissure location, number of fissures, a sentinel pile, or an infected fissure associated with a fistula. Anterior or atypical location should suggest associated pathology. Rectal examination can also assess internal sphincter function. Anoscopy is useful to exclude other pathology but should be done under anesthesia.

Treatment

Treatment can be classified into surgical and nonsurgical.

Nonsurgical treatment. Nonsurgical management includes the following measures:

- High-fiber diet to soften stool followed by adequate fluid intake.
- Sitz bath using warm water that may relief internal sphincter spasm.
- Local administration of ointments that may contain local anesthetics, calcium blockers, nitroglycerine, or other agents.
- Botulinum toxin injections to lower internal sphincter spasm that last up to 3-4 months. Healing rate is up to 60%-80% after 2 months of administration.

Among the agents used in ointments to help fissure healing, we mention:

- Nitroglycerin—as well as other nitrates (glyceryl trinitrate or isosorbide dinitrate) act as a vasodilator and improve local blood flow. Frequent side effects have been reported—most common being headache (up to 90% of patients). Many studies reported 70%-80% healing rate and a 50% decrease rate of recurrence (8 weeks of use).
- Calcium blockers—similar to diltiazem, nifedipine have been used with a healing rate of 88% (for diltiazem) and 94.5% (for nifedipine), but with more side effects for nifedipine. Both had less side effects compared to nitroglycerine. Oral nifedipine has lower healing rate and a higher side effects rate.
- Other agents used—bethanechol (with a healing rate of 60% without side effects), minoxidil (with a healing rate of 30%), and sildenafil (but without a good literature review for anal fissure treatment).

Surgical treatment. Surgical treatment is closed or open internal sphincterotomy. Both techniques have similar healing results, recurrence rate, and complications. It can be performed under any type of anesthesia, but local has a higher rate of recurrence. This procedure can be done in day surgery and involves transection of the lower one-third of the internal sphincter, below the dentate line. This technique has a 99% pain relief rate and a recurrence rate of 3%. Side effects are incontinence for flatus or feces, infections and fistula, hematoma, or ecchymosis.

Another surgical option along with sphincterotomy is excision of the fissure, but the complication rate and delayed healing should be taken into account.

Posterior sphincterotomy is not recommended due to a poor blood supply in that area and a higher risk of postoperative complications and recurrence.

Lord procedure (anal dilation or stretch)—still a favorite method among many surgeons—is done with two to four fingers and stretches both sphincters and leads pain relief and temporarily paralysis of sphincters.

Fissurectomy—can be combined with a stretching or a lateral sphincterotomy. This procedure has a higher healing time, up to 4-6 weeks.

Another surgical option is the V-Y mucosal advancement graft that has limited indications such as low-pressure sphincters where sphincterotomy has no indication or benefit.

Internal anal sphincterolysis—described by Gupta (2007)—requires a finger fracture of internal sphincter with a pain relief rate of 86%, healing rate of 91% at 4 weeks, and recurrence rate of 6%.

Retained Anorectal Foreign Bodies

After unsuccessful attempts to remove the retained foreign body at home, these patients will present to the emergency department, and many of them have rectal injury at presentation (**Figure 19.9**).

Assessment and Diagnosis

Obtain a plain x-ray of the abdomen and pelvis to assess the nature and position of the foreign object. This can also identify the presence of pneumoperitoneum, raising the diagnosis of hollow viscus perforation. A rectal examination can be performed to assess the size of the foreign body and possibility of bedside removal.

Treatment

Nonoperative management. In many cases, using a retractor, the retained foreign body (if it can be seen) can be removed at bedside in the emergency department (**Figure 19.9**). Blind grasping and attempted removal of the foreign body is not recommended because it can cause further mucosal bleeding and injury.

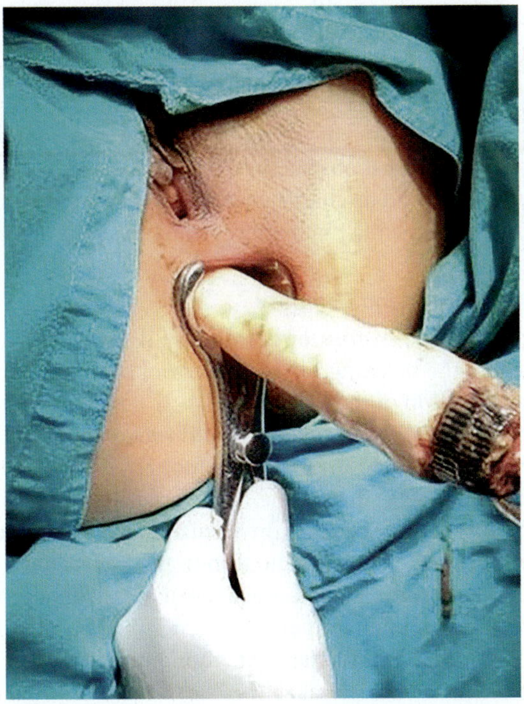

Figure 19.9 A retained foreign body.

Operative management. This is necessary for patients with sigmoid migrated retained objects or in patients with peritonitis. For the patient with a sigmoid migrated retained object, the object often can be grasped and removed under regional spinal anesthesia or general anesthesia with an anoscope. For large objects or objects that cannot be grasped under these conditions, a laparotomy is indicated. Milking the object distally is a safe method if possible. For a large object, colotomy might be required to extract the foreign body. A flexible or rigid proctoscopy should be done after object removal to assess mucosal injury.

For sharp objects such as glasses that can break during extraction or already broken inside rectum, a laparotomy is required. Removal of sharp objects with assessment of mucosal injury using rigid or flexible sigmoidoscope is mandatory. After assessment, a primary repair with or without loop colostomy can be performed.

BLEEDING EMERGENCIES

Bleeding Hemorrhoids With Vascular Fistulae

Hemorrhoids develop in up to 75% of adults at some time in their lives. Bleeding can occur as a complication.

Assessment and Diagnosis

Patients with bleeding hemorrhoids usually present with a history of bleeding for several days. Initial investigations include history taking, clinical examination that can reveal hemorrhoids with an active bleeding fistula, and blood samples that can reveal anemia. At presentation, the patient can be stable or unstable, with or without severe anemia. Most patients require operative treatment. Hemodynamically unstable patients with severe anemia require initial resuscitation followed by immediate surgery.

Treatment

After initial assessment and resuscitation, the patient should be sent to the OR. In the OR, bleeding should be controlled with minimal surgery (absorbable stitch or stitches) under anesthesia (local/spinal or general). Severe anemia should be corrected before discharge and a programmed operative management of hemorrhoids should be planned to prevent recurrences. Anticoagulant medication should be reassessed before discharge.

Thrombosed Hemorrhoids

This is another common complication of hemorrhoidal disease. It occurs due to a clot formation at the level of the external hemorrhoidal plexus.

Assessment and Diagnosis

The patient presents with severe pain, swelling, inflammation, and a very sensitive tumor in the perianal region (**Figure 19.10**). Initial investigations include history taking, clinical examination, and digital rectal examination if possible. Clinical examination should distinguish between a simple thrombosed external hemorrhoid and a prolapsed thrombosed internal hemorrhoid.

Treatment

Nonoperative management. General and local treatment is possible. General treatment is based on diosmin, with a regular dose (2 × 500 mg/day) to decrease bleeding and local pain and also prevent recurrences. Stool softeners, increased dietary fibers, increased liquid intake, warm baths, and analgesia are useful adjuncts. Local treatment includes different ointments. Recent studies suggest that ointments containing nifedipine have better results comparing to lidocaine ointments. Ointments should be used daily. If general and local treatment do not improve symptoms over several days, operative management should be considered.

If nonoperative management improves local conditions, then a delayed or elective surgery should be taken into consideration to prevent recurrences.

In case of a prolapsed thrombosed internal hemorrhoid, local treatment should be first: ointment and manual reduction of the prolapse to reduce pain and inflammation. Treatment includes diosmin, followed by nifedipine, lidocaine, and heparin ointment with regular medical clinical examination to assess for recurrence, necrosis, or resolution. Delayed or elective operative management should be considered.

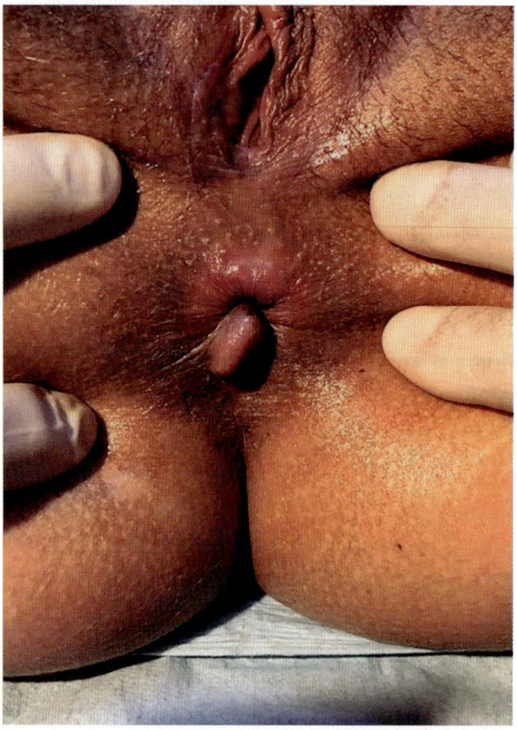

Figure 19.10 Thrombosed hemorrhoids.

Operative management. Operative management should be considered in severe cases: severe pain, nonresponse to oral and local medication, extreme inflammation, anal sphincter spasm or necrosis of the prolapsed mucosa. Operative management should be performed under local, spinal anesthesia (preferred due to better relaxation of anal sphincter) or general anesthesia.

Procedures include the following:

- A small incision with clot evacuation and an absorbable suture stitch to close the incision
- The Milligan-Morgan procedure—with removal of the thrombosed hemorrhoid
- Removal of the prolapsed thrombosed internal hemorrhoid with a mucosal absorbable suture

Bleeding Anorectal Tumor

Patients with local advanced anorectal tumors may present with one of the following common symptoms: intestinal obstruction, rectal bleeding, rectal pain, or rectal discharge. Bleeding tumors may lead to severe anemia that requires initial resuscitation.

Assessment and Diagnosis

A complete history of the disease is necessary to assess the bleeding history and stool changes with progression of the disease.

Clinical examination should include a digital rectal examination to assess tumor circumference, location, and if possible, size (length). Inguinal lymph node examination is mandatory. Flexible endoscopy can assess the tumor and provide palliative treatment. It can also be used to obtain a tumor specimen for pathology examination and to plan radiation therapy or chemotherapy.

Contrast-enhanced computed tomography will provide data about not only local extent of the tumor, local invasion of neighboring organs, but also distant metastases (peritoneal, hepatic, lung, lymphatic).

Pelvic MRI can also be used to assess the local extent of tumor and can provide more details compared to CT scan. Although endoanal sonography has appropriate specificity and sensitivity in evaluation of muscularis propria invasion, rectal wall and perirectal structure invasion, lymph node invasion, MRI has been proven superior in such evaluation.

Treatment

The main focus for advanced local rectal tumors should be symptom relief. Because surgical extirpation of local advanced tumors leads to increased postoperative disability, an experienced surgeon should assess tumor resectability. Contraindications to resection of locally advanced tumors include sciatic nerve pain, bilateral ureteral invasion with obstruction, fixation to lateral pelvic wall, venous thrombosis or lymphoedema (bilateral), multiple peritoneal or organ metastases (fixed to vital organs), or sacral involvement (above S2). Taking these conditions into account, treatment can be planned as operative or nonoperative.

Nonoperative management. Laser ablation has been successfully used in advanced rectal tumors where the main symptom is rectal bleeding. Coagulation is achieved in two to five sessions with a success rate of 80%-90%. The complication rate is low (2%-15%), mostly minor, but perforation that requires urgent laparotomy has been reported. Laser ablation does not improve survival, and further palliative therapy is required. This technique is low cost, minimally invasive, and offers acceptable results for high-risk patients.

Argon plasma coagulation is used in recent years due to its results on superficial diffuse bleeding. It has a low penetration (of 2-3 mm) compared with laser ablation; therefore, the risk of perforation is decreased. Due to superficial penetration, this technique cannot be used for obstructive tumors.

Chemotherapy has been demonstrated to provide symptomatic relief in 1-2 weeks after the initial dose but should not delay surgical treatment in cases with imminent obstruction or bleeding.

Radiotherapy is used in patients with advanced pelvic tumors involving pelvic nerves and bleeding. It has been proved effective in up to 75% of patients with a median survival of 6-9 months. This method does not improve survival and is used for patients with short life expectancy (6 months).

Operative management. Surgical options for bleeding are similar to those for obstruction. Despite large tumors, the setting of obstructive advanced rectal cancer, bleeding can occur in much smaller tumors; tumors that may be resectable—either through open or transanal excision. Transanal endoscopic surgery has been successfully used for such tumors. Surgery may not be curable but can relieve local symptoms.

OBSTRUCTIVE EMERGENCIES

Obstructive Anorectal Tumors

Many cases of local advanced anorectal tumors present as obstructive tumors (**Figure 19.11**).

Assessment and Diagnosis

Patients with obstructive anorectal tumors often present with a long history of stool modification, weight loss, anorectal bleeding, and in the immediate past days absence of stool and gas transit, onset of vomiting, and even fecaloid vomiting.

Clinical examination can identify a palpable mass in the lower abdomen and a distended abdominal wall. Auscultation of abdomen confirms the absence of intestinal sounds. Digital rectal examination can assess the anorectal tumor that cannot be overpassed. There may be associated bleeding.

A plain abdominal x-ray can be performed in lateral decubitus. Distended small bowel loops and large bowel loops can be observed. In case of an obstructive anorectal cancer, perforation may be at

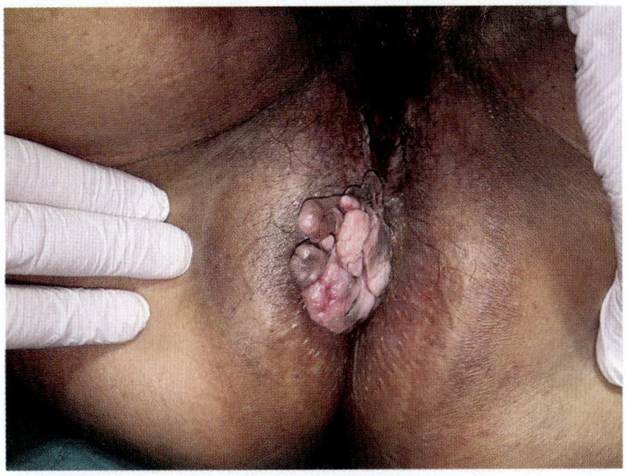

Figure 19.11 Obstructive rectal tumor.

the site of the tumor or more proximally (cecum); free air in the peritoneal cavity can be observed.

Abdominal ultrasound is easy to use and can be performed at bedside. Suggestive signs include distended intestinal loops without peristaltic movement, air-fluid levels in intestinal loops, peritoneal free fluid, or air in case of bowel perforation.

Computed tomography (contrast enhanced) can be used to determine the local extent of anorectal tumor, perforation (peritoneal free fluid and/or air in the peritoneal cavity), distant peritoneal, liver or lung metastases, their number and relationship to other structures. CT assessment of the tumor and its relationships locally should guide the surgeon's decision.

MRI is not often used in obstructive anorectal tumors but can provide useful details including the relation of the tumor to nearby organs and detection of pelvic invasion.

Treatment

Nonoperative management. For patients with obstructive local advanced anorectal tumor placing a self-expanding metallic stent is a viable option, either as a palliative measure in patients with widespread disease or as a bridge to relieve obstruction and ultimately allow a surgical resection.

Correct assessment is necessary to choose the most appropriate stent (based on length and location of tumor). These devices are well tolerated and can be placed under endoscopic or fluoroscopic guidance. Minimal sedation is required. Recent studies describe a success rate over 90% and relief of symptoms in 92%. Complication and mortality rates are lower than surgery. Failure includes inability to pass guidewire and stent-related complications such as bleeding, malposition, reobstruction, perforation, or stent migration. Perforation has a high morbidity. High-risk surgery is required in these patients.

Operative management. Preoperative assessment should guide the surgeon to decide on surgery with primary anastomosis or a colostomy or, in case of unresectable tumor, a diverting colostomy and palliative treatment.

For patients with obstructive locally advanced anorectal cancer, diverting colostomy is the method of choice. Loop colostomy can be performed laparoscopically or open. A tumor biopsy guides palliative treatment. Radiotherapy can be used as palliative treatment only or can be used as

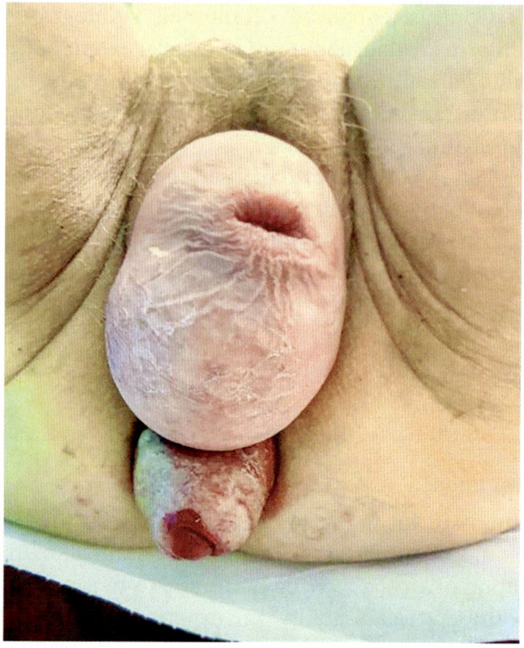

Figure 19.12 Rectal and uterine prolapse.

a tumor downstaging method to make it surgically amendable.

Primary resection of locally advanced rectal tumors can require extensive resection or pelvic exenteration. This surgery has a high rate of morbidity and mortality and does not significantly improve survival. Recent guidelines do not recommend such an approach in emergency cases. Elective surgery should be performed after initial resuscitation and complete evaluation of risks.

Obstructive Intussusception

Rectal intussusception is a telescoping of rectal wall during defecation that subsequently obstructs the rectal lumen (**Figures 19.12** to **19.15**). Urgent

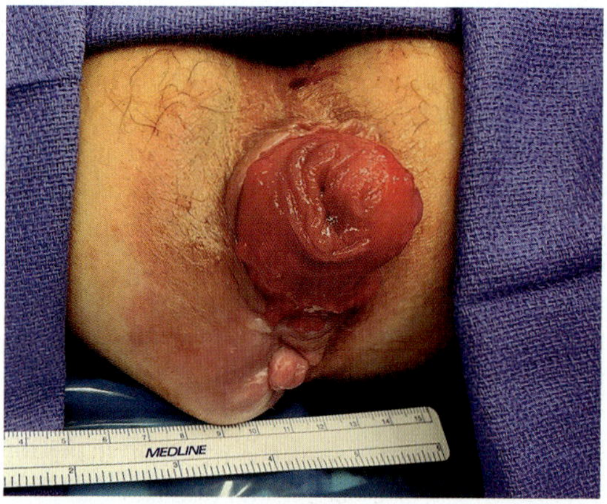

Figure 19.13 Rectal prolapse.

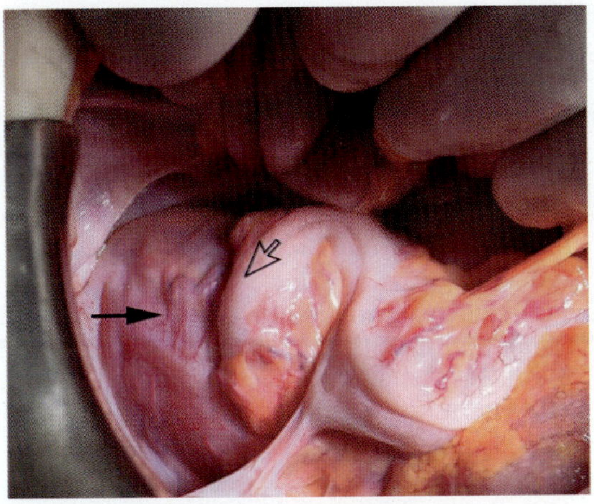

Figure 19.14 Intraoperative view of rectal intussusception (*black arrow*, rectum; *arrowhead*, sigmoid colon).

medical treatment remains the primary treatment. Urgent surgery is rarely needed.

Diagnosis and Assessment

Clinical examination can easily identify rectal prolapse or detect low-lying obstructive rectal lesions.

Clinical examination should note the appearance of the rectal intussusception (normal appearance, edema, ulceration, or necrosis), and a digital rectal examination should note the status of anus and surrounding tissue and test the anocutaneous reflex and anal sphincter tonus.

Proctoscopy should be performed to complete the assessment. Associated multiple lesions may include, to varying degrees, anal fissures, hemorrhoidal prolapse, rectal prolapse, rectal intussusception, rectal mucosal ulceration, edema, and in severe cases, necrosis.

Obstructive defecation is associated with rectal prolapse. Colonic transit time (assessed by wireless motility capsule or scintigraphy) can differentiate between slow colonic transit constipation and obstructive defecation.

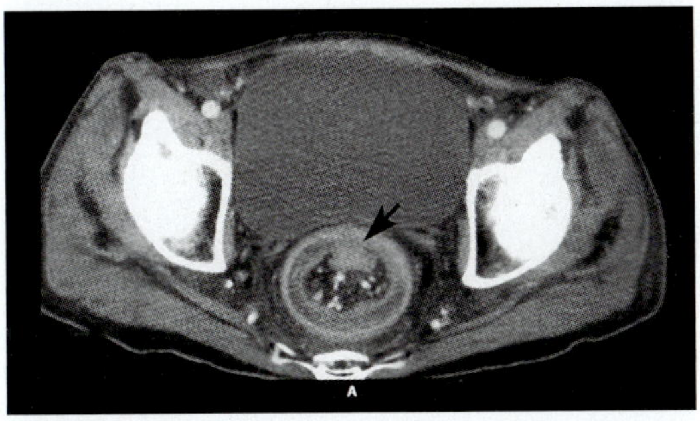

Figure 19.15 CT demonstration of rectal intussusception (*arrow*).

Anorectal manometry is essential for the diagnosis of obstructive defecation. Parameters for assessment include resting and squeezing pressure, rectal compliance, and assessment of internal and external sphincters.

Rectal balloon expulsion test may be used to assess anorectal coordination and can be performed single or in conjunction with anorectal manometry.

Evaluation of pelvic floor and anal sphincter tonus is by electromyography.

A more complex method to evaluate the region is by defecography or dynamic MRI defecography and is used for assessment how the rectum empties its contents.

Vaginal ultrasound can evaluate the anorectal region as an alternate to MRI defecography.

Treatment

Nonoperative management. Conservative medical management includes high-fiber diet, adequate hydration, and laxatives/enema in case of obstructive defecation. Patients can benefit also from electromyography biofeedback (at least two sessions). Almost two-third of patients who follow biofeedback electromyography respond and do not require surgery. Patients who fail this combination are directed for surgical treatment.

Operative management. Surgical treatment options include the Delorme transrectal mucosal excision (complete mucosal incision above the dentate line, resection of mucosa and plication of muscularis mucosae, and reanastomosis of mucosa), stapled transanal rectal resection (STARR or Longo procedure), and abdominal rectopexy.

SUMMARY

Perianal diseases can have a diverse spectrum of pathologies, which can result in significant morbidity with persistent symptoms. These conditions are common and can present with advanced disorder with the extent of the pathology may not reflecting the symptomatology. Differentiation of these conditions varies from benign pathology to cancer, disease that require conservative treatment with lifestyle change or surgical therapy. This chapter summarizes accepted evidence-based modern recommendations for the management of perianal abscess, anal fistula, anorectal trauma, foreign bodies, bleeding hemorrhoids with vascular fistulae or thrombosed hemorrhoids, bleeding anorectal tumor, or obstructive emergencies from an anorectal tumor or anorectal intussusception.

SUGGESTED READINGS

Beck DE, Steele ST, Wexner SD. *Fundamentals of Anorectal Surgery*. Springer; 2019.

Bevans DW, Westbrook KC, Thompson BW, et al. Perirectal abscess: a potentially fatal illness. *Am J Surg*. 1973;126:765-768.

Blaker K, Anandam JL. Functional disorders: rectoanal intussusception. *Clin Colon Rectal Surg*. 2017;30:5-11.

Bosarge PL, Como JJ, Fox N, et al. Management of penetrating extraperitonealrectal injuries, An Eastern Association for the Surgery of Trauma practice management guideline. *J Trauma Acute Care Surg*. 2016;80(3):546-551. doi:10.1097/TA.0000000000000953

Cameron JL, Cameron AM. The Management of Anorectal Abscess and Fistula, 2017. Current Surgical Therapy.

Chennamsetty A, Khourdaji I, Burks F, Killinger KA. Contemporary diagnosis and management of Fournier's gangrene. *Ther Adv Urol*. 2015;7(4):203-215.

Chowdri NA, Parray FQ. *Benign Anorectal Disorders—A Guide to Diagnosis and Management*. Springer; 2015.

Fabrizio AC, Alimi Y, Kumar AS. Methods of evaluation of anorectal causes of obstructed defecation. *Clin Colon Rectal Surg*. 2017;30:46-56.

Fajdic J, Bukovic D, Hrgovic Z, et al. Management of Fournier's gangrene. Report of 7 cases and review of the literature. *Eur J Med Res*. 2007;12:169-172.

Givel JC, Mortensen NJ, Roche B. *Anorectal and Colonic Disease: A Practical Guide to their Management*. Springer; 2010.

Gupta PJ. Internal anal sphincterolysis for chronic anal fissure: a prospective, clinical, and manometric study. *Am J Surg*. 2007;194(1):13-6. doi:10.1016/j.amjsurg.2006.11.020.

Jayne N, Stuto A. *Transanal Stapling Techniques for Anorectal Prolapse*. Springer; 2009.

Lee DK. *Practices of Anorectal Surgery*. Springer; 2019.

Ronnekleiv-Kelly SM, Kennedy GD. Management of stage IV rectal cancer: palliative options. *World J Gastroenterol*. 2011;17(7):835-847.

Schein M, Rogers PN, Leppaniemi A, Rossin D, Efron JE. *Schein's Common Sense Emergency Abdominal Surgery*. TFM Publishing Limited; 2016.

Wexner SD, Fleshman JW. *Colon and Rectal Surgery—Anorectal Operations*. Wolters Kluwer; 2018.

Zutshi M. *Anorectal Disease—Contemporary Management*. Springer; 2016.

CHAPTER

20 Vascular Emergencies

Alan Biloslavo, Marina Troian, Andrea Costanzi, and Michela Monteleone

CASE PRESENTATION

A 76-year-old Caucasian overweight male was referred to the emergency department with hematemesis and hypotension. His past medical history was remarkable for primary arterial hypertension, peptic ulcer disease treated endoscopically, previous sigmoidectomy for diverticular disease, and open surgical repair of an abdominal aortic aneurysm (AAA) 2 years earlier.

At the time of clinical evaluation, the patient had pale, clammy skin and an altered mental status (GCS 12). His heart rate was 125 beats/min, arrhythmic, with a blood pressure of 90/60 mm Hg. Blood tests showed anemia (hemoglobin 7.2 g/dL) and leukocytosis (white cell count 11 700/μL). The remainder of the labs, including electrolytes, renal function, coagulation, and liver enzymes, were normal. Abdominal examination was positive for tenderness in the upper quadrants, with no palpable masses.

After initial resuscitation, upper GI endoscopy was performed, showing a large amount of fresh blood in the stomach and duodenum, although no definitive source of bleeding could be identified. Despite massive blood transfusion and fluid resuscitation, the patient remained hemodynamically unstable. Therefore, about 3 hours after admission, the general surgeon on call performed an exploratory laparotomy. At the time of surgery, the duodenum and stomach appeared distended, without any free blood in the peritoneal cavity. A gastrotomy was performed along the greater curvature and fresh and clotted blood was drained. Still, no active source of bleeding was detected, and intraoperative upper GI endoscopy failed to provide additional information. The gastrotomy was closed followed by closure of the abdomen. Postoperatively, as the patient continued to have fresh bleeding through the nasogastric tube, a CT angiogram was performed. Imaging revealed a dense adhesion between the fourth part of the duodenum and the aortic graft, near the anastomosis (**Figure 20.1**). Enhanced blood in the duodenum suggested a communication between the aorta and the intestinal tract. The vascular team was consulted, and the patient returned to the operating room for a second exploratory laparotomy. After obtaining proximal and distal control of the aorta, the duodenum was carefully freed from the aorta; a 1-cm defect was identified in the duodenal wall. The graft was resected, the duodenal fistula was closed in two layers, and an axillobifemoral bypass procedure was performed. In the postoperative period, the patient developed severe sepsis and died on the 2nd postoperative day.

Question: *What would you consider in the differential diagnosis of a patient presenting in the emergency room for hematemesis and hypotension?*

Answer: *Bleeding peptic ulcer, bleeding esophageal varices, Mallory Weiss tear, Dielafoy lesion, bleeding gastric cancer.*

Question: *What is the classic triad of presentation of secondary aortoenteric fistula?*

Answer: *Gastrointestinal bleeding, abdominal pain, and sepsis.*

INTRODUCTION

General surgery has historically encompassed a wide variety of subspecialty procedures, especially in the emergency setting. However, the last decades have witnessed a shift toward increasingly subspecialized and focused training programs, potentially restricting younger surgeons' experience in the subspecialty procedures once usually associated with general surgery.

In this context, the separation of vascular surgery as an independent specialty from general surgery, as well as the ongoing centralization of vascular services to high-volume hospitals is of particular relevance for everyday clinical practice.

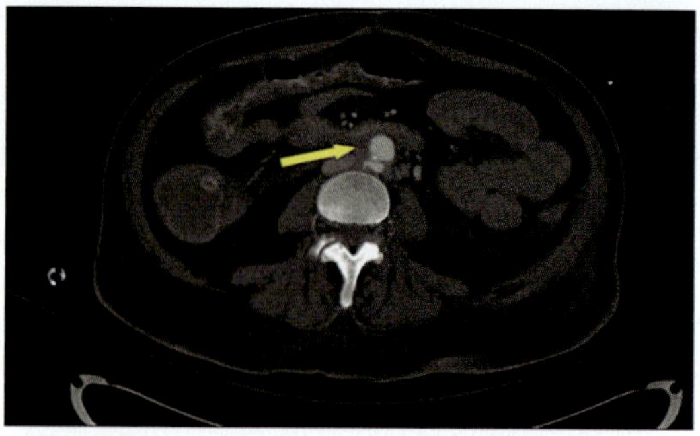

Figure 20.1 CT shows findings suggestive of an aortoenteric fistula. There is effacement of the fat plane between the aortic graft and the overlying 4th portion of the duodenum, with soft tissue thickening surrounding the graft (*yellow arrow*). (Reprinted from Chung J. Management of aortoenteric fistula. *Adv Surg* 2018;52:155-177, with permission from Elsevier.)

In addition, the recent advancements in new technologies and endovascular procedures have further narrowed the common ground between vascular and general surgeons. Of note, vascular surgical emergencies represent time-critical threats to life and/or limb, and their incidence is common among an ever-growing elderly population. This gives rise to a paradox where nonvascular surgeons no longer have the necessary skills to treat patients requiring either elective or emergency vascular procedures, but in many institutions, the general surgeons are the first line caring for patients who present with acute vascular conditions. The vascular surgeon is either not present or not readily available.

Although most cases allow time for urgent transfer to referral centers, at times, an immediate intervention may be required, as prompt recognition and treatment of the vascular condition can diminish the resultant morbidity and mortality. Indeed, delay in limb reperfusion increases the risk of amputation. In addition, for the patient with a ruptured abdominal aortic aneurysm, delay in treatment due to transfer time is a well-established predictor of mortality.

Because of the frequency of vascular emergencies in the general population, acute care and general surgeons will often be called to evaluate and manage patients referred to the emergency department with a vascular condition. Consequently, acute care and general surgeons still need to be adequately trained in order to be sufficiently skilled in the recognition and management of the most common vascular emergencies.

Among the various teaching strategies, simulation-based courses, cadaveric laboratories, and dedicated workshops are the most common training methods to improve knowledge of anatomy and operative skills. Although nothing can replace hands-on practice, the aim of this chapter is to provide the theoretical knowledge to deal with the most commonly encountered vascular emergencies, including ruptured aortic aneurysm and acute limb ischemia (ALI).

RUPTURED ABDOMINAL AORTIC ANEURYSM

Abdominal aortic aneurysm (AAA) is the most common form of true aneurysm, with an estimated 200 000 new cases diagnosed and more than 50 000 surgical procedures performed each year in the United States. AAA is usually located below the renal vessels. Thoracoabdominal aneurysms are less common.

Patients presenting with a ruptured AAA (rAAA) present a clinical challenge for everyone involved in their care. Ruptured AAA is often a lethal event, and mortality rates range up to 85%, with more than half of these patients dying before reaching the hospital. In the United States, rAAA accounts for about 15 000 deaths per year and represents the 13th cause of death overall.

Therefore, identification and treatment of the AAA is essential to reduce mortality from rAAA. Few other surgical emergencies derive more benefit from immediate diagnosis and treatment than rAAA.

General Principles

- The underlying cause of AAA is unknown in the majority of cases, and no specific mechanism has been found for its development. The most known risk factors for AAA are summarized in **Table 20.1**.
- According to the current literature, an AAA diameter of 5.5 cm or greater should be considered for surgical repair.
- The risk of rupture of small AAA is much higher in women than in men; thus, repair is recommended for a diameter ≥5 cm in women.
- Aneurysms of more than 6 cm have a rupture rate of ~10% per year.
- A rapid increase in size should be taken into account when evaluating the indication for elective surgical repair (ie, more than 0.7 cm in 6 months or 1 cm in a year).
- Only 30% of patients presenting to the emergency department for rAAA are previously known to have an aortic aneurysm.

TABLE 20.1 ■ Risk Factors for Abdominal Aortic Aneurysm

Risk Factor	Odds Ratio	95% CI
Increased risk		
• Smoking history	5.1	4.1-6.2
• Family history of	1.9	1.6-2.3
AAA	1.7	1.6-1.8
• Older age	1.5	1.4-1.7
• Coronary artery	1.4	1.3-1.6
disease	1.2	1.1-1.4
• High cholesterol	1.2	1.1-1.3
• COPD		
• Height (per 7 cm interval)		
Decreased risk		
• Abdominal imaging	0.8	0.7-0.9
within 5 y	0.7	0.5-0.8
• Deep venous	0.5	0.5-0.6
thrombosis	0.5	0.4-0.7
• Diabetes mellitus	0.2	0.1-0.5
• Black race		
• Female gender		

CI, confidence interval; COPD, chronic obstructive pulmonary disease; odds ratio indicates relative risk in comparison to patients without that risk factor.

Data from Lederle FA, Johnson GR, Wilson SE, et al. The aneurysm detection and management study program: validation cohort and final results. Aneurysm detection and management Veterans Affairs Cooperative Study Investigators. *Arch Intern Med*. 2000;160:1425.

- Approximately 10%-20% of patients with an infrarenal AAA have concurrent involvement of the common or internal iliac arteries.
- Aneurysms rupture most frequently through the left posterolateral aortic wall, but rupture into the abdominal cavity, the inferior vena cava (aorto-IVC fistula), or the gastrointestinal tract is described as well.
- The literature highlights better outcomes when patients are managed by vascular surgeons and treated by endovascular techniques.

Diagnosis

Diagnosis of a symptomatic AAA relies on an accurate medical history and physical examination, as well as a high index of suspicion. The diagnostic pathway will be tailored according to the patient's hemodynamic stability or instability. It is worth noting that clinical examination *per se* carries a sensitivity of 68% and a specificity of 75%.

One of the most common symptoms of rAAA is diffuse back or flank and/or abdominal pain. This can be associated with hypotension, shock, and the presence of a pulsatile mass (this triad is usually present in 50% of cases). However, presentation can be more subtle, with a latent appearance of symptoms. This is often the case when the rupture occurs into the retroperitoneum (in which case, bruising may be found in periumbilical, scrotal, leg, or flank areas), or when only a small leak is present. At clinical evaluation, checking the peripheral pulses is mandatory. Their absence may be explained by the presence of concomitant thromboembolic events.

The classical presentation of a rAAA remains an indication for proceeding directly to the operating room (OR). However, the ready availability of computerized tomography (CT), which not only has a near 100% diagnostic accuracy for this condition but also provides essential anatomical information for the potential deployment of an endovascular stent, makes this the first choice in most cases. A good-quality CT angiogram (CTA) is of paramount importance to properly assess the feasibility of endoluminal repair and graft sizing. However, taking a potentially unstable patient to the CT suite and delaying final treatment remain cause of concern and debate among clinicians. On the other hand, in 2004, Lloyd and colleagues demonstrated that only 13% of patients who died from rAAA did so within 2 hours of admission. Thus, it seems reasonable that patients with suspected rAAA and a systolic pressure above 80 mm Hg should be preoperatively investigated with CTA.

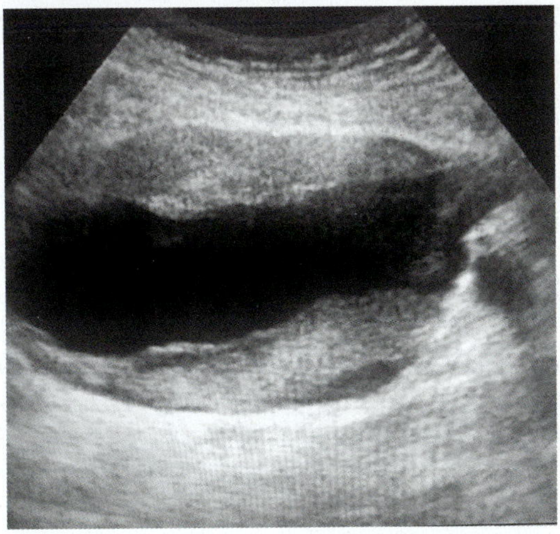

Figure 20.2 Longitudinal view of an abdominal aortic aneurysm on ultrasound.

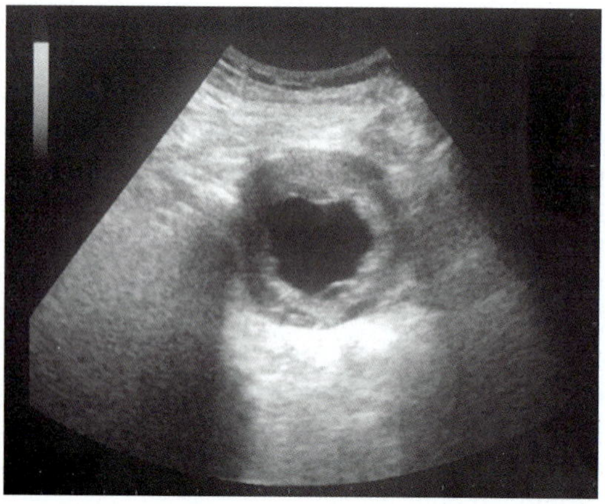

Figure 20.3 Transverse view of an abdominal aortic aneurysm on ultrasound.

Ultrasound (US) may also be a useful diagnostic tool and expedite the decision-making process. It is easy to use, can be performed at the bedside, and has a high sensitivity and specificity (both up to 100%) for detection of AAA and the presence of free fluid (**Figures 20.2 and 20.3**). However, its main pitfall is the inability to reliably define the relationship between the AAA and renal arteries—essential when considering the option of endovascular intervention.

Resuscitation

We suggest that each unit has a carefully designed, clinical protocol and pathway for the management of patients with rAAA that are tailored to local facilities and resources.

Preoperative resuscitation should follow the concept of "permissive hypotension," with the aim of maintaining consciousness and preventing ST changes on electrocardiography. A systolic blood pressure between 70 and 80 mm Hg is recommended to preserve adequate blood flow to the heart, brain, and lungs, until operative control of the bleeding can be obtained. However, in elderly patients, the goal systolic blood pressure may need to be higher. This goal is achieved by limiting fluid infusion and reducing blood pressure where necessary.

Standard perioperative care includes use of large-bore IV lines, central venous access, airway control, and urinary output monitoring by means of a bladder catheter. Perform arterial blood gas and blood sample examination including cross-matching, to ascertain the availability of blood products.

Surgical Treatment

The patient should be prepared in a standard fashion from the neck to knees and ideally draped prior to induction of anesthesia. Essential equipment includes straight and bifurcated 16- to 22-mm Dacron prostheses, vascular clamps (ie, Satinsky and DeBakey types), double-armed 3-0 Prolene sutures, retractors, and complete general and vascular surgery instrument sets.

When endovascular skills are available, a preoperative CTA can be obtained in most cases. Mehta and colleagues have reported a prospective analysis of the Albany Vascular Group standardized protocol for endovascular aneurysm repair (EVAR) of rAAA (**Figure 20.4**). According to this protocol, unstable patients went emergently to the OR for EVAR without preoperative CT imaging. The operating surgeon performed a femoral artery cut-down allowing the placement of a long (12- to 14-French) arterial sheath. A guidewire was then advanced into the juxtarenal aortic position, to perform an angiogram and support the placement of an aortic occlusion balloon, that could be inflated in case of persistent hemodynamic instability. This maneuver effectively replaced the standard open supraceliac aortic cross-clamping and permitted the anesthesiology team to resuscitate the patient. Subsequent technical improvements now allow a 7-French balloon catheter to be passed percutaneously into the femoral artery without the need for a cut-down.

Endoluminal balloons provide an alternative method to traditional atraumatic clamps. First described as Foley catheters deployed through the aneurysm, aortic occlusion catheter kits are now available that facilitate blind insertion and aortic control (although not recommended in case of patients with rAAA still in the emergency department).

Once the bleeding is controlled, perform an angiogram to evaluate the neck of the aneurysm and determine the feasibility of EVAR. Current commercially available endografts require a 10- to 15-mm proximal neck and a 20-mm iliac landing to complete the procedure successfully.

When the patient's anatomy is not suitable for EVAR, either an open or retroperitoneal approach is required, keeping in mind that the briefer the operation, the better the outcome.

A midline laparotomy provides exposure of the entire peritoneal cavity. A retroperitoneal approach can be employed if there is a known supraceliac extension of the aneurysm, a battle-scarred abdomen, or in patient with atypical anatomy (eg, horse-shoe kidney).

Once the peritoneal cavity is entered and the retroperitoneal hematoma identified, the first step is to obtain proximal vascular control. This can be

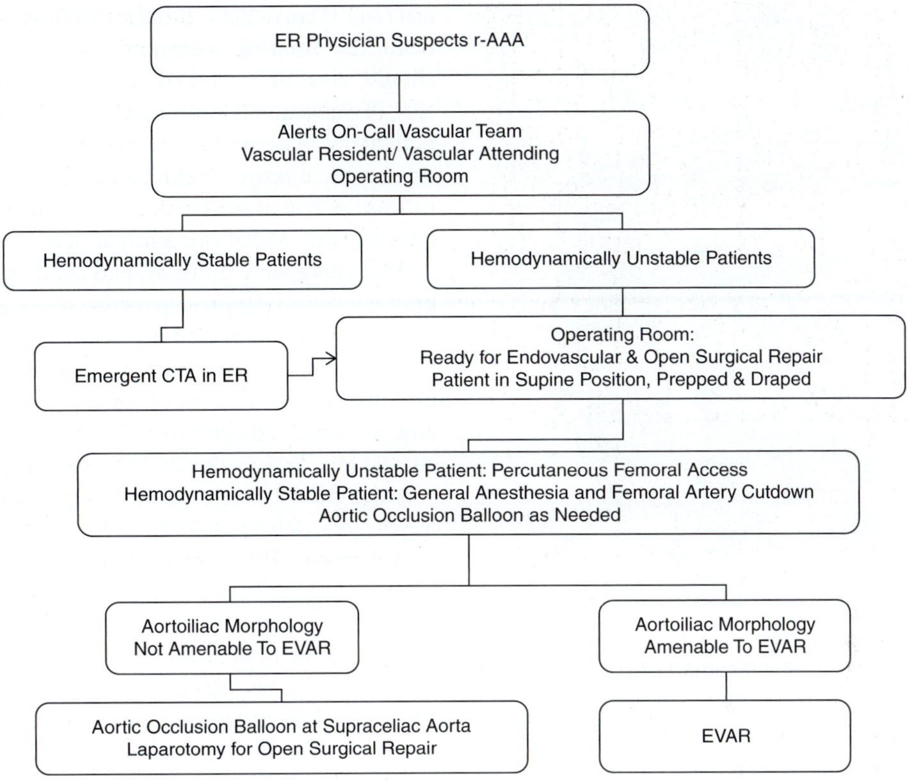

Figure 20.4 Albany Vascular Group standardized protocol for endovascular aneurysm repair (EVAR) of a ruptured abdominal aortic aneurysm (rAAA). BP, blood pressure; CTA, computed tomographic angiography; ER, emergency room. (Reprinted from Mehta M, Kreienberg PB, Roddy SP, et al. Ruptured abdominal aortic aneurysm: endovascular program development and results. *Semin Vasc Surg*. 2010;23:206-214, with permission from Elsevier.)

achieved by eviscerating the small bowel to the right and incising the retroperitoneum up to the left of the ligament of Treitz, until reaching the white and smooth surface of the aorta. If necessary, the ligament of Treitz can be divided (**Figure 20.5**).

Blunt dissection on both sides of the aorta is then performed with the index and middle finger of the right hand, until the renal vessels are visualized (remember that the left renal vein is posterior to the aorta in 5% of cases). Ideally, the neck of the rAAA is infrarenal. Although systemic anticoagulation prior to placement of the aortic clamp is routine in elective operations for AAA, this practice is controversial in the setting of a rAAA. Once adequate space is created, the clamp should be placed to achieve satisfactory bleeding control. Attention must be paid to the gonadal and inferior mesenteric veins, since an injury to these vessels worsens prognosis. In cases where an aortic balloon was previously positioned, remember to deflate and remove it before placement of the clamp.

When uncontrollable bleeding is encountered during dissection, or when the aneurysm extends above the renal vessels, this maneuver can be challenging and difficult to accomplish. In these cases, a good alternative option is the manual compression of the aorta against the spine, followed by the clamping of the subdiaphragmatic aorta through a space created by dividing the left triangular ligament of the liver and by opening the lesser sac. Caution is, however, required not to cause injury to the esophagus or the vagus nerve (remember to feel the gastric tube).

The distal extent of the aneurysm is assessed after dissection of the distal aorta. The aortic bifurcation and iliac arteries are assessed, as their status determines the choice of using either a bifurcated or a straight tube graft for the aortic replacement.

Once the distal aorta or iliac arteries are clamped, the aneurysm is opened longitudinally (**Figures 20.6 and 20.7**). The thrombus is removed from the aneurysmal sac, and the ostia of the lumbar arteries are oversewn with sutures placed from the inside (there are usually three pairs of lumbar

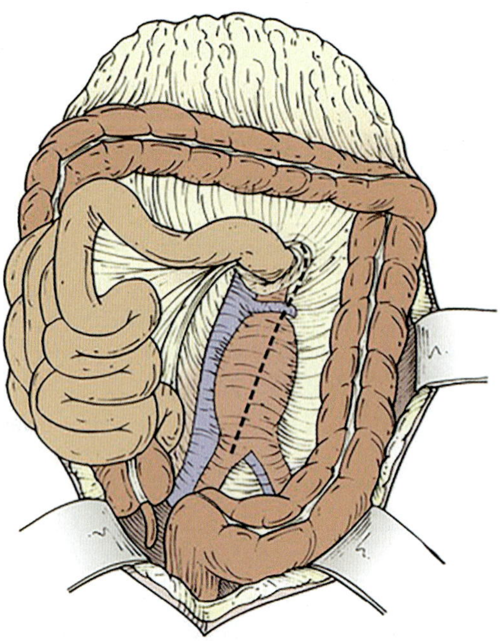

Figure 20.5 The small intestine is displaced cephalad to the patient's right. Left and sigmoid colon are retracted to the patient's left. The aorta is exposed by incising the posterior peritoneum overlying the aorta. (From Woo EY, Damrauer SM. Abdominal aortic aneurysms: open surgical treatment. In: Sidawy AN, Perler BA, eds. *Rutherford's Vascular Surgery and Endovascular Therapy*. 9th ed. Philadelphia, PA: Elsevier; 2019.)

arteries) (**Figure 20.8**). If back bleeding is detected from the inferior mesenteric artery, its orifice should also be occluded, keeping in mind the risk of subsequent bowel ischemia especially for patients with a previous bowel resection, superior mesenteric artery (SMA) occlusive lesion, or significant pelvic occlusive disease. Consider replantation of the IMA if the colon appears ischemic.

An adequately dimensioned synthetic Dacron graft is sewn to the proximal edge of the aorta with a running double-armed 3-0 Prolene suture. Once the proximal anastomosis is accomplished, the proximal clamp should be moved to the prosthesis and the distal anastomosis performed in a similar fashion. Before closing the distal anastomosis, it is mandatory to release the clamp to allow clearing of clots, debris, and air from within, to prevent embolization. This is particularly important when the patient is neither systemically nor peripherally heparinized (**Figure 20.9**).

If no leak is detected from the anastomoses, the aneurysm sac can be approximated over the graft, and the retroperitoneum should be closed whenever possible (**Figure 20.10**). When this is not feasible, a tongue of omentum is prepared and rotated to cover the aortic repair and prevent later fistulization to the bowel.

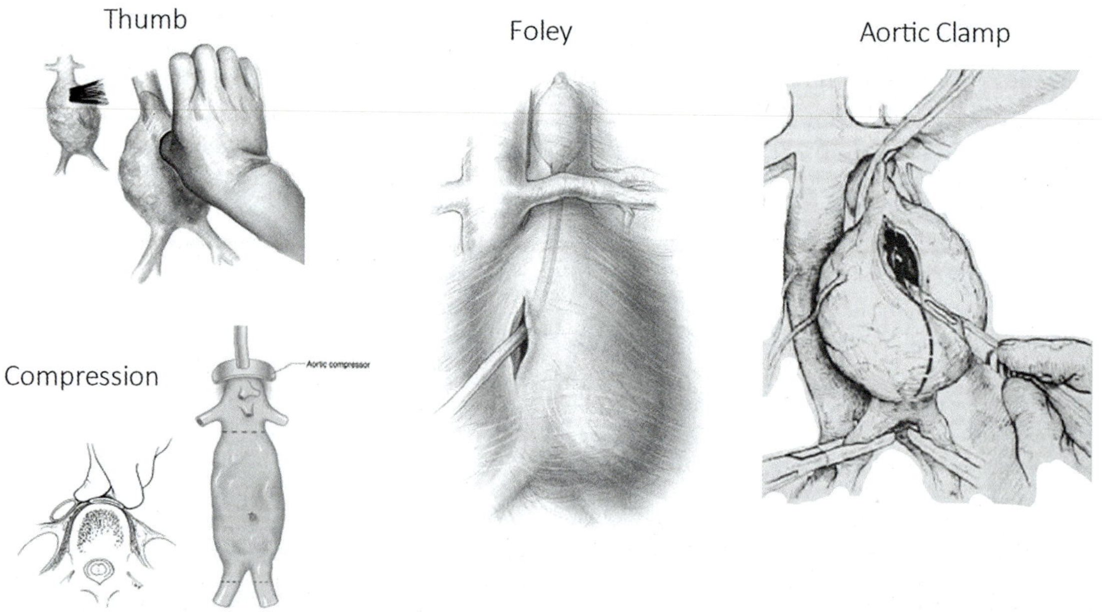

Figure 20.6 Options for proximal control of a ruptured abdominal aortic aneurysm. (Modified from Luis Filipe Pinheiro and Fischer JE. *Fischer's Mastery of Surgery*. 5th ed. Wolters Kluwer; 2007.)

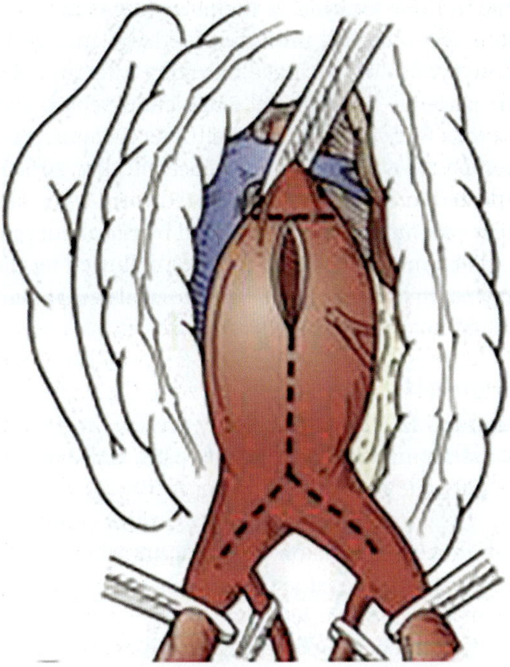

Figure 20.7 With proximal and distal control secured, the aneurysm is opened. (From Woo EY, Damrauer SM. Abdominal aortic aneurysms: open surgical treatment. In: Sidawy AN, Perler BA, eds. Rutherford's Vascular Surgery and Endovascular Therapy. 9th ed. Philadelphia, PA: Elsevier; 2019.)

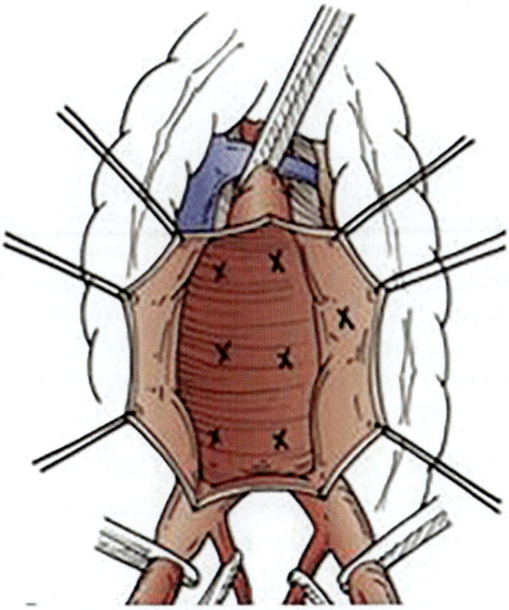

Figure 20.8 The lumbar arterial orifices are oversew from within the hernia sac. (From Woo EY, Damrauer SM. Abdominal aortic aneurysms: open surgical treatment. In: Sidawy AN, Perler BA, eds. *Rutherford's Vascular Surgery and Endovascular Therapy.* 9th ed. Philadelphia, PA: Elsevier; 2019.)

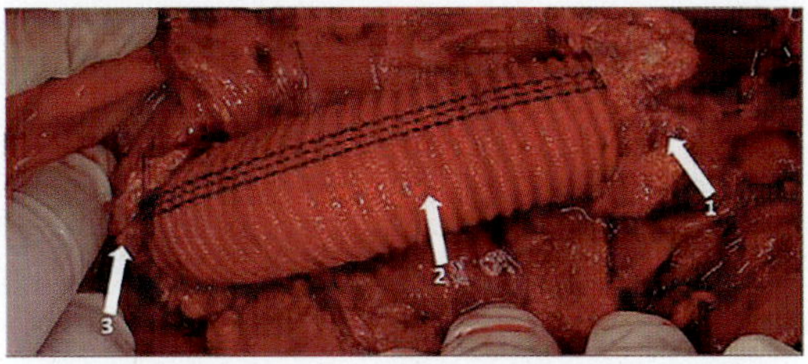

Figure 20.9 Aortoaortic Dacron interposition graft. Infrarenal aorta and proximal end-to-end anastomosis (*arrow 1*). Dacron graft (*arrow 2*). Terminal aorta and distal end-to-end anastomosis (*arrow 3*). (From Baila S, Parnia A, Panaite C, et al. Arterial bypass-a surgical method in treatment of peripheral arterial obstructive disease of the lower limbs. *Romanian J Cardiol*. 2015;25:158-169.)

When closing the abdomen, always remember that an abdominal compartment syndrome (ACS) is not rare in such patients, due to fluid shifts associated with aggressive resuscitation, bowel edema, and the presence of the hematoma. Indeed, about 50% of patients will exhibit an

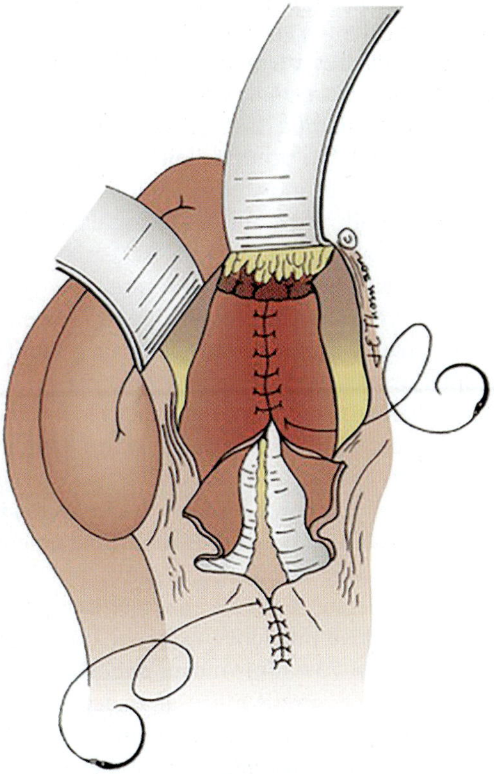

Figure 20.10 The aneurysm sac and posterior peritoneum are closed over the graft. (From Woo EY, Damrauer SM. Abdominal aortic aneurysms: open surgical treatment. In: Sidawy AN, Perler BA, eds. *Rutherford's Vascular Surgery and Endovascular Therapy*. 9th ed. Philadelphia, PA: Elsevier; 2019.)

elevated postoperative intra-abdominal pressure. Therefore, an open abdomen with delayed fascial closure should always be considered. In this context, it is worth noting that although EVAR has the obvious advantage of avoiding a laparotomy, it also carries a high risk of ACS (18%, mainly occurring in patients with preoperative hemodynamic instability).

Postoperative Measures

Mortality reaches up to 50%, and patients require careful monitoring in an intensive care unit (ICU). Primary end points of resuscitation include maintenance of a normal temperature, repletion of the coagulation system, as well as of correction of acidosis and electrolyte imbalance, optimization of the renal function, and hemodynamic normalization. Appropriate restoration of volume and use of blood products will optimize patient outcomes. Antibiotic prophylaxis can be continued for 24 hours after the end of the surgical procedure.

The physicians caring for these patients must be alert for the development of surgical complications including anastomotic leaks, bowel ischemia (especially colonic), and abdominal compartment syndrome. Bladder pressures should be measured routinely as a vital sign.

Colonic ischemia (see Chapter 12: Mesenteric Ischemia) can occur following elective aortic operations, but more commonly after surgery for rAAA (both open and endovascular repair). The risk of postoperative colonic ischemia is more common with aneurysmal rupture (5%-20%), hypotension, prolonged cross-clamp time, open vs endovascular repair, and improper management of the inferior mesenteric artery. Symptoms include bloody diarrhea, abdominal pain, and leukocytosis. Fifty percent of cases present within 24 hours postoperatively, nearly all within 7 days. Perform prompt flexible sigmoidoscopy when ischemic colitis is suspected. The finding of normal mucosa at sigmoidoscopy has 100% negative predictive value. If moderate to severe mucosal ischemia is seen, the positive predictive value for transmural necrosis is 55%-73%. This means endoscopy cannot differentiate severe mucosal ischemia alone from transmural necrosis. Laparotomy or laparoscopy is necessary to determine if colonic ischemia is transmural.

RUPTURED ILIAC ANEURYSM

As with AAA, iliac artery rupture occurs in the setting of preexisting iliac artery aneurysm (IAA). Due to their location in the pelvis, IAAs are usually not discovered until they are large enough to cause symptoms. Average mortality rates are 28% for patients undergoing emergency repair and 5% for elective cases. Isolated IAAs are quite rare (0.4%-1.9%), while a prevalence of 10%-20% is reported in case of IAA associated with AAA. The most common segment involved by the aneurysm is the common iliac artery (70%), followed by the internal iliac artery (20%), and contralateral aneurysmal involvement is reported.

Diagnosis

Ruptured IAA most frequently presents with sudden abdominal, groin, or thigh pain, and a palpable pulsatile mass. However, only 50% of patients are symptomatic before rupture. In this context, a high index of suspicion is paramount when examining patients. Bedside US imaging is a potentially useful tool for the detection of this form of vascular emergency. However, CTA remains the standard for diagnosis.

Surgical Treatment

Open repair is often the approach for ruptured IAA, because of profound hemodynamic instability. Recent trends and society guidelines support an endovascular approach as the preferred option where available and appropriate. Open elective repair may be preferred if compressive symptoms are caused by a large IAA, as this approach allows decompression of the aneurysmal sac. The sac generally should not be excised due to risk of injury to adjacent structures. In cases of common iliac artery involvement, the aneurysm should be repaired by interposition of a graft, but when confined to the internal iliac artery, an aneurysm can be dealt with by either interposition of a graft or ligation. If the contralateral internal iliac artery is not patent, restoration of flow should be the operative goal. Preservation of the pelvic arterial blood supply must be considered.

VISCERAL ARTERY ANEURYSMS

Ruptured visceral arteries are rare with a mortality ranging between 8.5% and 75% in literature depending on the artery involved. In most cases, the rupture results from an unrecognized preexisting aneurysm, and it represents a surgical emergency in 20%-70% of patients.

The visceral arteries most commonly involved include the splenic artery, the hepatic artery, the superior mesenteric artery, and the celiac artery.

Other sites include the renal and pancreaticoduodenal arteries.

Diagnosis

Prior to rupture, most patients are asymptomatic, and diagnosis is usually made incidentally. Clinical presentation depends on the pattern of rupture. A free rupture into the peritoneal cavity presents acutely with hypotension or shock. However, the most common symptom is pain. The detection of a palpable pulsatile mass depends on the location and size of the aneurysm. Other reported symptoms include gastrointestinal bleeding and hemobilia. Not uncommonly, the final diagnosis is made in the OR during emergency exploration of a patient with a hemoperitoneum. However, CTA is highly accurate in detecting ongoing bleeding and contrast extravasation can direct the surgery so every effort should be made to perform a CTA before an exploratory laparotomy whenever possible (**Figure 20.11**). An endovascular approach should always be considered particularly for a hemodynamically stable patient with a preoperative diagnosis. Patients with nonruptured but symptomatic aneurysms are diagnosed by CTA, US, or angiography.

The vast majority of ruptured visceral aneurysms are pseudoaneurysms, not true aneurysms. A visceral artery pseudoaneurysm should be treated, no matter the size.

Surgical Treatment

The surgical approach depends on the vessel involved and the overall physiological status of the

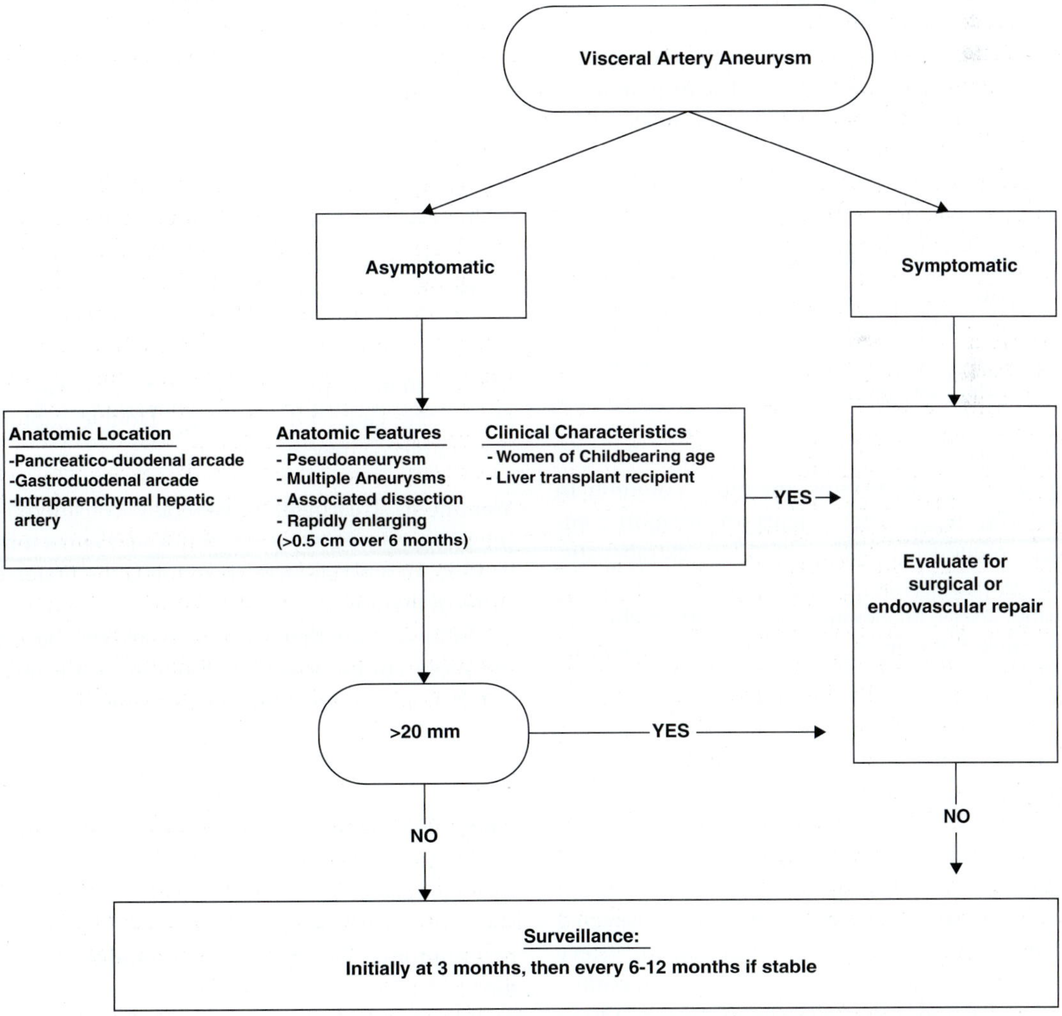

Figure 20.11 Approach to the management of visceral artery aneurysms. (Reprinted by permission from Springer: Springer Nature. Ibrahim F, Dunn J, Rundback J, et al. Visceral artery aneurysms: Diagnosis, surveillance, and treatment. *Curr Treat Options Cardiovasc Med*. 2018;20. https://doi.org/10.1007/s11936-018-0696-x.)

patient. Traditionally, treatment of ruptured visceral arteries consists of an open surgical approach with ligation and bypass or reconstruction of the vessel. When the rupture involves the splenic artery, proximal ligation and splenectomy may be performed. An endovascular approach should always be considered based on patient stability and local expertise.

Splenic Artery Aneurysms

Splenic artery aneurysm are more common in women than men, 4/1. Splenic artery aneurysms are generally true aneurysms and associated with pregnancy, medial fibrodysplasia, portal hypertension, post liver transplant, and pancreatitis. The majority are asymptomatic. They may present with vague abdominal discomfort or in extremis with severe left upper quadrant pain if freely ruptured. The patients may present with a "double rupture" where the initial bleeding contained in the lesser sac followed by free intraperitoneal rupture. Splenic artery rupture associated with pregnancy carries a 75% maternal and 95% fetal mortality.

Treatment. Treat a splenic artery aneurysm when >2 cm, in the pregnant patient, s/p liver transplant, or if symptomatic. Treatment options include aneurysm resection with interposition graft or primary anastomosis; splenectomy with excision of the aneurysm; percutaneous transcatheter embolization; or endovascular stent graft exclusion of splenic artery aneurysm.

Hepatic Artery Aneurysms

Hepatic artery aneurysms are more common in men (3/2). Hepatic artery aneurysms are more commonly pseudoaneurysms; most are extrahepatic, most commonly the common hepatic artery. Most hepatic artery aneurysms are asymptomatic but may cause right upper quadrant pain and epigastric pain or can produce free intraperitoneal hemorrhage. Large aneurysms of hepatic artery can cause obstructive jaundice. Hemobilia may result with rupture into a bile duct. A ruptured hepatic artery aneurysm carries 35% mortality.

Treatment. Treat a true hepatic aneurysm if larger than 2 cm or symptomatic. Intervene on all patients with a pseudoaneurysm or suspected inflammatory condition. Common hepatic artery aneurysms are generally treated with aneurysmorrhaphy, ligation, or aneurysm exclusion. Other treatment includes percutaneous transcatheter obliteration of the hepatic artery aneurysm with a balloon or embolization.

Superior Mesenteric Artery (SMA) Aneurysms

SMA aneurysms are the third most common visceral aneurysm. Mycotic aneurysms are the most common etiology—often in association with bacterial endocarditis. SMA aneurysms present with abdominal pain, nausea, vomiting, or gastrointestinal bleeding. Intestinal ischemia may produce hemodynamic instability.

Treatment. Repair true SMA aneurysms >2.5 cm; repair all SMA pseudoaneurysms. Aneurysm rupture is common with mortality rates from 30% to 90%. Ligation and aneurysmorrhaphy is the most common management. Aneurysmectomy or simple ligation of branches of the SMA aneurysm may necessitate intestinal revascularization (aorto-mesenteric bypass). Endovascular treatment is an option for certain SMA aneurysms (saccular) or in high-risk patients without infection, as is stent graft or obliteration by coils.

Celiac Artery Aneurysms

Celiac artery aneurysms account for 4% of visceral aneurysms.

Atherosclerosis/medial degeneration is the most common etiology, but they may be associated with spontaneous dissection. Celiac artery aneurysms are generally saccular, located in the distal trunk. Rupture occurs in 13% of the aneurysms with mortality up to 50%. Rupture results in life-threatening intra-abdominal hemorrhage but rarely may cause GI bleeding. "Double rupture" (herald bleed) may also occur.

Treatment. Treatment is generally considered if the aneurysm size is > 2.5 cm. Aneurysmectomy, ligation, or arterial reconstruction is the preferred surgical therapy.

Endovascular therapy of celiac artery is becoming more common with embolization, thrombin or ethanol injection, and stent placement.

Pancreaticoduodenal and Gastroduodenal Arteries

Aneurysms of the pancreaticoduodenal and gastroduodenal arteries are at higher risk of rupture compared to other splanchnic lesions, and should be addressed, regardless of the presence of symptoms. Pancreatitis is commonly the etiology of these visceral aneurysms. They are generally pseudoaneurysms, with an average size of only 1.27 cm when ruptured. They present with epigastric pain, emesis, hemoperitoneum, and shock.

Treatment. Treat all pancreaticoduodenal and gastroduodenal aneurysms. An endovascular approach is preferred if possible—coil embolization or thrombin injection. Open repair is by ligation, partial pancreatectomy, or pancreaticoduodenectomy.

AORTIC DISSECTION

Aortic dissection is the most common aortic catastrophe, accounting for 5-30 cases for every million people each year. The peak incidence is between the ages of 40 and 70 years. The high mortality results from insufficient tissue perfusion or from rupture of the aortic wall. Dissection may also arise in the setting of a preexisting aneurysm, but the term "dissecting aneurysm" is considered obsolete and not used in clinical settings.

From a pathophysiological point of view, the lesion begins at the level of the intimal layer with the formation of a tear and, subsequently, a flap. The systolic pressure forces blood into the flap and cleaves the intimal and medial layers of the aortic wall longitudinally, creating a separation of the vessel into a true lumen and a false lumen.

Various classification systems have been used to describe aortic dissection. Based on the duration of symptoms, aortic dissection can be divided into hyperacute (<24-hour duration), acute (2-7 days), subacute (8-30 days), and chronic (>30 days). Another classification is the DeBakey system, which is an anatomical description of the aortic dissection and categorizes the condition into three groups based on where the original intimal tear is located and how far it extends. Currently, however, the most commonly used system is the Stanford classification, which divides the patients into two groups (A and B) depending on whether the ascending aorta is involved or not (**Figure 20.12**). According to the Stanford system, type A aortic dissection involves the ascending aorta and/or aortic arch, and possibly the descending aorta. Type B involves the descending aorta or the arch, distal to the left subclavian artery, without involvement of the ascending aorta. This classification is particularly useful as it directs clinical management: type A dissection generally requires primary surgical treatment, whereas type B dissection may undergo successful nonoperative treatment. Indeed, type A dissections are reported to have a 91% mortality rate if not treated within a week. Type B dissections generally carry better outcomes, with most series reporting 85%-100% success rates.

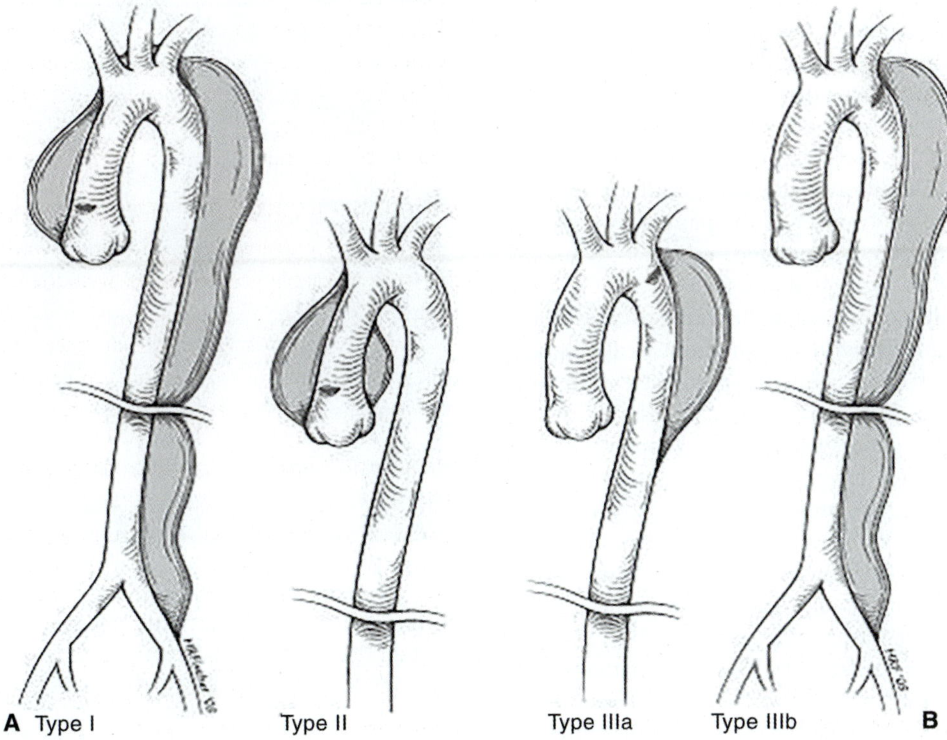

Figure 20.12 The Stanford and DeBakey classifications for aortic dissections. (From Mulholland MW. *Greenfield's Surgery*. 6th ed. Wolters Kluwer; 2017. Figure 85.9.)

Even though general surgeons are rarely called to deal with patients presenting with aortic dissection, they should be prepared to provide an immediate response to improve patient outcomes when a vascular surgery service is not readily available. Moreover, ischemic complications due to aortic dissection (ie, visceral and/or lower limb ischemia) are still generally managed by acute care and general surgeons.

Diagnosis

Most patients present to the emergency department complaining of sharp or tearing pain, with an abrupt onset that can be located at the thorax either anteriorly (Stanford type A) or in the back with radiation to the interscapular area or to the abdomen (Stanford type B).

Often patients arrive hypertensive and have a past medical history of chronic hypertension. Other presentations depend on the site of dissection and include myocardial infarction, pericardial tamponade, visceral and/or limb hypoperfusion (with possible discrepancies in pulse examination), and cerebrovascular ischemia.

CTA is the imaging modality of choice for suspected aortic dissection.

Treatment

When a Stanford type A aortic dissection is detected, urgent operative intervention by an expert team is required and replacement of the ascending aorta is considered the treatment of choice. When the diagnosis is made in a hospital without a readily available cardiothoracic surgeon, an immediate transfer of the patient to a specialized center is recommended.

Stanford type B dissections present a more favorable outcome, and patients are usually treated nonoperatively with maximal medical management, consisting of antihypertensive and anti-impulse medications. Surgical intervention is reserved for patients developing symptoms of poor perfusion (ie, lower extremity ischemia, acute renal failure, mesenteric ischemia, paralysis) or those with aneurysmal degeneration and rupture.

Thanks to recent technological advancements, the endovascular approach has become increasingly popular and, whenever feasible, it represents the treatment of choice for patients with aortic dissection. However, open repair, consisting of either a segmental aortic graft replacement or an open fenestration and excision of the intimal flap to restore a normal blood flow, is reserved for patients who are deemed not suitable for the minimally invasive technique or in case of ischemic complications.

AORTOENTERIC FISTULA

Life-threatening hemorrhage is the most common presentation when a fistulization of the aorta into viscera occurs. Most often, this results from the loss of the retroperitoneal plane between the aorta and the duodenum (involved in 75% of cases) (**Figure 20.13**).

Primary aortoenteric fistula (AEF) is associated with an AAA or IAA. Secondary AEF develops in patients who have undergone previous aortic surgery. The reported incidence is 1%-2% in patients who have previously undergone open AAA repair.

Diagnosis

The classic triad of secondary AEF comprises gastrointestinal bleeding, sepsis, and abdominal pain. Patients usually present with gastrointestinal

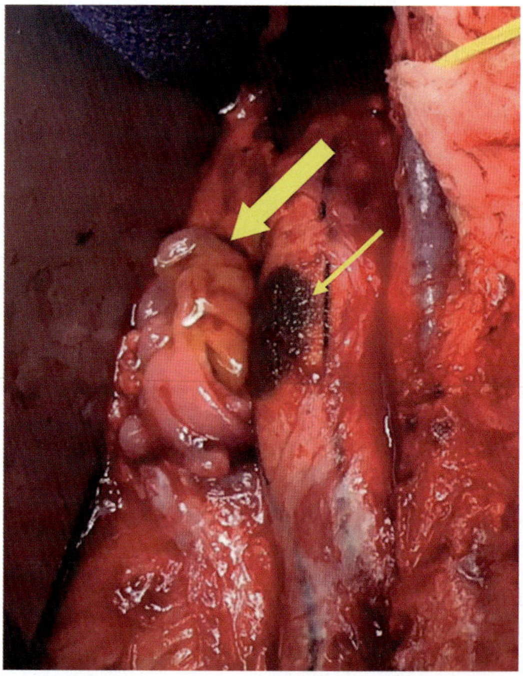

Figure 20.13 Aortoenteric fistula involving the body of an aortobifemoral graft, and the 4th portion of the duodenum. Note the dark stain on the graft (*thin yellow arrow*) indicative of exposure to bile. The adjacent bowel defect (*large yellow arrow*) was managed with resection and anastomosis. (Reprinted from Chung J. Management of aortoenteric fistula. *Adv Surg*. 2018;52:155-177, with permission from Elsevier.)

bleeding, with or without hemodynamic compromise, and have a previous history of AAA repair. In up to 50% of cases, there is graft infection, and the most commonly isolated bacteria are *Streptococcus, Escherichia coli* and *Staphylococcus aureus*. Pain and fever are also typical symptoms at presentation.

Esophagogastroduodenoscopy (EGD) may allow direct visualization of the fistula (diagnostic in ~30%) or another source for the GI bleeding, but other suggestive signs include duodenal compression by an extrinsic mass, mucosal ulceration and bleeding, and visualization of the prosthesis.

CT presents a diagnostic sensitivity and specificity of 94% and 85%, respectively. Other potentially useful diagnostic tools include aortography, nuclear scan, and colonoscopy.

Treatment

The main goal of treatment is to eradicate the infection while preserving the blood flow to target organs. Hemodynamically stable patients have time to be transferred to tertiary centers to be managed by a specialty team. In contrast, unstable bleeding patients require prompt surgical intervention. In these cases, emergent repair consists of graft excision and formation of an extra-anatomical bypass. (An endovascular stent as a temporizing bridge to future repair has been described.) The open procedure follows the same steps described for open repair of a rAAA. Proximal and distal vascular control allows the excision of the prosthesis. After repairing or resecting the involved viscera, an axillobifemoral bypass is constructed to restore extremity perfusion.

Mortality rates reach 50% and limb amputation is reported in up to 30% of cases when an extra-anatomical bypass is created.

Another key point in management of aortoduodenal fistula is reconstruction of the duodenum. Complications of the enteric repair carry high risk of morbidity and mortality. Based on the size of the defect in the duodenum, options include simple oversew, resection and anastomosis, and on occasion, pyloric exclusion. If resection is required, derotation of the small intestine with a side-to-side handsewn duodenojejunostomy widely separates the enteric anastomosis from the aortic suture line. Omental interposition between the aortic suture line and the intestine is also a critical step in the operation. Antibiotics are continued months postoperatively based on operative cultures.

ACUTE LOWER EXTREMITY ISCHEMIA

Most emergency vascular interventions are performed for arterial ischemia. Although the basic mechanism is always the same (ie, interruption of arterial blood flow), the potential causes are varied and include embolism, thrombosis, trauma, dissection, and inadequate cardiac function.

In 2007, the Transatlantic Intersociety Consensus Working Group redefined ALI as "any sudden decrease in limb perfusion causing a potential threat to limb viability." The incidence of ALI is reported to be 9-14 cases per 100 000 people, with a peak incidence in patients older than 90 years.

The most common cause is embolism (30%-40% of cases). It usually occurs in healthy arteries, and generally, the embolic source can be easily identified (eg, atrial fibrillation in 80%-90% of patients). Embolic ischemia produces an immediate arrest in the blood flow to the extremity and urgent vascular restoration is required. In this context, the introduction of the Fogarty embolectomy catheter has dramatically decreased mortality and limb loss.

Another common cause of ischemia is arterial thrombosis. This condition usually occurs in patients with preexisting chronic arterial disease of the lower extremities. However, it is worth noting that when an embolus overlaps a chronic situation stopping blood flow in an atherosclerotic artery, limb salvage rates are lower due to the difficulty encountered when performing the embolectomy.

Diagnosis

Acute lower extremities ischemia is still a clinical diagnosis and, irrespective of the cause, signs and symptoms are classically defined by the "6 P's":

- *Pain*: initially localized to the toes and feet, it is the most common symptom to be first reported by patients, usually continuous and of high intensity.
- *Paresthesia*: as ischemia progresses, paresthesia develops because of reduced perfusion to large sensory nerves.
- *Paralysis*: in the terminal phase of nerve hypoperfusion, motor nerves are involved resulting in loss of extension and flexion of toes, followed by loss of foot dorsiflexion and plantarflexion, to complete loss of passive movements. After 6-8 hours of acute ischemia, the muscles become rigid and contracted, and the limb may be considered unsalvageable.

- *Pallor*: the lower extremity appears pale, waxy, with absent capillary refill. At a late stage, pallor is replaced by cyanosis, indicating that limb recovery is highly unlikely.
- *Pulselessness*: absence of pulses appears to be the most important alerting sign in cases of suspected acute ischemia. However, they may not always be easy to detect (eg, diabetic foot, obese patients). Unilateral pulse deficit with normal contralateral palpable pulses suggests embolism, whereas bilateral pulse deficit usually results from atherosclerotic conditions. Indirect signs of thrombosis may be represented by thickened toenails.
- *Poikilothermia*: low skin temperature localized in the context of surrounding warm skin is a good predictor of ischemia.

Good clinical practice includes a careful physical examination, including complete evaluation of pulses and measurement of the ankle/brachial index (ABI). ABI < 0.8 suggests moderate to severe arterial disease. CTA is highly sensitive and specific in aiding the diagnosis. When the diagnosis is made, the severity of ischemia is graded according to Rutherford criteria (**Table 20.2**).

Treatment

The mainstay of treatment is to restore any circulating volume deficit and promptly initiate anticoagulant therapy to prevent clot propagation or further embolic events.

Arterial embolism is usually best treated by embolectomy, while arterial thrombosis may require more sophisticated vascular techniques, including endovascular approaches and thrombolysis. Patients presenting with an immediately threatened, but potentially viable, limb warrant expeditious surgical treatment.

When the limb is considered irreversibly damaged, the best option remains urgent amputation. Depending on local resources and individual experience, careful consideration should be given to whether to immediately treat the condition or transfer the patient to a specialized center. In the latter case, the patient should be started on systemic heparinization prior to transport.

Embolectomy is the most common vascular operation, applying basic techniques of vascular surgery. However, if balloon embolectomy fails, a vascular reconstruction or a bypass is indicated.

Before starting the procedure, particular attention must be paid to equipment preparation. The balloon catheters must be available in various sizes and checked for possible leaks by preemptive insufflation of saline. Availability of self-retaining retractors and clamps is mandatory.

The surgeon needs to have a basic anatomical knowledge of the arterial anatomy. In general, the aortic bifurcation is located at the level of the umbilicus, and the popliteal trifurcation is found ~10 cm below the knee. It is important to remember that the Fogarty catheter is marked with a centimetric scale; pay attention to the distances as the catheter advances within the artery.

All patients should receive full systemic heparinization while being prepared for the procedure. Sterile skin prep should extend from the xiphoid and include the entire limb.

A longitudinal or oblique skin incision is performed to obtain femoral artery exposure. The

TABLE 20.2 ■ Rutherford Criteria to Grade Extremity Ischemia

Category	Description	Prognosis	Sensory Loss	Motor Deficit	Arterial Doppler	Venous Doppler
I	Viable	No immediate threat	None	None	Audible	Audible
IIA	Marginally threatened	Salvageable if promptly treated	Minimal (toes) or none	None	Inaudible	Audible
IIB	Immediately threatened	Salvageable if immediately revascularized	More than toes, rest pain	Mild/ moderate	Inaudible	Audible
III	Irreversible	Major tissue loss, permanent nerve damage inevitable	Profound, anesthetic	Profound, paralysis (rigor)	Inaudible	Inaudible

Modified from Rutherford RB, et al. Recommended standards for reports dealing with lower extremity ischemia: revised version. *J Vasc Surg*. 1997;26:517-538.

artery usually lies approximatively two fingerbreadths lateral to the pubic tubercle, and the incision should begin above the inguinal ligament and continued through the fibers of the external oblique aponeurosis. Once the superficial fascia is opened, tributaries of the great saphenous vein are encountered and divided to facilitate arterial exposure. Avoid lymphatic injury. The deep fascia is then incised longitudinally and the common femoral artery will be noted. Sharp and blunt dissection on both side of the vessel are necessary to obtain optimal vascular control.

The dissection is then continued distally, and the femoral bifurcation is identified. The superficial and deep femoral arteries are isolated for vascular control. At this time, the patient should be given a bolus of heparin, and after waiting 3 minutes, a 15-mm arteriotomy is performed. The arteriotomy may be made transversely or longitudinally. Transverse arteriotomy over the bifurcation helps avoid narrowing the artery after closure. A longitudinal arteriotomy adds the advantage of facilitating an endarterectomy if a thrombus is suspected. The arteriotomy may be closed with a patch with any concern for narrowing the artery.

Typically, a 4- to 5-Fr Fogarty catheter is repeatedly passed proximally, until thrombotic clots are no longer retrieved. Attention should be paid during this maneuver because of the sudden gush of blood flow while releasing the proximal clamp. Heparinized saline is then injected, and the artery is reclamped.

A similar process is repeated for the distal limb, utilizing a 4-Fr catheter followed by a 3-Fr catheter as necessary, until an acceptable back flow is obtained. Avoid forcing the Fogarty catheter to advance or overinflating the balloon.

The goal is to "scrape" the balloon against the arterial wall without excessive force. A gentle traction parallel to the vessel axis is mandatory. Fluoroscopy and other adjunctive procedures may be required to retrieve clots that extend into the tibial vessels.

After a successful embolectomy, both limbs of the artery are flushed with 20 mL of heparinized warm saline. Finally, the arteriotomy is closed with a 5-0 Prolene running suture, catching the distal intima to prevent further dissection. Before completion of the intervention, an on-table angiogram is highly recommended, as unsuspected technical flaws are reported in 10% of cases.

The basic principles of embolectomy are the same also for upper extremity ischemia. In this case, the brachial artery is exposed by means of a medial incision performed at the middle-third of the arm, parallel to the biceps gutter. Once proximal and distal control is achieved, the arteriotomy is performed transversely.

Postoperative Measures and Four-Compartment Fasciotomy

Despite the advancements in surgical techniques and resuscitation, comorbidities of patients presenting with ALI add an intrinsic burden on the prognosis. Common complications related to surgery include hypotension, myocardial infarction, stroke, acute renal failure, infection, bleeding, compartment syndrome, and death. The limb must be frequently checked postoperatively for any changes. Indeed, amputation rate after a first successful revascularization attempt is reported in 15%-30% of cases.

Anticoagulation should be started with intravenous or low molecular weight heparin (LMWH) and then converted to oral anticoagulants that should not be discontinued until the primary source of embolism has been diagnosed and eradicated if possible. With persistent atrial fibrillation, anticoagulation is continued.

One of the most dreaded complications occurring in patients successfully revascularized is reperfusion syndrome. This condition is explained by the large load of myoglobin, free hemoglobin, creatine kinase, potassium, and lactic acid released from the venous system at the time of reperfusion. This leads to the development of acidosis, renal failure, and hyperkalemia, potentially causing life-threatening cardiac arrhythmias. The best way to avoid reperfusion syndrome is prompt restoration of blood flow and adequate systemic support with aggressive resuscitation. In selected cases, techniques to control reperfusion have been described. These are based on proximal femoral artery/vein occlusion, cannulation of the saphenous/femoral junction and superficial femoral artery, intra-arterial infusion of heparinized warm saline, retrieval of blood clots from the venous bed, ligation of the saphenous/femoral junction, and open clamp closure of the arteriotomy. However, the best way to prevent reperfusion syndrome is the restoration of blood flow as soon as possible.

Another challenging condition secondary to acute inflammation following reperfusion is compartment syndrome (CS). It usually develops after a prolonged delay in restoring blood flow. In this context, patients with more than 6 hours of ischemia prior to reperfusion need to be considered for preemptive fasciotomy. Typical signs and symptoms of CS include spontaneous and induced intense pain, paresthesia, tension, taut and bright skin, and absence of motor function. Evaluation and detection of peripheral pulses have low sensitivity in the diagnosis of CS.

These signs and symptoms are, however, difficult to assess in unconscious or sedated patients referred to critical care units. In these instances, the intracompartment pressure should be routinely and constantly measured, and fasciotomy is advocated when a muscle perfusion pressure (the difference between diastolic blood pressure and the intracompartment pressure) <30 mm Hg is detected. In case of doubt, the decision to perform a four-compartment fasciotomy should be based on the level of suspicion.

Performing an adequate fasciotomy is of utmost importance to reduce the complications related to CS. Proper placement of the incisions is essential (mark them), as well as knowledge of the main landmarks (ie, lateral malleolus and fibular head identify the course of the fibula). Here, we present a short description of the correct technique. Widely used during World War II, the two-incision (medial and lateral) four-compartment fasciotomy (**Figure 20.14**) is the standard treatment for decompression when more than one leg compartment is involved. The main anatomical concepts to remember are as follows:

- The anterior compartment contains the anterior tibial artery and vein and the deep peroneal nerve.
- The lateral compartment contains the superficial peroneal nerve.
- The superficial posterior compartment contains the soleus and gastrocnemius muscles.
- The deep posterior compartment contains the posterior tibial and peroneal vessels and the tibial nerve.

The lateral incision is made one fingerbreadth anterior and in front of the fibula, ~25-30 cm long, extending from two fingerbreadths below the head of the fibula to two fingerbreadths above the malleolus. Once the subcutaneous tissue is dissected, the intermuscular septum—dividing the anterior and lateral compartments—will be identified. The fascia is now classically open using an H-shaped incision. The crosspiece of the "H" is usually incised by using a scalpel and exposing in this way both the compartments and septum. Anterior and lateral compartments are then opened using scissors, 1 cm in front and behind the septum, respectively. Care should be taken to preserve the superficial peroneal nerve laying just below the fascia.

The medial incision is made one thumbbreadth posteriorly to the palpable medial edge of the tibia, for about 25-30 cm in length. Attention should be paid to the great saphenous vein. Once the fascia is exposed, it should be open from the tibial tuberos-

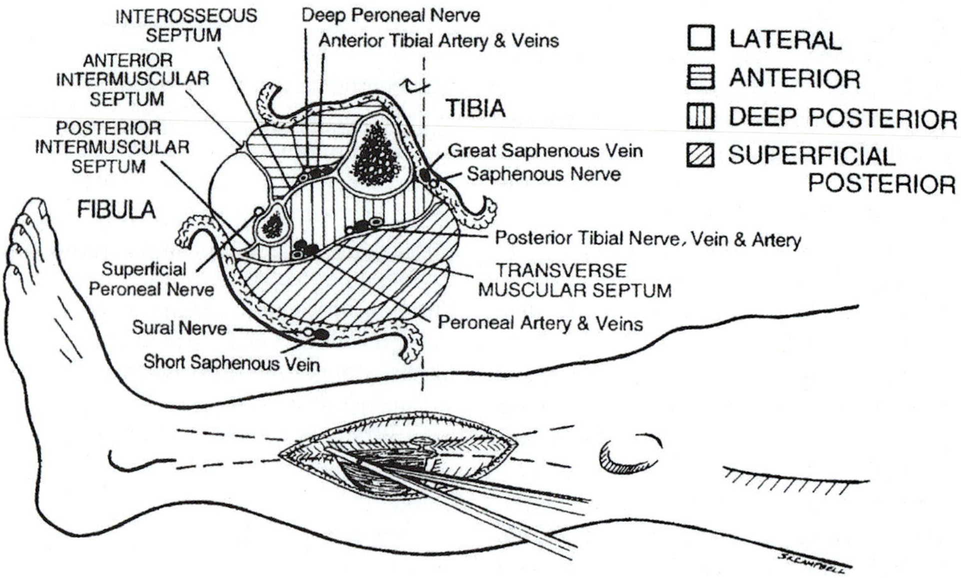

Figure 20.14 Surgical approach for four-compartment fasciotomy in the lower leg. (Reprinted from Ombrellaro MP , Steven SL . Compartment syndrome: a collective review. In: Maull KI , Cleveland HC , Feliciano DV , et al., eds. *Advances in Trauma and Critical Care*. Vol. 10. St. Louis, MO: Mosby—Year Book; 1995:100. Figure 2, with permission from Elsevier.)

ity to the medial malleolus using partially opened scissors. The soleus muscle needs to be separated from the medial edge of the tibia to ensure entry into the deep posterior compartment. The identification of the posterior tibial neurovascular bundle confirms the correctness of the maneuver.

Once the incisions are completed, each compartment should be assessed for muscle viability. Usually every 24-72 hours, the patient will be brought back to the operating room for reassessment and progressive gradual closure of the wounds.

SUMMARY

- Prompt identification and treatment of rAAA is of paramount importance, as mortality rates are high.
- Only 30% of patients with rAAA are previously known to have an aortic aneurysm, and in ~10%-20% of cases, there is concurrent involvement of iliac arteries.
- Whenever possible, patients suspected of having rAAA should have a preoperative CTA to plan appropriate treatment.
- EVAR should be considered for rAAA according to local expertise and resources.
- Bedside US has high specificity and sensitivity for detecting AAA and free fluid, but it cannot reliably determine the relationship between the AAA and renal arteries, which is essential when considering EVAR for an option.
- Aortic dissection is the most common aortic catastrophe, with high mortality rates due to either insufficient tissue perfusion or aortic rupture.
- CTA is the imaging of choice for aortic dissection and allows for classification of patient depending on whether the ascending aorta is involved (Stanford type A) or not (type B).
- Type A aortic dissection requires urgent surgical intervention by a cardiothoracic team, which may require immediate transfer to a specialized center.
- Type B aortic dissection can be managed nonoperatively, but complications may require surgical intervention (ie, distal malperfusion, aneurysmal degeneration, and rupture).
- Aortoenteric fistula is a rare but highly lethal condition, usually associated with AAA. However, it can also occur in patients with previous vascular surgery, and surgical intervention may require extensive vascular surgery skills.
- Acute limb ischemia is a relatively common vascular emergency, and it is most commonly caused by arterial embolism or thrombosis. The mainstay of treatment is to restore any circulating volume deficit and introduce anticoagulant therapy to prevent clot propagation or further embolic events.
- Peripheral arterial embolism is usually best treated by embolectomy, which does not require specific experience or highly specialized skills. However, in case of failure, vascular reconstruction and/or a bypass may be required.
- Peripheral arterial thrombosis usually occurs in arteriosclerotic vessels and may require specific vascular techniques, including endovascular and thrombolysis.
- When the limb is considered irreversibly damaged, the best option remains urgent amputation.

SUGGESTED READINGS

Acosta S, Wanhainen A, Björck M. The open abdomen in non-traumatic vascular emergencies. In: Coccolini F, Ivatury R, Sugrue M, Ansaloni L, eds. Open Abdomen. *Hot Topics in Acute Care Surgery and Trauma.* Cham: Springer; 2018. https://doi.org/10.1007/978-3-319-48072-5.

Ang ZH, Brown K, Rice M, Fisher D. Role of rural general surgeons in managing vascular surgical emergencies. *ANZ J Surg.* 2020;90(7-8):1364-1368.

Benzoni C, Benini B, Pirozzi C. Intestinal derotation in emergency surgery. *Eur J Trauma Emerg Surg.* 2010;36:495-498.

Boutros J, Sechon MS, Webber EM, Sidhu RS. Vascular surgery training, exposure, and knowledge during general surgery residency: implication for the future. *Am J Surg.* 2007;193:561-566.

Chaer RA, Abularrage CJ, Coleman DM, et al. Society for Vascular Surgery clinical practice guidelines on the management of visceral aneurysms. *J Vasc Surg.* 2020;72:3S-39S.

Chaikof EL, Dalman RL, Eskandari MK, et al. The Society for Vascular Surgery practice guidelines on the care of patients with an abdominal aortic aneurysm. *J Vasc Surg.* 2018;67:2-77.

Chopra A, Cieciura L, Modral JG, et al. Twenty-year experience with aorto-enteric fistula repair: GI complications predict mortality. *J Am Coll Surg.* 2017; 225:9-18.

Chung J. Management of aortoenteric fistula. *Adv Surg.* 2018;52:155-177.

Dos Santos CR, Casaca R, De Almeida JCM, et al. Enteric repair in aortoduodenal fistulas: a forgotten but often lethal player. *Ann Vasc Surg.* 2014;28:756-762.

Gahtan V, Costanza MJ. *Essentials of Vascular Surgery for the General Surgeon*. Springer New York, Heidelberg Dordrecht London; 2015.

Ibrahim F, Dunn J, Rundback J, et al. Visceral artery aneurysms: diagnosis, surveillance, and treatment. *Curr Treat Options Cardiovasc Med*. 2018;20(12):97. https://doi.org/10.1007/s11936-018-0696-x.

Jalalzadeh H, Indrakusuma R, Koelemay MJW, et al. Nationwide analysis of patients undergoing iliac artery aneurysm repair in the Netherlands. *Eur J Vasc Endovasc Surg*. 2020;60:49-55.

Mehta M, Kreienberg PB, Roddy SP. Ruptured abdominal aortic aneurysm: endovascular program development and result. *Semin Vasc Surg*. 2011;23:206-214.

Panagiotopoulou IG, Pilgrim S, Sengupta N, et al. What vascular skills do general surgery trainees need to learn? *Ann R Coll Surg Engl*. 2014;96:308-311.

Peitzman AB, Yealy DM, Fabian TC, et al. *The Trauma Manual: Trauma and Acute Care Surgery*. 5th ed. Wolters Kluwer; 2020.

Pereira BMT, Chiara O, Ramponi F, et al. WSES position paper on vascular emergency surgery. *World J Emerg Surg*. 2015;10:49.

Rehman ZU, Moosa MA, Riaz Q. Knowledge gain of the non-vascular surgeons after attending a course on traumatic vascular emergencies. *J Pak Med Assoc*. 2020;70(2 suppl 1):S6-S9.

Stewart B, Khanduri P, McCord C, et al. Global disease burden of conditions requiring emergency surgery. *Br J Surg*. 2014;101:e9-e22.

Wanhainen A, Verzini F, Van Herzeele I, et al. European Society for vascular surgery 2019 clinical practice guidelines on the management of aorto-iliac artery aneurysms. *Eur J Vasc Surg*. 2019;57:8-93.

CHAPTER

21 Necrotizing Soft Tissue Infections

Sharon Henry, Sonlee West, and Alexandra Briggs

CASE PRESENTATION

A 59-year-old man presented to his community emergency department (ED) with a history of fevers and shortness of breath. He reported a rash on his anterior leg for 10 days. The area became painful over the last 2 days. On evaluation in the ED, he had a temperature of 102 °C and erythema and woody induration of the calf. There were bullae noted over the calf. His vital signs were blood pressure (BP) 80/50 mm Hg and heart rate (HR) 96/min. Blood cultures were sent, and he was given multiple antibiotics, including vancomycin, clindamycin, doxycycline, and cefepime. He complained of chest pressure, and an electrocardiogram (EKG) showed ST-segment elevations. Cardiac catheterization demonstrated minimal left anterior descending disease. Computed tomography (CT) scan and magnetic resonance imaging (MRI) of the lower extremity were obtained. Edema of the tissues found on CT and MRI was thought to be compatible with cellulitis (**Figure 21.1A and B**). He was transferred to a tertiary referral center for further management on hospital day 3. On evaluation, his vital signs were normal with BP 108/64 mm Hg, HR 91/min, RR 34/min, T 38.2 °C, and oxygen (O_2) saturation 93% on 2-L nasal cannula. His labs demonstrated a white blood cell (WBC) 52 × 10^9 cells/L, hematocrit (Hct) 29.8%, hemoglobin (Hgb) 10.3 g/dL, blood urea nitrogen (BUN) 50 mg/dL (17.85 mmol/L), creatinine (Cr) 1.54 mg/dL (136.17 μmol/L), sodium (Na) 132 mmol/L, glucose (Glu) 100 mg/dL (5.55 mmol/L), C-reactive protein (CRP) 33.7 mg/dL (330 mg/L), erythrocyte sedimentation rate (ESR) 87/hour, and hemoglobin A1c (HbA1c) 6.3% (45.4 mmol/mol). His COVID-19 was negative as were his blood cultures. The calculated Laboratory Risk Indicator for Necrotizing Fasciitis (LRINEC) score was 10.

The right leg had dense dusky erythema circumferentially to the calf. There was purple-gray discoloration of the tissue over the ankle. There were ruptured bullae on the distal leg (**Figure 21.2A**). The erythema extended to the hip but was less diffuse proximally (**Figure 21.2B**).

Question: *Based upon the presentation and data in the following case scenario, what is the optimal management of this patient?*

Answer: *This patient has a presentation, laboratory findings and clinical exam consistent with a Necrotizing Soft Tissue Infection (NSTI). Prompt surgical debridement is indicated along with aggressive medical management with antibiotics and resuscitation.*

He was taken to the operating room urgently. Extensive necrosis of the subcutaneous tissue, superficial, and portions of the deep fascia was found on exploration. He was returned to the operating room again after 24 hours for a reevaluation of the wound. The wound measured 85 cm by 14 cm by 1 cm after maximal debridement (**Figure 21.3**). His hospital course was uncomplicated.

The WBC was slow to resolve but finally decreased to 12 x 10^9 cells/L after his initial debridement. He received hyperbaric oxygen treatments beginning on postoperative day (POD) 1. Initial treatment was 2-2.4 atmospheres absolute (ATA) for 120 minutes three times, followed by 2.0 ATA for 120 minutes twice daily for 10 treatments. His cultures grew Group A *Streptococcus* (GAS), and his antibiotics were de-escalated on POD 3. He received a 14-day course of antibiotics. He was discharged on hospital day 14 to acute rehabilitation. He returned weekly for dressing changes (**Figure 21.4**) and was readmitted at 4 weeks and underwent split-thickness skin grafting (STSG) (**Figure 21.5**). He has required readmission with cellulitis twice in 6 months since his discharge but is now home with family.

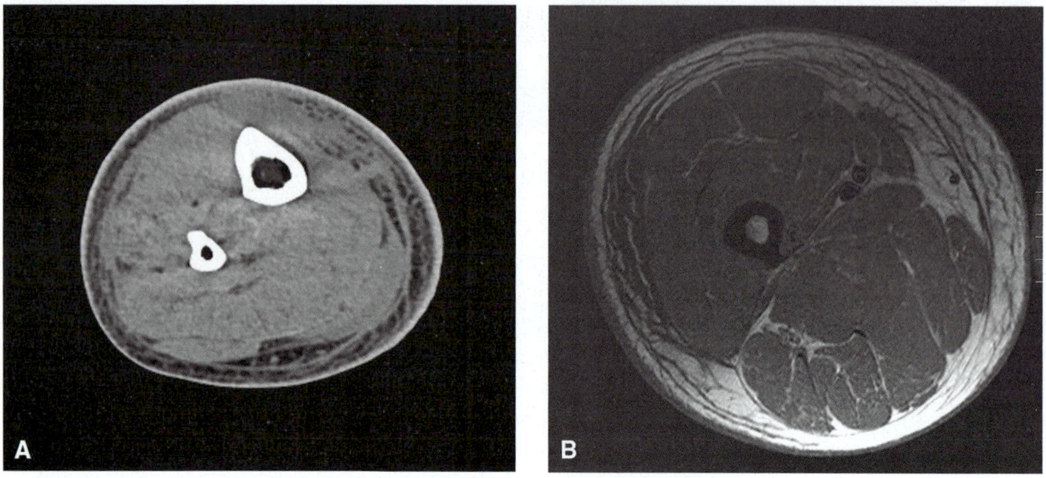

Figure 21.1 **A.** CT scan from the day of presentation. Evidence of edema in the subcutaneous tissue. No fascial thickening fluid or air. Read as compatible with cellulitis. **B.** MRI diffuse abnormal signal throughout the subcutaneous fat of the entire thigh, leg, foot, and ankle compatible with diffuse cellulitis.

INTRODUCTION

Necrotizing soft tissue infections (NSTI) are characterized as rapidly advancing, potentially fatal infections involving the dermis, subcutaneous tissue, fascia, or muscle. They may affect any part of the body and have multiple causes, risk factors, and pathogenic mechanisms, but all result in widespread tissue destruction.

Historically, necrotizing soft tissue infections have been recognized since the time of Hippocrates. They were first defined as such by Jones in 1871 over a century ago. Numerous terms have been used to describe NSTIs. Wilson introduced the term necrotizing fasciitis in 1951. The term NSTI has now predominately replaced necrotizing fasciitis as the preferred term as it is inclusive of all

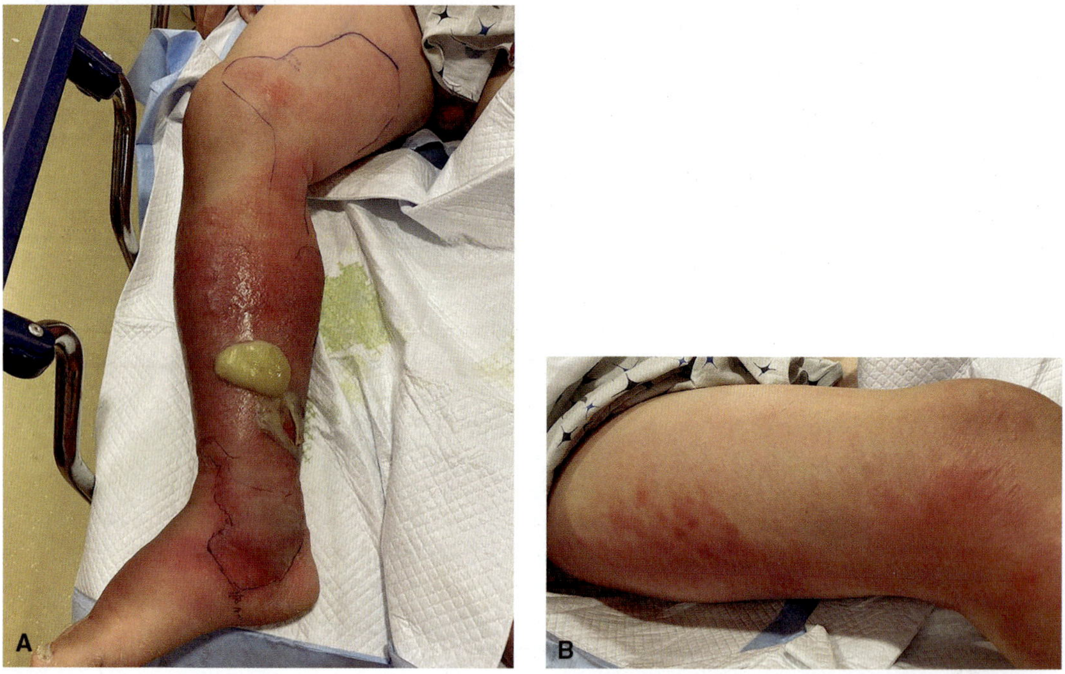

Figure 21.2 **A.** Photograph of the right leg taken the day of transfer to tertiary care and 3 days after admission to index hospital. There is diffuse swelling with brawny erythema. A ruptured and partially intact blister on the medial calf are seen. The swelling is tense, and the erythema is not sharply demarcated. **B.** Photograph of the right leg taken the same time as **(A)** showing the lateral thigh and knee. There is erythema without blistering.

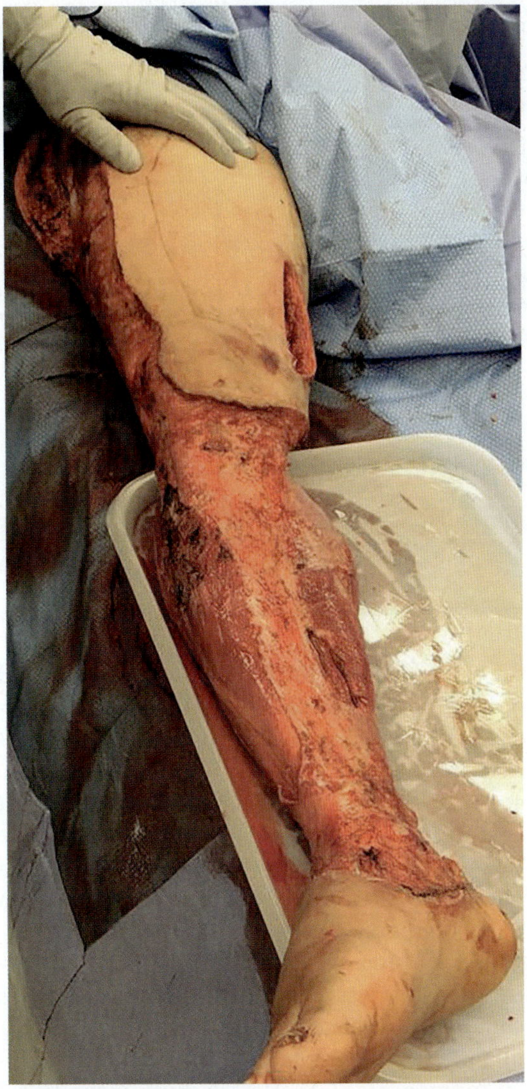

Figure 21.3 Intraoperative image of the right leg after debridement. Note the extensive resection of skin and subcutaneous fat portions of deep fascia. Medial thigh exploratory wound.

diagnoses since the management requires a similar approach regardless of the anatomic location or depth of involvement.

EPIDEMIOLOGY

NSTIs are rare, with an estimated incidence that ranges from 8 to 10 cases per 100 000 population

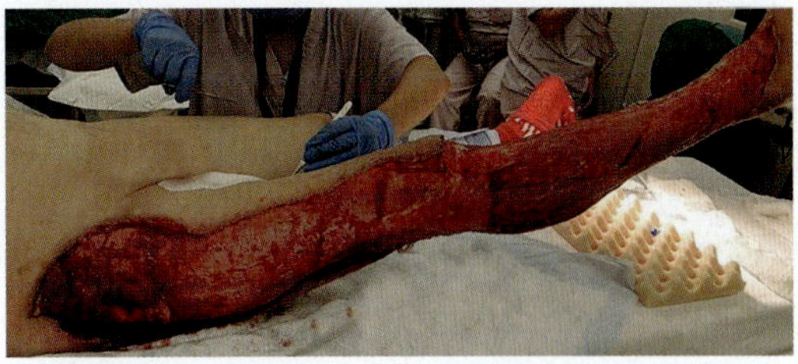

Figure 21.4 Dressing change performed in the operating room 26 days after admission. The wound is clean with viable wound bed. STSG performed.

in the United States but lower rates internationally. The incidence has increased, although mortality rates have mainly improved. The increased prevalence is likely multifactorial with greater awareness of the condition, rising use of immunosuppression, and increasing incidence of obesity and diabetes as recognized associations. In early reports, mortality ranged from 46% to 76%. Contemporary reports state mortality ranges from 10% to 30%, depending on the causative agent and associated factors. In 67 studies that included over 3000 patients from 1980 to 2008, the overall mortality was 23.5%. Improvements in outcomes continue to require early diagnosis, early and aggressive surgical debridement, early administration of appropriate empiric antibiotics, and optimization of underlying comorbidities.

PATHOPHYSIOLOGY

NSTIs develop when microbes gain access to subcutaneous tissues and can replicate, injure tissue, and travel along fascial planes. **Figure 21.6** illustrates the level of involvement of necrotizing and nonnecrotizing infections. Tissue destruction can be massive. There are host and pathogen factors that lead to the development of these infections. The inoculum of the microbe must overwhelm the host response to generate infection. NSTI, unlike uncomplicated soft tissue infection, generates tissue destruction rather than localized purulence. Pathogens produce toxins that cause local tissue necrosis creating an environment for replication. Toxins also facilitate the loss of tissue adhesion allowing movement of the infection along fascial

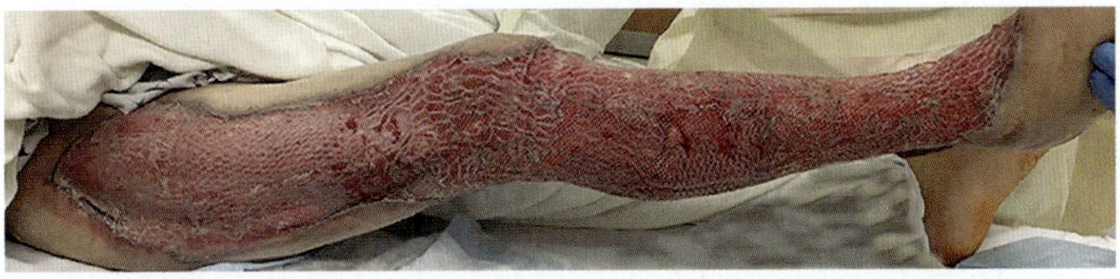

Figure 21.5 Dressing change 6 days after STSG meshed 6:1 with excellent graft adherence.

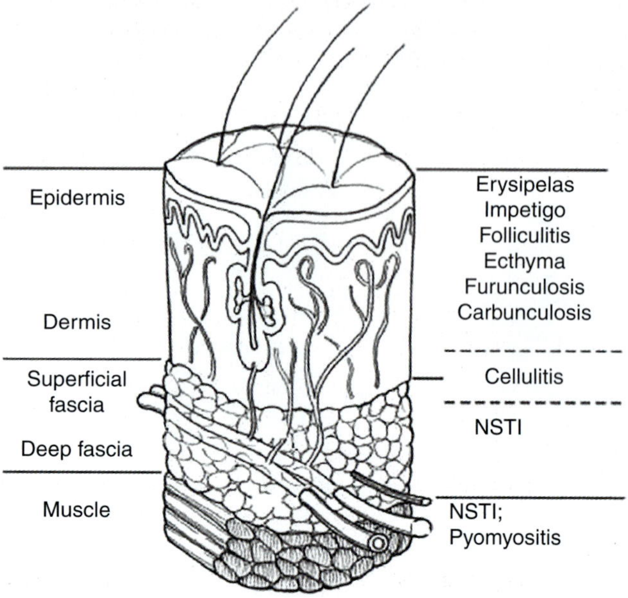

Figure 21.6 Skin diagram illustrating depth of soft tissue infections. NSTIs involve the superficial and deep fascia. They can extend deeper to involve muscle. NSTI, necrotizing soft tissue infection. (Figure modified from Henry S. Soft tissue infection. In: Asensio JA, Trunkey DD, eds. *Current Therapy of Trauma and Surgical Critical Care*. 1st ed. Mosby Elsevier; 2008:580, Figure 1, with permission from Elsevier.)

planes. Toxins also elicit a systemic response through cytokine and complement activation that can result in fever, hypotension, and organ dysfunction. **Figure 21.7** outlines the process.

CLASSIFICATION/BACTERIOLOGY

A variety of classification systems have been used to describe necrotizing soft tissue infections. Terms such as necrotizing fasciitis and myonecrosis refer to classification by the depth of infection. Historically, necrotizing infections were classified according to the anatomic site; for example, Fournier gangrene involving the perineum and Ludwig angina involving the submandibular space.

The extremities are the most commonly reported location of NSTI, accounting for 60%-80%. Perineal/Fournier gangrene represents 12%-16% of these infections and the torso another 10%-12%. Head and neck locations for NSTIs are the least common and represent 0.9%-8.9% of sites. The American Association for the Surgery of Trauma (AAST) developed grading scales for the seven most commonly treated emergency general surgery (EGS) diseases. The scale for skin and soft tissue infections was based on the expert consensus opinion of AAST members and included anatomical, clinical, radiographic, operative, and pathological components (**Table 21.1**). A multi-institutional

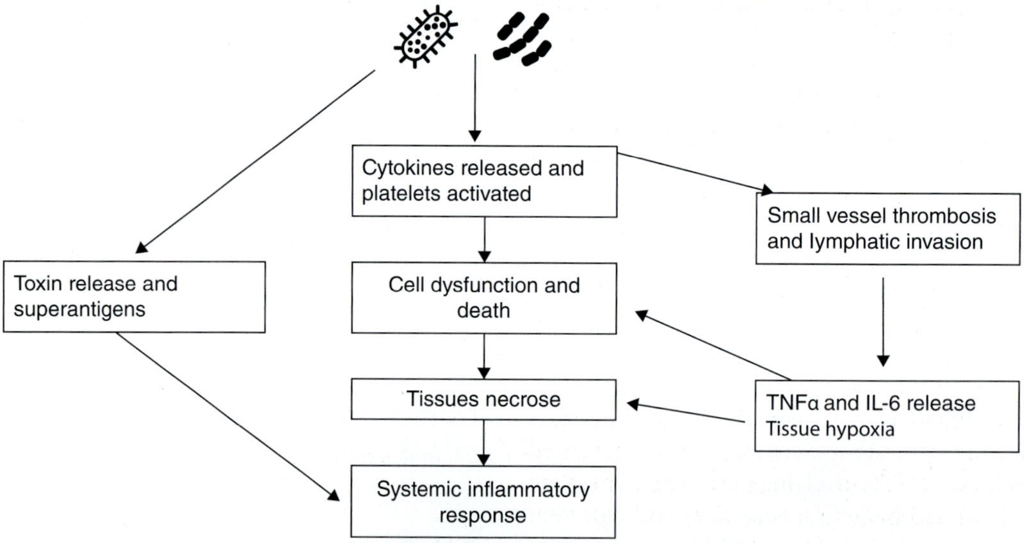

Figure 21.7 Pathogenesis of necrotizing soft tissue infections.

TABLE 21.1 ■ The American Association for the Surgery of Trauma Grading Scale for Soft Tissue Infections

AAST Grade	Description	Clinical Criteria	Radiologic Criteria	Operative Criteria	Pathologic Criteria
I	Cellulitis	Folliculitis, erysipelas, impetigo, cellulitis	Superficial inflammation, no subcutaneous stranding	N/A	Acute inflammation of epidermis
II	Superficial liquefaction or necrosis	Necrotizing, blistering, or bullous cellulitis	Subcutaneous stranding, no abscess	N/A	Acute inflammation of epidermis and dermis
III	Subcutaneous abscess	Abscess	Well-defined subcutaneous fluid	Well-defined fluid collection	As above and subcutaneous fat, cultures +
IV	Fasciitis	Fasciitis	Inflammation to fascia, +/– gas	Clear fascial involvement, viable muscle	As above and fascia, cultures +
V	Myonecrosis	Myonecrosis	Gas deep to fascia, poor perfusion of muscle	Necrosis into muscle and deep tissues	As above and muscles/deep tissues, cultures +

Reproduced from AAST data dictionary for EGS conditions. NST represented in grades IV and V and Savage SA, Li SW, Utter GH, et al. EGS grading scale for skin and soft tissue infections is predictive of poor outcomes: a multicenter validation study. *J Trauma Acute Care Surg*. 2019;86(4):601-608.

validation study demonstrated patients with grade IV and V had higher mortality, longer hospital lengths of stays, and more complications.

Microbiology is the basis of the most commonly used classification system. Type 1 NSTIs are polymicrobial with cultures yielding a mixture of aerobic and anaerobic organisms, averaging four isolates per specimen. At least one anaerobic species (most commonly *Bacteroides* or *Clostridium*) is isolated in combination with aerobic isolates (*Streptococcus*, *Staphylococcus*, *Enterococcus*, Enterobacteriaceae family–*Escherichia coli*, *Enterobacter*, *Klebsiella*, *Proteus*). Type 1 infections are considered the most prevalent form of NSTIs, occurring in 55%-75%. Type 1 infections typically occur on the perineum and trunk of immunocompromised individuals. The most common predisposing factor is diabetes, but other associated comorbidities include obesity, chronic kidney disease, HIV infection, alcohol, and IV drug use. **Table 21.2** lists several associations and risk factors. There is frequently an inciting event associated with these infections. These events range from merely a crack in the skin related to tinea pedis to bowel perforation. Some commonly cited mechanisms are listed in **Table 21.3.** NSTIs involving the head and neck are usually caused by mouth anaerobes and represent another presentation of type 1 NSTI.

Type 2 NSTIs are monomicrobial and are less common than the polymicrobial variety. However, geographically, the frequency may vary as some studies describe type 1 infections as more prevalent and some describe similar incidence between the

TABLE 21.2 ■ Patient Factors Associated With Diagnosis of NSTI

Risk Factors Associated With NSTI
Immunosuppression
Posttransplant
Steroid or other immune-modulating drug use
• Diabetes
• Cirrhosis
• Neutropenia
• HIV infection
• Malignancy
Malnutrition
Obesity
Peripheral vascular disease
Chronic kidney disease
Alcoholism/IV drug use
Chronic skin ulcers

TABLE 21.3 ■ Inciting Mechanisms

Chronic skin ulcer Arterial Venous Diabetic Neuropathic Vasculitic
Dermatopathy Psoriasis Eczema
Surgical procedures
Childbirth
Perforated cancer, diverticulitis, or appendicitis
Skin cracks, abrasions, and lacerations
Abscesses Furuncles Carbuncles
Bites and stings
Injections
Hematoma

An inciting cause is identified in 70%-80% of patients. Bacteria gain access to deeper tissue through breaks in the skin

two types. Unlike type 1 infections, type 2 infections may occur in any age group and without any underlying illness. There is often a history of minor trauma associated with type 2 NSTIs. Group A strep (GAS) or other β-hemolytic streptococci and *Staphylococcus aureus* (SA) remain the most common pathogen, but there is an increasing incidence of community-acquired methicillin-resistant *S aureus* (MRSA) as the causative agent. The community-acquired MRSA that is overwhelmingly associated with NSTI is clone USA300 containing the Panton-Valentine leukocidin cytotoxin. This cytotoxin destroys leukocytes and causes tissue necrosis. Since toxin-producing bacteria (*Streptococcus pyogenes* and *S aureus*) are pathogens in type 2 NSTIs, toxic shock syndrome is common. GAS remains one of the most common organisms isolated in NSTIs. The toxicity of NSTIs caused by GAS is severe and more fulminant, with an average mortality of 29%. Mortality increases with associated toxic shock and septic shock syndromes (38% and 45% mortality). Specific proteins produced and expressed at the GAS surface are implicated in its virulence and adherence to target tissues. The M protein is the most extensively studied. The M protein, encoded by the *emm* gene, is considered a significant virulence factor because of its ability to resist phagocytosis.

Although there are over 80 M protein types and not all GAS carry the M protein, specific disease manifestations are commonly associated with particular M protein types. For example, the M-1 and M-3 subtypes have been associated with toxic shock syndrome and necrotizing soft tissue infections. Superantigens are key exotoxins that cause the excessive systemic inflammatory response of the host. Streptococcal superantigens include streptococcal pyrogenic exotoxins (Spe). For many years, superantigens were known as pyrogenic toxins based on their association with fever. Marrack and Kappler suggested the term superantigen to highlight these exotoxins' ability to induce T-cell stimulation. Although studies have shown that tissue preference or disease manifestations may be linked to a particular protein strain, the outcome of infection depends not only on bacterial factors but also on the host's immune status.

Some classification systems describe monomicrobial infections by *Clostridium* species, *Vibrio*, or other gram-negative bacteria as type 3 NSTI and fungal etiology as type 4 NSTI. Infections with *Clostridium septicum* or *Streptococcus bovis* may indicate that the patient harbors a gastrointestinal or hematologic malignancy, requiring further investigation once the acute problem resolves. *Vibrio vulnificus* and *Aeromonas hydrophila* typically occur in the setting of a break in the skin exposed to seawater or freshwater, respectively. These infections are reported more commonly in Southeast Asia. Mucormycosis is an uncommon but potentially devastating cause of NSTI. These fungi are ubiquitous and found in soil, manure, plants, and decaying material. *Candida* is not infrequently found in polymicrobial NSTI (Type 1). Fungal pathogens most commonly found alone in human infections are *Mucor*, *Rhizopus*, *Aspergillus*, and *Cunninghamella*. Cutaneous mucormycosis is associated with diabetes, especially poorly controlled, but immunocompetent patients with trauma or burn wounds have also been described (**Figure 21.8A and B**). Mortality rates range from 38% to 80%.

Good-quality pre- or intraoperative tissue or fluid cultures are the basis of the microbiological diagnosis. Blood cultures are positive in as many as 25% of cases, while cultures obtained from the site of infection during surgical debridement are positive in the majority of cases (>75%).

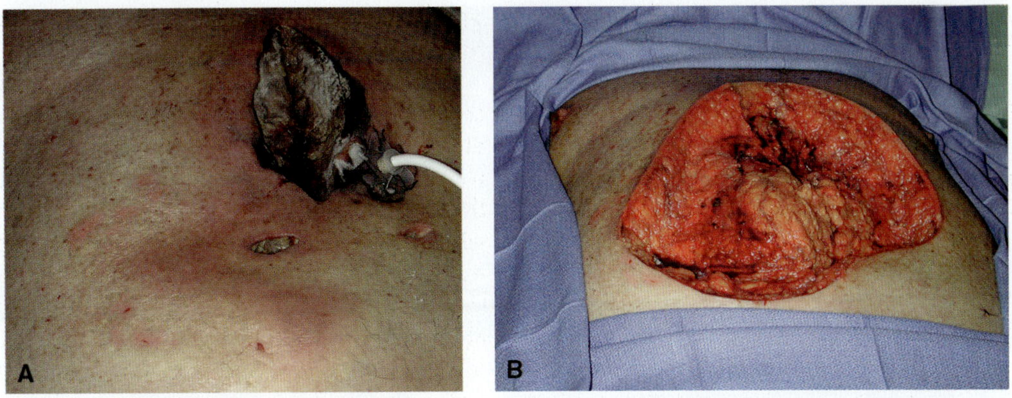

Figure 21.8 **A.** Fungal infection in a debilitated patient with complicated course following cardiac bypass. Note the classic appearance of fungus in the wound. **B.** After excisional debridement of the infected area and removal of the feeding tube and gastric repair.

DIAGNOSIS

No one clinical finding is diagnostic for NSTI. Patients can present with a wide range of clinical findings. A variety of factors affect the presentation. These include the time from onset of infection to treatment, bacterial virulence, and host susceptibility. NSTI is often not recognized during the initial examination due to a lack of skin findings and absence of systemic symptoms. Signs of systemic sepsis, including hypotension and tachycardia, may be present, although they are usually late occurrences. The most common findings associated with NSTI, unfortunately, are woefully nonspecific. **Figure 21.9A–D** demonstrates a spectrum of clinical findings seen in patients with NSTIs. This variation has led to a search for reliable aids or scoring systems to differentiate NSTI from less-lethal infections. Some frequently noted physical examination signs identified in patients with NSTI are nonspecific. The classical findings used to differentiate NSTI from other skin and soft tissue infections are unfortunately less regularly found (**Table 21.4**). Localized pain may be the earliest finding and should raise suspicion. Hemorrhagic bullae, crepitus, foul odor, and "dishwater" drainage are late manifestations and are usually associated with systemic sepsis and organ dysfunction (**Table 21.5**).

Laboratory values are also often utilized to aid in the diagnosis. The LRINEC score was devised retrospectively by Wong et al. based on six clinical parameters: serum CRP, WBC, HGB, Na, Cr, and Glu. According to the authors, a score of 6 is associated with necrotizing fasciitis, with a positive predictive value of 92% and a negative predictive value of 96% (**Table 21.6**). Since the development of the LRINEC score, several studies have attempted to validate its clinical use to diagnose NSTI. A recent meta-analysis evaluated the LRINEC score at two different thresholds. They concluded that an LRINEC score ≥6 was poorly sensitive for diagnosis and only moderately specific. A score ≥8 increased the specificity but at a considerably reduced sensitivity. They cautioned that the score itself had poor diagnostic accuracy for NSTI, and a low score is insufficient to rule out the diagnosis. They did note that individual components of the score (such as WBC or Na) may have better individual accuracy and represent an area for future research. Elevation of serum lactate above 2 mmol/L and creatine phosphokinase (CPK) >600 IU/L have also been found in patients with NSTI. Plain x-ray, ultrasound, and CT scans may all display findings that are associated with NSTI. Unfortunately, none are pathognomonic. Plain x-rays demonstrate nonspecific findings, and most authors find that they are not helpful. Radiographic findings on plain film are more apparent in advanced disease. Unexpected fractures, foreign bodies, and osteomyelitis can be seen. Air in the tissues usually represents infection, although other causes may occur. Subcutaneous gas is present in only 25% of cases, and therefore, obtaining x-rays to demonstrate this finding may delay operative intervention. Ultrasound is widely available in many emergency departments. Although operator-dependent, there is a potential for demonstration of edema, air, or fascial thickening. Although computed tomography and magnetic resonance imaging have a higher sensitivity than plain radiography, they lack specificity for the diagnosis of NSTI, and their use can lead to significant delays in definitive treatment. Findings commonly seen on CT scan in patients with NSTI include fat

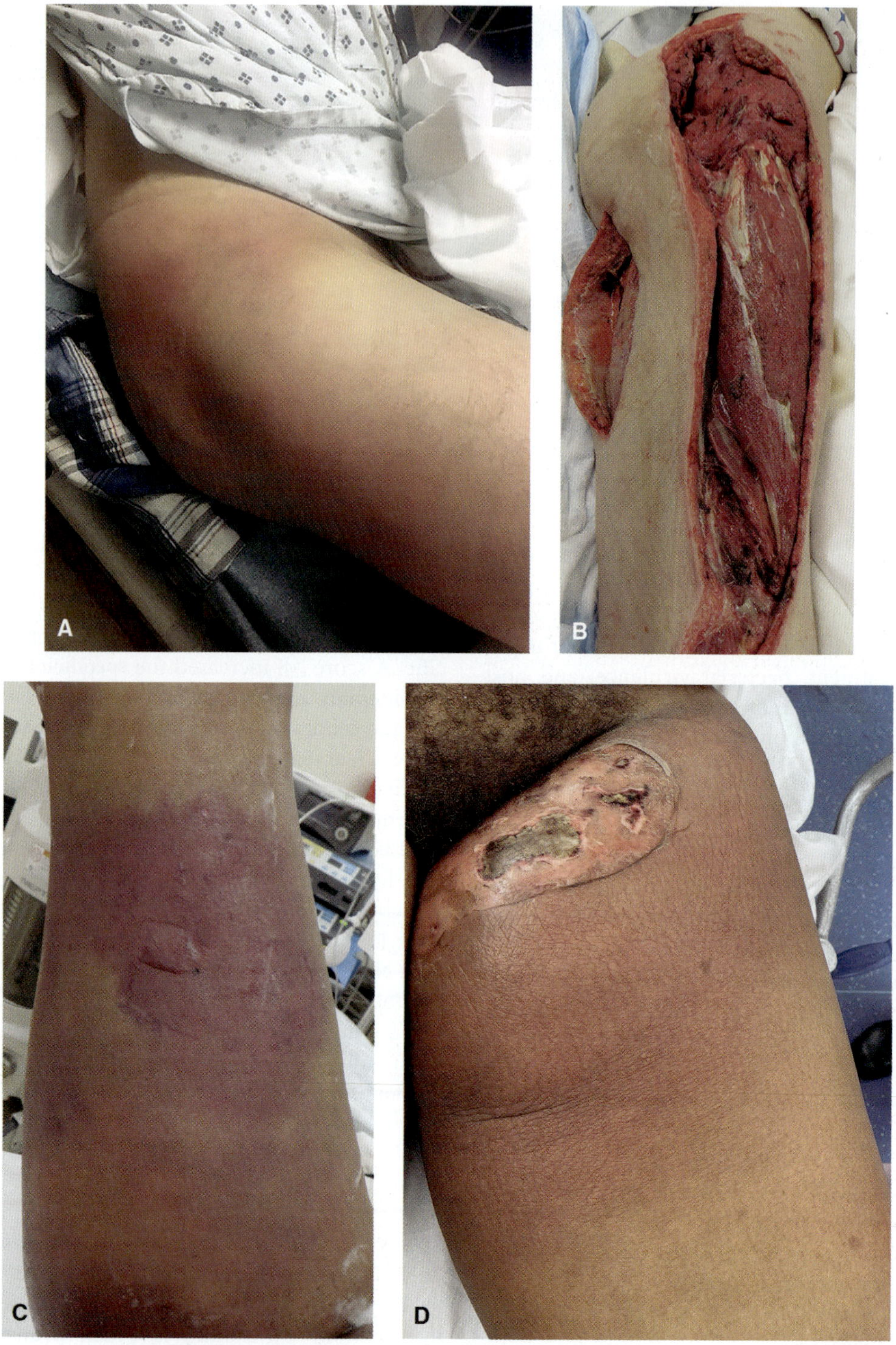

Figure 21.9 Spectrum of clinical findings in NSTI. **A.** Minimal skin changes. A 41-year-old intravenous drug user with seizure disorder suffered seizure 1 week prior and after noted swelling and tenderness from right hip to knee transferred for management. **B.** Note the extensive debridement of deep fascia and skin. **C.** Violaceous skin discoloration and edema. A 68-year-old man with a history of CAD and HTN. One-day history of pain in the medial thigh above the knee. While under evaluation, he developed a large area of ecchymosis and crepitus. Operative cultures grew *Clostridium septicum*. Colonoscopy performed during hospitalization revealed ascending colon mass pathology revealed adenocarcinoma. **D.** Frank skin necrosis.

TABLE 21.4 ■ Clinical Skin Manifestations of NSTI With Frequency of Finding

Clinical Manifestation	Percentage of Patients With Symptom
Pain beyond area of erythema	73%-98%
Erythema	75%-100%
Soft tissue edema	92%-75%
Induration	12%-45%
Fluctuance	11%
Fever	53%-32%
Skin bullae	11%-57%
Necrosis	14%-30%
Crepitus	6%-36%

stranding and fluid or air in the fascial planes. Unfortunately, the absence of these findings does not reliably exclude the diagnosis of NSTI. CT is about 80% sensitive for detecting NSTI. CT adds the advantage of illustrating the extent and depth of infection. Also, areas of infection remote from areas of skin abnormalities may be demonstrated. This is particularly valuable in intra-abdominal or retroperitoneal sources of infection, as seen in **Figure 21.10** where CT scan demonstrates retroperitoneal NSTI in a patient with diverticulitis. MRI is considered to be the most sensitive radiographic modality for diagnosing NSTI. However, it is often not the most practical. MRI is rarely available for emergent use and is not a safe environment for the critically ill patient. T1 images can detect areas of fascial necrosis with lack of enhancement, and T2 images display hyperintense signaling. **Table 21.7** summarizes the imaging findings associated with NSTI.

TABLE 21.6 ■ Laboratory Risk Indicator for Necrotizing Fasciitis (LRINEC) Score

Variable (Units)		Points
C-reactive protein		
mg/L	mg/dL	
<150	<15	0
>150	>15	4
White blood cell count (cells/mm^3)		
<15		0
15-25		1
>25		2
Hemoglobin (g/dL)		
>13.5		0
11-13.5		1
<11		2
Sodium (mmol/L)		
>135		0
<135		2
Creatinine		
mg/dL	µmol/L	
<1.6	<141	0
>1.6	>141	2
Glucose		
mg/dl	µmol/L	
<180	<10	0
>180	>20	1

Variables included in Laboratory Risk Indicator for Necrotizing Fasciitis Scoring System.
Wong CH, Khin LW, Heng KS, et al. The LRINEC (Laboratory Risk Indicator for Necrotizing Fasciitis) score: a tool for distinguishing necrotizing fasciitis from other soft tissue infections *Crit Care Med*. 2004;32:1535-1541.

TABLE 21.5 ■ Early and Late Findings

	Skin Findings	Pain Character	Systemic Signs
Early	Erythema Swelling Warmth Serous blisters	Extends beyond area of erythema	Fever Tachycardia Malaise Nausea Diarrhea
Late	Induration Hemorrhagic bullae Dusky skin discoloration Skin necrosis Drainage of "dishwater" fluid	Anesthesia	Hypotension Tachypnea AKI Coagulopathy Thrombocytopenia Altered mentation

Early findings in NSTI are nonspecific. Late findings are found less frequently.

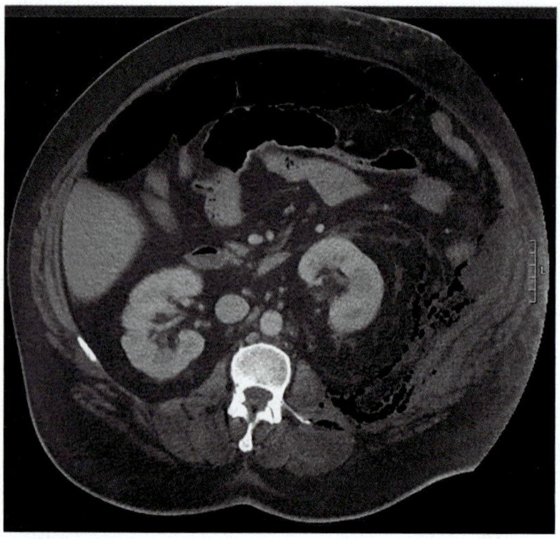

Figure 21.10 CT demonstrating retroperitoneal NSTI in patient with diverticulitis.

Because early diagnosis is associated with improved mortality but may be confounded by numerous factors, a high index of suspicion is required. Clinical history and physical features that raise suspicion of NSTI should prompt surgical exploration for a definitive diagnosis and treatment. Despite the availability of many options to augment diagnostic accuracy, our best tool is frequently operative exploration. Surgical exploration remains the gold standard in diagnosis of NSTI. A recent publication from a single center found that 20% of explorations for NSTI were negative. Furthermore, they found that 14% of those with negative explorations developed classic findings of NSTI requiring reexploration and debridement. Other groups rely on frozen section evaluation of tissue for patients who lack classical findings at exploration. Specimens for both culture and pathology were obtained from the fascia. They found that 75% of patients with only fascial edema on exploration had either positive fascial tissue cultures or microscopic evidence of NSTI, producing an overall 22% negative exploration. Mortality did not differ based on the presence or absence of macroscopic infection, but the ICU length of stay was longer in those with apparent infection.

TREATMENT

Initial Resuscitation and Antibiotic Therapy

While the principle treatment of NSTI is based upon prompt surgical debridement, concurrent medical management of these often critically ill patients is also required. Ensure adequate intravenous access and appropriate hemodynamic monitoring upon initial identification of a patient with suspected NSTI. Initiate intravenous fluid resuscitation to correct hypovolemia and improve overall perfusion. Utilize goal-

TABLE 21.7 ■ Imaging for NSTI

Imaging Technique	Sensitivity % (95% CI)	Specificity % (95% CI)
Plain radiography		
Soft tissue gas	48.9 (24.9-73.4)	94 (63.8-99.3)
Ultrasound		
Diffuse thickening of the subcutaneous tissue and a layer of fluid accumulation >4 mm along the deep fascia	88.2 (63.6-98.5)	93.3 (58.6-96.4)
Computed tomography		
Fascial enhancement, edema, gas	94.3 (81.2-98.5)	76.6 (21.3-97.5)
Magnetic resonance imaging		
Abnormal signal intensity on T2 images >3 mm	86	70
Extensive involvement of intermuscular fascia	100	61
Air	43	74
Focal or diffuse absence of postcontrast signal enhancement within fascial abnormalities seen on T2 images	86	74

Radiographic findings associated with NSTI and relative sensitivity and specificity. Confidence intervals omitted with small sample sizes.

CI, confidence interval; NSTI, necrotizing soft tissue infection.

directed therapy, titrating to signs of adequate end-organ perfusion and tailored to individual patient needs. In patients with persistent hypotension despite fluid resuscitation, use vasopressors to maintain mean arterial pressures >65 mm Hg.

Early administration of antibiotics is also essential in the treatment of NSTI, with an empiric regimen providing broad coverage of gram-positive, gram-negative, and anaerobic organisms until the causative organism is identified. Include coverage for MRSA. Several therapeutic combinations effectively cover these organisms and can be tailored to known local susceptibility patterns. The 2014 Infectious Diseases Society of America (IDSA) guidelines recommend vancomycin or linezolid, plus either piperacillin-tazobactam or a carbapenem, or ceftriaxone and metronidazole. Clindamycin should be added to inhibit toxin production in gram-positive bacteria. If *Vibrio* infection is suspected, doxycycline should be added to the empiric regimen. **Table 21.8** provides a summary of common bacteria and rational antimicrobial options.

TABLE 21.8 ■ Microbiology and Antimicrobial Options

Classification	Microbe	Antimicrobial Class	Antimicrobial Agent	Adult Dosage
Type 1 (polymicrobial)	Streptococci *Staphylococcus aureus* *Escherichia coli* *Bacteroides* species	β-Lactam/β-lactamase inhibitor or Carbapenem or Third-generation cephalosporin and Nitroimidazole All with lincomycin	Piperacillin/tazobactam	4.5 g every 6 h
			Meropenem	1-2 g every 8 h
			Ceftriaxone or Cefotaxime	2 g daily 1-2 g every 4-6 h
			Metronidazole	500 mg every 8 h
			Clindamycin	600-900 mg every 6-8 h
Type 2 monomicrobial	Group A *Streptococcus* ± *Staphylococcus aureus* or Methicillin-resistant *S aureus*	Penicillins β-Lactam First-generation cephalosporin Oxazolidinone or glycopeptide All with lincomycin	Penicillin G or Nafcillin or oxacillin Cefazolin Linezolid Vancomycin Clindamycin	2-4 million units every 4-6 h 1-2 g every 4 h 1 g every 8 h 600 mg every 12 h 30 mg/kg/d in 2 divided doses adjust based on trough levels 600-900 mg every 6-8 h
Type 3	*Clostridium* species *Aeromonas hydrophila* *Vibrio vulnificus* Extended-spectrum β-lactamase–producing Enterobacterales	Penicillins All with lincomycin Tetracycline + Fluoroquinolone Tetracycline + Third-generation cephalosporin Carbapenems Glycylcycline	Penicillin G or ampicillin Clindamycin Doxycycline Ciprofloxacin Doxycycline Cefotaxime or Ceftriaxone Meropenem Tigecycline	2-4 million units every 4-6 h 1-2 g every 4-6 h 600-900 mg every 6-8 h 100 mg every 12 h 500 mg every 12 h 100 mg every 12 h 1-2 g every 8 h 1-2 g daily 1-2 g every 8 h 50-100 mg every 12 h
Type 4	*Candida* species *Mucorales* *Aspergillus*	Polyene Polyene or Echinocandin Triazoles	Liposomal amphotericin B Liposomal amphotericin B or Micafungin Voriconazole	3-5 mg/kg/d 3-5 mg/kg/d 100 mg daily 6 mg/kg every 12 h for 2 doses then 4 mg/kg every 12 h

Adapted from Stevens DL, Bisno AL, Chambers HF, et al.; Infectious Diseases Society of America. Practice guidelines for the diagnosis and management of skin and soft tissue infections: 2014 update by the Infectious Diseases Society of America. *Clin Infect Dis*. 2014;59(2):e10-e52.

Hyperbaric Oxygen

Hyperbaric oxygen therapy (HBO) emerged in the literature in the 1980s as an adjunctive treatment for NSTI. This treatment uses 100% oxygen at a pressure of 2-3 absolute atmospheres (ATA) to achieve hyperoxia and, therefore, significantly increases tissue oxygen tension. HBO's benefits in wound healing are attributed to improvements in leukocyte function, suppression of bacterial toxins, and HBO's bactericidal effect for specific organisms. Even these early studies had conflicting results regarding any benefit in mortality or number of debridements. However, the theoretical benefit and small series describing improved outcomes prompted continued use.

More recent work continues to provide conflicting results regarding the benefit of HBO. A 2012 retrospective study using over 20 years of data from the Nationwide Inpatient Sample demonstrated a mortality benefit for patients receiving HBO. In reviewing cases treated at University Health Consortium institutions, a 2014 study also described a decreased mortality with HBO, particularly in patients with "extreme" severity of illness. In contrast, other institutional studies have not seen any such mortality difference from HBO. Given the interest surrounding the efficacy of HBO in NSTI, attempts have been made to provide a comprehensive review of the existing literature to form evidence-based guidelines for us. An early review of HBO was limited by poor study quality, an issue also encountered by a Cochrane review performed in 2015, which identified 673 studies on the topic but found that zero met inclusion criteria. A more recent systematic review performed with PRISMA guidelines demonstrated that the available studies on HBO have significant risk for bias and lack the quality required to provide clear guidance on the use and outcomes related to this therapy. The 2018 World Society of Emergency Surgery/Surgical Infection Society Europe Guidelines provide a 2B recommendation (weak recommendation, moderate-quality evidence) that HBO be considered after surgical debridement of NSTI based upon available data.

Overall, HBO therapy is well tolerated, although described risks have included temporary myopia, middle ear rupture and other barotrauma-related complications, and infrequent reports of seizures. The main limitation to the use of HBO is the specialized equipment and expertise required to implement such therapy. The Undersea and Hyperbaric Medical Society has an accreditation for hyperbaric facilities throughout the United States, with 183 currently listed nationwide. In facilities with hyperbaric capabilities, this therapy can be used as an adjunct in the management of NSTI. While facilities without hyperbaric chambers can consider transferring patients for such therapy, it should not delay the most crucial component of NSTI treatment, namely initial surgical debridement. The course and intensity of HBO can vary between protocols, with most providing 30- to 90-minute sessions twice to three times daily at 2-3 ATA, continuing until the infection has improved.

Intravenous Immunoglobulin and Emerging Therapies

Intravenous immunoglobulin (IVIG) has also been used in the medical management of NSTI, based upon evidence that IVIG combats severe invasive group A streptococcal infections by providing opsonizing antibodies, counteracting the effects of superantigens, and decreasing the severe cytokine response to infection. Early studies on IVIG focused on efficacy in streptococcal toxic shock syndrome (STSS), with comparative and case-control studies demonstrating an association with survival and investigations describing the inhibitory ability of plasma taken from patients treated with IVIG. A randomized controlled trial in Europe of IVIG in STSS was attempted but stopped early due to poor recruitment. However, analysis of the 21 patients enrolled demonstrated a nonstatistically significant 3.6-fold higher mortality rate in placebo patients while also demonstrating improvement in sequential organ failure assessment (SOFA) scores.

When analyzing the effects of IVIG in the larger NSTI population, the available evidence has not shown any mortality benefit in patients treated with IVIG. A propensity-matched and risk-adjusted analysis of NSTI patients treated with IVIG vs without IVIG demonstrated, that only a small percentage of patients (4%) received IVIG therapy, and there was no difference in mortality or length of stay in these patients. The "Immunoglobulin G for patients with necrotizing soft tissue infection" (INSTINCT) trial published in 2017 was a prospective randomized trial of 100 patients given 25 g of IVIG daily for 3 days upon admission to the ICU. There was no mortality benefit at 6 months and no difference in self-reported physical function. Despite this, some continue to argue to consider using IVIG in patients with GAS infection.

The "Improving Outcome of Necrotizing Fasciitis" (INFECT) study is a prospective multicenter trial enrolling patients with NSTI, aiming to better understand the pathophysiology and outcomes of NSTI patients. This group has accrued many patients specifically with streptococcal NSTI, and in analyzing this cohort, the authors demonstrated that the lack of IVIG use was associated with mortality in patients with group A *Streptococcus* infection. Further investigation is needed to clarify the utility of IVIG in the NSTI population.

Given the morbidity and mortality of NSTI, a novel therapeutic option has recently been investigated. A multicenter phase 3 randomized trial of reltecimod, a compound that inhibits T-cell stimulation through CD28 binding, was recently completed. In the study, therapy was administered within 6 hours of diagnosis, and the primary end point was the previously described Necrotizing Infection Clinical Composite Endpoint (NICCE). This end point includes four elements: alive at 28 days, three or fewer debridements before day 14, no amputation after the first debridement, and modified sequential organ failure assessment score ≤1 at day 14. Improvement in NICCE was seen in the per-protocol analysis, but not in the modified intention to treat analysis, with the authors noting significant benefit in the resolution of multisystem organ dysfunction. These findings merit further investigation in the NSTI population, and the U.S. Food and Drug Administration has recently accepted the New Drug Application for this intervention.

SURGICAL TREATMENT

General Principles

To date, the only modifiable risk factor to impact the outcome of patients with NSTI is timely and adequate operative debridement of the infection. The general principles of debridement are the same regardless of the site, but with nuances and considerations specific to the infection's location. Four steps have been advocated by Wong. These are to confirm the diagnosis, determine the extent, excise nonviable and infected tissue, and provide wound care. Place the incision over the area of maximal skin abnormality.

The incision should extend through the area of necrosis, erythema, and induration. Incisions should extend vertically. It may be necessary to raise subcutaneous flaps. Excessively wide or thin flaps may cause skin ischemia making debridement necessary. Parallel incisions may avoid this. Extend the dissection through the superficial and deep fascia. Blunt dissection between the subcutaneous fat and deep fascia may reveal that the tissues give way easily. This hallmark of NSTI is the so-called finger test. The overlying tissues are opened until normal adherence is encountered. It is not necessary to remove normal tissue that demonstrates good perfusion. The deep fascia is incised to evaluate the underlying muscle. Grossly necrotic subcutaneous fat and fascia are characteristically seen with NSTI. It can be gray, green, or black (**Figure 21.11**). At times, the fat is indurated and does not bleed when incised. Thrombosed veins are frequently present. The debridement should remove all abnormal tissue. The debridement should follow any tracks of purulence or abnormal tissue adherence to identify areas of extension that may be contiguous or more remote from the area explored. Make additional incisions as needed to explore all suspicious areas. Obtain cultures of fluid and tissue. Swabbing the tissue with cotton tip applicators produces inadequate samples. Send both aerobic and anaerobic samples. Special cultures for fungus or mycobacteria should be sent with unusual appearance or not, with presentations, or with immunocompromised patients.

When there is little skin involvement, positioning the incision can be challenging. Choose areas of induration if present. If not, creating incisions as for fasciotomy is a good starting place on extremities.

Assess the muscle for viability once the deep fascia is incised. Nonviable muscle takes on a few appearances. Involved muscle can appear pale or deep burgundy, and involvement can be patchy and

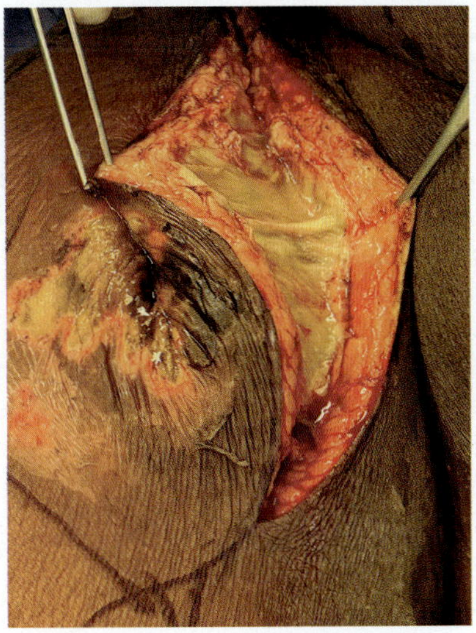

Figure 21.11 Typical operative findings of necrosis involving the superficial fat and fascia.

incomplete. There may be no bleeding, or in a muscle that is a deep burgundy, venous thrombosis may be evident with venous bleeding when divided. The consistency of the muscle is abnormal. There will be little resistance to traction, and the muscle will tear and can be removed bluntly. The muscle will not contract with stimulation. Zones of infection have also been described. In zone 1, the tissue is necrotic. Zone 2 contains tissue that is infected but potentially salvageable, and zone 3 contains uninvolved tissue. Zone 1 tissue should be excised entirely. The tissue in zone 2 should be meticulously assessed as described above and may require removal of some of it, whereas zone 3 does not need to be debrided (**Figure 21.12**).

Pay attention to the position of critical nerves and blood vessels. The anatomy is often distorted, swollen, or covered with exudate compromising visualization of critical structures. Use the knowledge of anatomy and structural relationships to avoid preventable injury.

Remember, pelvic and retroperitoneal infections can drain into the thigh or leg and vice versa. The thigh and retroperitoneum can communicate infection along the psoas muscle or directly along the femoral vessels through the inguinal canal.

The psoas can provide the conduit of spread or contain infection within its robust fascia. Abdominal or flank pain associated with findings of extremity NSTI should be investigated with imaging when the patient's physiology permits. Leg weakness or sciatic symptoms may be present.

Head and Neck

NSTI localized to the head and neck occurs in about 5% of cases. Dental infections, glandular infections, aerodigestive perforations, and superficial skin and surgical sites are all potential origins for infections in the head and neck. Spread follows anatomic fascial layers. The superficial fascia invests the neck muscles, surrounds the sternocleidomastoid and trapezius muscles, and extends from the inferior mandible posteriorly to the occiput. Inferior extension to include the manubrium, clavicles, and scapula is possible. Infections originating more deeply involving the middle fascia can extend from the hyoid bone to the pericardium and posteriorly to the prevertebral fascia. The deep fascia surrounds the paraspinous and perivertebral muscles and runs from the skull base to the coccyx. Anteriorly, the retropharyngeal space extends into the mediastinum. Classic neck skin incisions are used to debride and explore these spaces. Oblique incisions on the SCM borders or collar incisions are starting points extending vertically to the upper mediastinum when necessary. A partial sternotomy may be necessary to access the upper mediastinum. Infection can rupture into the pleural space resulting in empyema. When the infection extends to the shoulder girdle or chest wall, additional incisions are required. Infraclavicular or supraclavicular horizontal incision can connect to limb incisions.

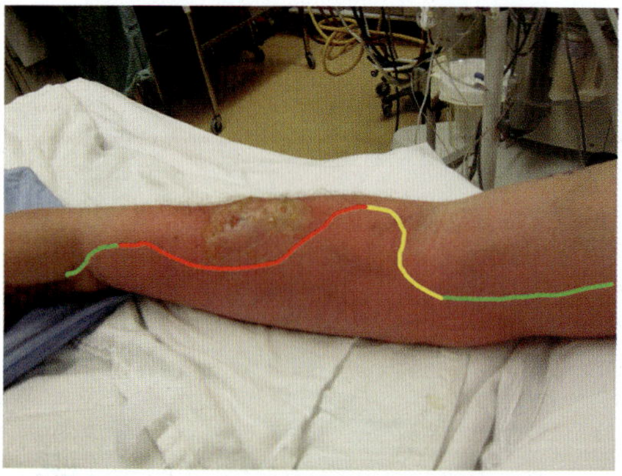

Figure 21.12 Zones of tissue involvement. *Red* is the area zone 1 involvement that will require resection; *yellow* represents zone 2 tissue is infected but may be salvageable; *green* represents normal tissue that does not need to be debrided.

Other Procedures

Patients with infections involving the perineum and/or buttock will sometimes require diversion with a colostomy. There is limited literature on indications for and outcomes specific to colostomy creation in NSTI patients. One recent retrospective review of 35 Fournier gangrene patients at a single center demonstrated that 77% of patients required fecal diversion. However, the vast majority of these patients were managed with endorectal tubes, and only a minority (six patients) required a colostomy. When the two groups were compared, there was no difference in length of stay, mortality, complications, or ultimate wound healing. With few exceptions, the literature indicates that colostomy formation does not appear to show specific benefit in outcome. It may be required if there is significant involvement of the anal sphincter or similar perineal destruction precluding any other approach. Otherwise, fecal diversion systems and wound VAC systems may adequately protect the open wound from fecal contamination. Urinary diversion has a similarly sparse presence in the literature, mentioned in case series and management discussions but without direct comparisons between patients with and without diversion. Similar to colostomies, urinary diversion may be

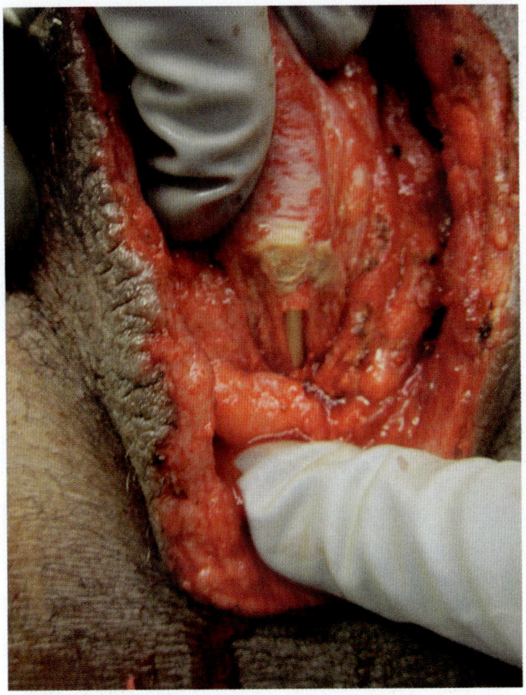

Figure 21.13 Patient with Fournier gangrene and a urethral necrosis and erosion.

required in specific clinical scenarios where there is extensive involvement and destruction of the urinary system. **Figure 21.13** shows urethral injury in patient with Fournier gangrene.

POSTOPERATIVE CARE

The postoperative care of patients with NSTI is multifaceted and often occurs in the intensive care unit for patients with severe infection. After initial surgical debridement, patients will often demonstrate improvement due to the source control obtained. However, persistent evidence of septic shock and end-organ dysfunction will require ongoing management. In addition to ongoing resuscitation and management of such conditions as respiratory failure and acute kidney injury/renal failure, other measures, including nutritional support, tailoring, and de-escalation of antibiotics, are also necessary for treatment. Once patients have improved from their initial critical illness, early physical and occupational therapy is initiated to aid with return to function.

Nutrition

Patients with NSTI require attention to their nutritional status to ensure adequate caloric and protein intake. With multiple and extensive surgical debridement, this population can have large wounds that will result in increased nutritional needs. In intubated patients, enteral feeds should be started via a nasogastric or orogastric tube as soon as possible postoperatively. In awake patients, the diet should be advanced promptly postoperatively, and supplementation via oral or nasogastric supplemental feeds should be considered in those who are unable to meet calorie needs. In patients requiring multiple returns to the operating room for additional debridement, care should be taken to minimize the time of NPO status or tube feed holds. Enteral nutrition is always preferred, but parenteral nutrition may be necessary if there is a contraindication or intolerance. Vitamin and mineral support in the form of vitamins A and C and zinc can be used to aid with wound healing.

Antibiotic Therapy and Duration

Once the results of intraoperative cultures are available, they are used to de-escalate and tailor antibiotics. In patients with *Streptococcus* infection, penicillin and clindamycin therapy should be adequate for treatment. Coverage for polymicrobial infections can be tailored based upon the identified organisms and their susceptibility patterns. For patients with *S aureus* infections, identification of methicillin sensitivity or resistance will guide antibiotic adjustments. *Vibrio* infections can be managed with doxycycline and a third-generation cephalosporin, while *Aeromonas* infections require doxycycline and either ceftriaxone or ciprofloxacin. Clostridium infections will be adequately covered by penicillin and clindamycin therapy. Additional adjustments in therapy or engagement with infectious disease services are helpful in patients with multidrug-resistant organisms. Duration of therapy is less clearly established and has been shown to vary significantly among institutions. In general, antibiotics continue until the wound is clean and the patient clinically improves. **Table 21.8** lists common bacterial pathogens and recommended antibiotics.

Wound Care

Management of the often-large, open wounds created by the necessary debridement of involved tissues can be a challenge. The use of negative pressure wound therapy (NPWT) has become commonplace and has simplified wound management in many cases. Important principles to consider are as follows:

1. NPWT is not an option for wounds that are incompletely debrided.

2. Patients with coagulopathy or incomplete hemostasis are poor candidates for NPWT.
3. Wounds in patients with vascular disease may deteriorate, and using lower target pressures or alternative dressings may be best.

Gauze dressings with or without antimicrobial impregnation are another option that is nearly uniformly available. Dressings may require frequent changes to manage drainage, particularly early on. Foams and alginates may be beneficial in managing exudative wounds.

Reconstruction of the soft tissue can begin once cellulitis has resolved, no necrotic or infected tissue remains in the wound, and the leukocytosis has resolved. Techniques for closure range from simple closure with or without drains to local tissue rearrangement (**Figure 21.14A and B**). Split-thickness skin grafts are commonly required. Dermal substitutes are increasingly used under autografts, particularly with exposed tendon or bone.

Tissue deficits that include bone may require rotational or free flap coverage. The timing of the more advanced closure techniques will depend on the patient's clinical recovery and comorbid conditions (**Figure 21.14C-E**).

LONG-TERM OUTCOME

Improvement in hospital mortality has occurred with improvement in critical care and wound management. Many modern reports document 6%-20% mortality substantially decreased from the 30% documented in studies from the 1980s and 1990s. Although an important end point, hospital survival fails to capture the impact the disease has on patients and their families or the resources that are utilized to control the infection and reconstruct the physical wound. A recent publication estimated that the 90-day risk of readmission was 24%-29%. More than 80% of those admissions were unplanned. Additionally, advanced age and

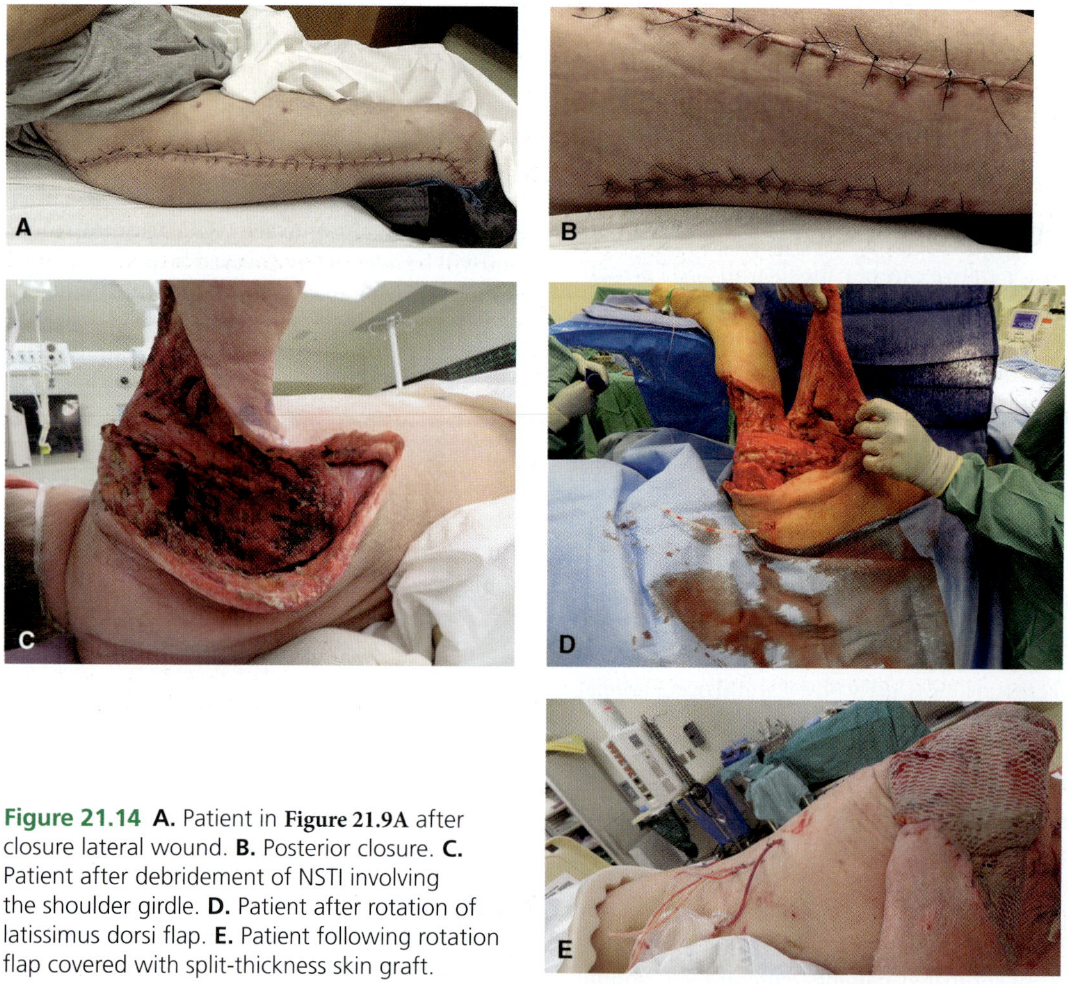

Figure 21.14 **A.** Patient in **Figure 21.9A** after closure lateral wound. **B.** Posterior closure. **C.** Patient after debridement of NSTI involving the shoulder girdle. **D.** Patient after rotation of latissimus dorsi flap. **E.** Patient following rotation flap covered with split-thickness skin graft.

comorbidities associated with NSTI make these patients at risk for postdischarge mortality. Some patients survive the infection only to develop chronic critical illness (CCI).

These patients have long lengths of hospital and ICU stay, require long-term care facility placement postdischarge, and have frequent readmissions to acute care. Risk factors for discharge to alternate care settings include increased age, comorbid conditions, and organ failure during hospitalization. The 1-year mortality of patients with CCI approaches 50%. The importance of providing patients and their families with realistic expectations of the potential trajectory for recovery and prognosis cannot be overemphasized.

A qualitative evaluation of the patient experience of the disease and recovery from it identified several factors that affected postdischarge functioning. Many experience depression, posttraumatic stress reactions, chronic pain, changes in sexual functioning, alterations in physical functioning, persistent fear of infection, changes in family dynamics, changes in activity levels, and social circles.

Many of those employed before injury lost their jobs or were unable to continue performing their job functions. Moving beyond survival as a measure of success, understanding the patient experience of necrotizing soft tissue infections is an underexplored area of study. As more patients survive this devastating disease, it is increasingly important to understand not just how to impact in-hospital mortality but which treatments can improve long-term survival and quality of life.

SUMMARY

NSTI can be a challenging problem to diagnose because the presentation varies from intense pain with subtle skin changes to frank necrosis with systemic signs of shock. Although some skin findings such as crepitus and violaceous skin are more specific for the infection, they are not uniformly present. Laboratory tests are also nonspecific. Imaging often fails to clarify questionable cases. Surgical exploration remains the mainstay of diagnosis. Treatment frequently requires removing large areas of tissue to gain control of the infection. Source control may involve the gastrointestinal or genitourinary tract and require supplemental procedures. Reconstruction can require plastic surgical expertise. Though the in-hospital mortality has decreased, ICU and hospital length of stays continue to be long.

SUGGESTED READINGS

Anaya DA, Dellinger EP. Necrotizing soft-tissue infection: diagnosis and management. *Clin Infect Dis.* 2007;44(5):705.

Bakleh M, Wold LE, Mandrekar JN, Harmsen WS, Dimashkieh HH, Baddour LM. Correlation of histopathologic findings with clinical outcomes in necrotizing fasciitis. *Clin Infect Dis.* 2005;40:410-414.

Bartram L, Aaron JG. Fungal necrotizing skin and soft tissue infections. *Curr Fungal Infect Rep.* 2019;13:146-156. https://doi.org/10.1007/s12281-019-00355-5

Bocking N, Matsumoto C, Loewen K, et al. High incidence of invasive Group A Streptococcal infections in remote indigenous communities in Northwestern Ontario, *Canada Open Forum Infect Dis.* 2016;4(1):ofw243.

Brown DR, Davis NL, Lepawsky M, Cunningham J, Kortbeek J. A multicenter review of the treatment of major truncal necrotizing infections with and without hyperbaric oxygen therapy. *Am J Surg.* 1994;167(5):485-489. doi:10.1016/0002-9610(94)90240-2.

Bruun T, Rath E, Bruun Madsen M, et al.; INFECT Study Group. Risk factors and predictors of mortality in streptococcal necrotizing soft-tissue infections: a multicenter prospective study. *Clin Infect Dis.* 2021;72(2):293-300. doi:10.1093/cid/ciaa027.

Bulger EM, May A, Dankner W, Maislin G, Robinson B, Shirvan A. Validation of a clinical trial composite endpoint for patients with necrotizing soft tissue infections. *J Trauma Acute Care Surg.* 2017;83(4):622-627. doi: 10.1097/TA.0000000000001564.

Bulger EM, May AK, Robinson BRH, et al.; ACCUTE study Investigators. A novel immune modulator for patients with Necrotizing Soft Tissue Infections (NSTI): results of a multicenter, phase 3 randomized controlled trial of reltecimod (AB 103). *Ann Surg.* 2020; 272(3):469-478.doi:10.1097/SLA.0000000000004102.

Chawla SN, Gallop C, Mydlo JH. Fournier's gangrene: an analysis of repeated surgical debridement. *Eur Urol.* 2003;43(5):572-575. doi: 10.1016/s0302-2838(03)00102-7.

Cocanour CS, Chang P, Huston JM, et al. Management and novel adjuncts of necrotizing soft tissue infections. *Surg Infect (Larchmt).* 2017;18(3):250-272. doi: 10.1089/sur.2016.200.

Darenberg J, Ihendyane N, Sjölin J, et al.; StreptIg Study Group. Intravenous immunoglobulin G therapy in streptococcal toxic shock syndrome: a European randomized, double-blind, placebo-controlled trial. *Clin Infect Dis.* 2003;37(3):333-340. doi: 10.1086/376630.

Elliott D, Kufera JA, Myers RAM. The microbiology of necrotizing soft tissue infections. *Am J Surg.* 2000;179:361-366.

Eucker J, Sezer O, Graf B, Possinger K. Mucormycoses. *Mycoses.* 2001;44:253-260.

Faraklas I, Yang D, Eggerstedt M, et al. A multicenter review of care patterns and outcomes in necrotizing soft tissue infections. *Surg Infect (Larchmt)*. 2016;17(6):773-778. doi: 10.1089/sur.2015.238.

Faunø Thrane J, Ovesen T. Scarce evidence of efficacy of hyperbaric oxygen therapy in necrotizing soft tissue infection: a systematic review. *Infect Dis (Lond)*. 2019;51(7):485-492. doi: 10.1080/23744235.2019.1597983.

Fernando SM, Tran A, Cheng W, et al. Necrotizing soft tissue infection: diagnostic accuracy of physical examination, imaging and LRINEC score: a systematic review and meta-analysis. *Ann Surg*. 2019;269(1):58-65.

George ME, Rueth NM, Skarda DE, Chipman JG, Quickel RR, Beilman GJ. Hyperbaric oxygen does not improve outcome in patients with necrotizing soft tissue infection. *Surg Infect (Larchmt)*. 2009;10(1):21-28. doi: 10.1089/sur.2007.085.

Gozal D, Ziser A, Shupak A, Ariel A, Melamed Y. Necrotizing fasciitis. *Arch Surg*. 1986;121(2):233-235. doi: 10.1001/archsurg.1986.01400020119015.

Hajdu S, Obradovic A, Presterl E, Vecsei V. Invasive mycoses following trauma. *Injury*. 2009;40:548-554.

Hau V, Ho CO. Necrotising fasciitis caused by Vibrio vulnificus in the lower limb following exposure to seafood on the hand. *Hong Kong Med J*. 2011; 17(4):335.

Jones J. *Surgical Memoirs of the War of the Rebellion: Investigation Upon the Nature, Causes, and Treatment of Hospital Gangrene as Prevailed in the Confederate Armies 1861–1865*. U.S. Sanitary Commission; 1871.

Kadri SS, Swihart BJ, Bonne SL, et al. Impact of intravenous immunoglobulin on survival in necrotizing fasciitis with vasopressor-dependent shock: a propensity score-matched analysis from 130 US Hospitals. *Clin Infect Dis*. 2017;64(7):877-885. doi: 10.1093/cid/ciw871.

Kao LS, Lew DF, Arab SN, et al. Local variations in the epidemiology, microbiology, and outcome of necrotizing soft-tissue infections: a multicenter study. *Am J Surg*. 2011;202(2):139-145. doi: 10.1016/j.amjsurg.2010.07.041.

Kaul R, McGeer A, Norrby-Teglund A, et al. Intravenous immunoglobulin therapy for streptococcal toxic shock syndrome—a comparative observational study. The Canadian Streptococcal Study Group. *Clin Infect Dis*. 1999;28(4):800-807. doi: 10.1086/515199.

Levett D, Bennett MH, Millar I. Adjunctive hyperbaric oxygen for necrotizing fasciitis. *Cochrane Database Syst Rev*. 2015;1(1):CD007937. doi: 10.1002/14651858.CD007937.pub2.

Lin HC, Chen ZQ, Chen HX, et al. Outcomes in patients with Fournier's gangrene originating from the anorectal region with a particular focus on those without perineal involvement. *Gastroenterol Rep (Oxf)*. 2019;7(3):212-217. doi: 10.1093/gastro/goy041.

Lina G, Pie'mont Y, Godail-Gamot F, et al. Involvement of Panton-Valentine Leukocidin–Producing *Staphylococcus aureus* in primary skin infections and pneumonia. *Clin Infect Dis*. 1999;29:1128-1132.

Linnér A, Darenberg J, Sjölin J, Henriques-Normark B, Norrby-Teglund A. Clinical efficacy of polyspecific intravenous immunoglobulin therapy in patients with streptococcal toxic shock syndrome: a comparative observational study. *Clin Infect Dis*. 2014;59(6):851-857. doi: 10.1093/cid/ciu449.

Madsen MB, Hjortrup PB, Hansen MB, et al. Immunoglobulin G for patients with necrotising soft tissue infection (INSTINCT): a randomised, blinded, placebo-controlled trial. *Intensive Care Med*. 2017;43(11):1585-1593. doi: 10.1007/s00134-017-4786-0.

Marrack P, Kappler J. The staphylococcal enterotoxins and their relatives. *Science*. 1990;248:705-711.

Massey PR, Sakran JV, Mills AM, et al. Hyperbaric oxygen therapy in necrotizing soft tissue infections. *J Surg Res*. 2012;177(1):146-151. doi: 10.1016/j.jss.2012.03.016.

May AK. Skin and soft tissue infections. *Surg Clin North Am*. 2009;89:403-420.

May AK, Talisa VB, Wilfret DA, et al. Estimating the impact of necrotizing soft tissue infections in the United States: incidence and readmissions. *Surg Infect (Larchmt)*. 2020. doi: 10.1089/sur.2020.099.

McHenry CR, Piotrowski JJ, Petrinic D, Malangoni MA. Determinants of mortality for necrotizing soft tissue infections. *Ann Surg*. 1995;221:558-565.

Miller LG, Perdreau-Remington F, Rieg G, et al. Necrotizing fasciitis caused by community-associated methicillin-resistant *Staphylococcus aureus* in Los Angeles. *N Engl J Med*. 2005;352:1445.

Narayanan S, Narayanan CD, Kindo AJ, Arora A, Haridas PA. Fatal fungal infection: the living dead. *J Surg Case Rep*. 2014;2014(10):rju104.

Nordqvist G, Walldén A, Brorson H, Tham J. Ten years of treating necrotizing fasciitis. *Infect Dis (Lond)*. 2015;47:319-325.

Norrby-Teglund A, Stevens DL. Novel therapies in streptococcal toxic shock syndrome: attenuation of virulence factor expression and modulation of the host response. *Curr Opin Infect Dis*. 1998;11(3):285-291. doi: 10.1097/00001432-199806000-00004.

Norrby-Teglund A, Kaul R, Low DE, et al. Plasma from patients with severe invasive group A streptococcal infections treated with normal polyspecific IgG inhibits streptococcal superantigen-induced T cell proliferation and cytokine production. *J Immunol*. 1996;156(8):3057-3064.

Olsen RJ, Musser JM. Molecular pathogenesis of necrotizing fasciitis. *Annu Rev Pathol*. 2010;5:1-31.

Ozturk E, Sonmez Y, Yilmazlar T. What are the indications for a stoma in Fournier's gangrene? *Colorectal Dis*. 2011;13(9):1044-1047. doi: 10.1111/j.1463-1318.2010.02353.x.

Riseman JA, Zamboni WA, Curtis A, Graham DR, Konrad HR, Ross DS. Hyperbaric oxygen therapy for necrotizing fasciitis reduces mortality and the need for debridements. *Surgery*. 1990;108(5):847-850.

Roden MM, Zaoutis TE, Buchanan WL, et al. Epidemiology and outcome of zygomycosis: a review of 929 reported cases. *Clin Infect Dis*. 2005;41:634-653.

Rosen DR, Brown ME, Cologne KG, Ault GT, Strumwasser AM. Long-term follow-up of Fournier's Gangrene in a tertiary care center. *J Surg Res.* 2016;206(1):175-181. doi: 10.1016/j.jss.2016.06.091.

Sartelli M, Guirao X, Hardcastle TC, et al. 2018 WSES/SIS-E consensus conference: recommendations for the management of skin and soft-tissue infections. *World J Emerg Surg.* 2018;13:58. doi: 10.1186/s13017-018-0219-9.

Shumba P, Shambat SM, Simens N. The role of Streptococcal and Staphylococcal exotoxins and proteases in human necrotizing soft tissue infections. *Toxins.* 2019;11:332.

Soh CR, Pietrobon R, Freiberger JJ, et al. Hyperbaric oxygen therapy in necrotising soft tissue infections: a study of patients in the United States Nationwide Inpatient Sample. *Intensive Care Med.* 2012;38(7):1143-1151. doi: 10.1007/s00134-012-2558-4.

Soltani AM, Best MJ, Francis CS, Allan BJ, Askari M, Panthaki ZJ. Trends in the incidence and treatment of necrotizing soft tissue infections: an analysis of the National Hospital Discharge Survey. *J Burn Care Res.* 2014;35:449-454.

Stevens DL. The Flesh-eating bacterium: what's next? *J Infect Dis.* 1999;179:S366-S374.

Stevens DL, Bryant AE. Necrotizing soft-tissue infections. *N Engl J Med.* 2017;377:2253.

Stevens DL, Bisno AL, Chambers HF, et al.; Infectious Diseases Society of America. Practice guidelines for the diagnosis and management of skin and soft tissue infections: 2014 update by the Infectious Diseases Society of America. *Clin Infect Dis.* 2014;59(2):e10-e52. doi: 10.1093/cid/ciu444. Erratum in: Clin Infect Dis. 2015 May 1;60(9):1448. Dosage error in article text.

Tibbles PM, Edelsberg JS. Hyperbaric-oxygen therapy. *N Engl J Med.* 1996;334(25):1642-1648. doi: 10.1056/NEJM199606203342506.

Wall DB, dc Virgilio C, Black S, Klein SR. Objective criteria may assist in distinguishing necrotizing fasciitis from nonnecrotizing soft tissue infection. *Am J Surg.* 2000;179:17-21.

Wallin TR, Hern HG, Frazee BW. Community-associated methicillin-resistant *Staphylococcus aureus. Emerg Med Clin North Am.* 2008;26:431-455.

Wang C, Schwaitzberg S, Berliner E, Zarin DA, Lau J. Hyperbaric oxygen for treating wounds: a systematic review of the literature. *Arch Surg.* 2003;138(3):272-279; discussion 280. doi: 10.1001/archsurg.138.3.272.

Weiss KA, Laverdiere M. Group A Streptococcus invasive infections: a review. *Can J Surg.* 1997;40:18-25.

Wilson B. Necrotizing fasciitis. *Am Surg.* 1952;18:416-431.

Wong CH, Chang HC, Pasupathy S, Khin LW, Tan JL, Low CO. Necrotizing fasciitis: clinical presentation, microbiology, and determinants of mortality. *J Bone Joint Surg Am.* 2003;85-A(8):1454.

Wong CH, Khin LW, Heng KS, et al. The LRINEC (Laboratory Risk Indicator for Necrotizing Fasciitis) score: a tool for distinguishing necrotizing fasciitis from other soft tissue infections. *Crit Care Med.* 2004;32:1535-1541.

Yaghan RJ, Al-Jaberi TM, Bani-Hani I. Fournier's gangrene: changing face of the disease. *Dis Colon Rectum.* 2000;43(9):1300-1308. doi: 10.1007/BF02237442.

Yen ZS, Wang HP, Ma HM, Chen SC, Chen WJ. Ultrasonographic screening of clinically suspected necrotizing fasciitis. *Acad Emerg Med.* 2002;9(12):1448-1451.

Young LM, Price CS. Community-acquired methicillin resistant *Staphylococcus aureus* emerging as an important cause of necrotizing fasciitis. *Surg Infect (Larchmt).* 2008;9:469-474.

CHAPTER

22 Abdominal Wall Hernias

Dorin Popa and Dzhendov Todor

CASE PRESENTATION

Case: A 60-year-old man came to the Emergency Room complaining of a lump localized in the right inguinal area that reduced when supine. He noticed it 4 years ago but related increasingly troublesome episodes of discomfort that are interfering with his employment and hobbies. For the past 4 days, the lump is no longer reducible, accompanied with increasing pain but no nausea or vomiting. The patient has no other medical history and enjoys good health.

Question: *Why did we choose TAPP technique instead of TEP or Lichtenstein?*

Answer: *TAPP allows inspection and treatment of both inguinal hernias. In addition we can correctly evaluate the viability of strangulated bowel.*

Clinical findings: Clinical examination revealed an incarcerated right inguinal hernia with a sac of ~4 × 4 cm. When asked to cough, examination detected a possible small inguinal hernia on the left side as well. The patient had no spontaneous/provoked abdominal pain. Based on this history and clinical examination, the diagnosis of incarcerated right inguinal hernia with possible uncomplicated left inguinal hernia was made (**Figure 22.1**).

Laboratory findings: WBC: 11 000/mm^3, CRP: 23 mg/L, Lactate: normal, Urea: normal, no fever.

Treatment plan: Laparoscopic transabdominal preperitoneal (TAPP) approach with suspicion of a hernia on the other side.

Intraoperative findings: Indirect right inguinal hernia with incarcerated greater omentum (**Figure 22.2A**). The defect was estimated at 2.5 cm^2 in diameter. Direct left inguinal hernia with a defect estimated at 1.5 cm in diameter. (**Figure 22.2B**). The peritoneum was dissected from the anterior superior iliac spine to the umbilical ligament on the same site, 3 cm over the hernia defect. Identification of inferior epigastric artery, Cooper ligament, space of Retzius, ductus deferens, and funiculus spermaticus was accomplished. A 15 × 10 cm mesh was applied to overlap the hernia defect with at least 3 cm in all the directions but also covering the femoral area as a precaution for a femoral hernia in the future. The mesh was fixed with fibrin glue (**Figure 22.2C**). The peritoneum was closed with a running suture.

Discharge: Next day in the morning. Postoperative recommendations were to avoid strenuous physical activities for the next 30 days.

One week after the surgery: Patient returned with a nonreducible bulge in the left inguinal area. No fever or signs of inflammation. Discrete local discomfort. Normal examination on the right side. Diagnosis: postoperative seroma, not a recurrence. The patient was reassured.

INTRODUCTION

A hernia is an abnormal protrusion of a peritoneal-lined sac through a defect in the abdominal wall. If the protruded contents can be returned to the abdomen (spontaneously or by pressure), the hernia is *reducible*. If the hernia contents cannot be pushed into the abdomen, the hernia is said to be *irreducible* (*incarcerated* hernia). In this case, there is a risk of intestinal obstruction and compromised blood supply, which results in tissue ischemia, called strangulation. *Strangulated hernia* is a surgical challenge, which is sometimes difficult to diagnose and requires emergent surgical intervention. Abdominal wall hernia frequency (from high to low) is inguinal, umbilical, linea alba, incisional, femoral, and the less common types. Seventy-five percent of abdominal wall hernias are groin hernias.

In their simplest taxonomy, groin hernias may be classified as **direct** (medial—abdominal contents protrude through the superficial inguinal ring), **indirect** (lateral—protrusion of abdominal

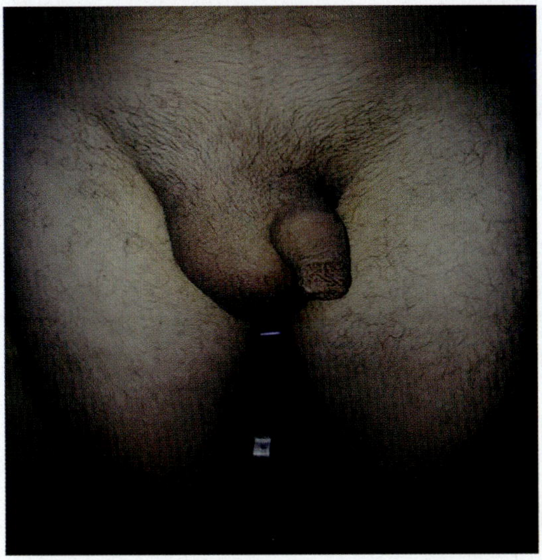

Figure 22.1 Incarcerated right inguinal hernia.

content through the deep inguinal ring), or **femoral hernia** (bounded by the Poupart ligament anterosuperiorly, Cooper ligament posteriorly, the femoral vein laterally, and the pubic tubercle/lacunar ligament medially) (**Figure 22.3**). The direct hernia passes through Hesselbach triangle, defined by the lateral edge of the rectus abdominis, the epigastric artery, and the inguinal ligament. The indirect inguinal hernia is the most common groin hernia in both males and females. Of groin hernias, 95% are inguinal and 5% femoral. They can be found concurrently, with a femoral hernia present on repair of 10% of inguinal hernias. The *pantaloon* hernia has both direct and indirect elements. Femoral hernias can be difficult to diagnose (female/male, 4/1), especially in obese patients. Up to 40% of femoral hernias may present as emergencies. Groin hernias are categorized into 2 main types: femoral and inguinal. Inguinal hernias are subdivided into direct and indirect (**Table 22.1**). Numerous classification for inguinal hernias have been described. The famous herniologist Nyhus offered an expanded classification to allow standardized description of the clinical and operative findings and this classification is now widely accepted by surgeons. The **sliding hernia** must also be recognized. In this case, the wall of the hernia sac is comprised of bladder, right colon, or sigmoid colon. This must be recognized to minimize risk to these organs during hernia repair.

True **umbilical hernias** may be congenital or acquired (especially in pregnancy), while **paraumbilical hernias** are associated with conditions of chronic increased intra-abdominal pressure, such as in obesity and cirrhosis with ascites. Umbilical hernias often close in young children. Thus, they generally are not repaired in children younger than 5 years. **Hernias of the linea alba** may be simple (eg, epigastric hernia) or present as multiple defects in the fascia. **Ventral (incisional) hernias** are acquired fascial defects, principally seen after laparotomy, especially in patients where recovery was complicated by wound infection. Occasional small incisional **"port site" hernias** result from laparoscopic access when fascial openings were not closed primarily or dehisced.

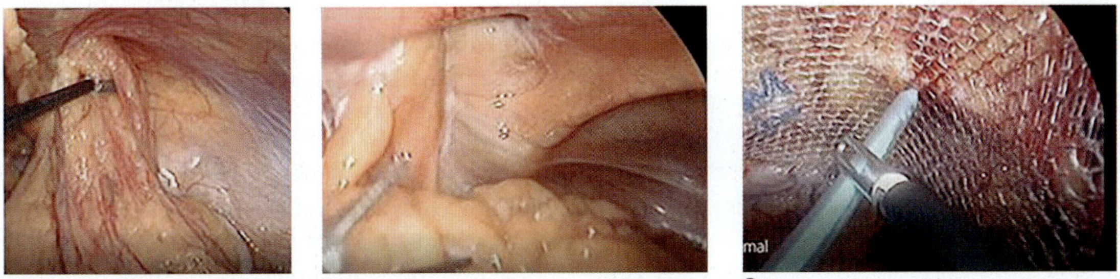

A B C

Figure 22.2 Greater omentum incarcerated in the right-sided inguinal hernia **(A)**, direct left inguinal hernia **(B)**, and mesh fixation with fibrin glue **(C)**.

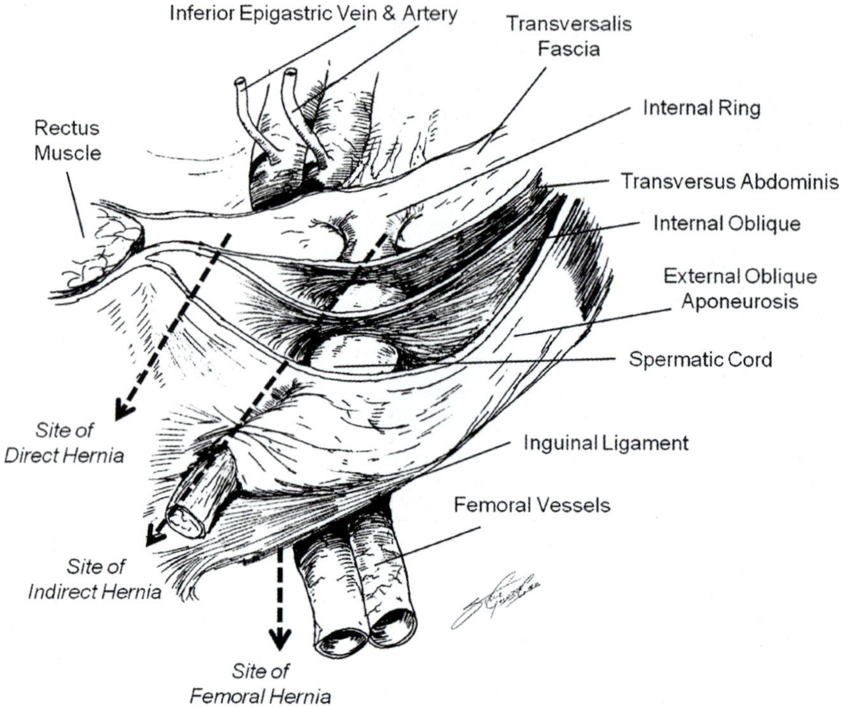

Figure 22.3 Inguinal anatomy and location of groin hernias. (From Peitzman AB, et al. *The Trauma Manual: Trauma and Acute Care Surgery*. 5th ed. Wolters Kluwer; 2020.)

DIAGNOSIS

While no randomized trials compare physical examination alone to imaging in securing the diagnosis of incarcerated abdominal wall hernia, examination remains the mainstay of diagnosis. Be certain to carefully exam the patient with a bowel obstruction for abdominal wall/groin hernias. With suspicion of a groin hernia, the patient should be examined in both the supine and standing positions. It is critically important to know when attempted reduction of a hernia is contraindicated, due to the high likelihood that infarcted intestine will be returned to the abdominal cavity (reduction en masse). Local skin changes of erythema or induration or signs of peritonitis require emergent operation without an attempt at reduction (**Figure 22.4**). The level of evidence that there is additional benefit in obtaining computed tomography (CT) or ultrasound (US) imaging for diagnosis of abdominal wall incarcerated hernia is poor and only applies to special circumstances: obese patients, and rarer defects such as Spigelian or obturator hernias. CT also has utility in planned repair of ventral hernias. Axial imaging facilitates localization of the abdominal wall defect, allows measurement of defect dimensions (for mesh planning), and may detect associated clinically occult hernias. Complications requiring emergency intervention may also be detected, such as an abrupt small bowel caliber transition suggestive of obstruction, abscesses in the hernia sac, and peritoneal enhancement. Reduced bowel wall enhancement has good specificity (94%) and sensitivity (56%) in predicting the risk of strangulation.

TABLE 22.1 ■ Classification of Groin Hernias
1. Indirect inguinal hernia
2. Direct inguinal hernia
3. Femoral hernia

Reprinted from Zollinger RM Jr. Classification systems for groin hernias. *Surg Clin North Am*. 2003;83(5):1053–1063, with permission from Elsevier.

SURGICAL DECISION-MAKING

The World Society of Emergency Surgery (WSES) offers recommendations for emergency repair of abdominal wall hernias in adults, providing evidence-based recommendations on the timing of intervention, laparoscopic approach, surgical repair according to the CDC wound classification, and antimicrobial prophylaxis on the topic of emergency repair of complicated abdominal wall hernias.

Early diagnosis of strangulation, reducing the time from onset to surgery, is the most important prognostic factor. Multivariate analysis has demonstrated that delayed presentation or intervention, with bowel necrosis, significantly increases mor-

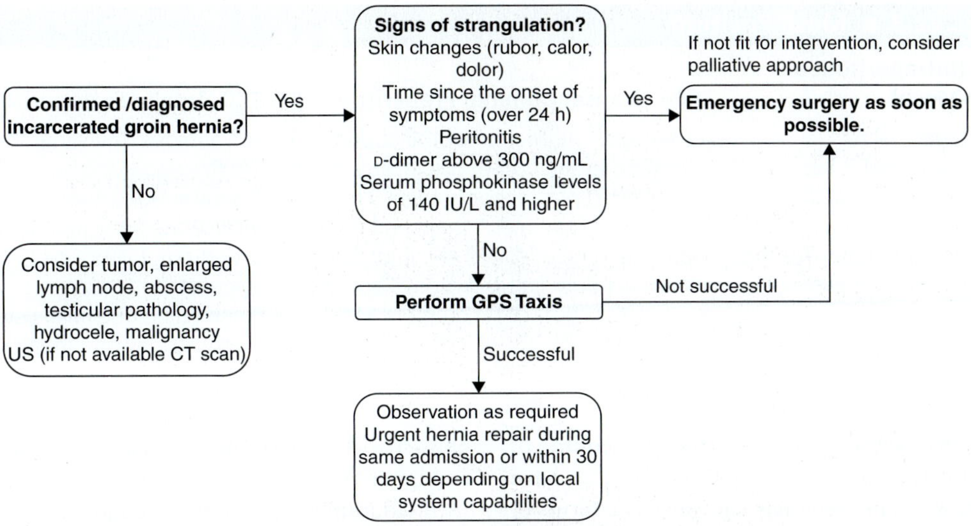

Figure 22.4 Management of the acute incarcerated inguinal hernia in adults. GPS Taxis: **G** be gentle. A constant steady pressure over the hernia for 5-15 minutes, avoiding forceful pushing. **P** be prepared. Appropriate environment with oxygen therapy, oxygen saturation and pulse monitoring, opioid and benzodiazepine antagonists at the bedside. **S** be safe. Careful titration of IV opioids and diazepines. (Reprinted by permission from Springer: Springer. Pawlak M, East B, de Beaux AC. Algorithm for management of an incarcerated inguinal hernia in the emergency setting with manual reduction. Taxis, the technique and its safety. *Hernia*. 2021;25:1253-1258.)

tality. The WSES guidelines thus stress that adverse elements of the history and physical examination, as well as laboratory findings (high serum lactate, D-dimer, and creatinine phosphokinase), as well as SIRS and contrast-enhanced CT signs are predictive of bowel strangulation and should prompt early operative intervention.

When strangulation is suspected, early emergency hernia repair is advised. Hernia repair may be performed open—still performed most commonly—or laparoscopically (**Table 22.2**). Strategic decision making for incarcerated or strangulated hernia raises several considerations. The priority is to save the incarcerated or strangulated organ, with mitigation of hernia recurrence as a secondary concern. Synthetic mesh placement is generally safe for abdominal wall reconstruction after reduction of an incarcerated or strangulated inguinal hernia.

The need for bowel resection is not an absolute contraindication to placement of synthetic mesh. The preferred mesh is a macroporous, monofilament polypropylene mesh, placed extraperitoneally. If a strangulated hernia is complicated by intestinal perforation or gross purulence/contamination, however, consideration should be given to avoidance of synthetic mesh placement. Instead, consider primary tissue repair, or a "damage control" approach with delayed repair of the hernial orifice. Interestingly, recent studies have shown little advantage to the use of biologic mesh compared to permanent synthetic mesh relative to infection, in addition to its high risk of recurrence.

INGUINAL HERNIAS

Surgery is the only effective treatment for patients with inguinal or femoral hernias. The *Shouldice* repair was considered the gold standard up to the 1990s. Since then, the *Lichtenstein technique*—

TABLE 22.2 ■ Surgical Approach Considerations

The Open Approach Is Recommended for	Laparoscopy Is an Alternative
• Unstable patients • Advanced laparoscopic surgical expertise is not immediately available • Have previously operated abdomen with midline incision • Have contaminated wounds (class III)/ dirty or infected wounds (class IV) • Have markedly distended bowel	• In the stable patient • For surgeons with experience in the laparoscopic approach for both elective and emergency hernia repair • For small bowel distension <4.5 cm in diameter or transition point closer to Treitz angle • In the absence of previous abdominal incision (other than open appendectomy) • Absence of signs of peritonitis

TABLE 22.3 ■ Mesh Position

IPOM (Intraperitoneal Onlay Mesh)	TAPP (Transabdominal Preperitoneal)	TEP (Totally Extraperitoneal)
Advantages: takes shorter time and is less demanding—no need to close the peritoneum. *Disadvantages:* it implies the usage of an intraperitoneal mesh.	*Advantages:* inspection of the abdominal cavity and evaluation of the incarcerated/strangulated part. Preperitoneal placement of the mesh that can be fixated with glue (so NO tackers). So, no contact between the organs and the mesh. This is the most complete MIS method.	*Advantages:* the same as for TAPP. *Disadvantages:* the incarcerated organ, once pulled out, cannot be evaluated. Open technique (also using mesh): on-lay and in-lay.

tension-free hernioplasty—is the procedure of choice for the open repair. Both approaches have been shown to be resolutely equivalent, in terms of recurrence (short-term and long-term follow-up) and complications.

Emergent laparoscopic repair of an incarcerated groin hernia is an alternative that should be limited to high-volume centers and experienced surgeons. Notwithstanding this, diagnostic laparoscopy may be a useful adjunct to assess bowel viability after spontaneous reduction of strangulated groin hernias, prior to open fascial re-approximation or mesh placement. Another technique to assess bowel viability is laparoscopically via the hernia sac during open groin exploration prior to the repair (hernioscopy). Several studies have shown that the laparoscopic hernia repair performed by a surgeon familiar with this technique is feasible and safe in patients with incarcerated incisional and ventral hernias. A minimally invasive approach—*TAPP (transabdominal preperitoneal)* or *TEP (totally extraperitoneal)*—is increasing in popularity, and acute care surgeons are becoming more facile with these techniques (**Table 22.3**).

Complication rates are similar to open approach in large series. Where appropriate expertise exists, laparoscopic repair of incarcerated/strangulated hernia is feasible even if bowel resection is needed. An apparent paradox exists in the advised approach to the elective management of recurrent incisional, inguinal, and femoral hernias. The open approach should be preferred if the initial technique was laparoscopic (the idea is to cut through unviolated tissues for repair). Conversely, the laparoscopic technique should be preferred if the initial approach was anterior (open).

VENTRAL HERNIAS

Ventral hernias, as a collective term, include incisional hernia, peri- and infraumbilical, and epigastric (linea alba) hernias. Factors contributing to higher risk for incarceration include increased intra-abdominal pressure (secondary to ascites, chronic cough, obesity, and obstipation). "Small" defects—3 to 4 cm in diameter—(for primary and incisional hernias), peri- and infraumbilical hernias (for primary hernias), female gender, and older age are also risk factors for incarceration.

Mesh placement provides superior results in ventral hernia repair. Mesh placement can be done in-lay (retromuscular or preperitoneal) or on-lay with the condition that an overlap of 5 cm is provided. Depending on the degree of contamination (gross contamination or purulence) and patient's general condition, there are situations when primary closure without mesh (if feasible) is favored. The abdomen can be left open with negative pressure and closed as soon as possible. WSES consensus recommendations for the placement of mesh differ according to the likelihood of surgical site contamination. In clean surgical fields, as already shown, mesh decreases recurrence rates without increasing the incidence of wound infection (but with a higher risk of seroma). Emergent hernia repair with a synthetic mesh can be performed in case of intestinal strangulation and/or concomitant bowel resection without gross enteric spillage (without any increase in 30-day wound-related morbidity) and is associated with a significant lower risk of recurrence, regardless of the size of hernia defect.

For the stable patient with a small defect (under 3 cm), a primary repair is advised. For unstable patients, however, damage control principles prevail, and abbreviated surgery with open abdomen and planned return to the OR is recommended. In this circumstance, abdominal fascial closure should be attempted as soon as physiologically possible due to the risk of fascial retraction, making the closure even more difficult. Although

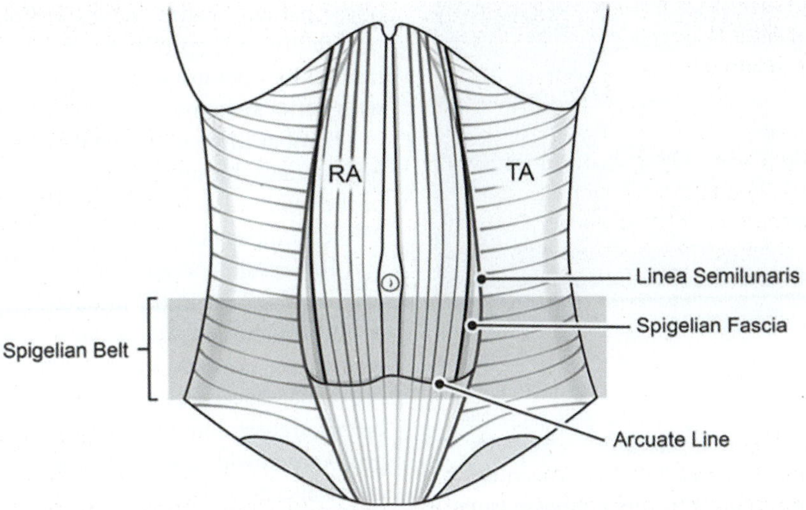

Figure 22.5 Area of appearance for Spigelian hernia. RA, rectus abdominis; TA, transversus abdominis. (Reprinted by permission from Springer: Springer. Webber V, Low C, Skipworth RJE, et al. Contemporary thoughts on the management of Spigelian hernia. *Hernia*. 2017;21:355-361.)

controversial, some recommend component separation techniques as an alternative when there is a significant abdominal wall retraction. Furthermore, component separation with transversus abdominis release in the emergency setting resulted in increased wound complications requiring intervention. When negative pressure devices are not available, skin-only closure is an option in the form of planned incisional hernia that can be treated later, when the conditions are better.

Repair of an incarcerated ventral hernia can be performed laparoscopically in the appropriate setting. With suspicion of bowel strangulation or the need for bowel resection, laparoscopy is not generally suitable and an open approach is preferable. For the laparoscopic approach, open abdominal access is recommended for initial camera placement and the creation of pneumoperitoneum. It is preferable to use nontraumatic graspers, if possible, silicone coated inside the jaws. Extreme attention is warranted when maneuvering the bowel loops to avoid iatrogenic perforation. A combination of gentle taxis, pushing (from outside) and pulling (from inside) should be used for reducing hernia content. Of note, because of adhesions, bowel damage may occur at this phase. Never pull on distended loops. A missed enterotomy is among the most feared complications following hernia repair.

Spigelian hernia accounts for just 1%-2% of all hernias. The "Spigelian hernia belt" is where most of the hernias occur: an area below the umbilicus and above the interspinal plane (**Figure 22.5**). Anatomic particularity explains why they are difficult both to palpate on examination and also to discover at operation (until the external oblique layer muscle is opened) (**Figure 22.6**). The laparoscopic approach facilitates identification of the Spigelian hernia compared to open surgery (**Figure 22.7**).

Pain is the most frequently described symptom, even years before coming to the emergency room. Depending on the hernia contents, other symptoms can be associated: nausea, vomiting,

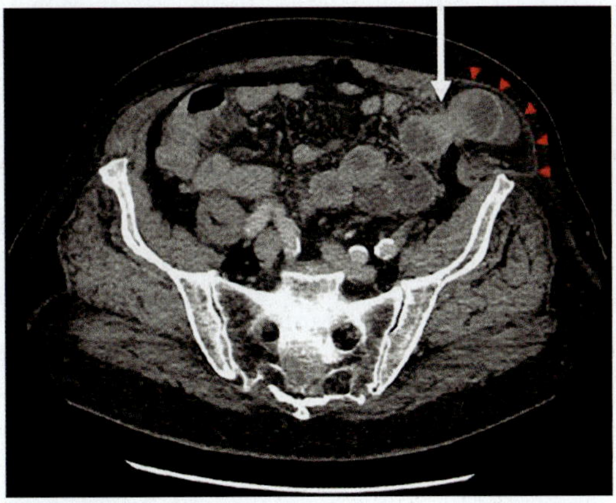

Figure 22.6 Spigelian hernia on CT. Abdominal CT demonstrates a left-sided Spigelian hernia with small bowel within the sac (*arrow*). Note the intact external oblique aponeurosis (*arrowheads*). (Reprinted by permission from Springer: Springer. Hanzalova I, Schafer M, Demartines N, et al. Spigelian hernia: current approaches to surgical treatment—a review. *Hernia*. 2021. https://doi.org/10.1007/s10029-021-02511-8. Open access.)

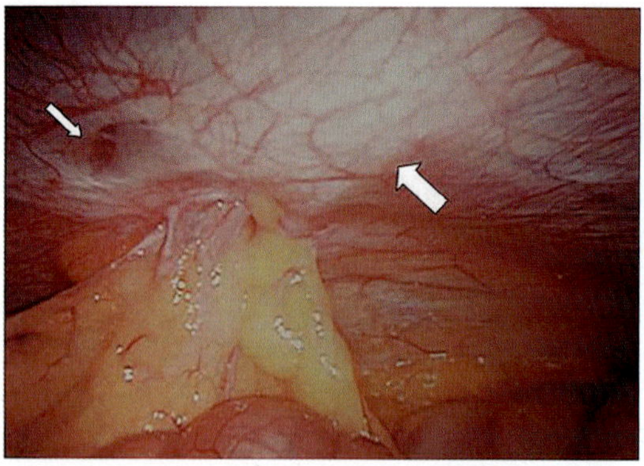

Figure 22.7 Moderate sized left Spigelian hernia with peritoneal sac, which is visible and treatable laparoscopically. Note that the defect is above the arcuate line (*large arrow*) and there is a second split in the Spigelian fascia further cephalad (*small arrow*). (Reprinted by permission from Springer: Springer. Webber V, Low C, Skipworth RJE, et al. Contemporary thoughts on the management of Spigelian hernia. *Hernia*. 2017;21:355-361.)

or abdominal distension. If the bowel is strangulated and the patient presents late, peritonitis can be observed (fever, tachycardia, and hypotension). Imaging augments the physical examination in small or occult Spigelian hernias, especially in obese patients. Ultrasound has the advantages of portability and reproducibility, but its reliability is limited by operator-dependence. CT is preferred, with better sensitivity and specificity.

Lumbar (dorsal) hernia is protrusion of abdominal contents through the superior (Grynfeltt hernia) or the inferior lumbar triangle (Petit hernia). About 25% of lumbar hernias lead to bowel incarceration, and 10% result in strangulation. A CT or MRI study will reveal defects in the musculofascial layer as well as the contents of the hernia. Repair can be performed via open or laparoscopic approach, which has similar success rates. In selected cases of lumbar hernia, transabdominal preperitoneal repair (TAPP) can be used with good outcome. A transabdominal or extraperitoneal laparoscopic approach is used predominantly in uncomplicated cases, as open repair is favored in complicated cases.

Obturator hernia generally occurs in elderly patients, female, multiparous, and often after weight loss. The obturator foramen contains the obturator nerve, artery, and vein, bound by the rami and pubic bones (**Figure 22.8**).

The obturator hernia is difficult to diagnose on physical examination. The patients often present with bowel obstruction. Delay in diagnosis

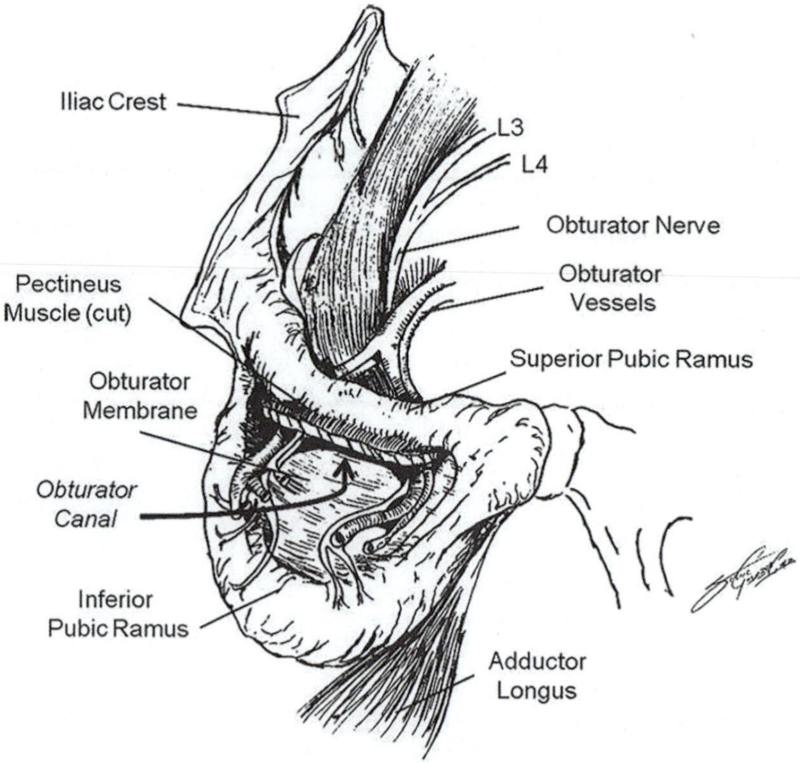

Figure 22.8 Obturator hernia. The obturator foramen is shown with its boundaries. (From Peitzman AB, et al. *The Trauma Manual: Trauma and Acute Care Surgery*. 5th ed. Wolters Kluwer; 2020.)

and operation is common, increasing morbidity and mortality. The patients may complain of hip or thigh pain or a palpable mass on the medial thigh. Patients with an incarcerated obturator hernia may have a positive Howship-Romberg sign (pain with external rotation and extension of the hip). CT is invaluable in confirming the diagnosis of obturator hernia (**Figure 22.9**). Treatment is immediate operation, with laparoscopy providing excellent exposure. A lower midline open approach may also be utilized. Defects <1 cm may be repaired primarily. Larger defects should be repaired with mesh (**Figure 22.10**). Examine the contralateral obturator canal as ~10% may be bilateral.

Sliding inguinal hernias comprise 5%-16% of groin hernias. They are far more common in males, left > right sided. With a sliding hernia, the bladder or retroperitoneal organ (sigmoid colon or cecum) with or without its mesentery comprises a portion of the peritoneal sac. The ureter may also be within the hernia. The internal ring may be quite large with a sliding hernia. With large sliding components, the entire posterior wall of the sac may be the mesentery of the bowel, which has slid caudally, often into the scrotum. Thus, without recognition of a sliding hernia, these viscera may be injured. In addition, recurrence of the hernia is higher after repair of a sliding groin hernia. A small sliding hernia can be repaired with a laparoscopic or open technique. Larger sliding hernias are best repaired with an open approach. With cecum or sigmoid colon as the sliding component, the hernia sac must be entered away from these structures. When the bladder is the sliding component, peritoneum should not be opened at that site. Reperitonealizing the cecum or sigmoid colon requires some innovation, as shown in **Figures 22.11 and 22.12.** For very large sliding hernias, restoring continuity of the peritoneum may not be feasible. Complete reduction of the hernia and its sliding components are more important than restoring the peritoneal covering. Once the hernia contents have been returned to the abdominal cavity, a Lichtenstein repair is generally performed.

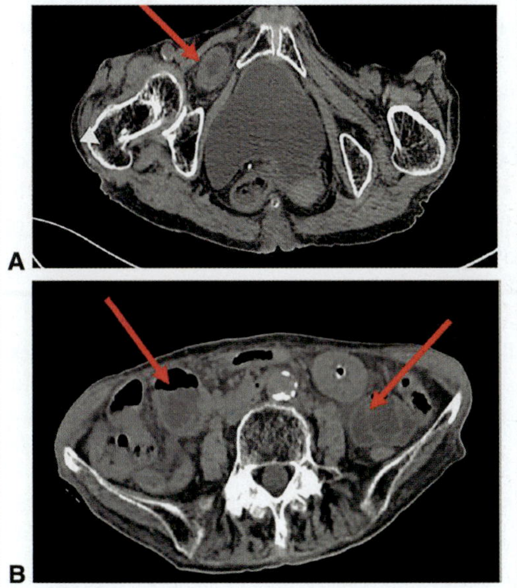

Figure 22.9 Obturator hernia. **A.** Abdominal CT shows an obturator hernia with incarcerated small intestine. **B.** Abdominal CT demonstrates the proximal dilated small bowel from the obstruction. (Reprinted by permission from Springer: Springer. Li Z, Gu C, Wei M, et al. Diagnosis and treatment of obturator hernia: retrospective analysis of 86 clinical cases at a single institution. *BMC Surg*. 2021;21:124. https://doi.org/10.1186/s12893-021-01125-2, open access.)

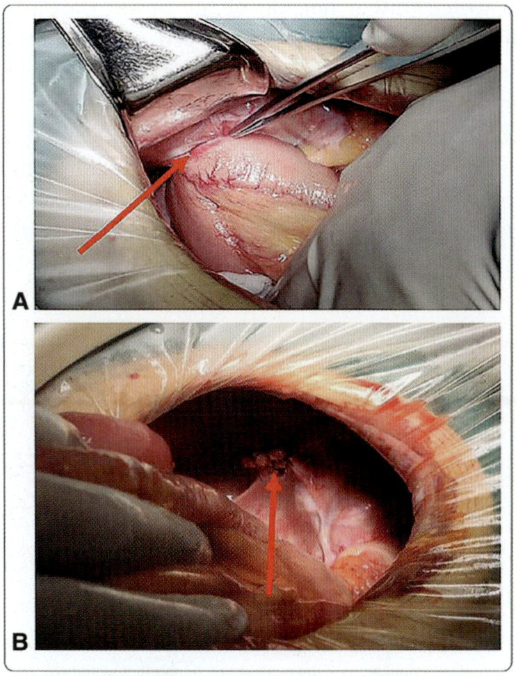

Figure 22.10 Obturator hernia. **A.** Intraoperative image showing small intestine incarcerated in the obturator foramen. **B.** Operative picture after reduction of the intestine, showing the obturator canal closed with an intermittent suture. (Reprinted by permission from Springer: Springer. Li Z, Gu C, Wei M, et al. Diagnosis and treatment of obturator hernia: retrospective analysis of 86 clinical cases at a single institution. *BMC Surg*. 2021;21:124. https://doi.org/10.1186/s12893-021-01125-2, open access.)

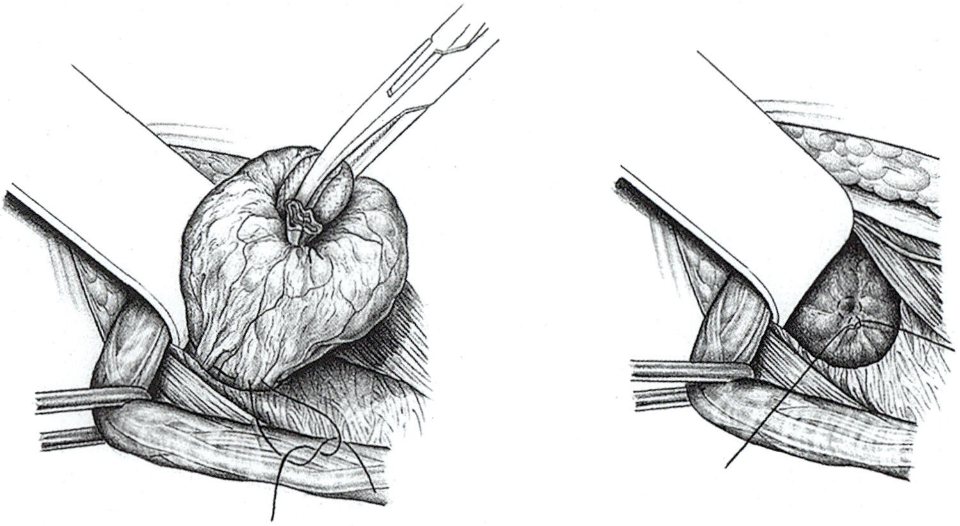

Figure 22.11 Sliding hernia. Repair by an external purse string suture, catching only peritoneum, avoiding incorporation and then dunking the viscera that comprise the sliding component. (From Special Hernias. In: Schumpelick V, Arlt G, Conze J, Junge K, eds. *Hernia Surgery*. Thieme; 2020. Figure 3.11.)

Richter hernia is worthy of mention. A Richter hernia is an abdominal wall or groin hernia in which only a portion of the bowel wall, usually antimesenteric, is entrapped in the hernia defect. Although a Richter hernia can occur with any hernia defect, high-risk hernias are femoral, obturator, and port site. As a Richter hernia does not produce a bowel obstruction, suspicion for an incarcerated hernia may be low. This can result in strangulation and perforation of the bowel wall and a septic patient.

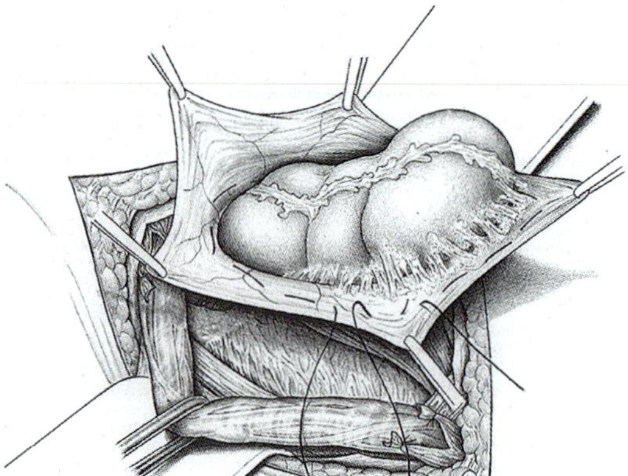

Figure 22.12 Sliding hernia. Repair by an internal purse string avoiding incorporation of the cecum in the purse string suture. The cecum is dunked and the purse string is tied. (From Special Hernias. In: Schumpelick V, Arlt G, Conze J, Junge K, eds. *Hernia Surgery*. Thieme; 2020. Figure 3.10.)

SUMMARY

Abdominal wall and inguinal hernias are commonly seen in emergency general surgery patients. Knowledge of the anatomic weaknesses that can lead to hernias is vital. Early diagnosis and reduction of incarcerated hernias are essential, ideally prior to the development of strangulation. Smaller defects can be repaired primarily. With larger hernia defects, placement of mesh will decrease the risk of recurrence. Be certain to search for an abdominal wall/groin hernia in any patient with a bowel obstruction. Remember that the patient with a Richter hernia may not have evidence of a bowel obstruction.

SUGGESTED READINGS

Alkhatib H, Tastaldi L, Krpata DM, et al. Outcomes of transversus abdominis release in nonelective incisional hernia repair: a retrospective study of the Americas Hernia Society Quality Collaborative. *Hernia*. 2019;23:43-49.

Andresen K, Bisgaard T, Rosenberg J. Sliding inguinal hernia is a risk factor for recurrence. *Langenbecks Arch Surg*. 2015;400:101-106.

Birindelli A, Sartelli M, Di Saverio S, et al. 2017 update of the WSES guidelines for emergency repair of complicated abdominal wall hernias. *World J Emerg Surg*. 2017;12:37.

Chihara N, Suzuki H, Sukegawa M, et al. Is the laparoscopic approach feasible for reduction and herniorrhaphy in cases of acutely incarcerated/strangulated groin and obturator hernia: 17-year experience from open to laparoscopic approach. *J Laparoendosc Adv Surg Tech A*. 2019;29(5):631-637.

Coccolini F, Montori G, Catena F, et al. The role of the open abdomen in non-trauma patient: WSES consensus paper. *World J Emerg Surg*. 2017;12:39. doi:10.1186/s13017-017-0146-1

Coccolini F, Roberts D, Ansaloni L, et al. The open abdomen in trauma and non-trauma patients: WSES guidelines. *World J Emerg Surg*. 2018;13:7. doi:10.1186/s13017-018-0167-4

De Simone B, Birindelli A, Ansaloni L, et al. Emergency repair of complicated abdominal wall hernias: WSES guidelines. *Hernia*. 2020;24(2):359-368.

Deeba S, Purkayastha S, Paraskevas P, et al. Laparoscopic approach to incarcerated and strangulated inguinal hernias. *JSLS*. 2009;13(3):327-331.

Di Saverio S, Coccolini F, Galati M, et al. Bologna guidelines for diagnosis and management of adhesive small bowel obstruction (ASBO): 2013 update of the evidence-based guidelines from the world society of emergency surgery ASBO working group. *World J Emerg Surg*. 2013;8(1):42.

Elsebae MM, Nasr M, Said M. Tension-free repair versus Bassini technique for strangulated inguinal hernia: a controlled randomized study. *Int J Surg*. 2008;6(4):302-305.

Gore RM, Levine MS. *Textbook of Gastrointestinal Radiology*. 3rd ed. Saunders Elsevier; 2008:2156-2165.

Hanzalova I, Schafer M, Demartines N, et al. Spigelian hernia: current approaches to surgical treatment—a review. *Hernia*. 2021. https://doi.org/10.1007/s10029-021-02511-8

Harris HW, Primus F, Young C, et al. Preventing recurrence in clean and contaminated hernias using biologic vs synthetic mesh in ventral hernia repair. The PRICE randomized clinical trial. *Ann Surg*. 2021;273:648-655.

Helgstrand F, Rosenberg J, Kehlet H, et al. Outcomes after emergency versus elective ventral hernia repair: a prospective nationwide study. *World J Surg*. 2013;37(10):2273-2279.

Jancelewicz T, Vu LT, Shawo AE, et al. Predicting strangulated small bowel obstruction: an old problem revisited. *J Gastrointest Surg*. 2009;13(1):93-99.

Köckerling F, Koch A, Adolf D, et al. Has Shouldice repair in a selected group of patients with inguinal hernia comparable results to Lichtenstein, TEP and TAPP techniques? *World J Surg*. 2018;42(7):2001-2010.

Koizumi M, Sata N, Kaneda Y, et al. Optimal timeline for emergency surgery in patients with strangulated groin hernias. *Hernia*. 2014;18(6):845-848.

Leibl BJ, Schmedt CG, Kraft K, et al. Laparoscopic transperitoneal hernia repair of incarcerated hernias: is it feasible? Results of a prospective study. *Surg Endosc*. 2001;15(10):1179-1183.

Li Z, Gu C, Wei M, et al. Diagnosis and treatment of obturator hernia: retrospective analysis of 86 clinical cases at a single institution. *BMC Surg*. 2021;21:124. https://doi.org/10.1186/s12893-021-01125-2

Lopez-Cano M, Garcia-Alamino JM, Antoniou SA, et al. EHS clinical guidelines on the management of the abdominal wall in the context of the burst or open abdomen. *Hernia*. 2018;22:921-939.

Martínez-Serrano MA, Pereira JA, Sancho J, et al. Specific improvement measures to reduce complications and mortality after urgent surgery in complicated abdominal wall hernia. *Hernia*. 2012;16(2):171-177.

Pawlak M, East B, de Beaux AC. Algorithm for management of an incarcerated inguinal hernia in the emergency setting with manual reduction. Taxis, the technique and its safety. *Hernia*. 2021;25:1253-1258.

Plastic Surgery Key. *Special Hernias*. Accessed December 7, 2021. https://plasticsurgerykey.com/special-hernias/

Reinke CE, Matthews BD. What's new in the management of incarcerated hernia. *J Gastrointest Surg*. 2020;24(1):221-230.

Sallinen V, Di Saverio S, Haukijärvi E, et al. Laparoscopic versus open adhesiolysis for adhesive small bowel obstruction (LASSO): an international, multicentre, randomised, open-label trial. *Lancet Gastroenterol Hepatol*. 2019;4(4):278-286.

Samra NS, Ballard DH, Doumite DF, et al. Repair of large sliding inguinial hernias. *Am Surg*. 2015;81:1205-1208.

Sneiders D, Yurtkap Y, Kroese LF, et al. Risk factors for incarceration in patients with primary abdominal wall and incisional hernias: a prospective study in 4472 patients. *World J Surg*. 2019;43(8):1906-1913.

Webber V, Low C, Skipworth RJE, et al. Contemporary thoughts on the management of Spigelian hernia. *Hernia*. 2017;21:355-361.

Wolf LL, Scott JW, Zogg CK, et al. Predictors of emergency ventral hernia repair: targets to improve patient access and guide patient selection for elective repair. *Surgery*. 2016;160(5):1379-1391.

CHAPTER

23 Complex Liver Masses

Ram Nirula and Miloš Buhavac

CASE PRESENTATION

A 78-year-old man presents to the emergency department with 5 days of upper abdominal/right upper quadrant/flank pain. He is accompanied by his daughter who states that over the last 4 weeks he has had intermittent fevers, chills, cough, weight loss, and malaise. The abdominal pain is new, and previous workup for pneumonia 2 weeks ago was unremarkable. Other than hypertension, which has been well controlled, he is healthy with no past medical or surgical history. On physical examination, blood pressure is 100/67 mm Hg, heart rate is 120/min, respirations are 26/min, and he is febrile to 39.1 °C. He does not appear jaundiced. He has diminished breath sounds at the base of the right lung. The emergency department administers an appropriate fluid bolus, draws blood cultures, and starts broad-spectrum antibiotics. An upright radiograph of the chest shows some consolidation/atelectasis of the right lower lobe with a possible effusion. A full set of labs is ordered, which reveals a leukocytosis of 26,000/mm^3, a creatinine of 2.3 mg/dL, and a lactate of 4 mg/dL. LFTs reveal a slight transaminitis but normal bilirubin. The remainder of his workup is unremarkable. A CT chest/abdomen/pelvis reveals no pneumonia. However, a rim enhancing mass in the liver consistent with a pyogenic abscess is found.

Questions: *What else does the differential diagnosis include? Which antibiotics are appropriate for this patient? Is there anything else that needs to be completed as part of the workup? How should the abscess be managed and what are the potential complications?*

Answers: *Please see the sections that follow for question answers.*

INTRODUCTION

For acute care surgeons, the liver is primarily an organ to be mastered and respected in the setting of trauma. However, liver masses, both benign and malignant, may present with acute symptoms. Due to advances in cross-sectional imaging technology and its more frequent use, liver lesions are recognized with increased frequency. These incidental liver lesions are detected in 30% of individuals older than 40 years of age. Most of these lesions are benign in nature, especially in the absence of chronic liver disease or known malignancy elsewhere. The lesions can be further subdivided into solid and cystic masses, with an estimated 5% of the population with cystic masses of the liver. Alternatively, patients can present with signs and symptoms consistent with an infectious process in the intra-abdominal cavity and be found to have a primary process in the liver driving this inflammatory response. Irrespective of the etiology of these liver masses, acute care surgeons must be familiar with their presentation, workup, including how these different masses appear on different imaging modalities and management strategies from antibiotic selection, radiographic drainage, open drainage, and surgery, as we are often the first port of call to manage these patients. In this chapter, we will discuss the most common benign solid and benign cystic masses likely to present and require immediate surgical evaluation. Management of hepatocellular cancer that presents with bleeding will also be reviewed.

CYSTIC LIVER MASSES

Pyogenic Liver Abscess

Liver abscesses are relatively uncommon, with an annual incidence of 2.3 cases per 100 000. The incidence is higher in men vs women, 3.3 vs 1.3 per 100 000, and reported as high as 17.6 per 100 000 in some South-East Asian populations. Liver abscesses are the most common visceral abscess, accounting for 48% of all visceral abscesses and 13% of intra-abdominal abscesses. Historically, acute appendicitis was the most common etiology of pyogenic liver abscess. Today, biliary disease, diverticulitis, benign strictures, malignancy, and congenital anomalies are the major causes of pyogenic liver abscess.

Liver abscesses can be divided into pyogenic, amoebic, parasitic, and fungal. Pyogenic liver abscess originates from a variety of routes including the biliary tree (50% of pyogenic liver abscesses), portal vein (pylephlebitis), hepatic artery, adjacent organ infections, and trauma to the liver, either from surgical/penetrating wounds or migrating foreign bodies. Rarely, pyogenic liver abscesses originate from hematogenous spread from the systemic circulation. Monomicrobial pyogenic liver abscesses arising from streptococcal or staphylococcal bacteria must trigger further workup to find the source of infection, specifically infective endocarditis. Pyogenic liver abscesses associated with *Klebsiella* pneumonia are strongly associated with underlying colorectal cancer, at least in patient populations from Asia. They most often involve the right lobe of the liver due to its large size and more robust blood supply. Risk factors include diabetes mellitus, hepatobiliary or pancreatic disease, chronic proton pump inhibitor use, chronic granulomatous disease, and liver transplantation. Mortality rates vary from 2% to 12%, with higher mortality associated with the need for open surgical drainage, presence of malignancy, and presence of aerobic infections. For the most part, pyogenic liver abscesses are polymicrobial, with mixed enteric facultative and aerobic species as the most common organisms. Due to the wide variety of causative organisms, cultures should always be sent to determine appropriate antibiotic selection. Causative bacteria include *Escherichia coli*, *Klebsiella pneumoniae*, *Streptococcus milleri* species, and *Staphylococcus* species. Similar to *K pneumoniae* in Asian populations, identification of *S milleri* should initiate a workup for metastatic infections from other locations. As in our case scenario, fever and abdominal pain (located in the right upper quadrant or upper abdomen) are the most common symptoms, occurring in 90% and 50% to 75% of patients, respectively. Patients also present with nausea, vomiting, anorexia, or malaise as with many other abscesses. Some patients may present with diffuse peritonitis. In these situations, the abscess may have ruptured freely into the peritoneal cavity. Risk factors for abscess rupture include diameter >6 cm and/or the presence of cirrhosis. Abscesses may also rupture locally, even into the pleural space. Additionally, patients can present primarily with respiratory complaints. Laboratory values will show an elevated white cell count and elevated liver function tests. Alkaline phosphatase can be elevated in up to 90% of cases, with bilirubin and aspartate aminotransferase elevated in up to 50% of cases. Unlike other surgical infections, where the merit of blood cultures can be discussed, blood cultures are essential in the workup of pyogenic liver abscesses as they identify a source of infection when particular organisms are identified in the liver abscess itself, as mentioned above. Although not essential to the diagnosis of pyogenic livers abscesses, patients should also have electrolytes and renal function measured to help quantify the degree of their illness and to ensure that an appropriate contrast load can be given for computerized tomography. Diagnosis is aided with abdominal imaging. CT is more sensitive than US in the identification of liver abscesses, 95% vs 85%, and carries the extra benefit of potentially helping identify sources of the infection. The appearance of pyogenic liver abscesses can be quite variable on ultrasound, ranging from hypoechoic most commonly to hyperechoic (**Figure 23.1**). Gas bubbles can be present. The addition of contrast-enhanced ultrasound will show wall enhancement during the arterial phase with washout during the portal and venous phases (**Figure 23.2**). Additionally, contrast-enhanced ultrasound allows characterization of septations, which if present, should lead the surgeon to consider surgical rather than percutaneous drainage. Of note, monomicrobial *Klebsiella* pneumonia abscesses may appear solid on ultrasound and mistaken for a solid hepatic tumor. In general, pyogenic liver abscesses appear as peripherally enhancing, centrally hypoattenuating lesions on CT, sometimes referred two as the double target sign (**Figure 23.3**). They too can be variable, sometimes appearing solid. Twenty percent of pyogenic

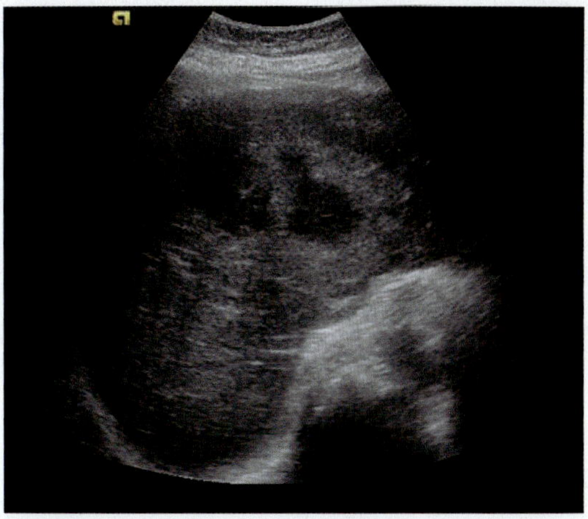

Figure 23.1 Pyogenic liver abscess.

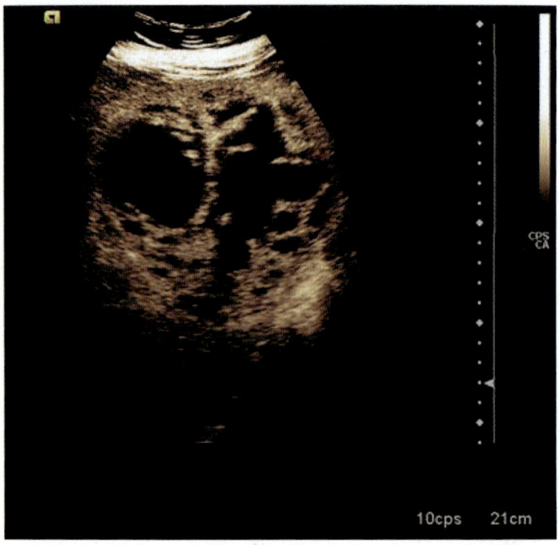

Figure 23.2 Contrast-enhanced pyogenic liver abscess on US.

liver abscess contain gas. Occasionally, when multiple abscesses are present, they can appear as one large, highly septated lesion or cluster sign. Although other imaging modalities, such as MRI (**Figure 23.4**) and tagged white blood cell scans, can be used, they are time consuming, costly, and less readily available. Other pathology that appears similar to pyogenic liver abscesses on imaging includes simple cysts, bilomas, and necrotic liver tumors. Definitive confirmation of a suspected pyogenic liver abscess requires aspiration, which can be both diagnostic and therapeutic. This also helps differentiate the pyogenic abscess from an

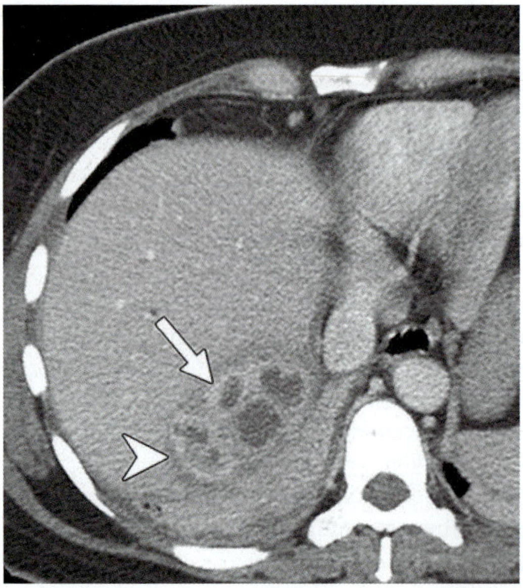

Figure 23.3 Arrows showing Pyogenic Live Abscess on CT image.

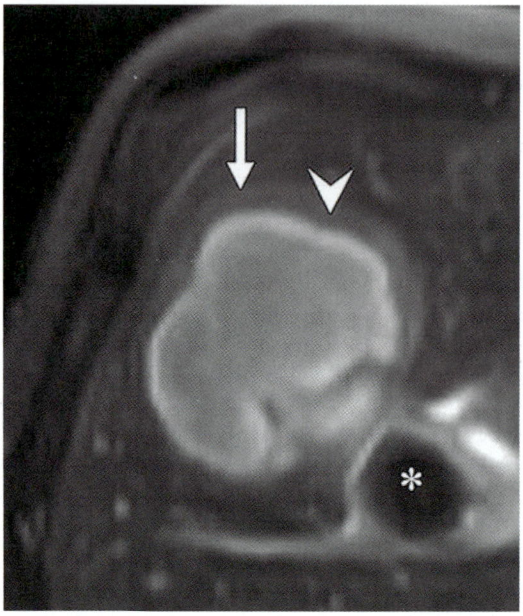

Figure 23.4 Arrows showing pyogenic abscess on T2 weighted MRI assocaited with acute gangrenbous cholecystitis. Asterisk denotes gllladder.

amebic liver abscess. Abscess size and location are key factors in determining if aspiration/catheter drainage is feasible. Posterior and superior location as well as proximity to major vessels increases risk of complications. Drainage can be performed via US-guided or CT-guided techniques. Other options include endoscopic retrograde cholangiopancreatography (ERCP) and endoscopic ultrasound-guided drainage. ERCP drainage is particularly helpful when abscesses communicate with the biliary tree from previous biliary procedures/disease (**Figure 23.5**). Endoscopic ultrasound-guided drainage is a novel method of treating pyogenic liver abscesses and has been

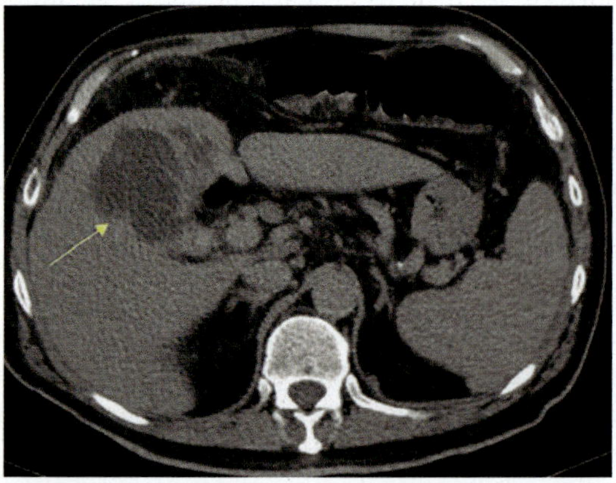

Figure 23.5 Arrow denotes pyogenic liver abscess from perforated cholecystitis.

shown to be helpful for abscesses in difficult locations for percutaneous drainage and in high-risk surgical patients. Patients with single and unilocular abscesses should undergo some form of nonoperative drainage. Even with abscesses <5 cm, we recommend attempting to leave a drain as repeat aspiration may be required in almost 50% of cases. Abscesses over 10 cm have also been treated successfully with catheter drainage but are more often associated with treatment failure and complications including pleural effusions, need for repeat drainage, and death from sepsis. In patients with multiple abscesses, multiloculated abscesses, failure to respond to nonsurgical drainage after 7 days, or inadequate drainage due to abscess size and fluid consistency, consider surgical drainage. Surgical approaches to pyogenic liver abscesses include open, laparoscopic, and robotic. Transthoracic, transdiaphragmatic approach to posterior and superior pyogenic liver abscesses has also been described. If the surgeon does not have adequate experience with liver surgery, the surgeon refers the patient to a tertiary center once stabilized. Some studies have shown that nonoperative drainage is still an option even when multiple and multiloculated abscesses are present. Send fluid for Gram stain and culture, fungal, and antigen or PCR testing for *Entamoeba histolytica*. Cultures should never be sent from preexisting drains since skin flora often contaminate the drain and lead to incorrect antibiotic therapy. The other essential component of managing pyogenic liver abscesses is antibiotic therapy. Currently, antibiotic regimens are based upon the common sources of the organisms and guided by local resistance patterns. Unless *E histolytica* can be excluded confidently, additional coverage with metronidazole should be added. Common empiric regimens include third-generation cephalosporins, β-lactam-β-lactamase inhibitors, and carbapenems. In patients with septic shock, obtain blood cultures as quickly as possible and start antibiotic treatment. If the patient has risk factors for a potential nosocomial source, add vancomycin. Once culture data and sensitivities from drainage are available, narrow the antibiotic treatment. Antibiotic therapy should last for 4-6 weeks. Switching from parenteral to enteral therapy is appropriate, negating the need for long-term intravenous access. A separate and unique form of pyogenic liver abscess is associated with gallbladder perforation. First described by Niemeier in 1934, three types of perforation have been proposed. Type 1: acute perforation resulting in generalized biliary peritonitis, type 2: subacute perforation resulting in pericholecystic abscesses and localized peritonitis, and type 3: chronic perforation resulting from cholecystoenteric fistulas. Type 2 perforation can lead to intraparenchymal, subcapsular abscesses from direct perforation of the gallbladder into the liver parenchyma (see **Figure 23.5**).

Cholecystohepatic fistulas can also form. As this is such a rare condition, no standardized treatment method exists. Other than antibiotic treatment, which should be initiated as soon as possible, several approaches have been described, including percutaneous drainage of the intrahepatic abscess followed by laparoscopic cholecystectomy or laparoscopic cholecystectomy and drainage of the abscess intraoperatively with subsequent drain placement. This surgery may be technically challenging and may necessitate the need for a subtotal cholecystectomy with drainage of the abscess or conversion to an open surgery (see Chapter 15, Figure 15.5).

Alternatively, in patients who are not able to tolerate surgery, percutaneous drainage of the abscess and percutaneous cholecystostomy tube may be appropriate.

Amebic Liver Abscess

Amebic liver disease is caused by *E histolytica*, the most common form of extraintestinal amebiasis. The amoeba ascends to the liver via the portal vein. They usually affect men in their 40s and 50s, despite equal gender distribution of colonic amebiasis. The abscesses are usually located in the right lobe of the liver. It commonly affects migrants and travelers from endemic areas, including Mexico, Central and South America, Africa, and India. It is transmitted via the feco-oral route, although there have been reports of sexual oral-anal transmission. Indeed, several studies have shown increased incidence of amebic liver disease in HIV-positive men, confounding whether immunosuppression is a potential risk factor. Much like pyogenic liver abscesses, abdominal pain, particularly right upper quadrant pain, and fever are the main presenting symptoms. Onset of these symptoms in returning travelers from endemic regions can range from 2 to 17 months, with most patients developing symptoms by 3 months. Other symptoms include weight loss, nausea, anorexia, and respiratory symptoms including cough and shortness of breath. As with pyogenic liver abscesses, amebic liver abscesses can rupture freely into the peritoneum, causing generalized peritonitis, local abscesses, or fistulas with adjacent organs. Rupture, however, is much more likely to extend into the pleural space than the peritoneal cavity. In these patients where rupture has occurred into the pleural or sometimes pericardial space (especially in the abscess involving the left lobe of the liver), patients will present with symptoms primarily affecting these two organ systems, including chest pain, hemoptysis, cough, and shortness of breath. When the abscess ruptures into the colon, an ameboma can form. This mass of granulation tissue can be confused for colon cancer. Due to the longer disease time, unlike patients with pyogenic liver abscesses, amoebic liver abscesses result in hepatomegaly. Laboratory values will show an elevated white blood cell count with normal eosinophils. Liver function tests demonstrate an elevated alkaline phosphatase in 80% of cases, with bilirubin and transaminase values varying greatly. As in pyogenic liver abscesses, renal function should be assessed to ensure that the patient is not systemically ill. Serologic and antibody testing should be performed but may be negative in the first 7 days of infection. Microscopic and serologic analysis of the stool is also warranted. Imaging studies identify the size and location of the abscess. With appropriate history and physical and serological testing, amoebic abscesses can be diagnosed without aspiration/drainage, but if serology is negative, aspiration/drainage can be both diagnostic and therapeutic. The ultrasound appearance of an amoebic hepatic abscess shows a hypoechoic lesson with no wall echoes. CT imaging demonstrates round lesions with attenuation values consistent with complex fluid. The wall is usually enhancing, and there is a peripheral zone of edema (**Figure 23.6**). If gas is present within the abscess,

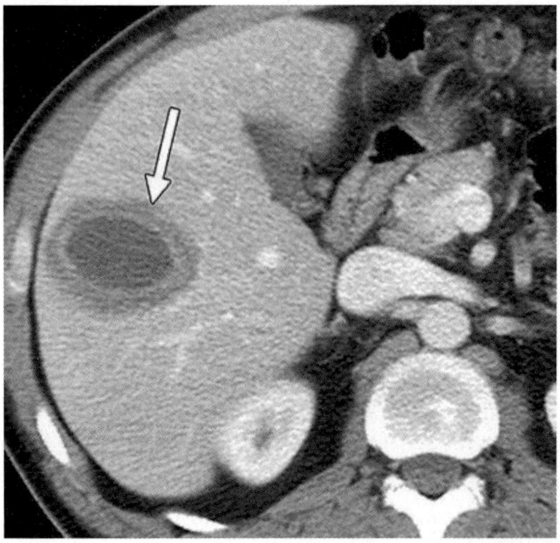

Figure 23.6 Arrow showing amoebic liver abscess.

this suggests a hepatocolic or hepatopulmonary fistula. MRI appearance depends on whether T1 or T2 imaging is utilized; T1 images show homogenous low signal intensity, while T2 images show homogenous high signal intensity with edema around the abscess in up to 50% of cases.

Other indications for drainage include abscesses >10 cm, risk of rupture (particularly lesions of the left lobe), or if there is clinical deterioration or failure to respond to empiric therapy. Drainage will reveal the classic "anchovy paste" appearance from necrotic hepatocytes. Trophozoites are rarely seen on microscopy, <20%. This fluid should be sent for antigen/PCR testing if a diagnosis has not already been established. Once the diagnosis has been confirmed or if there is high clinical suspicion, the mainstay of treatment is with metronidazole or tinidazole, curing more than 90%. Usual regimens include metronidazole 500-750 mg orally three times a day for 7-10 days or tinidazole 2 g daily for 5 days. Once this therapy has been completed, patients should undergo treatment for intraintestinal luminal cysts, even though stool serology/microscopy is negative. Infectious disease physicians should be consulted for appropriate agents and regimens. Surgery is generally not indicated for this disease. Surgery can be considered in patients who do not adequately respond to antiamoebic therapy or percutaneous drainage, those who are deteriorating clinically, large abscesses (over 8 cm), impending risk of rupture, or those who have already ruptured, especially if the cardiopulmonary cavities have been affected. Choice of surgical approach depends on the stability of the patient, the area affected, and the surgeon's comfort level with the different approaches available. Several small case series have shown that even in the setting of rupture, patients can be treated safely with drains and continued antiamoebic therapy.

Hydatid/Echinococcal Cysts

Echinococcus granulosus larvae cause hydatid liver cysts. This is a canine parasitic tape worm that is endemic to the Mediterranean, Africa, the Middle East, South America, Asia, and Europe where sheep farming is prevalent. Any dog species can be the primary host for the tapeworm, with sheep and many other animals being the intermediate host. Transmission to humans is via the feco-oral route. Infections in America are primarily from migrants from endemic areas. Ova penetrate the intestinal wall and travel to the liver via the portal circulation, although the lungs, brain, and bones can be seeding sites. Other forms of the tapeworm, such as *Echinococcus multilocularis*, are transmitted via elk and caribou and cause a hepatic infiltrative, potentially lethal form of the disease.

The hydatid cyst has a very distinct appearance on imaging, comprising a two-layer cyst. The inner wall is active and comprised a single-cell germinal layer where the daughter cysts develop and is often referred to as "hydatid sand." The outer layer is a reactive fibrous layer called the pericyst and is calcified in 50% of patients. Currently, a World Health Organization Informal Working group on Echinococcus (WHO-IWGE) has developed a classification system found below (**Table 23.1**). Patients with hydatid disease are usually asymptomatic and are found incidentally on cross-sectional imaging. However, as cysts expand and sometimes rupture, patients may become symptomatic. They can present with right upper quadrant pain, fever, or hepatomegaly. If the biliary tree is involved, obstructive jaundice and cholangitis may develop. Cysts can erode through the diaphragm and rupture into the pleural cavity causing pleuritic chest pain, cough, and shortness of breath. If the cysts rupture freely into the peritoneum, which is uncommon, patients can experience anaphylactic shock.

Diagnosis is based on history and clinical examination, imaging, and serology and confirmed by protoscoleces on direct microscopy or changes in ultrasound appearance as described in **Table 23.1**. A CBC will show eosinophilia in only 40% of patients. Liver function tests can vary in their results and can show mild elevation of transaminases, alkaline phosphatase, and gamma-glutamyl transferase. Enzyme-linked immunosorbent assay (ELISA) has 64%-100% sensitivity and has replaced Casoni skin and Weinberg complement fixation test. Immunoelectrophoresis is diagnostic in 90% of hepatic hydatid cysts and 70% of pulmonary hydatid cysts. The US appearance of the cysts has been detailed above. CT can also be used to aid in the diagnosis of the disease and gives additional information on the location and depth of the cyst, which is crucial for operative planning (**Figure 23.7**).

MRCP will provide additional information on cyst characteristics and the presence of associated abscesses. ERCP is helpful when there is involvement of the biliary tree or when cholangitis or jaundice is initially present, which can occur in up

TABLE 23.1 ■ WHO-IWGE Classification System

Cyst Type	Status	Ultrasound Features	Remark	Treatment Approach
Cystic lesion	None	Unilocular, anechoic Usually round Cyst wall not visible	Early, not fertile Needs additional diagnostic tests	Needs diagnosis
Cystic *Echinococcus* 1 (type 1)	Active	Unilocular, anechoic Round or oval Cyst wall visible Hydatid sand (snowflake)	Usually fertile Pathognomonic	<5 cm = ABZ >5 cm = PAIR + ABZ
Cystic *Echinococcus* 2 (type 2)	Active	Multivesicular, septated Round or oval Cyst wall visible Rosette, honeycomb	Usually fertile Pathognomonic	PT or surgery + ABZ
Cystic *Echinococcus* 3 (type 3)	Transitional	Detached floating membrane Less round, complex mass Water lily sign	Starting to degenerate Pathognomonic	PT, PAIR, or surgery + ABZ
Cystic *Echinococcus* 4 (type 4)	Inactive	Heterogeneous, hypoechoic degenerating membrane No daughter cyst Ball of wood	Most not fertile Needs additional diagnostic tests	Surgery + ABZ, or watch and wait
Cystic *Echinococcus* 5 (type 5)	Inactive	Thick, calcified wall Arch shaped Cone-shaped shadow	Most not fertile Highly suggestive Needs diagnostic confirmation	Surgery + ABZ, or watch and wait

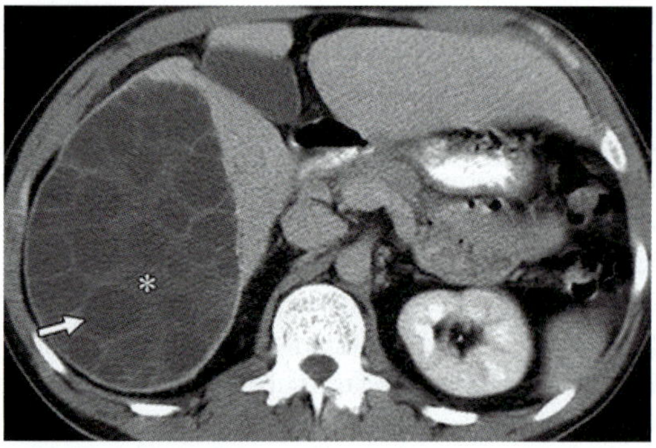

Figure 23.7 Hepatic hydatid cyst showing daughter cysts (*arrow*) with lower attenuation at cyst matrix (*asterisk*).

to 25% of cases; but it is controversial. The mainstay of treatment is early intervention to prevent the complications mentioned above caused by cyst expansion and rupture. Patient overall health and stability, cyst characteristics, and the presence of complications are key factors in choosing which treatment to pursue. Currently, there is no "gold standard" of care, but several options exist. Systemic chemotherapy; puncture, aspirate, injection, and reaspiration (PAIR) (**Figure 23.8**); percutaneous drainage, surgery, and watchful waiting.

Antihelminthic drugs, such as albendazole (ABZ), are the medical treatments of choice for echinococcal disease. It is absorbed in the gut and metabolized into its active form in the liver where it accumulates in the cystic fluid. Specific dosing and duration are not standardized. These drugs are ineffective if the cysts are in their inactive or calcified phase. It is crucial to monitor the patient's CBC and LFTs during treatment as side effects include neutropenia and hepatotoxicity. New studies suggest that the addition of the antiparasitic praziquantel is more effective than albendazole alone. The side effects make this a poor choice for immunocompromised patients and patients with underlying liver disease. Chemotherapy alone leads to only 30% success rate in small, <5-cm type 1 cysts. Ideally, it should always be combined with percutaneous or surgical drainage. PAIR is the most common form of percutaneous drainage. It either destroys the germinal layer or evacuates the entire endocyst via catheter drainage. Surgical drainage is usually reserved for giant, >10 cm, unilocular cysts, and the drain is left in place until output is <10 mL/d. Current guidelines recommend PAIR for high-risk patients, those who refuse surgery, failure of medical management alone, cysts that have been infected with bacteria, and cysts that recur after surgery. Cysts most likely to respond to PAIR and benzimidazoles are type 1 and 3 cysts that are >5 cm. Patients with biliary fistulas, inaccessible or high-risk locations (superficial), type 2, 4, and 5 cysts, and inactive or calcified cysts are

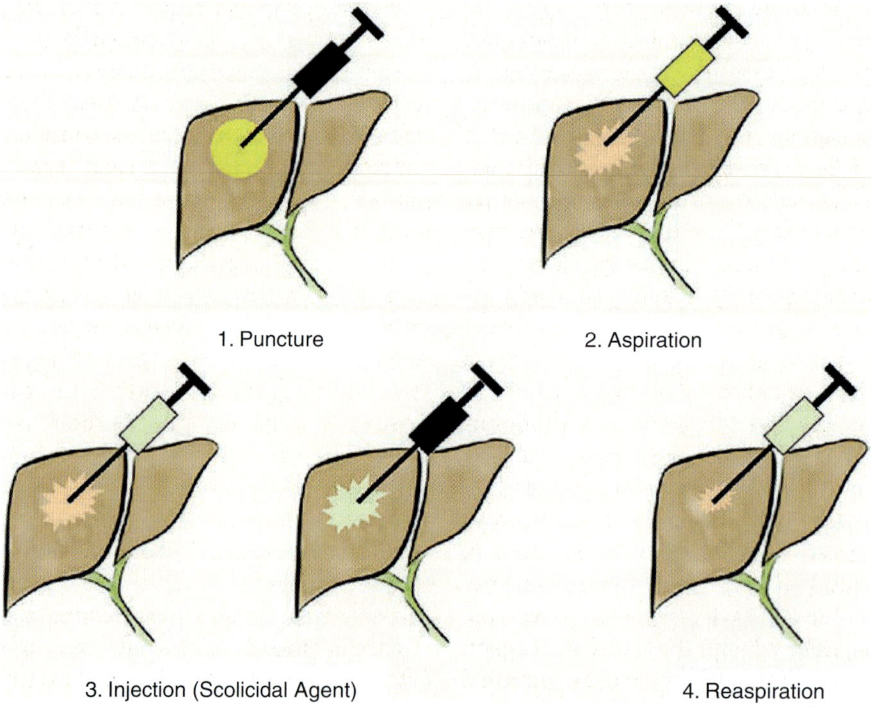

Figure 23.8 PAIR technique.

not candidates for PAIR. It is vital that benzimidazoles are administered 4 hours before PAIR and continued for 1 month after. At this time, no good data exist comparing PAIR and benzimidazoles with surgery and benzimidazoles. Indications for surgical intervention include large type 2 and 3 cysts with multiple daughter cysts, superficial cysts at risk of rupture, cysts with biliary fistulas, and cysts compressing adjacent organs. Contraindications include small cysts, poorly located cysts, inactive cysts, and patients who are poor surgical candidates. Regardless of which option the surgeon chooses, the tenants of surgery are to completely inactivate the scolices, eliminate the parasite and viable cyst contents, prevent spillage or recurrence, manage the cyst cavity, and prevent complications. To achieve these goals, appropriate preoperative workup includes US, CT, MRI, and possibly ERCP. Intraoperative ultrasound is also crucial to ensure no vital structures are damaged. As with PAIR, it is imperative that benzimidazoles are administered well before surgery and for 1 month after. Open and laparoscopic approaches have been described and we will look at them in detail. Choice of technique will depend on surgeon experience, size of cyst, location, and presence of complications. Regardless of which option is used, it is strongly recommended that scolecoidal agents are used. Current recommendations are that 20% hypersonic saline be placed in contact with the germinal layer of the cyst for at least 15 minutes. The scolecoidal agent should not be injected prior to cyst aspiration as the cyst is already a high-pressure system and may rupture. Other agents have been used in the past, but no data on their efficacy exist. Patients with biliary fistulas should not have hypertonic saline or other chemical agents injected into the cyst as they may cause chemically induced sclerosing cholangitis. Other complications of hypertonic saline administration include hypernatremia. Open cyst evacuation is the classic approach to managing these cysts and is best suited to superficial cysts. If the cysts are located in anterior segments, an abdominal approach via a midline or subcostal incision is best. If the involved segments are in the right lateral segments, 6 and 7, a flank incision is probably advantageous. After entry into the abdomen, the field should be lined with hypertonic saline-soaked gauze. The cyst cavity is then aspirated and, if appropriate, injected with the scolecoidal agent. After at least 15 minutes, the cyst can be unroofed and the contents aspirated with a high negative-pressure suction device. At this time, daughter cysts are removed, the active cyst lining is resected, and all debris within the cavity is cleared, taking care not to spill any of the contents.

Once again, the cyst cavity can be irrigated with scolecoidal agents if no bile staining was present within the cavity. If encountered, any biliary connection can be closed with simple interrupted absorbable sutures. The cyst cavity should then be packed with a pedicled tongue of omentum or the entire omentum and sutured into place. Alternatively, if the cystobiliary fistula cannot be closed, place a closed suction drain. In experienced hands, laparoscopic cyst evacuation is an option. Patients with noncalcified superficial cysts and cysts located in segments 6 and 7 are good candidates to this approach. A 11- or 12-mm trocar is placed directly over the cyst, and sponges with scolecoidal agents are packed around the cyst. The cyst is then punctured and aspirated and can be injected with scolecoidal agents at this time if appropriate. The trocar above the cyst is then exchanged for an 18-mm trocar to allow aspiration of the thick germinal layer. The camera is then inserted directly into the cyst to identify any daughter cysts or bile staining, after which the cavity can be irrigated with scolecoidal agents. The cyst wall is then excised, and similar to the open approach, either an omentoplasty is performed or a closed-suction drain is left. However, this technique remains the tool of experienced centers due to the potentially life-threatening risk of anaphylactic shock that results from cyst spillage. More radical approaches exist for managing hydatid cysts. Open and laparoscopic cyst evacuation is considered conservative. Pericystectomy, formal liver resections, and even transplantation have been described as options. Although probably outside the scope of practice for most general and acute care surgeons, it is important to know that these patients can be referred for more aggressive surgery with hepatobiliary and transplant surgeons if necessary. Benefits of pericystectomy include decreased risk of cyst spillage and anaphylactic shock as well as disease recurrence. Unfortunately, this is balanced by increased risk of bleeding and damage to biliary structures. Formal resection is indicated when there are multiple cysts, large biliary fistulas, proximity to important vascular, and biliary structures or large cysts confined to anatomic sectors. Liver transplantation is reserved for cases of *E multilocularis* where fulminant liver failure from sclerosing cholangitis, Budd-Chiari, or biliary sclerosis occurs. Patient outcomes are centered on whether the disease is uncomplicated or complicated (biliary obstruction, biliary fistulas, or rupture of any kind). If patients rupture freely into the peritoneum, an open surgical approach is warranted with appropriate care for anaphylactic shock in the OR and ICU subsequently. With pleural and lung involvement, thoracic consultation should be sought immediately as free rupture can result in anaphylactic shock and lung resection may be warranted. Outcomes of these various approaches vary, with postoperative morbidity ranging from 8% to 13% for PAIR, 8%-25% for laparoscopic surgery, and 12%-63% for open surgery of any kind, with open evacuation techniques having less associated morbidity. Mortality is only 0.1% for PAIR and between 0% and 3% for open and laparoscopic surgery. As long as spillage is avoided, adequate long-term treatment can be achieved in 90%-95% of patients who undergo a drainage procedure plus benzimidazoles.

Fungal Liver Abscess

Fungal hepatic infections are rare in the nonimmunocompromised population, accounting for <2% of the total isolates from hepatic abscesses (**Figure 23.9**). The most at-risk population are those patients with hematologic malignancies and those undergoing hematopoietic stem cell transplantation. The most common fungus identified is *Candida*, secondary to intestinal colonization and dissemination. Risk factors include neutropenia and mucositis. However, since the use of widespread antifungal prophylaxis in these patients, the incidence of this disease has decreased, from 10% before prophylaxis to between 5% and 7%. *Candida* is also an important cause of liver abscess after orthoptic liver transplantation. *Aspergillus* is the most common mold found in hepatic abscesses in oncohematologic setting. High mortality rates are seen in patients in whom fungemia is identified, so initiate early treatment with appropriate antifungals. These abscesses are at risk of superinfection with bacteria and have a low threshold to treat patients concomitantly with appropriate antibiotics. Similar to pyogenic liver abscesses, patients who fail to respond to treatment should undergo percutaneous drainage. Surgery is rarely a good choice in these immunocompromised patients. Imaging appearance is similar to pyogenic liver abscesses.

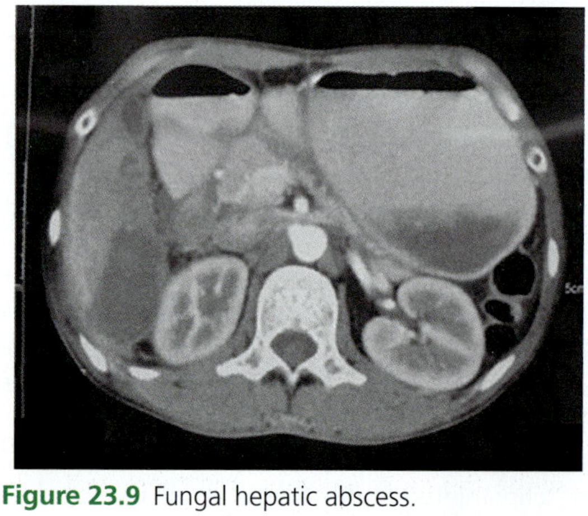

Figure 23.9 Fungal hepatic abscess.

CYSTIC DISEASE OF THE LIVER

Although we have discussed the main cystic masses that may warrant surgical consultation, surgeons should be aware of these other cystic diseases of the liver and include them in the differential diagnosis. Due to the increased utilization of cross-sectional imaging, up to 5% of the population is diagnosed with one or multiple cysts. Cysts can be asymptomatic or present with abdominal/right upper quadrant pain along with other signs and symptoms, with or without derangements in liver function tests. Depending on the size of the cyst and its location, patients may present with early satiety, gastric outlet/intestinal obstruction, or jaundice. If intracystic rupture occurs, patients may have sudden onset pain as Glisson capsule is stretched. Rarely do cysts rupture, and the majority are benign and asymptomatic. If the infective cysts that we discussed previously have been confidently excluded, then the next important step is to rule out malignancy. No reliable laboratory values differentiate these noninfectious cysts, and aspiration is rarely helpful. Imaging is the best way to differentiate cysts characteristics. Ultrasound, CT, and MRI are all reasonable modalities to evaluate cysts. **Table 23.2** describes the appearance of benign and malignant cysts.

Ultrasound by an experienced sonographer has a >90% sensitivity and specificity. CT imaging should include IV contrast so the arterial/portal venous and delayed venous phases can be assessed to see the proximity of the cyst to the surrounding vasculature. MRI/MRCP can assess whether biliary communication is present. Both CT and MRI carry the advantage of detailing the exact size and depth/relation of the cyst to adjacent structures. The most common cysts are simple cysts. These cysts are congenital and present in 5% of the

TABLE 23.2 ■ Imaging Appearance of Benign and Malignant Solid Liver Masses

Imaging Modality	Benign	Malignant
US	Homogenous, anechoic lesions with smooth boarders	Nodules, septations with echogenic areas that do not move with the patient
CT	Low-density fluid, smooth, regular boarder	High-density fluid, nodules, septations, irregular thickened walls
MRI	Hypointense on T1 Hyperintense on T2	Varied appearance depending on cyst type

population, arising from aberrant intrahepatic bile ducts. Fortunately, these cysts have no malignant potential and do not communicate with the biliary tree. They are usually asymptomatic but can cause pain when they are larger than 5-8 cm, pedunculated, or when intracystic hemorrhage occurs. Aspiration may help identify what type of cyst is in question, but it is not therapeutic and can lead to complications of infection. Mucin in the cyst aspirate indicates the presence of a cyst adenomas or cystadenocarcinoma, which we will discuss shortly. If bile is encountered, MRCP or ERCP is warranted. Treatment of large, symptomatic cysts is via open/laparoscopic/robotic marsupialization in patients who can tolerate surgery and where the cysts are not deep within the hepatic parenchyma. As much of the cyst wall should be removed without performing a hepatic resection. This allows the peritoneum to reabsorb the fluid; any suspicious areas can be biopsied and allows the cavity to collapse over time. As with hydatid cysts, an omentoplasty can be performed at the end of the procedure to ensure that the cavity does not close and the cyst recurs. If bile leak is encountered, it can be oversewn at this time. The laparoscopic approach has the added benefit of decreasing mortality and improving visualization in some difficult liver segments. When multiple cysts or a large cyst is present, a formal hepatic resection or enucleation may be necessary. Anything beyond a simple unroofing is probably best referred to a hepatobiliary specialist, although these surgical approaches do not have a clear benefit over simple unroofing. Although aspiration alone is not an appropriate treatment option, aspiration followed by injection of sclerosing agents is associated with only a 5%-10% symptomatic recurrence rate and may be an appropriate treatment modality in patients who are not good surgical candidates. As mentioned above, indications for surgery include multiple cysts; however, one must first rule out polycystic liver disease. This is a rare condition, with no standard definition, but a family history and the presence of kidney and brain cysts is suggestive. Most patients have enough healthy liver parenchyma and are usually asymptomatic. However, patients can present with liver failure, hepatomegaly causing intestinal obstruction, portal obstruction, and inferior vena cava obstruction/Budd-Chiari syndrome. The role of the acute care/general surgeon in this setting is to perform laparoscopic or open fenestration and refer the patient for formal resection or even potential liver transplantation. The other important cyst to be aware of is the traumatic cyst. Blunt trauma can cause parenchymal hematomas and bilomas, which develop into false cysts as they do not have an epithelial lining. They can usually be observed; however, if the cyst enlarges and causes pain, compresses adjacent structures, or a bile leak is present, intervention may be warranted. For bile leaks, attempt ERCP and sphincterotomy before surgical ligation. For patients with compressive symptoms, the cyst can be unroofed in a similar fashion to other simple liver cysts. Finally, some cysts are neoplastic, including cystadenomas and cystadenocarcinomas, which account for 5% of hepatic cysts. They are seen most commonly in women in their 40s and 50s. The management of these entities is beyond the scope of this chapter, but surgeons should have a high suspicion of these premalignant and malignant entities. If there is diagnostic uncertainty, a hepatobiliary specialist should be consulted.

BENIGN SOLID LIVER MASSES

Solid masses of the liver are encountered incidentally or when they become symptomatic from bleeding, increases in size, or compression of adjacent structures. These masses have a distinct appearance from cystic lesions on imaging and should be included on a surgeon's differential of liver masses. Although the differential diagnosis for benign solid masses is extensive, we will describe the most common and those that may require acute surgical intervention.

Hemangioma

The most common benign solid tumors of the liver are hemangiomas. Autopsy studies have shown that their incidence ranges from 0.4% to 20%. They are three times more common in women and thought to arise from congenital proliferation of vascular endothelial cells. They can vary in size and are often referred to as giant when >5 cm. Their predominance in females suggests hormonal influence and explains the growth that is seen with steroids, pregnancy, and use of the oral contraceptive pill. Hemangiomas are most commonly diagnosed in the 40-60 age range. They are usually found in the right lobe of the liver and multiple in up to 40% of cases. They are sometimes referred to as cavernous due to their histologic appearance rather than their size. Most patients remain asymptomatic once the mass is identified. In up to 15% of cases, the hemangiomas may actually regress and decrease in size. Patients can present either with symptoms due to the presence of the hemangioma or an increase in its size. Symptoms vary but are most commonly right upper quadrant pain and fullness. This has been attributed to thrombosis, infarction, and stretching of Glisson capsule. Often, this pain is either nonspecific and located in the epigastrium or mistaken for acute/chronic cholecystitis. Rarely, patients can present with fever, nausea, or vomiting. If the hemangioma is large, obstructive symptoms can occur including jaundice and bowel obstruction. Giant hemangiomas can lead to arteriovenous shunting, congestive heart failure, and the associated symptoms. If hemangiomas are pedunculated and on the surface of the liver, they may be difficult to distinguish from tumors of adjacent organs. Rupture is uncommon, <1%, and patients can present with symptoms of shock, including tachycardia, hypotension, and localized or diffuse abdominal pain. In fact, rupture is so uncommon that unlike other liver masses we have talked about in this chapter, size and risk of rupture alone are not indications for surgical intervention. Lab values are variable in the presence of hepatic hemangiomas and depend on what complications have occurred. If the biliary tree is obstructed, bilirubin and alkaline phosphatase will be elevated. Kasabach-Merritt syndrome is characterized by thrombocytopenia and low fibrinogen due to consumption within the hemangioma. Although this syndrome is usually found in children, it can occur at any age. Hepatic hemangiomas are associated with many vascular syndromes beyond the scope of this chapter.

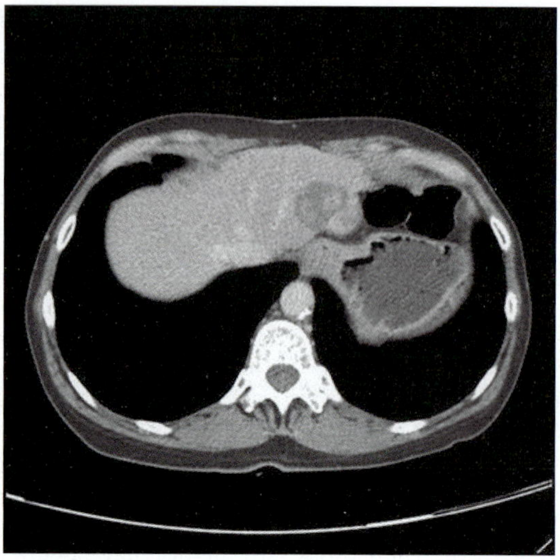

Figure 23.10 Hepatic hemangioma.

Hepatic hemangiomas are readily diagnosed on imaging. They have a characteristic appearance on CT and MRI. For CT imaging, it is crucial to obtain a delayed phase in addition to arterial and venous phases to identify the late contrast puddling that is unique to hemangiomas. Through the three phases, the mass will enhance peripherally on the arterial phase, centripetally fill on the portal venous phase, and retention of contrast on the delayed phase (**Figure 23.10**).

On MRI, the hemangioma has low signal intensity on T1 images and bright signal on T2 noncontrast images (**Figure 23.11**). With the addition of contrast, MRI images are similar to CT, with early peripheral enhancement and delayed centripetal filling. Other imaging modalities include ultrasound, angiography, and tagged red blood cell scan but are far less sensitive and specific in comparison to CT and MRI. As the vast majority of hemangiomas remain asymptomatic or at such low risk

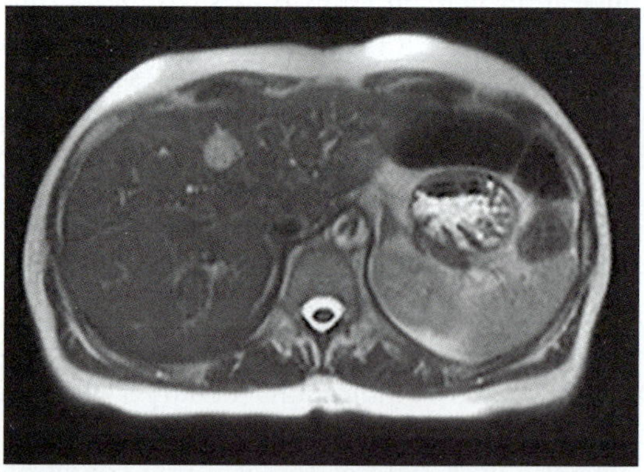

Figure 23.11 MRI hepatic hemangioma.

of rupture, hemangiomas are generally managed with serial imaging. However, there are instances when intervention is needed. Some hemangiomas, such as those associated with Kasabach-Merritt syndrome, traumatic or spontaneous rupture, or hemorrhage leading to shock, require acute intervention. In this setting, arterial embolization is the mainstay of therapy but must be followed by definitive resection. In patients who are symptomatic, or in whom malignancy cannot be ruled out, elective resection is also indicated. As with all liver masses, size, location, and severity of symptoms must be weighed against risk of surgical morbidity and mortality. Various approaches include open, laparoscopic, and robotic. Peripherally located hemangiomas are best approached using the laparoscopic approach. Enucleation is the favored surgical procedure as it leads to decreased blood loss, OR times, and complications compared to larger liver resections. Regardless of the surgical approach, dissection along the plane of the pseudocapsule is essential to minimize blood loss and rupture of the hemangioma. Identify and control the feeding vessels. Before the dissection is started, the hepatoduodenal ligament should be encircled or a clamp should be readily available to perform a Pringle maneuver, and occlude hepatic inflow to decrease blood loss if the dissection drifts away from the pseudocapsule, or if the hemangioma is inadvertently entered. Transarterial embolization, radiofrequency, and microwave ablation have been described but do not have the same efficacy as surgery in the resolution of symptoms. Complete ablation, regardless of the technique, is often not possible due to the proximity of vital vascular and biliary structures.

Focal Nodular Hyperplasia

Focal nodular hyperplasia (FNH) entity is composed of nodular, polyclonal cells from all hepatic subtypes. The risk of malignant potential and the risk of rupture or hemorrhage are low, but these masses can enlarge. They are either discovered incidentally or patients can present with symptoms of pain, weight loss, or early satiety. FNH is more common in premenopausal women, but 10% of cases have been described in male patients. In 20% of cases, the lesions may be multiple or occur in tandem with other liver masses, most commonly hemangiomas. FNH is usually seen in the 30-50 age range and occur equally in both lobes of the liver. FNH can occur *de novo* after chemotherapy treatment with oxaliplatin. The arterial supply is from the hepatic artery and the venous drainage to the hepatic veins. These masses do not have a connection with the portal venous system. They can be subdivided into typical and atypical variants (**Table 23.3**).

Laboratory findings are usually normal. When the mass is discovered incidentally, no further workup or treatment is required and surveillance with serial imaging is not necessary. Fortunately, these lesions have distinctive features on imaging that allow differentiation from other hepatic masses. Ultrasound is not a reliable imaging modality to identify FNH. Only 20% of cases will have lesions that demonstrate the pathognomonic central scar of peripheral vasculature on Doppler ultrasound. On CT, the lesion will appear hypo- or isointense on the noncontrast phase (central scars are seen in 60% of cases if the lesion is smaller than 3 cm), with homogenous enhancement except for the central scar on the arterial phase and finally hypo/isointense appearance during the portal venous phase (**Figure 23.12**).

TABLE 23.3 ■ Focal Nodular Hyperplasia

	Macroscopic Appearance	Histologic Appearance	Malignant Potential
Typical	Large, well-circumscribed margins, poorly encapsulated. Has central scar with radiating fibrous septa (absent in over 50% of cases). Large central artery with spoke-wheel–like centrifugal flow.	Abnormal nodular architecture, malformed vessels, cholangiolar proliferation. Hepatocytes are arranged in plates. Bile ductules are present at the junction of the hepatocytes and fibrous areas. Kupffer cells are present.	None
Atypical	No central scar or artery. Pseudocapsule present. Heterogeneous appearance, with nonenhancement of central scar and the presence of intralesional fat.	No abnormal nodular architecture or malformed vessels but presence of abnormal cholangiolar proliferation. Kupffer cells are present.	Appear similar to other lesions that may have malignant potential so harder to differentiate, but itself nonmalignant

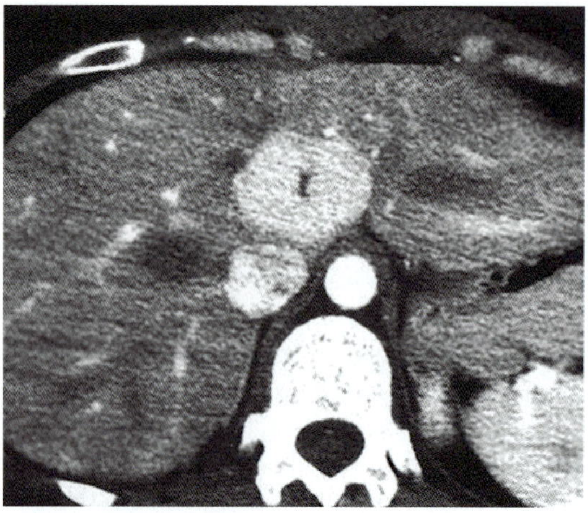

Figure 23.12 Focal nodular hyperplasia.

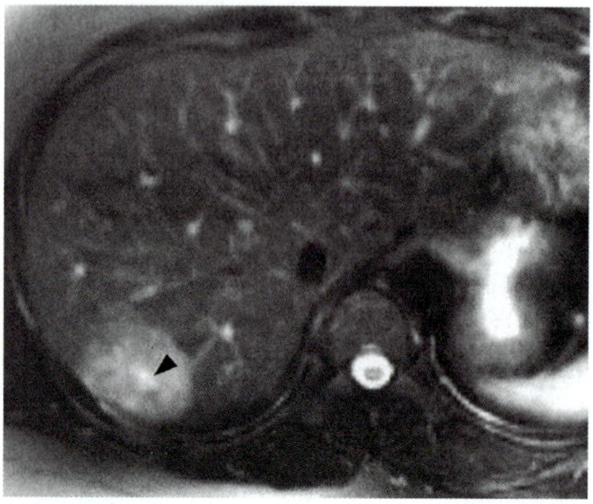

Figure 23.13 Arrow showing focal nodular hyperplasia.

MRI imaging is also useful, with similar appearance to CT, depending on whether T1 or T2 imaging is utilized. On T1, the lesions appear hypo- to isointense with a hypointense central scar. On T2 imaging, they inverse is true with the lesion appearing hyper- to isointense and the central scar is hyperintense (**Figure 23.13**).

Finally, a sulfur colloid scan can differentiate FNH from hepatic adenomas, hepatocellular carcinoma (HCC), or hepatic metastases. This is due to the presence of Kupffer cells in FNH that are not present in these other masses, which allows increased uptake by the lesion (**Figure 23.14**).

In patients who are persistently symptomatic or in whom malignancy cannot be ruled out, surgical resection is warranted. If masses are smaller than 5 cm, additional steps should be taken to find an alternative source of abdominal pain. If conservative management is not appropriate, then surgery, radio frequency/microwave ablation, or transarterial embolization can be used. Surgical management for

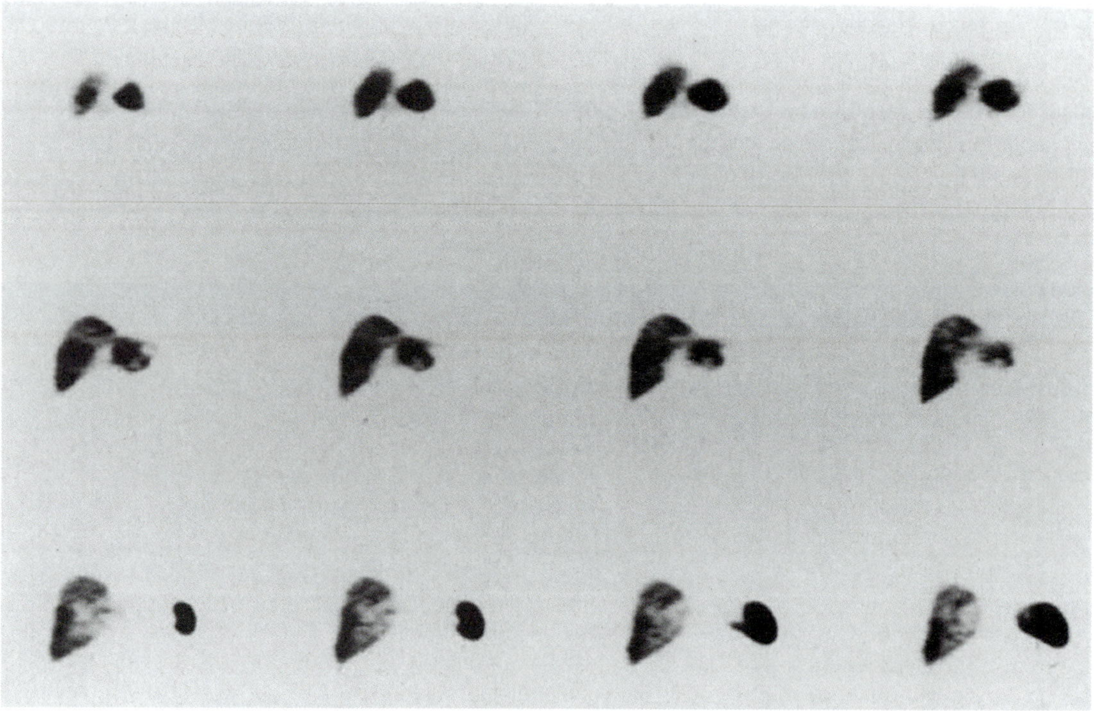

Figure 23.14 Sulfur colloid scan showing increased activity in the anterior aspect of the lateral segment of the left lobe of the liver.

TABLE 23.4 ■ Hepatic Adenomas

	Epidemiology	MRI Features
Hepatocyte nuclear factor-1 alpha mutation	35%-50% of hepatic adenomas. Only found in women. Low risk of complication if <5 cm	Moderate arterial enhancement that does not extend into portal venous phase
Inflammatory	40%-55% of hepatic adenomas, mostly in women	Intense arterial enhancement that persists into portal venous and delayed phase
β-Catenin	10%-15% of hepatic adenomas, more common in men. Increased risk of malignant transformation	No specific features on MRI

FNH includes enucleation or anatomical resection. Both approaches are safe, with low morbidity and mortality and low transfusion rates.

Hepatic Adenoma

Hepatic adenoma is the most common cause of nontraumatic hepatic bleeding in regions where hepatocellular cancer is not prevalent. Sometimes referred to as hepatocellular adenomas, these lesions are usually solitary, hormone-induced masses found in young women using estrogen-containing medications. Indeed, the incidence of hepatic adenoma is up to 40 times higher in users of oral contraceptives compared to nonusers. Hepatic adenomas often regress after oral contraceptives are discontinued and return if the medication is restarted. Other risk factors include exogenous anabolic androgen steroids, glycogen storage diseases, and obesity/metabolic syndrome. Hepatic adenomas have clear margins of variable size, even being pedunculated in rare instances. They are often located in the right lobe of the liver and appear tan, soft, and smooth. Unlike FNH, complications such as hemorrhage or necrosis can occur due to a lack of a fibrous capsule and robust arterial supply to the hepatic sinusoids within the mass. Microscopically, they are composed of large plates of adenoma cells that are arranged in trabeculae interspersed with blood vessels and sinusoids. Kupffer cells may be present but in small amounts. Several different subtypes exist and are described in the table below (**Table 23.4**).

The spectrum of presentation varies widely from asymptomatic, incidentally found individuals to those who present with abdominal pain and even patients in extremis from massive intraperitoneal hemorrhage. When symptoms are present, some form of upper abdominal pain from bleeding, necrosis, or stretching of the hepatic capsule is present. If the pain is accompanied by hypotension, a rapid workup and treatment must be initiated as mortality rates as high at 20% have been described. In ~25%-30% of patients, an abdominal mass or hepatomegaly may be palpated on examination. Similar to other masses, hepatic masses, compression of the bile ducts, can rarely occur and lead to jaundice as well. Liver function tests are usually normal, but alkaline phosphatase and gamma-glutamyl transpeptidase can be increased if bleeding is present. If hepatic adenoma is suspected, alpha-fetoprotein can be elevated if there is malignant transformation. The ultrasound appearance of hepatic adenomas is usually a well-demarcated, heterogeneous mass that is solitary. When contrast-enhanced ultrasound is used, similar to FNH, the mass appears hypervascular during the arterial phase but shows centripetal filling during the portal and delayed phase, unlike FNH, which shows centrifugal filling. On CT, hepatic adenomas appear as well-demarcated isoattenuating lesions. The actual attenuation depends on whether there has been recent hemorrhage, in which case the mass will appear hyperintense (**Figure 23.15**).

MRI imaging can vary in appearance; however, on T1 and T2 imaging, hepatic adenomas

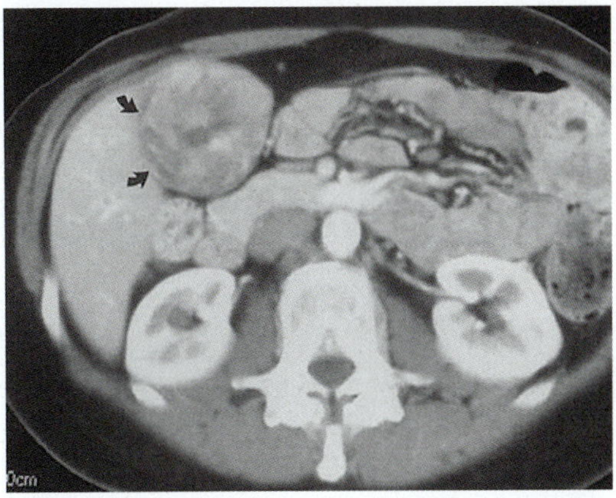

Figure 23.15 CT scan of a hepatic adenoma with the presence of a pseudocapsule (*arrows*).

are usually hyperintense. Biopsy is rarely needed as samples are often inadequate and diagnosis can be made on imaging. Management is based on multiple factors including presents of symptoms, size, gender, and whether the lesion changes over time. All female patients regardless of presentation should discontinue the use of oral contraceptive pills. As obesity is a risk factor, weight loss can also be indicated. In female patients who are asymptomatic with lesions <5 cm, serial imaging can be performed to ensure that the lesion is not enlarging and therefore at risk of rupture. Interval of imaging can be between 6 and 12 months. However, if patients are symptomatic or with lesions >5 cm, surgical resection with minimal margins may be necessary. Other options include transarterial embolization and radiofrequency ablation. Radiofrequency ablation appears to only be beneficial for hepatic adenomas <3 cm in size, with many of these patients requiring multiple ablations. It cannot be used in the acute setting. Transarterial embolization on the other hand has been used for lesions larger than 5 cm in both acute bleeding adenomas and elective procedures. In asymptomatic women with adenomas >5 cm, following with serial MRI every 6-12 months to ensure no progression may be a reasonable option. In male patients, however, the presence of a hepatic adenoma should always prompt intervention due to the higher incidence of β-catenin subtypes, which have a much higher malignant potential (**Figure 23.16**). Bleeding is the most feared consequence of hepatic adenomas and bears separate discussion. Patients can either bleed into the lesion or free rupture into the intraperitoneal cavity. Initial management follows the standard ABC approach of all critically ill patients. Massive transfusion may be necessary. The choice of whether to go to the operating room will depend on the patient's hemodynamic status and available resources and personnel. Surgical resection for bleeding hepatic adenomas is associated with greater blood loss and complications. Transarterial embolization is a reasonable alternative; however, it may not be feasible in unstable patients. If available, a combined approach in a hybrid OR may lead to the best outcomes in select patients with large-volume bleeding.

MALIGNANT LESIONS

Hepatocellular Carcinoma

Hepatocellular carcinoma (HCC) is the third most common tumor worldwide and the second leading cause of cancer-related death. The incidence is on the rise in the United States. Certain risk factors should alert the surgeon to the possibility that the mass in question is not benign. Eighty percent of HCC occurs in cirrhotic livers. Other risk factors include primary malignancy elsewhere, hepatitis B and C, long-term alcohol and tobacco use, nonalcoholic steatohepatosis, obesity, diabetes, and genetic conditions such as alpha-1 antitrypsin

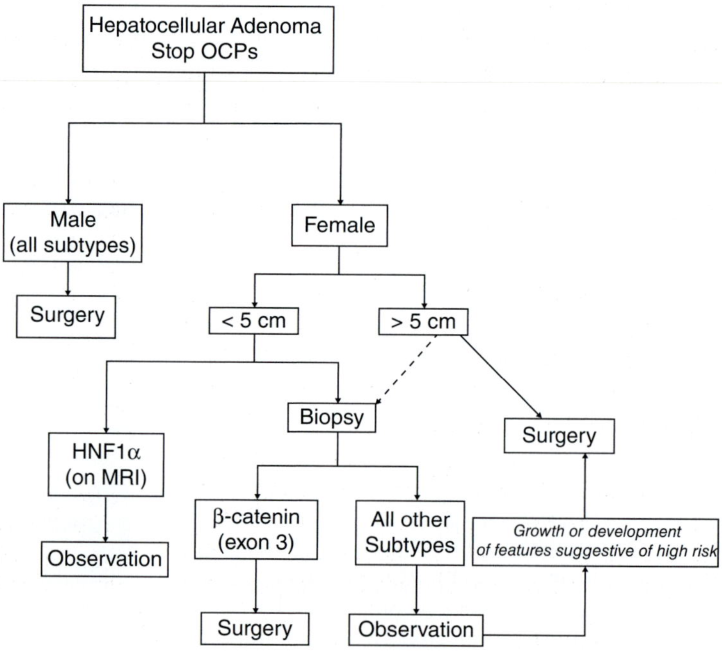

Figure 23.16 Management of hepatic adenoma in the elective setting. (Reprinted by permission from Springer: Springer Nature. Krause K, Tanabe KK. A shifting paradigm in diagnosis and management of hepatic adenoma. *Ann Surg Oncol.* 2020;27:3336(16).)

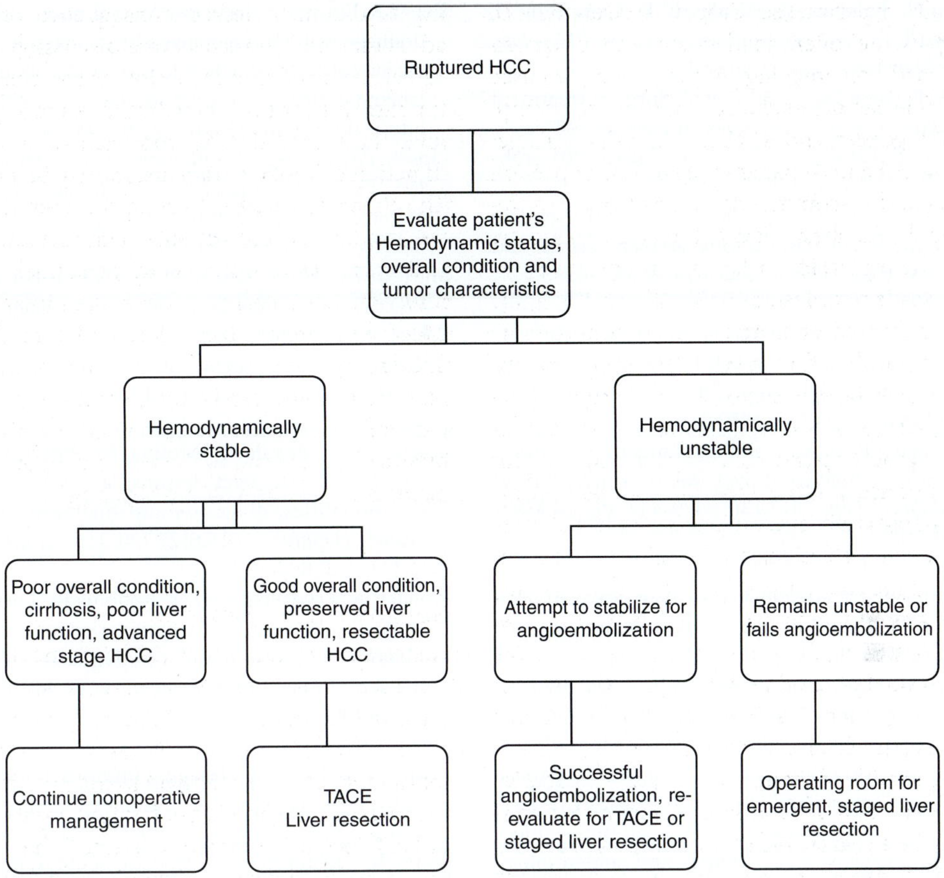

Figure 23.17 Algorithm for the management of ruptured hepatocellular cancer (HCC). (TACE, transarterial chemoembolization). (Courtesy of Dr. Andrew B. Peitzman.)

deficiency or Wilson disease. Up to 20% of HCC will present with bleeding as the initial symptom. In regions where HCC is endemic, it is the most common cause of nontraumatic hepatic bleeding. Larger HCC size, peripheral location, exophytic morphology, and severity of underlying cirrhosis increase the risk of HCC rupture. HCCs enhance on the arterial phase of CT with evidence of washout on the venous phase. A pseudocapsule may be noted on CT. With active bleeding, a contrast blush may be detected.

Based on hemodynamic status of the patient, management of the ruptured HCC (**Figure 23.17**) should start with bland angioembolization. Perform the embolization with Gelfoam, to allow later chemoembolization. Transcatheter arterial chemoembolization (TACE) at the index presentation is also an option. If hemodynamic instability necessitates operative management of a ruptured HCC, achieve hemostasis without resection at the index procedure. This can be followed by a later elective resection. Operative resection of the ruptured HCC at the index operation results in 25%-40% mortality.

SUMMARY

The liver is a complex organ that can be affected by multiple pathologies. It is necessary for acute care surgeons to know the most common masses, what complications can arise and the safest way to manage them. If diagnostic uncertainty exists or management questions, both surgical and nonoperative, arise, early consultation with a hepatobiliary specialist is warranted.

SUGGESTED READINGS

Aeberhard P, Fuhrimann R, Strahm P, Thommen A. Surgical treatment of hydatid disease of the liver: an experience from outside the endemic area. *Hepatogastroenterology*. 1996;43(9):627-636.

Bächler P, Baladron MJ, Menias C, et al. Multimodality imaging of liver infections: differential diagnosis and potential pitfalls. *RadioGraphics*. 2016;36(4):1001-1023.

Bajenaru N, Balaban V, Săvulescu F, Campeanu I, Patrascu T. Hepatic hemangioma—review. *J Med Life*. 2015;8 Spec Issue(Spec Issue):4-11.

Balik AA, Başoğlu M, Çelebi F, et al. Surgical treatment of hydatid disease of the liver: review of 304 cases. *Arch Surg*. 1999;134(2):166-169. doi:10.1001/archsurg.134.2.166.

5. Baranes L, Chiaradia M, Pigneur F, et al. Imaging benign hepatocellular tumors: atypical forms and diagnostic traps. *Diagn Interv Imaging*. 2013;94(7–8):677-695.

Bayrak M, Altıntas Y. Current approaches in the surgical treatment of liver hydatid disease: single center experience. *BMC Surg*. 2019;19:95. https://doi.org/10.1186/s12893-019-0553-1

Cheng Z, Liang P, Yu X, et al. Percutaneous microwave ablation for benign focal liver lesions: initial clinical results. *Oncol Lett*. 2017;13(1):429-434. doi:10.3892/ol.2016.5409

Cho SW, Marsh JW, Steel J, et al. Surgical management of hepatocellular adenoma: take it or leave it? *Ann Surg Oncol*. 2008;15:2795. https://doi.org/10.1245/s10434-008-0090-0

Doherty GM, Way LW. *Current Surgical Diagnosis & Treatment*. McGraw-Hill Medical; 2006.

Filippou D, Tselepis D, Filippou G, Papadopoulos V. Advances in liver echinococcosis: diagnosis and treatment. *Clin Gastroenterol Hepatol*. 2007;5(2):152-159.

Fiore M, Cascella M, Bimonte S, et al. Liver fungal infections: an overview of the etiology and epidemiology in patients affected or not affected by oncohematologic malignancies. *Infect Drug Resist*. 2018;11:177-186. doi:10.2147/IDR.S152473

Grazioli L, Federle MP, Brancatelli G, Ichikawa T, Olivetti L, Blachar A. Hepatic adenomas: imaging and pathologic findings. *RadioGraphics*. 2001;21:877-892.

Grazioli L, Morana G, Kirchin MA, Schneider G. Accurate differentiation of focal nodular hyperplasia from hepatic adenoma at gadobenate dimeglumine-enhanced MR imaging: prospective study. *Radiology*. 2005;236:166-177.

Zalaquett E, Menias C, Garrido F, et al. Imaging of hydatid disease with a focus on extrahepatic involvement. *Radiographics*. 2017;37:901-923. 10.1148/rg.2017160172.

Huang CJ, Pitt HA, Lipsett PA, et al. Pyogenic hepatic abscess. Changing trends over 42 years. *Ann Surg*. 1996;223(5):600-609.doi:10.1097/00000658-199605000-00016.

Hussain T, Adams M, Ahmed M, Arshad N, Solkar M. Intrahepatic perforation of the gallbladder causing liver abscesses: case studies and literature review of a rare complication. *Ann R Coll Surg Engl*. 2016;98(6):e88-e91. doi:10.1308/rcsann.2016.0115

Kammula US, Buell JF, Labow DM, et al. Surgical management of benign tumors of the liver. *Int J Gastrointest Cancer*. 2001;30:141-146. https://doi.org/10.1385/IJGC:30:3:141

Kouzu K, Einama T, Nishikawa M, et al. Successful surgical drainage with intraoperative ultrasonography for amebic liver abscess refractory to metronidazole and percutaneous drainage: a case report. *BMC Surg*. 2020;20:112. https://doi.org/10.1186/s12893-020-00776-x

Lipsett PA, Huang CJ, Lillemoe KD, Cameron JL, Pitt HA. Fungal hepatic abscesses: characterization and management. *J Gastrointest Surg*. 1997;1(1):78-84. doi: 10.1007/s11605-006-0013-y.

Marrero JA, Ahn J, Reddy R; FACG3 on behalf of the Practice Parameters Committee of the American College of Gastroenterology. ACG clinical guideline: the diagnosis and management of focal liver lesions. *Am J Gastroenterol*. 2014;109(9):1328-1347. doi: 10.1038/ajg.2014.213.

Mavilia MG, Pakala T, Molina M, Wu GY. Differentiating cystic liver lesions: a review of imaging modalities, diagnosis and management. *J Clin Transl Hepatol*. 2018;6(2):208-216. doi:10.14218/JCTH.2017.00069.

Mohajer K, Frydrychowicz A, Robbins JB, Loeffler AG, Reed TD, Reeder SB. Characterization of hepatic adenoma and focal nodular hyperplasia with gadoxetic acid. *J Magn Reson Imaging*. 2012;36(3):686-696. doi:10.1002/jmri.23701.

Mortelé KJ, Praet M, Van Vlierberghe H, Kunnen M, Ros PR. CT and MR imaging findings in focal nodular hyperplasia of the liver: radiologic-pathologic correlation. *Am J Roentgenol*. 2000;175(3):687-692.

Rubin R, Lichtenstein G. Hepatic scintigraphy in the evaluation of solitary solid liver masses. *J Nucl Med*. 1993;34:697-705.

Serraino C, Elia C, Bracco C, et al. Characteristics and management of pyogenic liver abscess: a European experience. *Medicine (Baltimore)*. 2018;97(19):e0628. doi:10.1097/MD.0000000000010628.

Sozuer E, Akyuz M, Akbulut S. Open surgery for hepatic hydatid disease. *Int Surg*. 2014;99(6):764-769. doi:10.9738/INTSURG-D-14-00069.1.

Srinivasan AJ, Peitzman AB. Nontraumatic liver hemorrhage. In: Coccolini F, Catena F, eds. *Textbook of Emergency General Surgery: Traumatic and Nontraumatic Surgical Emergencies*. Springer; 2021.

Strasberg SM, et al. Subtotal Cholecystectomy–"Fenestrating" vs "Reconstituting" subtypes and the prevention of bile duct injury: definition of the optimal procedure in difficult operative conditions. *J Am Coll Surg*. 2016;222(1):89-96.

Syed MA, Kim TK, Jang HJ. Portal and hepatic vein thrombosis in liver abscess: CT findings. *Eur J Radiol*. 2007;61(3):513-519.

Verma GR, Bose SM. Laparoscopic treatment of hepatic hydatid cyst. *Surg Laparosc Endosc*. 1998;8(4):280-282.

Koculen V, Jayarajah U, Ambawatte AP. Intrahepatic type II gall bladder perforation secondary to acute acalculous cholecystitis. *Case Rep Surg*. 2020;2020:5435921 https://doi.org/10.1155/2020/5435921.

Virgilio E, Cavallini M. Managing focal nodular hyperplasia of the liver: surgery or minimally-invasive approaches? A review of the preferable treatment options. *Anticancer Res.* 2018;38(1):33-36. doi:10.21873/anticanres.12188.

Wuerz T, Kane JB, Boggild AK, et al. A review of amoebic liver abscess for clinicians in a nonendemic setting. *Can J Gastroenterol.* 2012;26(10):729-733. doi:10.1155/2012/852835.

Yang DM, Kim HN, Kang JH, et al. Complications of pyogenic hepatic abscess: computed tomography and clinical features. *J Comput Assist Tomogr.* 2004;28(3):311-317.

Yoon JH, Kim JY. Atypical findings of focal nodular hyperplasia with gadoxetic acid (Gd-EOB-DTPA)-enhanced magnetic resonance imaging. *Iran J Radiol.* 2014;11(1):e9269. doi:10.5812/iranjradiol.9269.

CHAPTER

24 Obstetric and Gynecologic Considerations in Acute Care Surgery

Karen Brasel and Chrissy Guidry

INTRODUCTION

Many obstetric and gynecologic diseases must be distinguished from those more frequently seen by the general surgeon. In many cases, due to patient factors and resource considerations, general surgeons may need to treat these conditions either on an occasional or routine basis. In addition, pregnancy may alter both presentation and treatment considerations of many general surgical conditions (**Table 24.1**). For all of these reasons, understanding the presentation, diagnosis, and treatment of these conditions is essential for the acute care surgeon. This chapter reviews common and life-threatening diseases that are seen and treated by acute care surgeons.

ECTOPIC PREGNANCY

CASE PRESENTATION

A 38-year-old woman presents to the emergency department with RLQ pain. Her pain started 18 hours ago in the RLQ and has been increasing in severity. She has had several episodes of pelvic inflammatory disease, most recently treated 4 years ago. She has unprotected sex with multiple partners. Her last normal menstrual period was 8 weeks ago, but she has had some spotting over the last week. She is afebrile and has a blood pressure of 130/80 mm Hg and HR of 120 beats/min.

Question: *What is the likely diagnosis? How is the diagnosis established? What is the recommended treatment?*

Answer: *Ectopic pregnancy must be excluded in the patient by measuring B-HCG and a transvaginal ultrasound if the B-HCG is elevated. Treatment is tailored based on hemodynamics and the ability to perform serial monitoring. Careful assessment of hemodynamics in any pregnant patient is necessary due to the normal physiologic changes that may mask shock.*

Ectopic pregnancy should be considered in female with lower abdominal pain in whom pregnancy is a possibility. The incidence worldwide is increasing and is particularly on the rise in the United States. Risk factors for ectopic pregnancy include prior ectopic pregnancy, history of pelvic inflammatory disease, prior tubal ligation, age >35 years, and prior ruptured appendicitis. Presentation and management differ based on whether rupture has occurred. The most common presenting symptoms include abdominal pain, amenorrhea, and abnormal vaginal bleeding. Dizziness and signs and symptoms of acute blood loss accompanying these symptoms raise concern for ruptured ectopic pregnancy. The most common location for an ectopic pregnancy is the fallopian tube (95% of all ectopic pregnancies); late presentation and rupture are more common when the ectopic pregnancy is in another location, including cervical, abdominal, interstitial, or ovarian (**Figure 24.1**).

Diagnostics

Measurement of B-HCG and transvaginal ultrasound forms the cornerstones of diagnosis. The presence of an elevated beta-HCG with an empty uterus confirms the diagnosis of ectopic pregnancy. An intrauterine pregnancy should be visible on transvaginal ultrasound at a B-HCG of >1000 mIU/mL. Serial measurements of B-HCG may be helpful early in pregnancy; in a normal pregnancy, doubling occurs every 2-3 days, with slower rates of doubling in ectopic pregnancy.

Characteristic ultrasound features of ectopic pregnancy in the fallopian tube include a hyperechoic ring around an extrauterine hypoechoic

TABLE 24.1 ■ Physiologic Changes of Pregnancy

Cardiac output	Increased
Heart rate	Increased
Peripheral vascular resistance	Decreased
Blood volume	Increased
Red cell mass	Increased
Hematocrit (physiologic anemia of pregnancy)	Decreased
Alveolar ventilation	Increased
$PaCO_2$	Decreased
Oxygen consumption	Increased

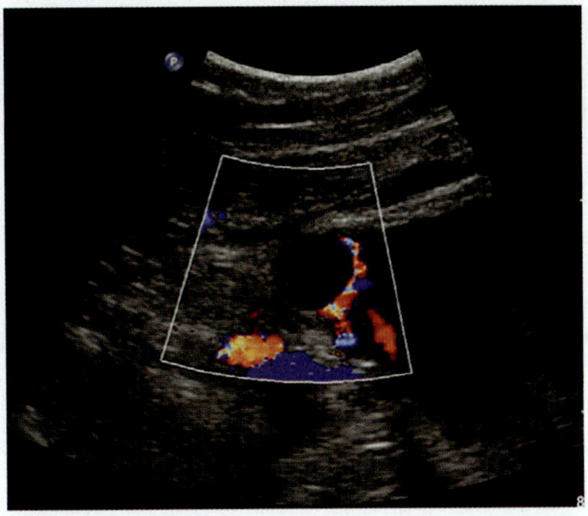

Figure 24.2 Ring of fire in ectopic pregnancy seen on Doppler ultrasound image. (From Lee R, Dupuis C, Chen B, et al. Diagnosing ectopic pregnancy in the emergency setting. *Ultrasonography*. 2018;37:81.)

gestational sac. The outermost portion of this ring demonstrates increased vascular flow by Doppler, the so-called ring of fire (**Figure 24.2**).

In an ectopic pregnancy not in the fallopian tube, ultrasound may demonstrate a fetus outside the uterus or simply intraperitoneal fluid and an empty uterus. In the presence of an elevated B-HCG, the latter establishes the diagnosis of a ruptured ectopic pregnancy and a surgical emergency.

Treatment

Once a surgical disease, earlier diagnosis of ectopic pregnancy has allowed some to be treated medically. The use of methotrexate has approximately an 80% success rate. Although an invasive procedure is avoided, there is an increased risk of rupture with failure of treatment. The effect on future fertility is unknown, as the fallopian tube is preserved but is scarred, increasing the risk of future ectopic pregnancy. Close monitoring with serial B-HCG and serial ultrasound is required, with success more likely if the initial B-HCG is <2000 mIU/mL and size <3.5 cm.

If treatment with methotrexate is not possible or not desired, laparoscopy is preferred to laparotomy in the hemodynamically stable patient. Salpingostomy should be performed if possible, with confirmation that all trophoblastic tissue has been

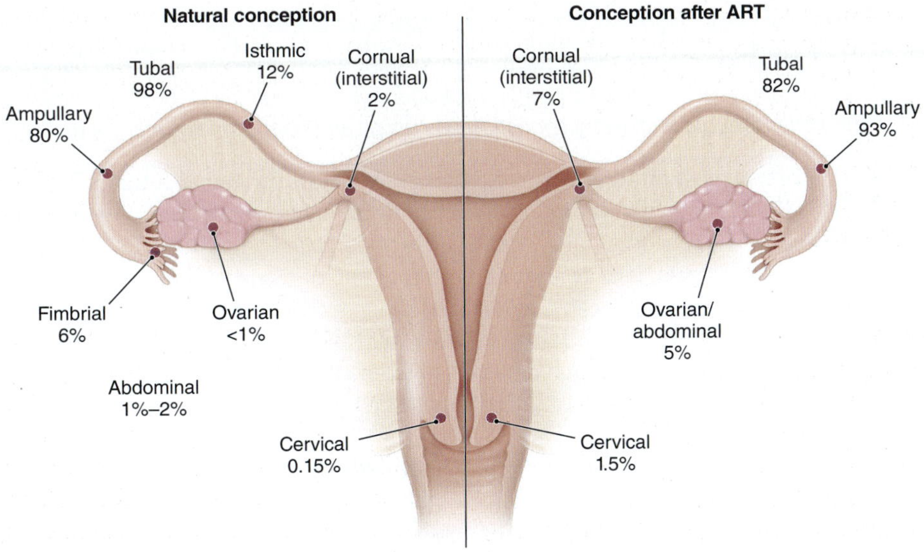

Figure 24.1 Incidence of types of ectopic pregnancy by location. ART, assisted reproductive technologies. (From Casanova R. *Beckmann and Ling's Obstetrics and Gynecology*. Wolters Kluwer; 2019. Figure 19.1).

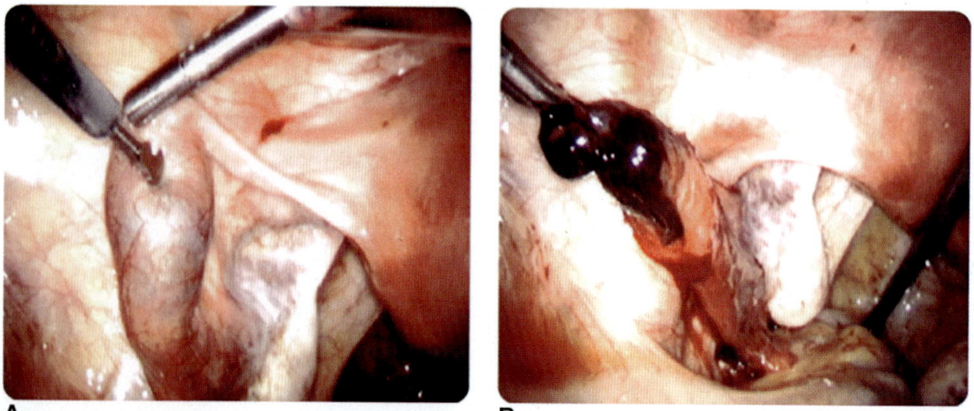
A B

Figure 24.3 **A, B.** Salpingostomy with removal of ectopic pregnancy. (Reprinted from Fylstra DL. Ectopic pregnancy not with the (distal) fallopian tube: etiology, diagnosis and treatment. *Am J Obstet Gynecol.* 2012;206(4):290, with permission from Elsevier.)

removed (**Figure 24.3**). The rate of persistent ectopic pregnancy is 5%-10% after salpingotomy, making monitoring of postprocedure B-HCG mandatory. Salpingectomy, done when salpingotomy is not possible, has a much lower rate of persistent ectopic pregnancy (essentially zero) but a much lower rate of subsequent intrauterine pregnancy.

Laparotomy is performed for ectopic pregnancy in locations other than the fallopian tube and ruptured ectopic pregnancy in the hemodynamically abnormal patient. Salpingectomy is the appropriate procedure for a ruptured tubal ectopic pregnancy. Ruptured ectopic pregnancy in other locations may require an emergent hysterectomy.

OVARIAN TORSION

CASE PRESENTATION

A 35-year-old woman presents to the emergency department with LLQ pain. She has had intermittent pain over the last several days, but it worsened acutely 6 hours ago. She has no bowel or bladder symptoms, and her last menstrual period was 3 weeks ago. She has been undergoing ovarian stimulation for *in vitro* fertilization and is otherwise healthy on no medications. She is afebrile and has a blood pressure of 110/85 mm Hg and HR of 110 beats/min. She has significant LLQ tenderness and normal laboratory tests.

Question: *What is the likely diagnosis? What is the recommended treatment?*

Answer: *In vitro fertilization is a risk factor for ovarian torsion, which is very likely in this patient without signs, symptoms, or laboratory evidence of other intra-abdominal pathology. Once confirmed with ultrasound or CT, this patient should undergo diagnostic laparoscopy and oophoropexy unless a tumor is found.*

Ovarian torsion occurs most often with an enlarged ovary—most commonly a tumor—and includes cysts or follicles in women undergoing ovarian stimulation for *in vitro* fertilization. Torsion presents as acute abdominal pain and can be intermittent in the case of partial/recurrent torsion. Nausea and vomiting can occur secondary to pain, with fever onset in the setting of tissue ischemia and necrosis due to vascular compromise. Ovarian torsion can occur during pregnancy as the enlarging uterus causes displacement of the ovaries anteriorly.

An enlarged ovary on physical examination must be differentiated from a tuboovarian abscess, ectopic pregnancy, and a tumor or cyst that has not undergone torsion.

Diagnostics

Ultrasound is the mainstay of diagnosis of ovarian torsion, with the absence of flow seen in the case of complete torsion. Increased flow seen on Doppler suggests either abscess or malignancy. In the setting of a normal ultrasound, CT may be helpful.

Treatment

The primary initial treatment of ovarian torsion is laparoscopic detorsion. Subsequent treatment depends on the status of the underlying ovary. In the setting of ischemia that persists after detorsion or frank necrosis, salpingo-oophorectomy is performed. Similarly, if the reason for torsion is due to a tumor, a salpingo-oophorectomy should be performed. However, if the ischemia resolves with detorsion and the ovary looks healthy with a simple cyst or follicle as the underlying etiology, cystectomy with oophoropexy is successful 90% of the time. This is particularly important for patients undergoing ovarian stimulation for *in vitro* fertilization, as it preserves the most options for future fertility.

BARTHOLIN ABSCESS

CASE PRESENTATION

A 28-year-old woman presents to the emergency department with perineal pain. She has had intermittent pain over the last several days, worse with sitting and with intercourse. She has no fever, no bowel or bladder symptoms, and her last menstrual period was 2 weeks ago. She is afebrile and has a blood pressure of 110/85 mm Hg and HR of 90 beats/min. She has exquisite perineal tenderness and a normal rectal examination.

Question: *What is the most likely diagnosis? What is the appropriate treatment?*

Answer: *Bartholin abscess is highly likely in a young woman with perineal tenderness and a normal rectal examination. Simple excision and drainage will take care of the acute problem, but the placement of a Word catheter to promote tract scarring is recommended to prevent recurrence.*

Bartholin abscesses are infections of the Bartholin gland, two glands just lateral to the vagina on the labia minora at the posterior introitus. Blockage of the internal opening of the gland results in a cyst, which may become infected. As these glands usually involute with age, this is most common in women <40 years of age.

Diagnostics

The diagnosis is based on history and physical examination, with perineal discomfort and dyspareunia as the most common symptoms.

Treatment

Incision and drainage is the first step in treatment, similar to most abscesses. The recurrence rate is high, and placement of a Word catheter is recommended to promote epithelialization of a fistula tract to prevent recurrence. The Word catheter is a small latex catheter with a 3-cc balloon placed into the abscess immediately after drainage. The end of the catheter can be placed into the vagina (**Figure 24.4**). Antibiotics are not recommended in the absence of cellulitis, similar to other skin abscesses. Cultures usually grow vaginal flora and are not usually helpful in guiding treatment. If a Word catheter is not available, simple packing with gauze strips can be utilized. Recurrence after initial treatment is treated with marsupialization, not recommended in the face of an acute abscess/infection.

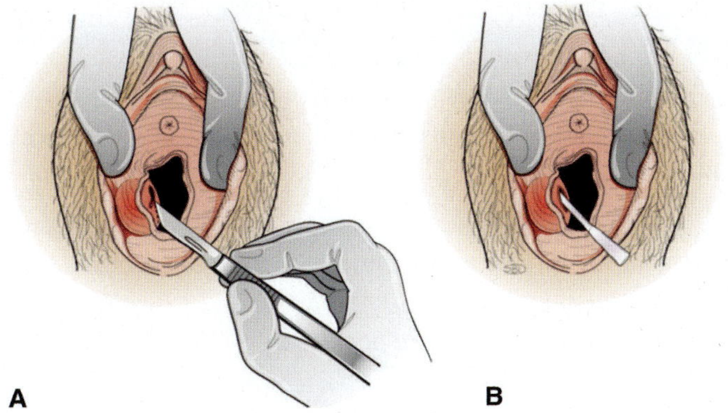

Figure 24.4 Treatment options of a Bartholin abscess. **A:** I&D of a Bartholin abscess: Make a vertical incision over the mucocutaneous junction on the vaginal mucosal side of the labia minora. **B:** Word catheter insertion: Make a 0.5-cm long stab incision into the duct or abscess, drain the cavity, insert the Word catheter as shown, and inflate the balloon with saline. (From Simon R, Ross C, Bowman SH, et al. Cook County Manual of Emergency Procedures. Philadelphia, PA: Lippincott Williams & Wilkins; 2011. Figure 8.27.)

TUBOOVARIAN ABSCESS

CASE PRESENTATION

A 29-year-old woman presents to the emergency department with lower abdominal and pelvic pain. She has had intermittent pain over the last several days, worse with sitting and with intercourse. She has unprotected sex with multiple partners, and her last menstrual period was 3 weeks ago. Her temperature is 38.9 °C, blood pressure 110/85 mm Hg, and HR is 120 beats/min. She has moderate tenderness in bilateral lower quadrants, worse on the right. She has R adnexal fullness and tenderness as well as cervical motion tenderness. Her WBC count is 15 700/mm^3.

Question: *What is the likely diagnosis? What treatment is required?*

Answer: *Tuboovarian abscess is most likely, or certainly most concerning. Intravenous antibiotics will be successful in most patients, with abscess drainage reserved for failure of conservative treatment or in those with severe sepsis who require immediate surgical sources control.*

Tuboovarian abscess is at the severe end of the spectrum of pelvic inflammatory disease, most commonly due to *Chlamydia trachomatis* and *Neisseria gonorrhea*. Although milder cases of pelvic inflammatory disease can be treated as outpatients, the diagnosis of tuboovarian abscess requires intravenous antibiotics and hospitalization. The majority resolve without further intervention. Those >7 cm are more likely to fail antibiotic treatment alone and require drainage.

Diagnostics

Diagnosis is based on a combination of physical examination and laboratory findings. Abdominal tenderness, adnexal tenderness, and cervical motion tenderness are all required for the diagnosis. In addition, one of the following is required: fever, leukocytosis, purulence from the cervical os, elevated erythrocyte sedimentation rate, Gram stain with gram-negative diplococci, culture of *Chlamydia trachomatis* or *Neisseria gonorrhea*, or pelvic abscess diagnosed by ultrasound or CT. Ultrasound has greater than a 95% sensitivity and specificity for the diagnosis of tuboovarian abscess.

Treatment

Initial antibiotic treatment should be intravenous cefoxitin or cefotetan along with doxycycline. In those patients with cephalosporin allergy, gentamicin and clindamycin can be used. In patients who do not improve with antibiotic therapy alone, percutaneous drainage of the abscess is recommended. If there is no option for percutaneous drainage, surgical drainage with either laparoscopy or laparotomy may be necessary. Drainage of the abscess is all that is required in the majority of patients, particularly in premenopausal patients. Salpingo-oophorectomy should be reserved for severely systemically ill patients, as it does have the advantage of complete source control.

APPENDICITIS

CASE PRESENTATION

A 36-year-old pregnant female, G1P0, currently 24 weeks pregnant, presents to the emergency department with RLQ pain. Her pain started 12 hours ago periumbilically and is now localized to the RLQ. She complains of mild nausea, no emesis. In the ED, she is afebrile and has a blood pressure of 130/80 mm Hg and HR of 105 beats/min.

Question: *What is the diagnosis? What is the next test that should be ordered to establish the diagnosis?*

Answer: *Appendicitis is the likely diagnosis. Care should be taken to promptly identify and work up causes for abdominal pain in the obstetric patient population.*

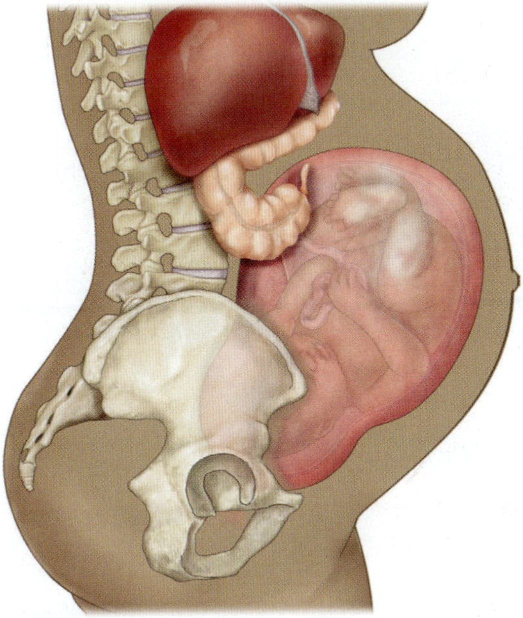

Figure 24.5 Displacement of the appendix by the gravid uterus.

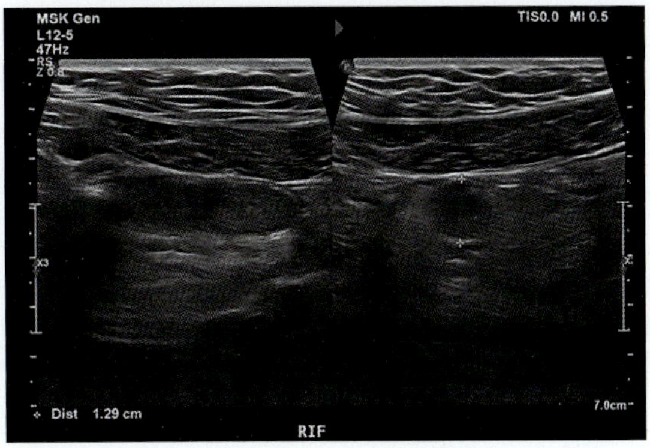

Figure 24.6 Appendicitis on ultrasound.

The acute abdomen in a pregnant patient remains one of the most difficult diagnostic and therapeutic challenges encountered in emergency general surgery. Laboratory changes occur throughout pregnancy, and anatomic displacement of internal organs by the enlarging uterus sometimes makes it difficult to make the correct diagnosis during pregnancy (**Figure 24.5**). Additionally, there is a high prevalence of nausea and vomiting in the obstetric patient population, making the diagnosis challenging.

Acute appendicitis is the most common nonobstetrical cause of an acute abdomen encountered in a pregnant patient.

Diagnostics

Maternal and fetal morbidity are usually related to delay in diagnosis. Ultrasound is the diagnostic imaging of choice in the obstetric patient population (**Figure 24.6**). The accuracy is higher in the first and second trimesters and lower in the third trimester based on the technical ability to perform the ultrasound in the gravid abdomen. If ultrasound is indeterminate, the next study to be ordered is an MRI. If MRI is unavailable, a CT may be ordered to help in diagnosing appendicitis. Fetal loss occurs in 3%-5% of pregnant patients without perforation but can be as high as 36% with perforation. Recent data suggest that negative appendectomy may be associated with an increase in fetal loss. Therefore, the importance of accurately early diagnosing of appendicitis in the obstetric population is critical. Pregnancy, however, should not influence the decision to perform an appendectomy in any patient once the diagnosis is highly suspected and/or confirmed.

Treatment

Antibiotics are recommended as an adjunct, but antibiotics alone are not recommended for appendicitis in the pregnant patient. Antibiotics should provide gram-negative and gram-positive coverage and coverage for anaerobes. A laparoscopic or open appendectomy can be performed in the pregnant patient. When using the laparoscopic approach, it is recommended to use the open (Hasson) technique and to avoid the Veress needle for insufflation to avoid injury to the uterus. A slightly lower intra-abdominal pressure (8-12 mm Hg) should be considered during laparoscopy. The pregnant woman undergoing an operation should have the uterus manually displaced to the left and a bump placed under the right hip to ensure that the inferior vena cava is not compressed. Trocar placement for laparoscopic appendectomy changes based on the size of the gravid uterus. **Figure 24.7** shows a guide to help in the placement of trocars during each trimester.

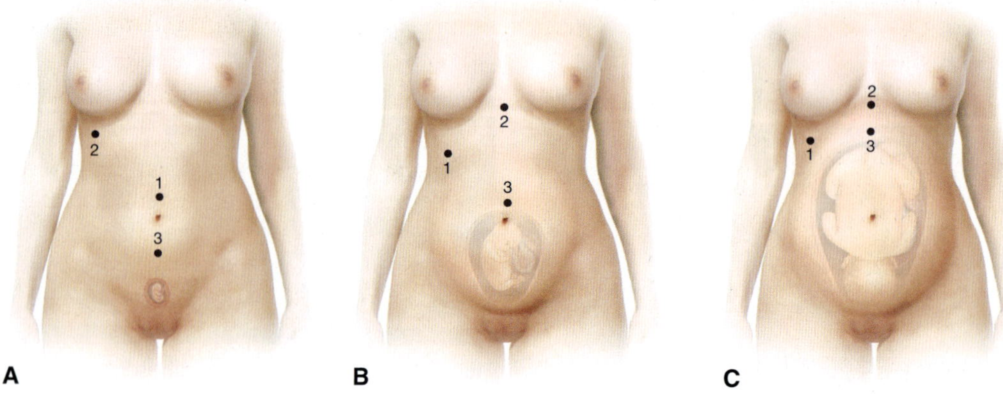

Figure 24.7 Trocar placement for laparoscopic appendectomy in the pregnant patient. **A.** 1st Trimester. **B.** 2nd Trimester. **C.** 3rd Trimester.

CHOLECYSTITIS

CASE PRESENTATION

A 21-year-old female who is 18 weeks pregnant, with a known history of hyperemesis gravidarum, is in the ED for RUQ pain and gallstones on bedside ultrasound. She has no fevers or other symptoms.

Question: *What is the suspected diagnosis? What is the recommended treatment?*

Answer: *Acute cholecystitis. Laparoscopic cholecystectomy.*

Biliary disease in the obstetric patient population is a frequently encountered problem in the hands of an acute care surgeon, as it is the second most common nonobstetric surgical disease requiring operation in the pregnant patient. Gallstones are more common during pregnancy due to decreased gallbladder motility and increased bile cholesterol saturation. Gallbladder pathology during pregnancy has been linked to increased preterm birth, maternal morbidity, and neonatal morbidity. In a pregnant patient with abdominal pain, fetal outcome depends on the outcome of the mother. Therefore, a risk-benefit discussion is important with discussing diagnosing and treatment strategies for all gravid patients with acute presentations of abdominal pain. Biliary disease presents on a spectrum, from symptomatic cholelithiasis to cholangitis and pancreatitis.

Diagnostics

Cholecystitis usually presents with colicky RUQ pain, nausea/vomiting, and low-grade fever. On physical examination, patients commonly have tenderness in the RUQ and sometimes will have a positive Murphy sign. Ultrasound is safe and effective in identifying the etiology of acute abdominal pain in obstetric patients. CT should be used when the diagnosis is unclear.

Treatment

Historically, treatment of biliary pathology was medical management and avoidance of operation until after parturition. However, newer data suggest that pregnant patients with symptomatic cholelithiasis should undergo cholecystectomy early due to decreased gravid complications, including decreased medication use, decreased recurrence of biliary symptomatology, shorter hospital stay, and decreased life-threatening complications during pregnancy. The treatment of choice is laparoscopic cholecystectomy. The Society of American Gastrointestinal Endoscopic Surgeons (SAGES) has provided the following important principles for laparoscopy in pregnancy.

1. Laparoscopy can be safely performed during any trimester of pregnancy when the operation is indicated.
2. Pneumatic compression devices must be used because of the enhancement of lower venous stasis with pneumoperitoneum and pregnancy-induced hypercoagulable state.

3. Fetal and uterine status, as well as maternal end-tidal CO_2 and arterial blood gases, should be monitored.
4. Use fluoroscopy selectively and protect the uterus with a lead shield if intraoperative cholangiography is possible.
5. Given an enlarged gravid uterus, abdominal access should be obtained using the open technique.
6. Dependent positioning should be used to shift the uterus off the inferior vena cava.
7. Pneumoperitoneum pressures should be minimized (8-12 mm Hg) and not allowed to exceed 15 mm Hg.
8. Obstetric consultation should be obtained before operation.

During the operation, the surgeon should avoid manipulation of the uterus. Additionally, postoperative fetal monitoring in all viable pregnancies of 24 weeks and older should begin immediately postoperatively.

POSTPARTUM HEMORRHAGE

CASE PRESENTATION

A 30-year-old female at 38 weeks without significant past medical history presents with signs of labor. She has an uncomplicated delivery with an estimated blood loss of 500 mL. Approximately 45 minutes after delivery, she has severe fatigue and light-headedness. Her blood pressure is 96/68 mm Hg, and her heart rate is 110 beats/min. On physical examination, she has a moderately firm uterus. Uterine massage is initiated, and she is taken to the operating room for an examination under anesthesia.

Question: *What is the working diagnosis and likely etiology in this patient? What are the next most appropriate steps in the management of this patient?*

Answer: *Primary postpartum hemorrhage (PPH) from uterine atony and vaginal lacerations should be the top differential diagnosis. Management should include initiating a massive transfusion protocol, starting balanced resuscitation, and administration of uterotonics. Additionally, maneuvers may include balloon tamponade of the uterus, angioembolization, resuscitative endovascular balloon occlusion of the aorta (REBOA), and surgical control of bleeding (see* ***Figures 24.8****).*

Definition

Postpartum hemorrhage is defined by the American College of Obstetricians and Gynecologists as the accumulation of blood loss ≥1 L of blood loss accompanied by signs or symptoms of hypovolemia within 24 hours after birth. This remains the leading cause of maternal mortality worldwide. Initial management is to diagnose the cause of bleeding while resuscitating the patient with blood products. After delivery, an atonic uterus is estimated to cause 70%-80% of primary postpartum hemorrhage and should be suspected as the cause of postpartum bleeding when recognized after delivery.

H—Ask for help and hands-on uterus (uterine massage)
A—ABCs
E—Establish etiology, ensure blood availability, oxytocin
M—Massage the uterus
O—Oxytocin infusion or prostaglandins
S—Shift to operating room, ideally hybrid
T—Tamponade. Balloon or packing. TXA
A—Apply compression sutures on the uterus
S—Systematic pelvic devascularization (uterine, ovarian, int. iliac arteries)
I—Interventional radiology (still in the operating room)
S—Subtotal or total hysterectomy

From Varatharajan L, Chandraharan E, Sutton J, et al. Outcome of the management of massive postpartum hemorrhage using the algorithm "Hemostasis". *Int J Gynaecol Obstet*. 2011;113(2):152-154.

Figure 24.8 Haemostasis mnemonic for hemorrhage control in Primary Postpartum hemorrhage. (From Varatharajan L, Chandraharan E, Sutton J, et al. Outcome of the management of massive postpartum hemorrhage using the algorithm "Hemostasis". *Int J Gynaecol Obstet*. 2011;113(2):152-154.)

In the United States, the rate of postpartum hemorrhage increased to 26% between 1994 and 2006 due to uterine atony. Maternal mortality, however, has decreased since the 1980s, likely related to improved resuscitation efforts with blood transfusion and observed increasing rates of peripartum hysterectomy.

Treatment

The initial assessment and evaluation of hemorrhage must be prompt. Resuscitative efforts must be ongoing with blood transfusions until definitive control of bleeding is done. Maintaining the principles of a primary survey is important. Make sure that the airway, breathing, and circulation are intact. Two large-bore IVs, at a minimum, should be in place. Coagulation labs should be sent to the lab, including an evaluation of thromboelastography (TEG) if available. A type and crossmatch should be sent to the lab but should not delay the transfusion of products. If blood is not typed and crossmatched and is needed for resuscitative efforts, type O negative blood should be used. Balanced resuscitation, including whole blood and tranexamic acid, should be used.

Since uterine atony is the leading cause of PPH, uterotonic agents should always be used in the setting of significant postpartum hemorrhage. Oxytocin is the most common medication used, but methylergonovine and misoprostol are also appropriate.

Along with medication and transfusion therapy, procedures to control bleeding may be needed. During the examination under anesthesia, if a vaginal laceration is noted, this should be sutured to control further bleeding. If an atonic uterus is noted to be the source of hemorrhage, uterine fundal massage stimulates the atonic uterus to contract using bimanual uterine massage compressing the uterus between the clinician's two hands. Massage should be maintained while uterotonic agents are given intravenously. If the uterus is fully contracted and the bleeding continues, a balloon for tamponade can be used to control bleeding. A Bakri balloon is inserted transcervically or through a C section incision and is inflated with saline. An Ebb uterine tamponade system has two balloons with both vaginal and uterine balloons for inflation. Additionally, uterine packing can be performed with a thrombin-soaked gauze for additional tamponade measures.

If local and conservative hemorrhage control measures are not effective, uterine embolization can be pursued if interventional radiology is available. Additionally, if noninvasive hemorrhage control fails or if the patient is hemodynamically unstable, surgical intervention should be pursued. The first approach would be bilateral uterine artery ligation. This technique helps to diminish blood flow to the uterus leading to a high success rate of hemorrhage control. However, when all conservative measures fail to stop hemorrhagic shock or if uterine rupture is identified, a hysterectomy is the definitive treatment for massive primary postpartum hemorrhage.

Resuscitative endovascular balloon occlusion of the aorta (REBOA) is an emerging, minimally invasive procedure to control noncompressible hemorrhage such as postpartum hemorrhage. Early studies are promising for using REBOA in obstetric hemorrhage, which revealed reduced blood loss, improved maternal outcomes, and decreased hysterectomy rates compared to traditional techniques previously described. For pelvic bleeding, the REBOA is inserted via the common femoral artery and deployed in zone III, which is above the aortic bifurcation and below the renal arteries. Once inserted, definitive surgical control of bleeding should be achieved within 30 minutes to avoid distal ischemia related to inflation of the REBOA.

PERIMORTEM C-SECTION

CASE PRESENTATION

A 42-year-old-female who was brought to the emergency department by EMS after involved in a high-speed motor vehicle collision is noticeably pregnant. She was the passenger and was restrained. You notice that her fundal height appears well above her umbilicus. In route, the patient was speaking in incomprehensible words with a blood pressure of 80/60 mm Hg, pulse 140 beats/min. When she was transferred to the bed in the resuscitation bay, she became unresponsive and lost a pulse.

Question: *What is the next step in management?*

Answer: *Perimortem cesarean (resuscitative hysterotomy, some refer to as "crash C-Section") should be considered as soon as possible along with resuscitation of the mother and search for identifiable sources of bleeding/shock.*

Definition

The perimortem cesarean section is the surgical delivery of the fetus, performed at or near the death of the maternal patient. It is also referred to as a resuscitative hysterotomy. A multidisciplinary team approach must be used to maximize the potential of both maternal and fetal survival. Maternal evaluation should be done expeditiously but not to delay the hysterotomy. Expected gestational age is usually not obtained in the emergency scenario. A uterine fundal height at the level of the umbilicus is correlated with a gestational age of 24 weeks. It is important to note that in a trauma situation, it is crucial to understand the main focus should be initially on resuscitating the mother, starting with the basics of Advanced Trauma Life Support (ATLS): airway, breathing, and circulation (ABCs).

Although consensus data from the American College of Obstetricians and Gynecologists (ACOG) is insufficient to make recommendations as to when to perform this procedure, most have agreed it should be performed with maternal arrest in pregnancy > 23 weeks of gestation. Additionally, although there is no optimal delivery timing in this setting, it is clear that fetal survival drastically decreases when the time from maternal death to delivery reaches 5 minutes.

ACOG recommendations:

1. If efforts to resuscitate a pregnant woman in cardiac arrest have been unsuccessful, resuscitative hysterotomy is recommended for maternal benefit in a woman with a uterine size at or above the umbilicus.
2. Consideration of resuscitative hysterotomy. It is recommended that the decision to perform a resuscitative hysterotomy should be considered as soon as there is a maternal cardiac arrest. Once the decision is made to proceed with the hysterotomy, the patient should not be moved to the operating room, but rather antiseptic is splashed (if available) and the resuscitative hysterotomy is performed.
3. Survival curves of women and neonates have shown 50% injury-free survival rates with perimortem cesarean delivery as late as 25 minutes after maternal cardiac arrest, so even if delivery does not occur within 4-5 minutes, there still may be a benefit, and resuscitative hysterotomy should be considered.

Technique

Frequently, the urgency of this operation limits the time of preparation. However, if EMS calls in a report of a pregnant female with periarrest findings, you should prepare for the worst-case scenario: a perimortem cesarean. With limited preparation time, you should prepare a team for the following immediate interventions: definitive airway (intubation), IV access, antiseptic solution, operative tray with a scalpel, hemostats, large scissors, gauze, retractors. Notify the obstetrics team as well as the neonatal intensive care team. All personnel involved should be working cohesively together for the best chances of effective resuscitative efforts for the patients.

If CPR is initiated in the ED, a newer recommendation proposes that the uterus be manually displaced with two hands to the patient's left while CPR is actively being performed. As CPR is started, operative team members should be preparing for the resuscitative hysterotomy. The procedure should be performed in the following manner:

1. Antiseptic solution splashed on the anterior abdomen.
2. Using a No. 10 blade, an incision is made from the level of the xiphoid to the pubic symphysis.
3. Once the peritoneal wall is encountered, scissors are used to cut the peritoneum vertically, and the uterus is delivered.
4. On the lower pole of the uterus, a small vertical incision is made and extended to the fundus superiorly with scissors until the fetus is exposed.
5. Once the fetus is exposed, the cord is clamped and cut. Once delivered, resuscitation of the infant should promptly follow with the neonatal intensive care team.
6. The maternal abdomen is then packed and further intervention is based on maternal response to resuscitative efforts.
7. Continue ACLS/ATLS until ROSC is achieved. If achieved, then damage control surgery should be implemented and further resuscitative efforts continue.

SUMMARY

- Gynecologic causes of the acute abdomen include ruptured ectopic pregnancy, ovarian torsion, and pelvic inflammatory disease, including tuboovarian abscess.
- Whenever a female of reproductive age presents with abdominal or pelvic pain, pregnancy should be ruled out.
- Any woman presenting with pain and bleeding in early pregnancy should be considered to have an ectopic pregnancy until proven otherwise.

- Ectopic pregnancy may present as a surgical emergency in case of rupture or uncontrolled bleeding.
- Ovarian torsion is a surgical emergency; laparoscopy confirms the diagnosis and permits the treatment in time.
- Tuboovarian abscesses may be managed with intravenous antibiotics first in the nontoxic patient. Patients who are not improving should be offered surgical exploration.
- Dealing with appendicitis or cholecystitis in pregnant women, the risk of miscarriage is higher with ongoing intra-abdominal infection or peritonitis than with early laparoscopy.
- A pregnant woman on the operating table should be rotated on the left side to decrease uterine compression on the inferior vena cava.
- Open laparoscopy is the gold standard.
- Fetal monitoring and early obstetrician involvement should be the mainstay of any surgical condition for which the gravid female seeks surgical attention.
- Postpartum hemorrhage should be approached similarly to a trauma resuscitation; massive transfusion, adjunctive medications (uterotonics), and bleeding control using manual compression, tamponade, and consideration of REBOA.

SUGGESTED READINGS

ACOG Practice Bulletin. No. 211: Critical care in pregnancy. *Obstet Gynecol.* 2019;133(5):e303-e319.

Bakhbakhi D, Gamaledin I, Siassakos D. Cardiopulmonary resuscitation of pregnant women. *Resuscitation.* 2015;91:A5-A6.

Bateman BT, Berman MF, Riley LE, Leffert LR. The epidemiology of postpartum hemorrhage in a large, nationwide sample deliveries. *Anesth Analg.* 2010;110:1368-1373.

Benson MD, Padovano A, Bourjeily G, Zhou Y. Maternal collapse: challenging the four-minute rule. *EBioMedicine.* 2016;6:253-257.

Bonney EA, Myers JE. Caesarean section: techniques and complications. *Obstet Gynaecol Reprod Med.* 2010;21:97-102.

Borgman MA, Spinella PC, Perkins JG, et al. The ratio of blood products transfused affects mortality in patients receiving massive transfusions at a combat support hospital. *J Trauma Acute Care Surg.* 2007;63(4):805-813.

Bouyou J, Gaujoux S, Marcellin L, et al. Abdominal emergencies during pregnancy. *J Visc Surg.* 2015;152:S105-S115.

Brenner M, Bulger EM, Perina DG, et al. *Trauma Surg Acute Care Open.* 2018;3:1-3.

Creanga AA, Berg CJ, Ko JY, et al. Maternal mortality and morbidity in the United States: where are we now? *J Womens Health (Larchmt).* 2014;23:3-9.

Dhupar R, Smaldone GM, Hamad GG. Is there a benefit to delaying cholecystectomy for symptomatic gallbladder disease during pregnancy? *Surg Endosc.* 2010;24:108-112.

Diegelmann L. Nonobstetric abdominal pain and surgical emergencies in pregnancy. *Emerg Med Clin North Am.* 2012;30:885-901.

Fylstra DL. Ectopic pregnancy not within the (distal) fallopian tube: etiology, diagnosis and treatment. *Am J Obstet Gynecol.* 2012;206(4):289-299.

Gilmandyar D, Thornburg LL. Surgical management of postpartum hemorrhage. *Semin Perinatol.* 2019;43:27-34.

Girard T, Morti M, Schlembach D. New approaches to obstetrical hemorrhage: the postpartum hemorrhage algorithm. *Curr Opin Anaesthesiol.* 2014;27:267-274.

Holcomb JB, Tilley BC, Baraniuk S, et al. Transfusion of plasma, platelets, and red blood cells in a 1:1:1 vs 1:1:2 ratio and mortality in patients with severe trauma: the PROPPR randomized clinical trail. *JAMA.* 2015;313(5):471-281.

Ibiebele I, Schnitzler M, Nippita T, Ford JB. Outcomes of gallstone disease during pregnancy: a Population-based Data Linkage Study. *Paediatr Perinat Epidemiol.* 2017;31(6):522-530.

Ito K, Ito H, Whang EE, Tavakkolizadeh A. Appendectomy in pregnancy: evaluation of the risks of a negative appendectomy. *Am J Surg.* 2012;203:145-150.

Kamaya A, Shin L, Chen B, et al. Emergency gynecologic imaging. *Semin Ultrasound CT MR.* 2008;29:353-368.

Kave M, Parooie F, Salarzaei M. Pregnancy and appendicitis: a systematic review and meta-analysis on the clinical use of MRI in diagnosis on appendicitis in pregnant women. *World J Emerg Surg.* 2019;14:37.

Lee R, Dupuis C, Chen B, et al. Diagnosing ectopic pregnancy in the emergency setting. *Ultrasonography.* 2018;37:78-87.

Masselli G, Derme M, Laghi F, Framarino-dei-Malatesta M, Gualdi G. Evaluating the Acute Abdomen in the Pregnant Patient. *Radiol Clin North Am.* 2015;53:1309-1325.

McWilliams GDE, Hill MJ, Dietrich CS III. Gynecologic emergencies. *Surg Clin North Am.* 2008;88:265-283.

Mercado J, Brea I, Mendez B, et al. Critical Obstetric and gynecologic procedures in the emergency department. *Emerg Med Clin North Am.* 2013;31:207-236.

Morel O, Malartic C, Muhlstein J, Gayet E, Judin P, Soyer P, et al. Pelvic arterial ligations for severe postpartum hemorrhage: indications and techniques. *J Visc Surg.* 2011;148:e95-e102.

Panici PB, Anceschi M, Borgia ML, Bresadola L, Masselli G, Parasassi T. Intraoperative aorta balloon occlusion: fertility preservation in patient with placenta accreta/increta. *J Matern Fetal Neonatal Med.* 2012;25:2512-2516.

Parry R, Asmussen T, Smith JE. Perimortem C-section. *Emerg Med.* 2016;33:224-229.

Pearl JP, Price RR, Tonkin AE, Richardson WS, Stefanidis D. Guidelines for the use of laparoscopy during pregnancy. Sages.org/publications/guidelines/guidelines-for-diagnosis-treatment-and-use-of-laparoscopy-for-surgical-problems-during-pregnancy. 2017.

Ramphal SR, Moodley J. Emergency gynaecology. *Best Pract Res Clin Obstet Gynaecol.* 2006;20:729-750.

Rigouzzo A, Louvet N, Favier R, et al. Assessment of coagulation by thromboelastography during ongoing postpartum hemorrhage: a retrospective cohort analysis. *Anesth Analg.* 2020;130(2):416-425.

Say L, Chou D, Gemmill A, et al. Global causes of maternal death: a WHO systematic analysis. *Lancet Glob Health.* 2014;2:e323-e333.

Shakur H, et al.; WOMAN Trial Collaborators. Effect of early tranexamic acid administration on mortality, hysterectomy, and other morbidities in women with post-partum haemorrhage (WOMAN): an international, randomized, double-blind placebo-controlled trial. *Lancet.* 2017;389(10084):2105-2116.

Soskin PN, Yu J. Resuscitation of the pregnant patient. *Emerg Med Clin North Am.* 2019;37(2):351-363.

Wang YL, Duan XH, Han XW, et al. Comparison of temporary abdominal aortic occlusion with internal iliac artery occlusion for patients with placenta accrete-A non-randomised prospective study. *Vasa.* 2017;46: 53-57.

Weisbrod AB, Sheppard FR, Chernofsky MR, et al. Emergent management of postpartum hemorrhage for the general and acute care surgeon. *World J Emerg Surg.* 2009;4:43. doi:10.1186/1749-7922-4-43.

Wu Q, Liu Z, Zhao X, et al. Outcome of pregnancies after balloon occlusion of the Infrarenal abdominal aorta during caesarean in 230 patients with placenta praevia accreta. *Cardiovasc Intervent Radiol.* 2016;39:1573-1579.

Yoong W, Ridout A, Memtsa M, Stavroulis A, Aref-Adib M, Ramsey-Marcelle Z, et al. Application of uterine compression suture in association with intrauterine balloon tamponade ('uterine sandwich') for postpartum hemorrhage. *Acta Obstet Gynecol Scand.* 2019;91: 147-151.

CHAPTER

25 Thoracic Emergencies

Morgan Schellenberg and Joseph Galante

CASE PRESENTATION

A healthy 30-year-old male with no past medical or surgical history presents to the emergency department with sudden onset of right-sided chest pain and shortness of breath. He denies antecedent trauma and states that the chest pain began suddenly while he was at rest. On physical examination, he does not appear to be in respiratory distress. His vital signs are within normal limits and his oxygen saturation is 96% on room air. Preliminary investigations include an upright chest x-ray, which demonstrates a large-volume right-sided pneumothorax without radiographic features of tension pneumothorax.

Question: *What is the patient's diagnosis and what is the most appropriate initial management?*

Answer: *This patient has a primary spontaneous pneumothorax (PSP), which is an atraumatic pneumothorax that occurs in patients without underlying lung disease. Although the traditional management of PSP involved chest tube decompression or aspiration of the accumulated air in the pleural space, contemporary literature supports noninterventional management for PSP, even with moderate or large pneumothoraces. In one large multicenter randomized noninferiority trial, noninterventional management was noninferior to chest tube drainage in terms of successful lung re-expansion by 8 weeks postpneumothorax. Additionally, noninterventional management was associated with fewer adverse events, reduced development of tension pneumothorax, and lower rates of recurrence. Analgesia, serial chest x-rays, and close clinical follow-up are cornerstones of management.*

LUNG AND TRACHEA

Emergency considerations of the lung parenchyma and trachea that are of particular interest to the general surgeon are tracheoinnominate fistulae and infectious pulmonary diseases, including tuberculosis, fungal balls, and other bacterial and viral causes of lung abscesses.

Tracheoinnominate Fistula: Principles of Management

Relevant Anatomy

The trachea is a relatively short segment of the upper airway that spans from the cricoid cartilage to the carina, where it bifurcates into the right and left primary bronchi. It is comprised of incomplete cartilaginous rings which are deficient posteriorly, such that the membranous posterior wall of the trachea allows esophageal expansion with the passage of food boluses. The trachea originates in the neck and terminates in the chest after traversing the thoracic inlet.

In coursing through the thoracic inlet and upper mediastinum, the trachea travels in close proximity to the innominate artery and it is this anatomic relationship which is relevant to the development of a tracheoinnominate fistula (TIF). The innominate artery, which is the first branch of the aortic arch, divides into the right subclavian artery and the right common carotid artery. In the upper mediastinum, the innominate artery travels anteriorly over the right lateral aspect of the trachea. Any inflammation in the area of this anatomy relationship can lead to erosion of the distinct tissue planes of these two structures and resultant catastrophic bleeding into the airway.

Clinical Presentation

The typical clinical presentation of a TIF occurs in the post-tracheostomy setting, although it can develop in the setting of malignancy, radiation, or infection in the involved field. Classically, most TIFs present 1-2 weeks after tracheostomy placement, although it can occur months later. There are several important risk factors that must be considered during tracheostomy placement and in the postoperative care to help prevent this potentially fatal complication. The tracheostomy ideally should be inserted between the second and third tracheal rings as a lower insertion site places the tracheostomy in closer proximity to the innominate artery and, therefore, erosion becomes more likely. Care should also be taken to avoid overfilling the tracheostomy tube cuff and to prevent frequent tracheostomy tube movement against the inner walls of the trachea, both of which contribute to tracheal wall erosion and TIF formation.

After routinely taking steps during tracheostomy tube placement to avoid TIF formation, the clinician must thereafter maintain a high index of suspicion for TIF in the setting of any bleeding from the tracheostomy. Although typically presenting 7-14 days after tracheostomy, bleeding from the tracheostomy >72 hours after insertion should be considered a TIF until proven otherwise. Many TIFs will present with a sentinel bleed, in which a small amount of blood will be shed through the tracheostomy days before the exsanguinating hemorrhage occurs. Mean time between the sentinel bleed and catastrophic hemorrhage is reported to be 3 days. It is for this reason that any amount of blood through the tracheostomy must be seriously evaluated when it occurs.

A tracheoinnominate fistula presents in one of two ways. It may manifest in a hemodynamically stable patient with small volume hemoptysis and then allows time for a deliberate work-up. Alternatively, TIF will present with exsanguination into the airway. The diagnosis and management depend upon which of these two scenarios occurs.

Diagnosis

Small-volume bleeding from a tracheostomy should immediately be assessed with close physical examination. Any blood not obviously originating from the skin or tracheal edges should be considered a TIF until this diagnosis is excluded. Hemodynamically stable patients undergo bronchoscopy to exclude lower respiratory causes of bleeding as well as a computed tomographic angiography (CTA) of the chest and neck to inspect the area of apposition between the innominate artery and trachea. Inflammation in this vicinity would suggest the diagnosis and active arterial extravasation from the innominate artery into the trachea would secure it.

Hemodynamically unstable patients require more decisive action and intervention, and it is these patients who are likely to come to the attention of the emergency general surgeon. The first step in the assessment of hemodynamically unstable patients with bleeding from the tracheostomy site is hyperinflation of the tracheostomy tube cuff. If TIF is the source of bleeding, hyperinflating the cuff may compress the innominate artery upward against the clavicle and assist in temporary hemorrhage control. Bleeding that abates with cuff hyperinflation is from a TIF. Although conceptually cuff hyperinflation is a logical maneuver to help tamponade bleeding, the reality is that modern tracheostomy tube cuffs are deliberately incapable of withstanding high pressures, a design feature intended to mitigate the risk of pressure necrosis of the tracheal wall and TIF. As a result, cuff balloons may simply be unable to produce enough pressure to aid in hemorrhage control. A recent case report described cuff hyperinflation assisting in abatement of bleeding directly into the airway after a TIF but that true tamponade of the bleeding did not occur until a Foley catheter balloon was introduced adjacent to the tracheostomy stoma.

If tracheostomy cuff hyperinflation has been unsuccessful at slowing the hemorrhage, intubate the patient orotracheally, remove the tracheostomy tube, and insert your finger through the stoma toward the right of the upper mediastinum. Lifting your finger up against the right clavicular head will compress the innominate artery against the bone and slow the bleeding.

Treatment

In the operating room, prepare the patient's neck and chest for surgical exploration. Once the airway is secured and hemorrhage is temporarily slowed, if the diagnosis remains unclear a quick bronchoscopy can be undertaken at this point to confirm tracheal erosion with associated bleeding. Otherwise, proceed with median sternotomy.

After dividing the sternum, locate and divide the innominate vein as it traverses the upper mediastinum. Although this can be simply retracted out of the way to gain access to the underlying great arterial vessels, in an exsanguinating patient it is most expedient to divide it. Next, identify the innominate artery and ligate it. The inflammation around the fistula site itself precludes safe dissection in that area and the TIF does not require formal division. In many patients, this is well tolerated and will not result in either right upper extremity ischemia or ischemic stroke.

In the hemodynamically stable patient with TIF detected after a sentinel bleed, cardiac surgery can proceed with the patient on cardiac bypass to isolate and divide the fistula itself. Any remaining abnormality of the innominate artery itself can be resected and patched or grafted. Any available tissue, such as strap muscle, thymic remnant, or an intercostal muscle flap can be placed between the innominate artery and the trachea to prevent fistula reoccurrence.

Complications

Ischemic stroke and right upper extremity ischemia as consequences of inadequate flow through the right common carotid or right subclavian artery, respectively, are feared complications of innominate artery ligation. With the alternative being death due to exsanguination, these are risks that must be incurred. Fortunately, these complications are infrequent, although admittedly survival after TIF is sufficiently rare that the short- or long-term sequelae after innominate artery ligation in these patients are not reliably known.

Infectious Pulmonary Diseases: Principles of Management

Relevant Anatomy

The lungs are paired organs within the thoracic cavities. The right and left lung are divided into lobes, which then subdivide into bronchopulmonary segments. The right lung consists of three lobes, comprised of a total of ten bronchopulmonary segments, while the left lung consists of two lobes and eight bronchopulmonary segments. Each bronchopulmonary segment is supplied by segmental bronchi and vasculature and contains clusters of alveoli, which are the unit where gas exchange occurs. Pneumonia, which can be bacterial, viral, or fungal, occurs when these alveoli become infected and accumulate pus.

Clinical Presentation

Although both community-acquired and nosocomial pneumonia are common, this review will focus on the specific pneumonia sequela of lung abscess. Although the emergency general surgeon is likely to encounter both community-acquired and nosocomial pneumonias in the course of surgical practice, lung abscesses may be referred for consideration of surgical resection and, therefore, the emergency general surgeon must be aware of the indications for intervention.

Diagnosis

When the history and physical examination provide clues to potential pneumonia with or without underlying pulmonary abscess, the next step in diagnosis is a complete blood count, blood cultures, chest x-ray, and a mini-bronchoalveolar lavage (mini-BAL) if the patient is intubated. If the patient is not intubated, an expectorated sputum sample is likely to be contaminated by oral flora, has low sensitivity and specificity for the true underlying pathogen, and is, therefore, low yield.

A quantitative culture of $>10^3$-10^4 colony forming units (CFUs)/cc on the mini-BAL is considered diagnostic. Although chest x-ray may demonstrate suggestive features of pulmonary abscess, such as a loculated fluid collection containing an air-fluid level (**Figure 25.1**), cross-sectional imaging is required to confirm this diagnosis. A rim-enhancing collection within the lung parenchyma in the context of infectious and/or pulmonary symptoms with a positive mini-BAL suggests the diagnosis of pulmonary abscess.

Because these abscesses can be the result of underlying bacterial, viral, or fungal infection, a thorough search for each type of infection is important. For vulnerable populations, such as homeless patients or the immunosuppressed, the mini-BAL sample should also be stained for acid fast bacilli to determine if tuberculosis is the underlying cause of infection.

If blood and mini-BAL cultures do not reveal the underlying infectious etiology, direct sampling of the pulmonary abscess may be necessary. Percutaneously, the lung abscess is aspirated and the fluid obtained is sent for culture and sensitivity. This will reveal the underlying infectious agent of the pulmonary abscess, which not only secures the diagnosis but helps guide antibiotic therapy.

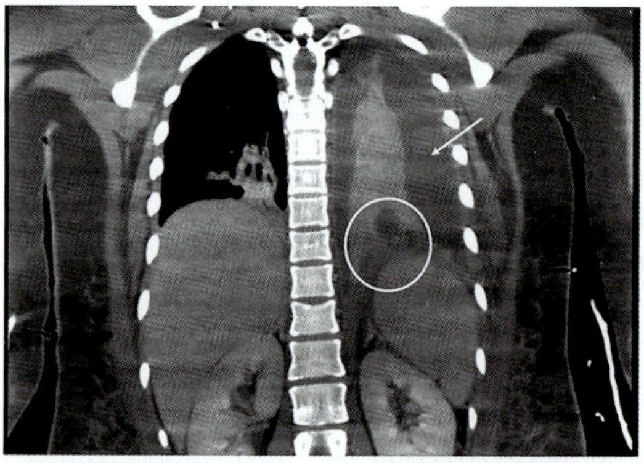

Figure 25.1 Lung abscess and empyema on CT scan of the thorax. A loculated pulmonary abscess containing air and pus is demonstrated in the left lower lobe (*circle*). An associated empyema is also visualized (*arrow*).

Treatment

The cornerstone of therapy for pulmonary abscess of any etiology is antibiotic administration. Appropriate empiric antibiotics will vary depending on local antibiograms but generally should cover streptococci and strict anaerobes if pulmonary abscess is suspected. As culture data become available, antibiotic therapy should be tailored to the appropriate offending agent. There is no clear consensus for duration of antibiotic administration to treat a pulmonary abscess, but several authors argue for prolonged antibiotic therapy, that is weeks to months of treatment, depending on symptomatic, laboratory, and radiographic evidence of improvement. In ~90% of cases of lung abscess, appropriate antibiotics alone are sufficient for complete resolution.

There are a number of established risk factors for nonresponse to antibiotic therapy alone. In these patients, percutaneous drainage or surgical resection is needed to obtain appropriate source control. Risk factors for inappropriate response to antibiotic therapy include large abscess size, slow or minimal reduction in size with antibiotic therapy, and associated bronchial obstruction with neoplasm or foreign body. In these patients who are not responding to antibiotic therapy alone, bronchoscopy and cross-sectional imaging should be obtained as the next steps, to exclude associated bronchial obstruction and to visualize the parenchymal abscess. A lung abscess that persists despite appropriate antibiotic therapy should always alert the clinician to the possibility of an underlying malignancy.

If bronchial obstruction is next identified, that should be managed accordingly as the next step. This may include bronchial stenting or, if an underlying tumor is identified, planned oncologic resection. Otherwise, when antibiotics alone have failed, the next step in therapy is percutaneous or bronchoscopic drainage. Most surgeons would only consider surgical resection if these interventions fail, although the optimal timing for operative intervention is currently unknown. Resection of a pulmonary abscess is typically accomplished via thoracoscopic nonanatomic resection. If concerns for underlying malignancy exist, a lobectomy or pneumonectomy may be the appropriate oncologic operation.

Complications

The primary concern in the treatment of a lung abscess is failure of antibiotic management. Early and adequate antibiotic therapy is critical to provide appropriate treatment from the beginning to give the patient the greatest chance at resolving the infection without requiring intervention. For some infections, such as tuberculosis, this can involve up to 26 weeks of antibiotic therapy to treat the acute infection. A parapneumonic effusion may also develop and can lead to an empyema, discussed below.

PLEURAL SPACE

Emergency general surgeons must be aware of emergent conditions involving the pleural space, including spontaneous pneumothorax or fluid accumulation of any type in the pleural space (empyema, hydrothorax, chylothorax, or nontraumatic hemothorax).

Spontaneous Pneumothorax: Principles of Management

Relevant Anatomy

The pleural space is formed between the parietal and visceral pleural in the bilateral thoracic cavities. The parietal pleura is a thin membrane that lines the inside of the chest wall and is continuous with the visceral pleura, which is closely apposed to the surface of the lung. With a spontaneous pneumothorax, air gains access to the pleural space via the lung parenchyma. When this occurs in a patient without underlying lung disease, this is termed a primary spontaneous pneumothorax and is thought to occur by way of a ruptured bleb. Although incompletely understood, a bleb is a collection of air that accumulates between the lung surface and the visceral pleura and is the result of overextension of the elastic fibers within the walls of alveoli. This overextension leads to alveolar rupture and subpleural coalescence of air spaces, forming a bleb. Blebs are most common in the apical regions of the lungs. The pathophysiology of a primary spontaneous pneumothorax is bleb rupture. Secondary spontaneous pneumothorax occurs in much the same fashion but arises in patients with underlying lung disease including chronic obstructive pulmonary disease (COPD) and cystic fibrosis.

Clinical Presentation

The accumulation of anything within the pleural space beyond the normal small amount of serous fluid will present in much the same way, with ipsilateral chest pain and/or shortness of breath. With spontaneous pneumothorax, these symptoms are typically sudden onset in nature, coinciding with bleb rupture. In a smaller spontaneous pneumothorax, the shortness of breath may be noted only with exertion. In a larger spontaneous pneumothorax, complete respiratory and circulatory collapse may occur if sufficient air accesses the pleural space to cause a tension pneumothorax, discussed further below under Complications.

Signs of pneumothorax include tachypnea, decreased or absent breath sounds over the affected hemithorax, and hypoxia. It is important to note that particularly in healthy individuals, these signs may be absent even in the presence of a large pneumothorax as patients with sufficient physiologic reserve can compensate accordingly.

Pulmonary blebs are most common in specific subsets of the population, and this information can be used by the clinician to provide epidemiologic suggestion that spontaneous pneumothorax is the etiology behind a patient's shortness of breath or respiratory distress. Male gender, tall stature, thin body types, family history, and smoking are known risk factors for blebs and primary spontaneous pneumothoraces. The history should also include full documentation of active and past medical conditions, with a specific focus on underlying pulmonary disease including those mentioned above as well as a history of lung infections including tuberculosis.

Diagnosis

In addition to a complete history and physical examination to detect the symptoms, signs, and epidemiologic and medical risk factors as discussed above, pursuing a diagnosis of spontaneous pneumothorax should begin with an upright chest x-ray. This imaging modality will detect a pneumothorax once approximately >50 mL of air have accumulated into the pleural space. In the majority of patients, an upright chest x-ray is sufficient to establish the diagnosis at the index presentation. For patients with a recurrent spontaneous pneumothorax, or those with underlying lung parenchymal disease, computed tomography (CT) scan of the chest with fine apical cuts is an important tool to identify apical blebs in primary spontaneous pneumothorax and to delineate underlying contributory lesions, such as a lung tumor or abscess, in secondary spontaneous pneumothorax.

Treatment

In the acute setting, a symptomatic spontaneous pneumothorax is generally treated with rapid insertion of a small bore chest tube or pleural drainage catheter. This allows external evacuation of the air within the pleural space and prevents progression of the pneumothorax to a tension pneumothorax. Although some guidelines recommend an attempt at needle aspiration of the pneumothorax alone as an alternative to chest drain placement, the reported failure rates of this technique are 20%-70%, rendering this an unreliable method of decompressing the pleural space. Newer literature is emerging that observation alone for a spontaneous pneumothorax may be the treatment of choice among patients who are hemodynamically stable and in no respiratory distress, even if the pneumothorax is large, as long as they can safely self-monitor symptoms after discharge and are reliable for close clinical follow-up.

Because the majority of patients with a single episode of spontaneous pneumothorax do not have a reoccurrence, surgical intervention is not recommended at the index presentation. Recurrence of a spontaneous pneumothorax is typically considered an indication for surgical intervention. Recurrence rates after a primary spontaneous pneumothorax are reported as 29% in the first year and 32% overall (Walker et al., 2018). Thus, nearly all recurrences occur in the first year after the index presentation and, therefore, patients who do not have a second episode within that year should be reassured that the likelihood of recurrence is exceedingly low thereafter.

Complications

Two important complications of spontaneous pneumothorax are development of tension pneumothorax and persistent air leak after chest drain placement. A tension pneumothorax is heralded by hemodynamic compromise as a result of a large pneumothorax. A tension pneumothorax presents with signs of obstructive shock, that is hypotension, tachycardia, and jugular venous distension. Additionally, absent breath sounds on the affected side will be noted as well as hyperresonance to percussion. Tracheal deviation away from the side of the tension pneumothorax is also a classic feature. Tension pneumothorax must be emergently decompressed with chest tube insertion to prevent cardiac arrest as a result of obstructive shock. If a tension pneumothorax is noted by prehospital providers prior to arrival in the emergency department, needle decompression may be attempted with a large-bore (14-18 gauge) angiocatheter inserted either into the second intercostal space in the midclavicular line, or, more contemporarily, into the fifth intercostal space in the anterior axillary line. A standard angiocatheter used for needle decompression is 5 cm long but has fails to reach the pleural space in 43% of patients when the second intercostal space at the midclavicular line is used as the decompression site. This failure rate is much lower (17%) when the fifth intercostal space at the anterior axillary line is used because the chest wall tends to be thinner at this point.

A persistent air leak after chest tube placement for a spontaneous pneumothorax is an indication for surgical intervention. Specifically, the intervention should consist of removal of the offending segment of lung parenchyma, which is typically resection of a bulla, followed by mechanical or chemical pleurodesis. Although the precise duration of air leak that mandates surgical intervention is not specifically defined by the current literature, surgical management is generally recommended after 5-7 days of persistent air leak in the patient with primary spontaneous pneumothorax. Similarly, in the patient with secondary spontaneous pneumothorax, postoperative complications after bullectomy and pleurodesis increase when surgical intervention is delayed beyond 5 days of air leak post chest tube insertion.

Pleural Effusions: Principles of Management

Relevant Anatomy

The pleural space contains a small amount of serous fluid in the physiologic state, which allows the lungs to expand smoothly with the chest wall during inspiration. In the pathologic state, this space can fill with an excessive amount of serous fluid, which is termed a *hydrothorax*; with pus, termed an *empyema*; with blood, termed a *hemothorax*, which can be either spontaneous or traumatic; or with lymphatic fluid, termed a *chylothorax*. These conditions together are referred to as pleural effusions.

Clinical Presentation

These patients present in much of the same way as patients with spontaneous pneumothoraces, reporting shortness of breath and/or chest discomfort. On physical examination, these patients may be tachypneic, have muffled breath sounds on auscultation and dullness to percussion over the affected hemithorax, and may have diminished oxygen saturation.

Diagnosis

The antecedent medical history is critically important to obtain as the first clue to the underlying diagnosis. Hydrothorax occurs in a number of disease states that involve abnormal regulation of fluid volumes. These include congestive heart failure (CHF), cirrhosis, and nephrotic syndrome, and therefore, a past medical history of any of these conditions is relevant. Empyemas are most commonly sequelae of bacterial pneumonia, particularly in immunosuppressed hosts such as patients with human immunodeficiency virus and malignancy. An empyema can also occur postoperatively following thoracic surgery. Spontaneous hemothorax occurs in patients taking anticoagulation, those with underlying hematologic disorders, and patients with malignancies that invade the pleural space. Lastly, a chylothorax is the result of an injured or obstructed thoracic duct. In the nontraumatic setting, this may be seen as a complication of thoracic surgery or as a result of malignancy.

Once suspicion of a pleural effusion occurs, an upright chest x-ray is the next step in securing the diagnosis. Fluid in the pleural space will present on x-ray in a variety of ways depending on the volume of fluid present. Blunting or absence of the costodiaphragmatic recess can occur with a small amount of fluid. A larger volume of fluid will result in progressive white opacification of the hemithorax with a meniscus sign (**Figure 25.2**).

The role for CT of the chest in diagnosing a pleural effusion is not well delineated. Practically speaking, an effusion that appears loculated on chest x-ray should undergo cross-sectional imaging so that an anatomic plan can be made for successful drainage. Effusions that occur in patients with underlying thoracic malignancies are likely to benefit from CT to image the underlying lesion.

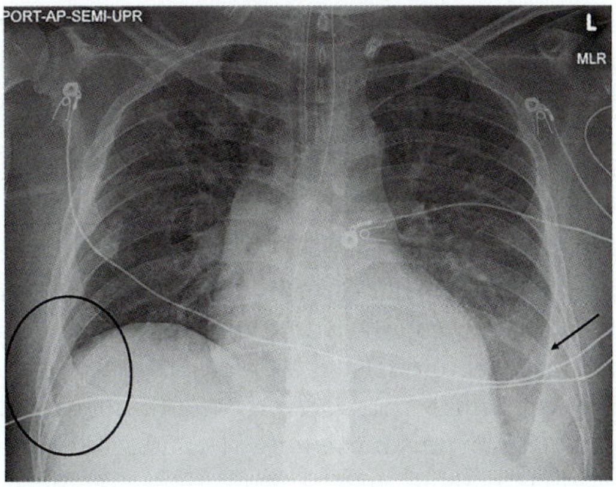

Figure 25.2 Appearance of pleural effusions on chest x-ray. A small pleural effusion appears radiographically as blunting of the costodiaphragmatic recess (*circle*). A larger pleural effusion may demonstrate a meniscus sign (*arrow*).

Chest CT scan can also be helpful in cases where the etiology is unclear.

The specific type of pleural effusion present may be suspected based on the history, physical examination, and imaging, but the diagnosis cannot be confirmed until the pleural fluid is sampled by either aspiration or chest drain placement. Much of the assessment of pleural fluid is visual. A hydrothorax is serous (thin, yellow) fluid, an empyema is purulent, a hemothorax is grossly bloody, and a chylothorax is milky. An empyema in its early stages, prior to appearing as pus, is an exudative fluid, which is indistinguishable on gross inspection from a transudative fluid as seen with a hydrothorax. For these patients, Light criteria must be established to determine diagnosis of transudative vs exudative fluid.

Determining Light criteria for a patient with pleural effusion involves sampling the patient's serum via blood draw and pleural fluid via aspiration or from the drain output. Fluids should be sampled at approximately the same time. Both fluids need to be tested for protein and lactate dehydrogenase (LDH). An exudative effusion meets at least one of the following criteria:

- The pleural fluid protein to serum total protein ratio is >0.5.
- The ratio of pleural fluid to serum LDH levels is >0.6.
- The pleural fluid LDH levels are greater than two thirds of the upper limit of normal serum LDH levels.

Although Light criteria have a sensitivity in the diagnosis of pleural exudate that approaches 100%, the specificity is closer to 75%. Put differently, if Light criteria are negative, the diagnosis of pleural exudate has been excluded. However, if Light criteria are positive for an exudative fluid, there is a chance that the fluid is truly a transudate.

Treatment

The initial treatment for most pleural effusions is pleural drainage via a small bore conventional chest tube or pigtail catheter. Some small pleural effusions, particularly hydrothoraces, can be monitored without drainage if asymptomatic. A hemothorax or empyema, however, is generally drained regardless of size, to treat infection and avoid fibrosis and underlying lung parenchymal scarring.

In terms of size selection of pleural drains, even blood from a hemothorax will drain easily via catheters as small as 14 French. Although there is no specific literature to guide the selection of an appropriately sized tube for each specific type of pleural effusion, it is clear that smaller-bore chest drains are sufficient to evacuate most fluid. Additionally, smaller chest tubes produce less patient discomfort without impeding drainage or impacting other clinical outcomes.

Removal of the chest drain should occur when the effusion has been evacuated. Most clinicians would use an upright chest x-ray showing fluid evacuation as visualized by demonstration of a clear view of the ipsilateral diaphragm, combined with decreasing daily output from the chest tube. Although there is no universally agreed upon volume of output that signals readiness for chest tube removal, most clinicians would remove a chest tube when output is <200-300 mL/daily if the upright chest x-ray is favorable. Zhang et al. reported that after lobectomy, discontinuation when output was <300 mL/24 hours resulted in shorter hospital length of stay without an increase in complications when compared to removal only when output was <100 mL/24 hours, suggesting that a more liberal threshold for chest tube discontinuation may improve patient outcomes.

Other treatment considerations apply specifically to types of pleural effusions. For example, a hydrothorax typically requires management of the underlying contributing condition in addition to pleural drainage. For patients with cirrhosis, this may involve more aggressive diuretic use or a transjugular intrahepatic portosystemic shunt (TIPS). With a spontaneous hemothorax, reversal of the contributing anticoagulant is needed as well as correction of the underlying coagulation abnormalities. In patients without anticoagulant use, a hematologic workup for underlying coagulation disorders is appropriate. For an empyema, appropriate antibiotic therapy must be paired with thorough pleural drainage. Lastly, a low output chylothorax (<1 L/day) is likely to resolve with pleural drainage, dietary modifications with a high-protein, low-fat diet that eliminates long-chain triglycerols, and adjuncts such as somatostatin. A high output chylothorax (>1 L/day) is less likely to be self-limited and early consideration of intervention such as thoracic duct embolization or surgical ligation paired with pleurodesis is prudent.

Complications

Re-expansion pulmonary edema is a concern during drainage of large-volume pleural effusions.

It appears that the risk of re-expansion pulmonary edema is likely much lower than classically described. Available data describe an incidence of <1%, even when draining large (<1 L) pleural effusions. Contemporary practice is to fully evacuate pleural effusions, even large ones, as long as the patient does not develop chest discomfort during drainage. If chest discomfort develops, the chest tube should be clamped and a chest x-ray obtained to investigate for signs of pulmonary edema. If none are present, drainage can be recommenced at a slower rate along with close clinical monitoring of the patient. If re-expansion pulmonary edema occurs, treatment is supportive and consists of administration of supplemental oxygen with or without mechanical ventilation.

Pleural effusions that reoccur or persist may necessitate chemical or mechanical pleurodesis to obliterate the pleural space and thereby prevent fluid accumulation. These procedures are typically performed thoracoscopically and the specific selection of type of pleurodesis is generally decided based on institutional and practitioner preferences as there is no clear evidence favoring one approach over another. For patients with short life expectancies or poor surgical candidates, or those with underlying medical conditions contributing to the effusion that may be optimizable, an indwelling pleural catheter may be considered instead of pleurodesis. For example, in a patient with cirrhosis who has undergone a TIPS procedure, one would not expect to see improvement in the patient's hydrothorax for several weeks post-TIPS. In these patients, temporary continued pleural drainage until the TIPS takes effect is a logical option.

MEDIASTINUM

Emergency conditions of the mediastinum of relevance to the emergency general surgeon include descending necrotizing mediastinitis and cardiac tamponade.

Descending Necrotizing Mediastinitis: Principles of Management

Relevant Anatomy

Although the majority of cases of mediastinitis occur postoperatively from cardiac surgery and, therefore, do not come to the attention of the emergency general surgeon, the anatomy of the upper mediastinum places it at risk for infection as a result of necrotizing soft tissue infections (NSTIs) originating in the oropharynx or from the teeth. Termed descending necrotizing mediastinitis, it is an important infection for general surgeons to be aware of as they may be called for emergent debridement of necrotic tissue, which can be lifesaving.

The mediastinum, spanning the area posterior to the sternum, anterior to the vertebral column, and bordered laterally the pleurae, contains the heart, great vessels, intrathoracic trachea, intrathoracic esophagus, thymic remnant, and the phrenic and vagus nerves bilaterally. Because the majority of these structures communicate freely with their cervical counterparts, oropharyngeal and odontogenic infections easily spread down the neck along tissue planes into the mediastinum.

Clinical Presentation

With oral cavity or cervical origin of these infections, patients typically present with pain in those regions accompanied by infectious symptoms, such as fever, and may have associated dysphagia or odynophagia. Infectious spread into the mediastinum can be associated with local thoracic symptoms including chest pain. However, due to the severe nature of infection in descending necrotizing mediastinitis, these patients are often so sick that they present to hospital obtunded. Because of the deep nature of these infections, there may be no cutaneous manifestation, although commonly the soft tissues of the neck and chest wall will be edematous and woody. Nonspecific infectious symptoms are the most common initial presentation.

The most reliable sign of descending necrotizing mediastinitis is septic shock. Hypotension, tachycardia, fever, evidence of end organ hypoperfusion, and positive blood cultures should be expected. A high index of suspicion for this specific infection should be maintained, because although it is rare, it is highly lethal. A recent history of dental or oropharyngeal procedures for infection may suggest descending necrotizing mediastinitis as the cause of sepsis.

Diagnosis

Blood cultures should be sent expeditiously and computed tomography (CT) scans of the head, neck, and chest rapidly obtained. These cross-sectional images are required to delineate the extent and spread of the infection through multiple body cavities (**Figure 25.3A and B**). As with any NSTI, the necrotizing nature of this infection is a clinical diagnosis that can merely be suggested

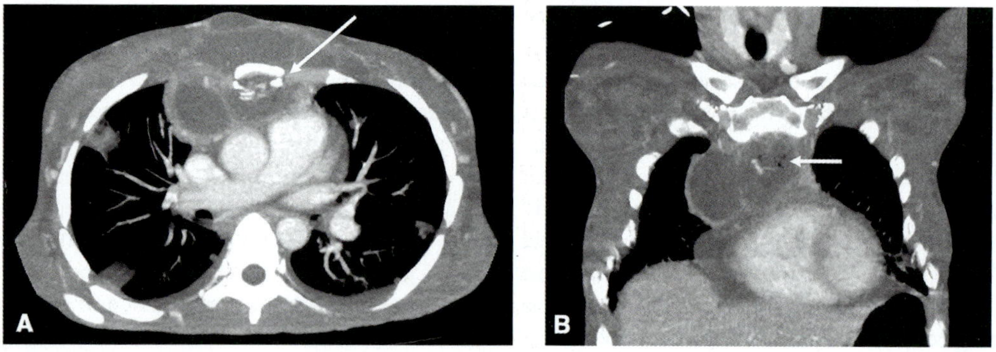

Figure 25.3 CT scan findings in descending necrotizing mediastinitis. **A.** Multiloculated abscess is seen surrounding the sternum, which demonstrates evidence of osteomyelitis (*arrow*). **B.** Multiloculated abscess in neck and upper mediastinum demonstrates air within the abscess (*arrow*), which is suggestive of necrotizing infection.

on imaging. CT findings may include soft tissue edema or emphysema, abscesses, lack of fascial enhancement, and/or osteomyelitis. A diagnosis of NSTI is suggested in a patient with infection with pain out of proportion on palpation of the affected areas or hemodynamic compromise. However, the diagnosis of NSTI is made in the operating room and on pathologic tissue examination.

Treatment

The surgical principles of descending necrotizing mediastinitis are identical to the NSTI debridement principles in any body region: immediate debridement of all devitalized tissue and wide drainage. Thorough operative intervention must be emergently pursued as mortality increases when debridement is delayed. Exploration must be broad to ensure no foci of infection are missed. In descending necrotizing mediastinitis, cervical or oropharyngeal debridement is likely to be required in additional to mediastinal debridement. Often, simply performing a sternotomy helps with infection control in these patients as this can be considered akin to unroofing an abscess, if the mediastinum itself is conceptualized as the abscess cavity. In severe cases, resection of the sternum and adjacent chest wall musculature and ribs may be required to remove all infection (**Figure 25.4**). Skin should be preserved if it is not involved to minimize wound morbidity if the patient survives.

Arrange planned return to the operating room within 24 hours for further debridement of any tissue that has declared itself as involved over the intervening hours. If the patient deteriorates prior to the planned re-exploration, the patient should be returned to the operating room immediately.

Although prompt removal of all infected tissue is the cornerstone of management, it is also critical that broad-spectrum antibiotics be administered immediately once the diagnosis is suspected. These empiric antibiotics should provide coverage of gram-positive and -negative organisms in addition to anaerobes, and specifically should include coverage for methicillin-resistant *S aureus*. Piperacillin/tazobactam with vancomycin would be one antibiotic regimen option. Additionally, the antibiotic regimen should include coverage for streptococcal and staphylococcal endotoxins, which is typically achieved with clindamycin administration. In addition to antibiotic therapy and prompt, complete surgical debridement, intravenous immune globulin (IVIG) is another therapeutic option. Among patients with NSTIs caused by group A *Streptococcus*, IVIG administration

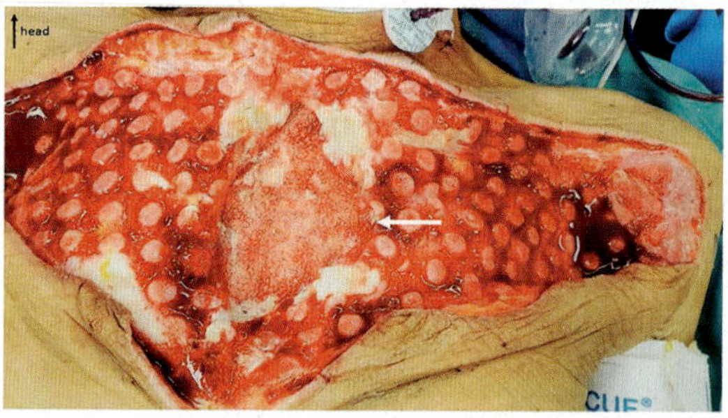

Figure 25.4 Intraoperative findings in descending necrotizing mediastinitis. Extensive mediastinal debridement was required to control the spread of infection in this patient with descending necrotizing mediastinitis. Resection of the sternum was required, leaving the pericardium exposed (*arrow*). Negative pressure wound therapy has been used on this patient and granulation tissue is seen to be accumulating.

reduces mortality. In practice, we consider the use of IVIG among patients with streptococcal NSTIs who remain in septic shock despite antibiotics and debridement, that is, those with severe NSTIs caused by group A *Streptococcus*.

If the patient survives the acute phase of infection, large soft tissue defects are frequently left. These patients require careful and deliberate wound care to preserve functionality and improve cosmesis of the affected body regions. Negative pressure wound therapy, particularly with instillation of antibacterial solution, can be extremely useful to expedite wound healing, encourage granulation tissue deposition, and to minimize soft tissue defects requiring skin grafting for coverage.

Complications

Because mortality is so high after descending necrotizing mediastinitis, there is limited literature on postoperative complications among patients who survive the index operations. From the available case reports and small case series, recurrent infection is common and should be anticipated. One study of three patients reported 100% developed postoperative abscesses requiring surgical or percutaneous drainage and 67% required tracheostomy placement for prolonged respiratory failure requiring mechanical ventilation.

Cardiac Tamponade: Principles of Management

Relevant Anatomy

The human heart is enclosed by bilayered connective tissue, similar to the lung with its two layers of pleurae. Surrounding the heart, intimately related to its surface, is the serous pericardium. The outer layer of connective tissue is the fibrous pericardium, which is a thickened and relatively inelastic layer. Under normal conditions, the space between these two layers of pericardium is filled with 15-35 mL of serous fluid. This provides lubrication that allows the heart to expand and contract to deliver cardiac output.

When the volume of fluid within the pericardial space increases, whether due to increased production of serous fluid as seen in acute pericarditis, certain malignancies, or autoimmune disorders, or due to accumulation of blood after trauma, the increased fluid in the pericardial space can be well or poorly tolerated. The pathophysiologic reaction to this increased fluid generally depends upon the speed with which it accumulates. Nontraumatic pericardial effusions are rarely brought to the attention of the emergency general surgeon as these tend to accumulate slowly over time, allowing the heart time to adapt to the increase in fluid volume and avoiding development of cardiac tamponade.

Clinical Presentation

As described above, nontraumatic cardiac tamponade is extremely rare. Because simple intervention with pericardiocentesis can be lifesaving, it is a condition and intervention that the emergency general surgeon should understand. Because nontraumatic pericardial effusions are chronic, ascertaining the antecedent history can be extremely useful. A history of any condition known to cause pericardial effusion in a patient with hemodynamic compromise should raise suspicion for nontraumatic cardiac tamponade. These conditions can be considered to be infectious and noninfectious in nature.

Infectious causes of nontraumatic pericardial tamponade include bacterial (eg, tuberculosis) and viral (eg, HIV) infection. Noninfectious causes include inflammatory disorders such as systemic lupus erythematosus, uremia, malignancy, and conditions related to cardiac and aortic pathology such as myocardial rupture following myocardial infarction or retrograde propagation of a type A aortic dissection.

In addition to clues provided on medical history, patients may also provide a history of exercise intolerance, in which the pericardial effusion was asymptomatic at rest but with exertion, the patient was unable to increase their cardiac output accordingly as a result of the extrinsic compression by the pericardial effusion.

The patient's physical examination is consistent with cardiac tamponade, with Beck triad eponymously describing the three classic findings: hypotension, jugular venous distension, and muffled heart sounds.

Diagnosis

With a suggestive history and physical examination, the next step is bedside echocardiography (**Figure 25.5**). This is an essential test, which can confirm the diagnosis within seconds with a sensitivity and specificity which approach 100%. Subxiphoid or parasternal views will demonstrate a pericardial effusion, which will be large and difficult to miss in nontraumatic cardiac tamponade. Because nontraumatic pericardial effusions develop gradually and are, therefore, well tolerated

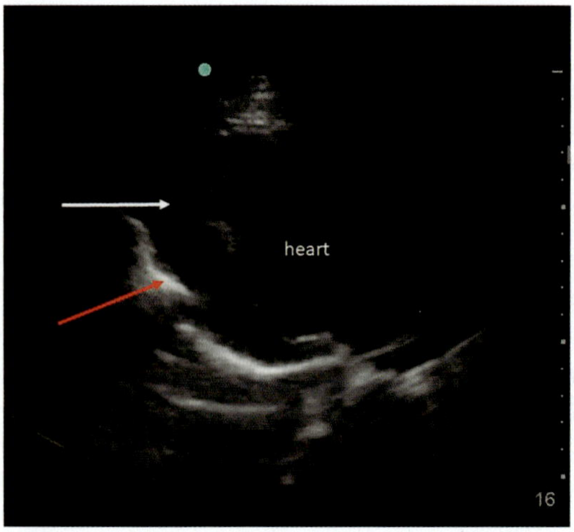

Figure 25.5 Bedside echocardiography of a patient with a large pericardial effusion and cardiac tamponade. Between the pericardium (*red arrow*) and the heart, a large pericardial effusion (*white arrow*) is visualized.

until >1 L in volume, they are apparent on bedside cardiac ultrasound. In addition to demonstration of a pericardial effusion, echocardiography findings specific to cardiac tamponade include cardiac chamber collapse. This occurs when the pericardial pressure exceeds the chamber pressure, which prohibits filling. Because the filling pressures are lower on the right side of the heart, particularly in the right atrium, this chamber will demonstrate collapse earliest. Next, the interventricular septum will be seen to bulge into the left ventricle on inspiration and into the right ventricle on expiration, demonstration of increased filling pressures within these chambers as a result of increased extrinsic compression. Ultimately, due to increasing degree of extrinsic compression, the filling pressures rise dramatically and then equalize between the four chambers, producing profound obstructive shock and then cardiac arrest without intervention.

Treatment

In nontraumatic cardiac tamponade, pericardiocentesis is often sufficient in the acute setting to relieve the cardiac tamponade. Subsequent interventions can be targeted toward medical optimization of the underlying condition contributing to the increase in pericardial fluid. To perform a pericardiocentesis, utilize a 18-gauge spinal needle and a syringe. After sterilizing the skin surrounding the xiphoid process, insert the needle through the skin immediately to the left of the xiphoid process and direct toward the left shoulder. Maintain negative pressure on the syringe throughout. Aspiration of air suggests pleural entry or penetration of lung parenchyma, both of which are unintended outcomes. A flash of fluid heralds entry into the pericardial effusion. This fluid should slowly be withdrawn until no additional fluid can be removed. In the setting of a nontraumatic pericardial effusion, a flash of blood suggests entry into a cardiac chamber. If this occurs, the needle should be withdrawn and repositioned. Pericardiocentesis under ultrasound guidance can assist in introducing the needle into the correct anatomic space.

Complications

The most important complication after evacuation of a pericardial effusion causing nontraumatic cardiac tamponade is reaccumulation of the fluid and tamponade reoccurrence. Placement of a pericardial drain allowing continued drainage will prevent this complication while medical optimization of the underlying contributing condition is pursued.

DIAPHRAGM

Although the diaphragm in and of itself is not a source of general surgical emergencies, abdominal viscera can become incarcerated and strangulated within a diaphragmatic hernia. Therefore, the emergency general surgeon must, therefore, be familiar with management principles of hiatal hernias.

Hiatal Hernias: Principles of Management

Relevant Anatomy

The diaphragm is a muscle that separates the thoracic and abdominal cavities. It functions primarily as a respiratory muscle, contributing to lung expansion on inspiration and chest wall recoil on expiration. The diaphragm also allows transient increases in intra-abdominal pressure, a function which is relevant for actions such as vomiting, defecating, and childbirth.

The diaphragm contains apertures to allow for the passage of the inferior vena cava, aorta, and esophagus. Of particular relevance to hiatal hernias is the esophageal hiatus. It is formed by the right crus, which is one of two crura that are tendinous attachments of the diaphragm to the vertebral column. Normally, the esophageal hiatus contains only the esophagus and paired vagus nerves. Herniation of abdominal contents through the esophageal hiatus is termed a hiatal hernia, of which there are four types.

A type I hiatal hernia accounts for the vast majority of hiatal hernias and is also referred to as a sliding hiatal hernia. In a type I hiatal hernia, the gastroesophageal (GE) junction is displaced superiorly from the abdomen, through the esophageal hiatus, and into the mediastinum. There are no additional structures herniated through the hiatus in a type I hernia; the GE junction is simply displaced from its normal anatomic confines in the abdomen.

Types II, III, and IV hiatal hernias are defined by a component of a true paraesophageal hernia, that is, the herniation of abdominal viscera alongside the esophagus via the esophageal hiatus and into the mediastinum. Type II has a normally positioned GE junction with partial herniation of the stomach, typically beginning with the gastric fundus, through the esophageal hiatus. Type III can be considered a combination of type I and type II, with herniation of both the GE junction and the gastric fundus through the esophageal hiatus. Lastly, a type IV hiatal hernia is defined by herniation of any abdominal viscera through the esophageal hiatus other than the stomach. The most common structure involved in a type IV hernia is the colon.

As paraesophageal hernias enlarge over time, gastric volvulus into the hernia can occur. Gastric volvulus involves rotation of the stomach along one of its axes, resulting in organoaxial or mesenteroaxial gastric volvulus. The axial rotation along with incarceration within the hiatal hernia can both result in vascular compromise and gastric ischemia.

Clinical Presentation

Hiatal hernias are frequently asymptomatic. When symptoms exist, however, they typically include symptoms of GE reflux disease, such as dysphagia and pyrosis; epigastric pain or discomfort; and early satiety. However, symptomatic hiatal hernias do not necessitate emergent intervention unless concern exists for hollow viscus ischemia. These patients may present with an antecedent history consistent with hiatal hernia, such as the symptoms described above. Patients with compromised viscera within the hernia will describe new or increased symptomatology, such as worsened epigastric or chest pain, progressively worsened dysphagia or odynophagia, and often describe complete PO intolerance. Large hiatal hernias can also produce signs of obstructive shock, as herniated contents can cause mediastinal compression and extrinsic limitation of cardiac filling and emptying, analogous to what is observed with pericardial effusions and cardiac tamponade. If herniated contents are necrotic, patients will also present with signs and symptoms of sepsis and/or septic shock, including fever, tachycardia, hypotension, and signs of organ failure.

Diagnosis

In the acute setting, diagnosis of a hiatal hernia begins with a chest x-ray. An air-fluid level within the mediastinum is consistent with a paraesophageal hernia, although the chest x-ray is unlikely to demonstrate signs of ischemia, such as pneumatosis. The chest x-ray may also be relatively normal, as a hiatal hernia may be obscured on plain radiographs by the cardiac silhouette. A high index of suspicion for a hiatal hernia should exist for patients presenting with an appropriate history and CT scan of the chest and abdomen should be the next step in diagnostic evaluation, even in the presence of a normal chest x-ray. IV contrast should be administered to allow assessment for ischemia. PO contrast is inadvisable because of the risk for aspiration. Although upper endoscopy plays a major role in patients with chronic hiatal hernias without visceral compromise, it has a relatively limited role in the diagnosis of hiatal hernias in the emergency settings.

Treatment

If a hiatal hernia is diagnosed with concern for compromise of the incarcerated contents, the general treatment principles are surgical exploration, reduction of the herniated contents back into the abdominal cavity, resection of nonviable tissue, and hernia repair. In the case of gastric volvulus, most surgeons would perform some type of gastropexy (eg, fundoplication or gastrostomy tube insertion) to help prevent recurrence.

Surgical exploration may proceed open or laparoscopically. Regardless, exposure of the upper abdomen and particularly of the esophageal hiatus is critical. Gentle, downward retraction of herniated contents allows reduction and inspection for tissue compromise. If restoration of gastrointestinal tract continuity is required as a result of necrotic tissue resection extent, this should occur next. Following this, hernia repair ideally involves resection of the hernia sac, although this is not absolutely necessary. Depending on the size of the hernia sac and physiologic condition of the patient, dissection of the sac from the mediastinum via the esophageal hiatus can be challenging and provides a risk of bleeding. If an expedient operation cannot be accomplished by removing the hernia sac, it may be left *in situ*. Emergent hernia repair is typically accomplished primarily, that is, without the use of mesh, and with a cruroplasty to narrow the aperture of the esophageal hiatus and thereby mitigate the risk of herniation.

Complications

The feared complications of hiatal hernias are strangulation of the hernia contents as well as gastric volvulus, both of which are discussed above. In the absence of these complications, hiatal hernias do not usually come to the attention of the emergency general surgeon. Although bleeding or ulceration are other complications of hiatal hernias that surgeons should be aware of, these are typically managed endoscopically.

SUMMARY

General surgeons often encounter thoracic emergencies in their practices outside of the setting of trauma. Being prepared to handle nontrauma emergencies such as tracheoinnominate fistulae (TIF), pulmonary infection, spontaneous pneumothorax, effusions, mediastinitis, cardiac tamponade, and hiatal hernia is critical for patient care, especially in settings without a thoracic surgeon. The definitive care of these emergencies may fall outside of a general surgeon's daily practice, but understanding the diagnosis and treatment allows a lifesaving intervention to facilitate the patient moving to a higher level of care. The chapter offers a guide to the principles of management for the various thoracic emergencies a general surgeon may be asked to see.

SUGGESTED READINGS

Ando K, Okhuni Y, Matsunuma R, et al. Prognostic lung abscess factors. *Kansenshogaku Zasshi.* 2010;84(4):425-430.

Bauman ZM, Kulvatunyou N, Joseph B, et al. A prospective study of 7-year experience using percutaneous 14-French pigtail catheters for traumatic hemothorax/hemopneumothorax at a level-1 trauma center: size still does not matter. *World J Surg.* 2018;42(1):107-113.

Bradley PJ. Bleeding around a tracheostomy wound: what to consider and what to do? *J Laryngol Otol.* 2009;123:952-956.

Brown SGA, Ball EL, Perrin K, et al.; The PSP Investigators. Conservative versus interventional treatment for spontaneous pneumothorax. *N Engl J Med.* 2020;382:405-415.

Bruun T, Rath E, Bruun Madsen M, et al.; INFECT Study Group. Risk factors and predictors of mortality in streptococcal necrotizing soft-tissue infections: a multicenter prospective study. *Clin Infect Dis.* 2021;72:293-300.

Carr JJ, Reed JC, Choplin RH, Pope TL Jr, Case LD. Plain and computed radiography for detecting experimentally induced pneumothorax in cadavers: implications for detection in patients. *Radiology.* 1992;183(1):193-199.

Donaldson L, Raper R. Successful emergency management of a bleeding tracheoinnominate fistula. *BMJ Case Rep.* 2019;12(12):e232257.

Feller-Kopman D, Berkowitz D, Boiselle P, Ernst A. Large-volume thoracentesis and the risk of reexpansion pulmonary edema. *Ann Thorac Surg.* 2007;84(5):1656-1661.

Garcia-Vazquez E, Marcos MA, Mensa J, et al. Assessment of the usefulness of sputum culture for diagnosis of community-acquired pneumonia using the PORT predictive scoring system. *Arch Intern Med.* 2004;164:1807-1811.

Gelbard RB, Ferrada P, Yeh DD, et al. Optimal timing of initial debridement for necrotizing soft tissue infection: a practice management guideline from the Eastern Association for the Surgery of Trauma. *J Trauma Acute Care Surg.* 2018;85(1):208-214.

Hirschtick RE, Glassroth J, Jordan MC, et al. Bacterial pneumonia in persons infected with the human immunodeficiency virus: pulmonary complications of HIV Infection Study Group. *N Engl J Med.* 1995;333(13):845-851.

Inaba K, Ives C, McClure K, et al. Radiologic evaluation of alternative sites for needle decompression of tension pneumothorax. *Arch Surg.* 2012;147(9):813-818.

Inaba K, Karamanos E, Skiada D, et al. Cadaveric comparison of the optimal site for needle decompression of tension pneumothorax by prehospital care providers. *J Trauma Acute Care Surg.* 2015;79(6):1044-1048.

Jeon HW, Kim YD, Choi SY, Park JK. When is the optimal timing of the surgical treatment for secondary spontaneous pneumothorax? *Thorac Cardiovasc Surg.* 2017;65(1):50-55.

Jones JW, Reynolds M, Hewitt RL, Drapanas T. Tracheo-innominate artery erosion: successful surgical management of a devastating complication. *Ann Surg.* 1976;184:194-204.

Light RW, Macgregor MI, Luchsinger PC, Ball WC. Pleural effusions: the diagnostic separation of transudates and exudates. *Ann Int Med.* 1972;77:507-513.

MacDuff A, Arnold A, Harvey J; BTS Pleural Disease Guideline Group. Management of spontaneous pneumothorax: British thoracic society pleural disease guideline 2010. *Thorax.* 2010;65(Suppl 2):18-31.

Nahid P, Dorman SE, Alipanah N, et al. Executive summary: official American Thoracic Society/Centers for Disease Control and Prevention/Infectious Diseases Society of America Clinical Practice Guidelines:

treatment of drug-susceptible tuberculosis. *Clin Infect Dis.* 2016;63(7):853-867.

Noppen M. Spontaneous pneumothorax: epidemiology, pathophysiology, and cause. *Eur Respir Rev.* 2010;19(117):217-219.

Papazian L, Thomas P, Garbe L, et al. Bronchoscopic or blind sampling techniques for the diagnosis of ventilator-associated pneumonia. *Am J Respir Crit Care Med.* 1995;152(6):1982-1991.

Porcel JM. Identifying transudates misclassified by light's criteria. *Curr Opin Pulm Med.* 2013;19(4):362-367.

Rahman NM, Maskell NA, Davies CWH, et al. The relationship between chest tube size and clinical outcome in pleural infection. *Chest.* 2010;137(3):536-543.

Schweigert M, Solymosi N, Dubecz A, et al. Predictors of outcome in modern surgery for lung abscess. *Thorac Cardiovasc Surg.* 2017;65(7):535-541.

Shamji FM, Deslauriers J, Nelems B. Recognition and management of life-threatening tracheovascular fistulae and how to prevent them. *Thorac Surg Clin.* 2018;28(3):403-413.

Singhal P, Kejriwal N, Lin Z, Tsutsui R, Ullal R. Optimal surgical management of descending necrotising mediastinitis: our experience and review of literature. *Heart Lung Circ.* 2008;17:124-128.

Vogiatzidis K, Zarogiannis SG, Aidonidis I, et al. Physiology of pericardial fluid production and drainage. *Front Physiol.* 2015;6:62-68.

Wali SO, Shugaeri A, Samman YS, Abdelaziz M. Percutaneous drainage of pyogenic lung abscess. *Scand J Infect Dis.* 2002;34(9):673-679.

Walker SP, Bibby AC, Halford P, Stadon L, White P, Maskell NA. Recurrence rates in primary spontaneous pneumothorax: a systematic review and meta-analysis. *Eur Respir J.* 2018;52(3):1800864.

Wang XL, Xu ZG, Tang PZ, Yu Y. Tracheo-innominate artery fistula: diagnosis and surgical\management. *Head Neck.* 2013;35:1713-1718.

Wong A, Galiabovitch E, Bhagwat K. Management of primary spontaneous pneumothorax: a review. *ANZ J Surg.* 2019;89:303-308.

Zhang Y, Li H, Hu B, et al. A prospective randomized single-blind control study of volume threshold for chest tube removal following lobectomy. *World J Surg.* 2014;38(1):60-67.

CHAPTER

26 Esophageal Emergencies

David T. Efron, Matthew Benns, and Lucy Zumwinkle Kornblith

CASE PRESENTATION

Sixty-four-year-old woman s/p multiple gunshot wounds to the face and abdomen. She underwent emergent exploratory laparotomy with right hemicolectomy, small bowel resection, ileostomy, mandible ORIF, and tracheostomy. This was complicated by anastomotic leak, multiple returns to the operating room, and prolonged ventilatory support. Progressive loss of volume resulted in over inflation of the tracheostomy balloon. On hospital day 35, the patient demonstrated sudden onset of massive subcutaneous emphysema. Computed tomography (CT) scan of the neck suggested loss of the tissue plane between the trachea and esophagus (**Figure 26.1**).

Diagnostic bronchoscopy demonstrated normal tissue but proximal bronchoscopy above the tracheostomy revealed visualization of the nasogastric tube through a posterior erosion confirming a fistula.

Question: *What is the optimal operative approach? What is the optimal repair?*

Answer: *Given the inferior cervical location of the fistula and the previous tracheostomy, a cervical collar incision was chosen. Dissection along the right tracheoesophageal groove revealed a 3 cm long by 1.25 cm wide erosion posteriorly spanning the first through third rings (**Figure 26.2**). Once dissected clear, the esophageal rent was closed longitudinally in two layers with an inner layer assuring meticulous mucosal apposition of running 3-0 PDS and an outer layer of interrupted 3-0 silk sutures. The sternocleidomastoid and strap muscles were ruled out as eligible flaps to buttress; therefore, a left pectoralis muscle flap was rotated to serve as a buttress to the esophageal repair and reconstruct the posterior wall of the trachea.*

ESOPHAGEAL ANATOMY

The esophagus is the conduit from the pharynx to the stomach positioned in the posterior mediastinum coursing anterior and parallel to the descending aorta. Its luminal surface is lined primarily by squamous epithelium, which generally transitions at the gastroesophageal junction to mucosal epithelium. It is generally 25 cm in length and is anatomically defined by the cricopharyngeal muscle proximally and the cardia of the stomach distally. Usually, the distal 2-3 cm of the esophagus is below the diaphragm. The esophagus is a muscular tube comprised of both striated muscle (more proximally) and smooth muscle (more distally); the esophagus is devoid of serosa.

The arterial blood supply to the cervical esophagus is from the inferior thyroid artery. The intrathoracic esophagus receives blood from branches of the bronchial arteries as well as direct branches from the thoracic aorta. The intra-abdominal esophagus is supplied by the left gastric artery.

Operative Approaches

Cervical Esophagus

The cervical esophagus is approached through the left neck. An incision along the anterior border of the sternocleidomastoid muscle is carried deep to the platysma. The sternocleidomastoid muscle body is retracted laterally exposing the omohyoid, which is then divided. The vascular bundle is then retracted laterally allowing access to the trachea anteriorly, the cervical vertebral bodies posteriorly, and the esophagus between. The esophagus can then be encircled; it is often safer and easier to begin this dissection along the prevertebral fascia. This allows full identification and repair of the esophageal injury. Alternatively, distal circumferential freeing of the esophagus allows lateral or end esophagostomy to enable diversion of oral secretions.

If both sides of the neck need to be explored, a cervical collar incision is used. This allows more complete access, for example, in the case of transcervical

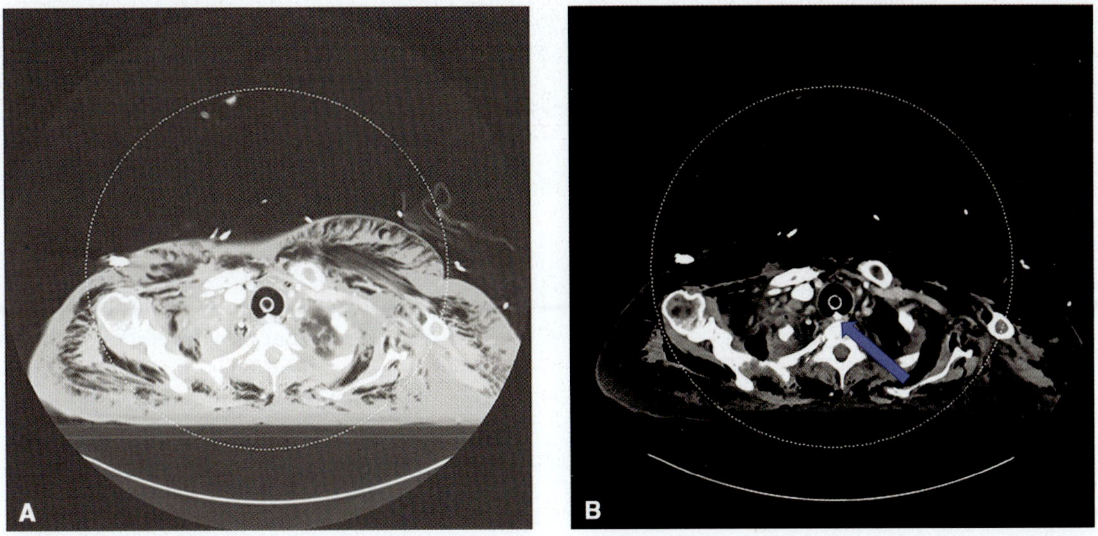

Figure 26.1 **A.** Massive subcutaneous emphysema. **B.** Loss of tissue plane between the posterior trachea and esophagus with NG tube in place (*blue arrow*).

gunshot wounds. On occasion, the addition of an upper sternal split can afford a few additional centimeters access distally on the esophagus.

Thoracic and Intra-abdominal Esophagus

The proximal thoracic esophagus is approached via a right posterolateral thoracotomy through the 4th or 5th intercostal space. Access to the lower thoracic esophagus is gained via a left posterolateral thoracotomy facilitated via the 7th or 8th intercostal space. For injuries at the diaphragm, the intra-abdominal esophagus can be accessed via radial incision of the diaphragm. Thorough inspection of the injury often includes lengthening the myotomy in a longitudinal orientation to assure identification of the mucosal rent. Repair of the esophagus entails meticulous mucosal apposition of the mucosa over a bougie (42-48 French) with primary repair ideally in two layers with an inner layer of absorbable material and the outer layer of 3-0 silk. The nasogastric be should be guided past the repair ensuring no disruption.

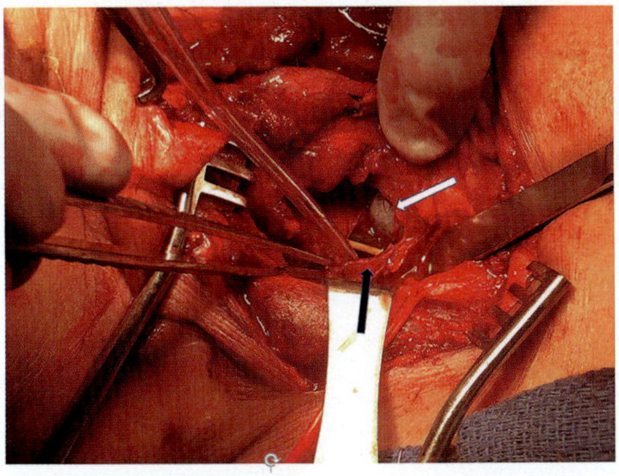

Figure 26.2 Tracheoesophageal fistula. *Black arrow* lateral wall of the esophagus with nasogastric tube visible; *white arrow*: posterior tracheal wall with endotracheal tube balloon visible.

Additional buttress with a vascularized tissue pedicle is usually indicated. In the cervical esophagus, this can consist of strap muscles, sternocleidomastoid, or even pectoral muscles. For buttress of thoracic esophageal repairs, a number of options exist. For the upper esophagus, a pedicle of intercostal muscle is often preferred, although other options include pericardial fat, pleural tissue, and even a latissimus dorsi flap. For very distal esophageal repairs, a flap of diaphragm may also be used to buttress the repair. When identified via laparotomy, esophageal repair at the gastroesophageal junction may be reinforced by partial or circumferential wrap of the gastric cardia or a pedicle of omentum. Wide drainage is important, especially for repair of the thoracic and mediastinal segments; closed suction drains are preferred. Occasionally, the injury is so destructive, or the patient physiology is so compromised as to preclude optimal primary repair or definitive resection. Placement of drains into the esophageal lumen as well as outside of the injured esophageal segment to create a controlled fistula may be warranted. Proximal diversion by means of a cervical esophagostomy may also be considered. The cervical esophagus is circumferentially mobilized to the thoracic inlet, divided (with a stapler), and the proximal end is brought to the subcutaneous tissue as an end stoma. A laparotomy is then performed for placement of a decompressive gastrostomy, with a distal enteric limb or separate jejunostomy tube for enteric feeding. The gastroesophageal junction may also be excluded to provide maximal protection from reflux into the esophagus.

ESOPHAGEAL PERFORATION

Esophageal perforation can occur in any location and encompasses a wide range of etiologies. The condition is relatively rare, occurring with a frequency of ~3 in 100 000 in the United States. The intrathoracic esophagus is the most common location (>50%), followed by the cervical esophagus and intra-abdominal locations. The majority of esophageal perforations are iatrogenic and can occur during a variety of diagnostic or therapeutic procedures. Esophageal endoscopy is the most common associated procedure. The risk of perforation is extremely low for strictly diagnostic procedures but is increased for therapeutic interventions. **Table 26.1** lists the common causes of iatrogenic perforation during esophageal endoscopy and their approximate risk. Other iatrogenic causes include surgery, transesophageal echocardiography, intubation, nasogastric tube insertion, bronchial artery embolization, and radiotherapy. Noniatrogenic causes of esophageal perforation include spontaneous rupture (Boerhaave syndrome), trauma, food/foreign body impaction, and neoplasia.

TABLE 26.1 ■ Common Esophageal Endoscopic Procedures and Approximate Risk of Perforation

Flexible esophagoscopy (diagnostic)	0.03%
Rigid esophagoscopy (diagnostic)	0.11%
Coagulation or photodynamic therapy	2%
Stent placement	2%
Dilation (stricture or achalasia)	0.09%-14%
Laser therapy of esophageal cancer	7%
Variceal sclerotherapy	0.5%-5%
Endoscopic mucosal resection	3%
Endoscopic submucosal dissection	6%

The diagnosis of esophageal perforation first requires a high index of suspicion based on recent history. Presenting symptoms vary depending on the location of the perforation and timing, but general signs of systemic sepsis may be seen. Atypical symptoms and delay in diagnosis are common. Radiographic studies for suspected esophageal perforation include plain imaging, computed tomography (CT), and contrast esophagography. CT imaging (with PO contrast) has the highest sensitivity and negative predictive value of any single study. CT findings of esophageal perforation may include extraluminal contrast or air, peri-esophageal fluid collection, or esophageal thickening. Contrast esophagography showing contrast extravasation at the site of injury is also confirmatory. Water-soluble contrast agents are generally preferred for suspected esophageal perforation, as barium carries a risk of tissue inflammatory reaction with extravasation. Barium mediastinitis can be particularly problematic, and even fatal. Barium studies are superior in terms of accuracy and specificity of diagnosis, however. Direct visualization of perforations with esophageal endoscopy is another option but is less common due to concerns that further dissection of the perforation may occur with direct instrumentation or air insufflation of the esophagus.

Esophageal perforation is a true emergency that requires emergent intervention. Even with prompt care, mortality can be >30%. **Table 26.2** lists the common interventions that should be performed for all patients with suspected or confirmed esophageal perforation.

Further management of esophageal perforation depends on patient-specific factors and physiology, but general options include the following:

TABLE 26.2 ■ General Interventions for Suspected or Confirmed Esophageal Perforation

Hospital admission (ICU if unstable or high-risk patient)	Volume resuscitation
NPO	IV broad-spectrum antibiotics and antifungals
Hemodynamic monitoring	IV proton pump inhibitors
Nutrition: TPN or tube feeds (if distal to perforation)	Assessment for invasive management

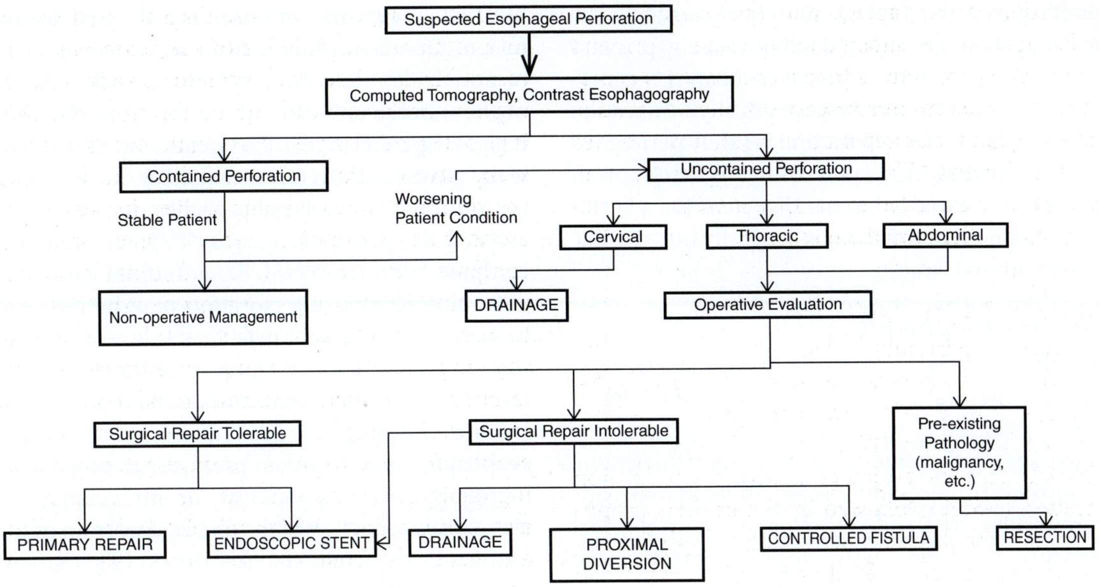

Figure 26.3 Algorithm for the evaluation and management of a suspected esophageal perforation.

nonoperative management, drainage, endoscopic management (closure, stenting, etc…), primary repair with vascularized flap coverage, resection, and diversion. Additionally, consideration of surgical or endoscopic enteral access should be given to all patients with esophageal perforation, as they may be unable to safely eat by mouth for prolonged periods of time. Specific interventions are most frequently guided by the location of the perforation along the esophagus. An algorithm for the evaluation and management of a suspected esophageal perforation is in **Figure 26.3**.

Cervical Esophagus

Disruptions of the cervical esophagus account for ~¼ of all esophageal perforations. Etiologies are predominantly iatrogenic as discussed. Surgical procedures in the neck, particularly anterior cervical spinal instrumentation, are other common etiologies. Traumatic neck injuries may also involve the cervical esophagus, with penetrating injuries significantly more common than blunt mechanisms.

Common symptoms of cervical esophageal perforation include neck pain, dysphagia, odynophagia, and dysphonia. Patients may also have palpable crepitus in the neck or report bloody regurgitation. The attachment of the cervical esophagus to the prevertebral fascia limits the spread of contamination, thus cervical perforations generally result in less severe manifestations of systemic sepsis.

Plain radiographs of the neck with cervical esophageal disruption may demonstrate subcutaneous emphysema, anterior displacement of the trachea, or prevertebral gas. CT scan with oral contrast is frequently confirmatory. Contrast esophagography may also be utilized for confirmation and can be particularly helpful in cases where CT findings are nonspecific. Water-soluble contrast is again most frequently used, but it should be noted that barium studies are more frequently employed in the cervical area to demonstrate perforations due to the rapid transit of liquid materials in the upper esophagus.

Perforations of the cervical esophagus are generally the most favorable, as they are more frequently contained than thoracic or intra-abdominal perforations. Stable patients with small and contained perforations can often be treated nonoperatively with the medical interventions outlined in **Table 26.2**. Contrast esophagography or CT imaging is then repeated prior to reinitiation of oral intake to ensure healing, usually after a minimum of 5-7 days. Patients with more significant perforations of the cervical esophagus are frequently treated with drainage procedures. This can be accomplished operatively or through percutaneous methods. The majority of cervical esophageal perforations will heal without further intervention, if drainage is adequate. Operative debridement and primary closure can also be undertaken but can be difficult to expose perforations of the very proximal and distal cervical esophagus. A flap of strap muscle or sternocleidomastoid should be utilized to buttress any primary repair. Stenting of the cervical esophagus is generally not an option due to issues of stent migration and patient comfort. Resection is rarely performed for the cervical esophagus with the exception of neoplasia. Formal proximal diversion for a cervical esophageal perforation is generally not possible due to limited length.

Thoracic Esophagus

The thoracic esophagus is the most frequent location for perforation, accounting for over 50% of cases. Etiology is most commonly iatrogenic as discussed, but spontaneous rupture (Boerhaave syndrome) is commonly seen. Spontaneous rupture results from sudden increases in esophageal pressure combined with negative intrathoracic pressure, often from forceful vomiting. The rupture is typically on the left side and in longitudinal fashion along the distal esophagus. Spontaneous rupture accounts for ~15% of all esophageal perforations. Traumatic injuries of the esophagus can occur in the thorax, more frequently with penetrating mechanisms. Traumatic esophageal injuries in the thorax can frequently be masked by more severe associated injuries such as the heart, great vessels, and trachea/bronchi.

Presenting symptoms of thoracic esophageal perforation include retrosternal chest pain, subcutaneous emphysema, dyspnea, and tachypnea. Symptoms associated with pleural effusion such as decreased breath sounds, dullness to percussion, and decreased fremitus are also common. Signs of systemic sepsis are frequently present, especially with any delay in presentation. Patients with Boerhaave syndrome will describe a history of emesis prior to the onset of their symptoms.

Chest x-ray will frequently show pneumomediastinum, pleural effusion (most often left sided), and mediastinal widening. CT imaging with oral contrast can be confirmatory and is useful to define the extent of mediastinal and thoracic contamination. Contrast esophagography is also a common confirmatory test, almost always with water-soluble contrast due to concerns of chemical mediastinitis with the use of barium.

Treatment of thoracic esophageal perforation begins with the interventions in **Table 26.2** and should occur rapidly, as even minor delays can significantly impact morbidity and mortality. Nonoperative management can be utilized in stable patients with small and contained perforations, but this is fairly uncommon for a thoracic perforation. Operative intervention with debridement of nonviable tissue, primary and separate closure of the mucosa and muscular layers, and flap buttress is the gold standard for treatment. This is typically performed via a posterolateral thoracotomy, but minimally invasive approaches such as video-assisted thoracoscopic surgery (VATS) or robotics have been described. Longitudinal myotomy at both ends of the perforation may be required to expose the mucosal defect, as it is often longer than the muscular tear. Options for buttress in the chest include intercostal muscle, pleura, pericardium, and diaphragm. Perforations in the thoracic esophagus may involve preexisting esophageal pathology, such as stricture or malignancy. In these cases, resection of the diseased portion of the esophagus to include the perforation (if proximal) is preferred. Reconstruction can proceed immediately if presenting early and without hemodynamic instability. Resection with proximal diversion or externalized t-tube drainage can be performed in cases requiring damage control options.

Endoscopic interventions are increasingly being utilized for thoracic esophageal perforations. Endoscopic clipping/suturing of defects can be successful if performed early and for easily apposable defects with healthy and compliant surrounding mucosa. The most success with endoscopic closure has been reported with iatrogenic endoscopic injuries that are identified and treated at the index procedure. Endoscopic vacuum therapy is another described treatment modality, but there are little comparative data to support widespread use. Endoscopic stent placement for thoracic perforation can be a good option for patients unlikely to tolerate chest surgery either due to extensive comorbidities or advanced sepsis. Adequate stent placement and seal of the perforation is usually confirmed with contrast esophagography. For patients with small perforations and minimal contamination, stent placement in conjunction with medical therapy may be all that is required. For patients with more extensive contamination, operative or percutaneous drainage can be performed in conjunction with stenting. If operative drainage is required, this can usually be accomplished in a minimally invasive fashion (VATS, etc.). Common short-term complications of stent placement include failure to adequately seal the perforation and stent migration. Stent migration risk is lower with metallic stents compared to plastic, but the long-term risk of stricture seems to be higher with metal. Duration of stenting can be variable but is generally <6 weeks. The use of stenting as a primary therapy in patients who are otherwise surgical candidates for primary repair remains controversial. There are no large randomized trials comparing esophageal stenting to surgery for thoracic esophageal perforation, but limited case series and retrospective reviews suggest similar rates of success with a potential for decreased morbidity and cost. Stenting is frequently employed after primary surgical repair if there is persistent leakage of the esophagus.

Intra-abdominal Esophagus

Perforation of the intra-abdominal esophagus is the least common location, representing <20% of all cases. Etiologies are again largely iatrogenic with an increased proportion of surgical injuries. Common operations involved are hiatal hernia repair, antireflux procedures, Heller myotomy, and bariatric surgery. Spontaneous rupture of the intra-abdominal esophagus can occur but is rarely isolated to only the intra-abdominal portion.

Presenting symptoms of intra-abdominal esophageal perforation include epigastric pain with radiation to the shoulder, nausea, and emesis. Uncontained perforations may present with localized or diffuse peritonitis. Systemic signs of sepsis are frequently present, especially with a delay in presentation or recognition.

Plain abdominal radiographs or chest x-ray may show free air under the diaphragm with intra-abdominal esophageal perforation. Suspected diagnosis can be confirmed with CT scan with oral contrast or contrast esophagography. CT scan is advantageous as it can effectively elucidate other etiologies if abdominal pain/peritonitis is the primary presenting symptom.

Treatment of intra-abdominal esophageal perforation utilizes the standard therapies illustrated in **Table 26.2**. Nonoperative management can be successful in stable patients with very minimal or contained perforations. Operative debridement and primary closure is the gold standard treatment option. This can be approached via a laparotomy, although many surgeons prefer the visualization afforded by laparoscopy or robotics. As in perforations elsewhere, primary repairs to the intra-abdominal esophagus should be buttressed with vascularized tissue. Common flap buttresses include mobilization of the fundus with either full or partial wrap, pedicled omentum, falciform, or diaphragm. Similar to thoracic esophageal perforations, preexisting pathology such as stricture or malignancy may be best treated with resection and either immediate or staged reconstruction. Proximal diversion and external drainage remain damage control options.

Endoscopic treatment of intra-abdominal esophageal perforation is similar to that of a thoracic perforation. Stenting is less commonly employed as a primary therapy, as many patients present with peritonitis and undergo more immediate surgery.

Conclusions

Esophageal perforation is a serious and life-threatening condition with a variety of etiologies and presentations. A high index of suspicion must be maintained to ensure timely diagnosis and management. Treatment modalities vary greatly depending on patient factors and location but include medical, endoscopic, and surgical modalities (**Figure 26.4**).

ESOPHAGEAL HEMORRHAGE

Esophageal hemorrhage can be primarily attributed to variceal bleeding in patients suffering from hepatic cirrhosis and associated portal hypertension. Although hepatic varices are common (50% of patients with cirrhosis), rates of hemorrhage depend on the severity of portal hypertension and decompensated cirrhosis, most common in those with elevated hepatic venous portal gradients. Life-threatening variceal hemorrhage in the setting of portal hypertension can occur at a yearly rate of 5%-15%, and a lifetime rate of 25%-70%. Further, despite many improvements of care, mortality rates remain at 20% overall due to rebleeding and difficulties effectively control bleeding.

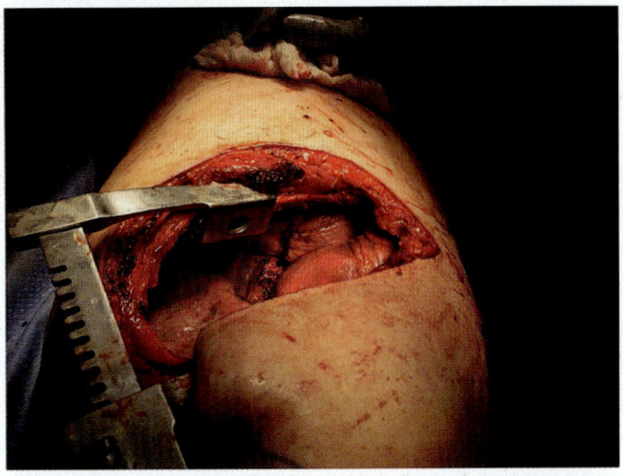

Figure 26.4 Esophageal repair with intercostal muscle buttress.

Details of prevention measures are not within the scope of this chapter. However, prevention of esophageal bleeding is a mainstay of management of patients at risk of life-threatening esophageal bleeding, including both pharmacologic (nonselective β-blockade, vasopressin, and somatostatin for purposes of decreasing cardiac output, increasing vasoconstriction splanchnic arterioles, and decreasing portal venous flow) and endoscopic surveillance and prophylactic interventions.

In the setting of variceal bleeding, treatment of hemorrhage is first and foremost includes blood product balanced resuscitation algorithms, followed by intravenous pharmacologic therapy to increase vasoconstriction of splanchnic arterioles (eg, vasopressin and octreotide). In addition, patients with variceal hemorrhage require antibiotic prophylaxis with either ceftriaxone or ciprofloxacin. Endoscopic diagnosis and treatment of bleeding esophageal varices is the mainstay of interventional treatment, focused on endoscopic variceal band ligation. Endoscopic variceal band ligation has primarily replaced endoscopic sclerotherapy given its effectiveness and more limited side effect profile (endoscopic sclerotherapy is associated with chest pain, dysphagia, and fevers, as well as risks of perforation). In the setting of esophageal variceal hemorrhage, EGD should be performed urgently after resuscitative efforts and often requires multiple sessions. Mechanical balloon tamponade using a Sengstaken-Blakemore or Minnesota tube may be required in patients who continue to hemorrhage despite resuscitative efforts, pharmacologic intervention, and endoscopic vein ligation. These balloons are effective at tamponade of the submucosal veins, however, are associated with rebleeding upon deflation, and complications of improper use. In the setting of ongoing massive hemorrhage, mechanical tamponade should be used to temporize for emergent shunting via transjugular intrahepatic portosystemic shunt (TIPS) or surgical intervention.

Transjugular intrahepatic portosystemic shunt is an intrahepatic diversion channel created under radiologic guidance between the hepatic vein and the portal vein using polytetrafluoroethylene (PTFE)-covered stents for longer term patency and is most commonly used in the setting of recurrent or failed control of variceal hemorrhage despite mentioned pharmacologic and endoscopic interventions. Early TIPS reduces rates of variceal hemorrhage treatment failure and ultimate morbidity and mortality. However, there are several contraindications including the presence of hepatic encephalopathy, congestive heart failure, and pulmonary hypertension. Further, preprocedural cross-sectional imaging of the abdominal anatomy in patients being considered for TIPS is important for assessment of patency of the portal vein and identification of anatomic variants of the hepatic vasculature. In general, with nonvariant hepatic vascular anatomy, most TIPS are created via a right hepatic vein approach through right internal jugular access. Once the portal vein is visualized, fluoroscopic-guided needle passes between the hepatic vein and portal vein are performed, a guidewire is then manipulated into the splenic vein or superior mesenteric vein with catheter exchange, followed by sheath and PTFE-covered stent graft placement. Further details on pressure measurements, portosystemic collateral identification, procedural details, and modified TIPS procedures such as direct intrahepatic portacaval shunt are beyond the scope of this chapter. However, TIPS for decompression of portal systemic hypertension for treatment of variceal bleeding decreases the bleeding risk by three-fold compared to endoscopic intervention. Despite higher rates of postprocedural encephalopathy, most reports suggest this encephalopathy can be controlled medically, and therefore, TIPS is the most common intervention for treatment of variceal hemorrhage that has failed endoscopic management, replacing previously commonly used surgical shunts described below. TIPS-related complications include TIPS dysfunction, markedly improved by use of PTFE-covered stents and close monitoring with duplex ultrasound for TIPS patency and development of stenosis and thrombosis. Further, development or worsening of encephalopathy occurs in up to 30% of patients, but only 5% fail to respond to medical therapy, requiring TIPS occlusion. Life-threatening complications of massive hemorrhage or heart failure are rare.

Surgical intervention for variceal hemorrhage was once a mainstay of treatment. However, modern advancements of pharmacologic, endoscopic, interventional radiologic procedures, as well as advances in liver transplantation have limited the need for surgical shunting to very rare cases (ie, noncirrhotic portal hypertension or total mesenteric venous occlusions). Surgical interventions for variceal hemorrhage can be grouped into decompressive operations (nonselective and selective) and devascularization procedures. Nonselective shunts divert the portal venous blood flow into the systemic circulation bypassing the liver, and selective shunts are intended to partially decompress the venous system while maintaining portal venous blood flow through the liver. Unlike these shunting procedures, devascularization procedures devascularize the esophagus (and stomach) rather than shunting portal venous blood flow, allowing separation of the esophageal and gastric drainage from the portal venous drainage.

Nonselective shunting is either total (end-to-side portacaval shunt, large side-to-side portacaval shunt, mesocaval shunts, and central splenorenal shunts) or partial. End-to-side portacaval shunts require division of the portal vein in the porta hepatis, and end-to-side anastomosis to the inferior vena cava with the splanchnic end of the portal vein, controlling variceal hemorrhage but not ascites, and risking hepatic encephalopathy or further hepatic decompensation. This shunt may be best used in patients with preserved hepatic synthetic function. Side-to-side portacaval shunts require mobilization of the portal vein from the pancreas to its bifurcation, and the inferior vena cava from the renal veins to the liver, followed by a side-to-side anastomosis (which may require a caudate hepatectomy or an interposition graft). These shunts are similarly complicated by hepatic encephalopathy in the setting of impaired liver function. Mesocaval shunts involve placement of an interposition graft between the superior mesenteric vein and the inferior vena cava and are at risk of thrombosis. Central splenorenal shunts physiologically behave like end-to-side portacaval shunts because they involve division of the distal splenic vein, splenectomy, and splenic vein to left renal vein anastomosis. Alternatively, selective shunting is intended to preserve some portal flow but separately decompress the splanchnic beds accounting for decreased post-procedural hepatic encephalopathy and improved control of ascites in the treatment of variceal hemorrhage. These shunts include the Sarfeh mesocaval shunt (side-to-side SMV to the IVC with a small Dacron or PTFE graft, preserving the porta for future hepatic transplantation), and the distal splenorenal shunt (mobilization of the splenic vein, anastomosis the splenic vein and left renal vein, division of collaterals at the pancreas, portal vein, and left gastric vein). The distal splenorenal shunt treats variceal hemorrhage, limits hepatic encephalopathy, and preserves the porta, but risks worsening medically refractory ascites due to the need for disconnection of the splenopancreatic branches.

Devascularization for variceal hemorrhage involves direct ligation of esophageal veins, short gastric veins, and veins of the lesser and greater gastric curves, preserving hepatopetal flows. Added esophageal transection and anastomosis with splenectomy can also be performed. Rebleeding and survival rates are variable, and devascularization should be reserved for refractory hemorrhage with extensive mesenteric and portal vein thrombosis, limiting TIPS. Modifications of devascularization with division of the esophageal plexus through the hiatus, splenectomy without esophageal transection, and selective vagotomy and pyloroplasty are also described. These procedures require preservation and presence of the left gastric vein so that portal and azygous collateral drainage can develop to reduce recurrent esophageal varices. Finally, splenopneumopexy can effectively decompress patients via the pulmonary veins in the setting of total mesenteric venous occlusion with an anastomosis between the parenchyma of a transected superior splenic pole and the left lower pulmonary lobe with pleurectomy through the left hemidiaphragm (requiring preoperative splenic arterial embolization). Finally, liver transplantation, beyond the scope of this chapter, is an effective treatment of portal venous hypertension associated variceal hemorrhage.

FOREIGN BODIES

Foreign body ingestion, commonly in children, afflicts ~100 000 individuals a year in the United States. In children, this is most often in the setting of accidental ingestion of small objects including noncaustic items such as toys and coins, and potentially caustic items including batteries and magnets. In adults, ingestions are often accompanied by behavioral conditions or impaired mental status due to intoxication, psychological disturbances, or cognitive decline. Determining the foreign body size and shape is important. Impacted foreign bodies are often stuck at the hypopharynx or within the thoracic esophagus at the level of the cricopharyngeus and aortic arch due to anatomy and the reduction in pressure at the site of striated to smooth muscle fiber transition. In nonobtunded adults and verbal children, identification of the area of impaction can be traced to symptoms and location of pain; however, in the young child or impaired adult, this may not be possible. Clinically, patients typically experience acute dysphagia and inability to swallow secretions. They may also experience odynophagia, throat pain, sensation of a foreign body, neck pain and tenderness, retrosternal pain, drooling, and emesis. In the setting of dyspnea, choking, and stridor, ruling out airway obstruction is of critical importance. There are often few physical exams findings in the acute phase, although in the setting of complications due to perforation of the esophagus, patients can have febrile illness, sepsis, cervical and thoracic subcutaneous emphysema, and general clinical manifestations of mediastinitis (see "Esophageal Perforation" section).

Evaluation beyond the patient's history and physical examination should include laboratory assessment of markers of infection and sepsis. In addition, plain radiographic films of the neck, chest, and abdomen can identify both the foreign body presence, appearance, and location, as well as possible evidence of perforation. However, the false negative rate of identification of perforation and identification of foreign bodies is up to 85% in some series, particularly in the setting of small or radiolucent foreign bodies. Prospective study of patients with symptomatic fish bone impaction found that plain radiographs had a sensitivity of 32%, but CT imaging had a sensitivity of 90%-100% and specificity of 94%-100%, highlighting that in all patient's plain radiographs should be followed by CT imaging if any suspicion of perforation or impaction that may require endoscopic and surgical intervention. Further, if clinical evidence or concern for mediastinitis or sepsis in this setting exists, CT imaging is useful to confirm. However, oral contrast CT should be avoided as patients with impaction and inability to clear secretions are at risk of aspiration of barium or gastrografin. Further, barium and gastrografin can impair endoscopic visualization and delivery for the purpose of imaging can delay needed endoscopic or surgical interventions.

The vast majority of esophageal foreign bodies will pass spontaneously through via gastrointestinal transit. If a patient remains symptomatic, however, even with negative CT imaging, the first-line therapy for impacted esophageal foreign bodies should be flexible endoscopy. For potentially caustic objects (batteries, magnets), sharp objects, and impaction with complete occlusion of the esophagus, emergent flexible endoscopy should be performed due to risk of pressure necrosis, electrical or chemical burns, perforation, and potential for aspiration. In patients with symptoms and concern for impaction without complete occlusion or caustic ingestions, then flexible endoscopy can be performed on a nonemergent, urgent basis. Technically, attempts to push the obstruction into the stomach should be the first technique employed for food impaction; however, if this is unsuccessful, retrieval should be attempted using careful passage of a balloon catheter beyond the foreign body for extraction. However, for sharp objects, grasping forceps, baskets, and snares should be used instead. Often, a combination of these procedures may be required. During the endoscopy, it is critical to evaluate the esophagus for an inciting factor of the impaction, as 25% of patients may have an esophageal disorder identified at the time of extraction including stricture, hiatal hernia, web or Schatzki ring, esophagitis, achalasia, and benign and malignant tumors. If flexible endoscopy is unsuccessful, rigid endoscopy can be used as a second approach and is often required for foreign body impaction within the upper esophagus or in settings where there is concern of concomitant airway obstruction. Meta-analysis data of flexible compared to rigid endoscopy for esophageal foreign body impaction confirms similar success rates and complications for retrieval.

If a foreign body is not retrievable, has caused perforation, has intimate proximity to vital structures such as the aortic arch, or has caused other complications, surgical intervention is indication. In the setting of esophageal perforation with significant neck, mediastinal, pleural, or abdominal contamination, emergent surgical intervention should be undertaken as the primary intervention. However, <5% of patients require operative intervention due to complications of foreign body. The surgical approach to esophageal foreign bodies holds true to the tenets of esophageal surgery and depends on anatomic location, as well as the baseline and physiologic status of the patient and degree of contamination. If there is limited contamination, in a stable patient, esophagotomy (using anatomic surgical principles addressed above for the approach) should be performed for foreign body extraction and primary closure. Taking care to be sure of vital edges, washout of contamination, and appropriate drainage are critical. This is described with both minimally invasive techniques as well as open techniques. Rarely, rescue esophagectomy with primary or delayed reconstruction may be required.

CAUSTIC INJURY

Although uncommon, ingestion of caustic and corrosive substances can be devastatingly morbid leading to complications resulting in ultimate death. Those who survive are plagued by difficulty eating and swallowing, poor quality of life, creating monumental burden on medical systems. As with most ingestions, those in children are often accidental resulting in less morbid outcomes, due to limited ingestion. Ingestions in adults, however, are often related to psychiatric illness and suicidal attempts. In these situations, patients are at risk of massive ingestions and ingestions of severe corrosive agents. These events are always emergencies and can be difficult to diagnose and manage because the clinical presentations and physical exam findings may not well correlate with the extent of esophageal and gastrointestinal tract damage. Absence of clear nasal or oral injury does not rule out life-threatening esophageal damage. Early diagnosis and intervention are, therefore, of utmost importance.

Both acids and alkalis can cause severe corrosive injury to the esophagus and gastrointestinal tract. The identification of the agent, its chemical and physical form, and the amount ingested are central in the early evaluation (**Table 26.3**). In addition, assessment of the events surrounding the ingestion, and the voluntary nature of them, is important for identifying concomitant injuries and ingestions, as well as care planning. One of the first steps after confirming a secure airway and hemodynamic stability of a patient is contacting the local poison control center to identify and treat any potential systemic toxicities of the ingested agents. Although both acids and alkalis cause necrosis of the esophagus, the phenotypes of injuries do vary based on ingested agent. For example, ammonia ingestion causes a particular hemorrhagic esophagitis and gastritis that requires monitoring. The most important prognostic factors for a patient with corrosive ingestion are the quantity of agent ingested, the physical form of the agent (ie, solids primarily injure the mouth and pharynx, while liquids primarily injure the esophagus and stomach), concomitant ingestion and vapor aspiration (ie, formaldehyde and ammonia), and agents that cause severe systemic effects (ie, phosphoric and hydrofluoric acids, and strong acids and alkalis).

Evaluation beyond the patient's history and physical examinations should include laboratory assessment of markers for evidence of perforation, mediastinitis, and sepsis but also electrolyte derangements. As part of the workup for transmural necrosis and its complications as well as systemic toxicities, a comprehensive panel of laboratory assays should include complete blood count, electrolytes, liver function tests, coagulation assays, pH, lactate, toxicology screens, and pregnancy tests in women of child-bearing age. Further, in this scenario, serial laboratory assessments should be considered as ini-

TABLE 26.3 ■ Caustic Agents (Commonly Found in)
Alkalis
Sodium hypochlorite (bleach, household cleaning products, swimming pool products)
Sodium or potassium hydroxides (drain cleaning products, oven cleaners, grease removers, hair products, washing powders)
Ammonium hydroxide (household cleaning products, grease remover)
Acids
Sulfuric acid (batteries, cleaning agents, drain cleaning products)
Oxalic acid (paint thinners, metal polishes)
Hydrochloric acid (solvents, metal cleaners, toilet cleaners, mildew/mold removers)
Phosphoric acid (toilet cleaners, rust remover)
Acetic acid (pickling, photographic baths)
Selenous acid (gun agent)
Other
Sodium carbonate (soap production)
Sodium polyphosphate and cationic detergents (detergents, cleaners, preservatives)
Potassium permanganate (disinfectants, hair dye)
Hydrofluoric acid (rust removers)
Phenols (surface cleaners)

Derived from Contini S, Scarpignato C. Caustic injury of the upper gastrointestinal tract: a comprehensive review. *World J Gastroenterol*. 2013;19:3919; Hoffman RS, Burns MM, Gosselin S. Ingestion of caustic substances. *N Engl J Med*. 2020;382(18):1739-1748.

tial normal laboratory values cannot be relied upon to rule out transmural necrosis. Derangements of laboratory values including the presence of severe acidosis, liver failure, elevated inflammatory markers, acute kidney injury, and leukocytosis or thrombocytopenia are all predictive of severe illness, transmural necrosis, and ultimate morbidity.

As with foreign body ingestion, plain radiographs can show evidence of free perforations requiring immediate intervention. However, the central imaging modality of importance is CT as data support that emergent CT, contrast-enhanced, is better at detecting transmural injuries after corrosive ingestion and of predicting long-term stricture formation than endoscopy. Specifically, contrast-enhanced CT of the neck, chest, and abdomen should be performed, and with appropriate contrast timing, the absence of postcontrast wall-enhancement at any location in the gastrointestinal tract is an indication for emergency surgery for transmural necrosis. In addition, CT grading is the gold standard grading technique (**Figure 26.5**).

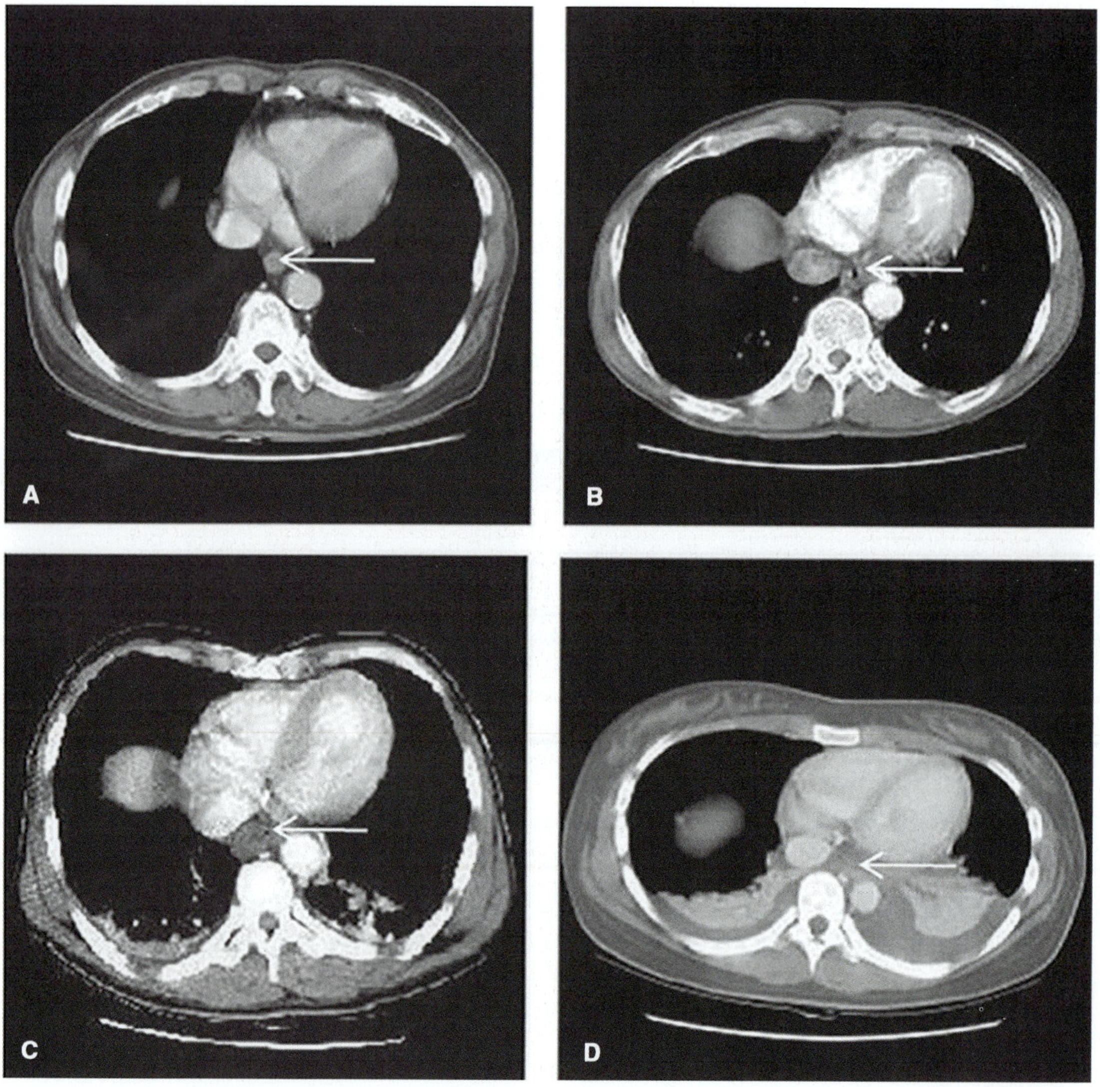

Figure 26.5 Computed tomography grading of esophageal caustic injuries. **A.** Grade 1, no definite swelling of the esophageal wall. **B.** Grade 2, edematous wall thickening without periesophageal soft tissue infiltration. **C.** Grade 3, edematous wall thickening with periesophageal soft tissue infiltration plus well-demarcated tissue interface. **D.** Grade 4, edematous wall thickening with periesophageal soft tissue infiltration plus blurring of tissue interface or localized fluid collection around the esophagus or aorta. *Arrows* indicate the esophageal wall. (From Ryu HH, Jeung KW, Lee BK, et al. Caustic injury: can CT grading systems enable prediction of esophageal stricture? *Clin Toxicol*. 2010;48:138. Reprinted by permission of the publisher (Taylor & Francis Ltd, http://www.tandfonline.com).)

The indication for emergent flexible endoscopy should be considered if CT is unavailable, the patient has a contraindication to contrast administration including kidney injury or allergy, the CT imaging is indeterminate, or to spare radiation in children. This is a change from historical practice in which endoscopy was first line for diagnosis and management of corrosive ingestions. However, endoscopy poorly identifies transmural necrosis leading to either under diagnosis and poor outcomes or over diagnosis and unnecessary operative interventions. In children, endoscopy remains a first-line diagnostic given the rarity of transmural necrosis, and the concerns of radiation with CT imaging. However, it should be stressed that the endoscopic classifications have been proven to be outperformed with CT grading (**Figure 26.6**). However, endoscopy remains the main diagnostic and intervention for the development of stricturing disease, the most common long-term complication of corrosive ingestions. These strictures generally form months after ingestions leading to dysphagia and reflux. Endoscopic dilation is the first-line management of these strictures and can be attempted several weeks from ingestion after healing of the acute injury, in patients with limited number and/or limited length strictures. These dilations can be done every few weeks, often require multiple sessions to improve symptoms. However, if failure of dilations, multiple, long, or irregular strictures, surgical intervention with esophageal reconstruction may be required.

Patients with more limited corrosive injuries who do not have transmural necrosis should still undergo close monitoring with a low threshold for performance of CT imaging as described if clinical decline. Once patients can swallow, trials of eating can be performed, and if patients cannot tolerate oral feeds, enteral feeding should be the mainstay of nutrition. In addition, it is recommended that all patients have psychiatric support prior to discharge due to the debilitating nature of these corrosive ingestions.

If a patient requires emergent surgery for transmural necrosis, all necrosis must be resected at the initial operation, and a feeding jejunostomy tube

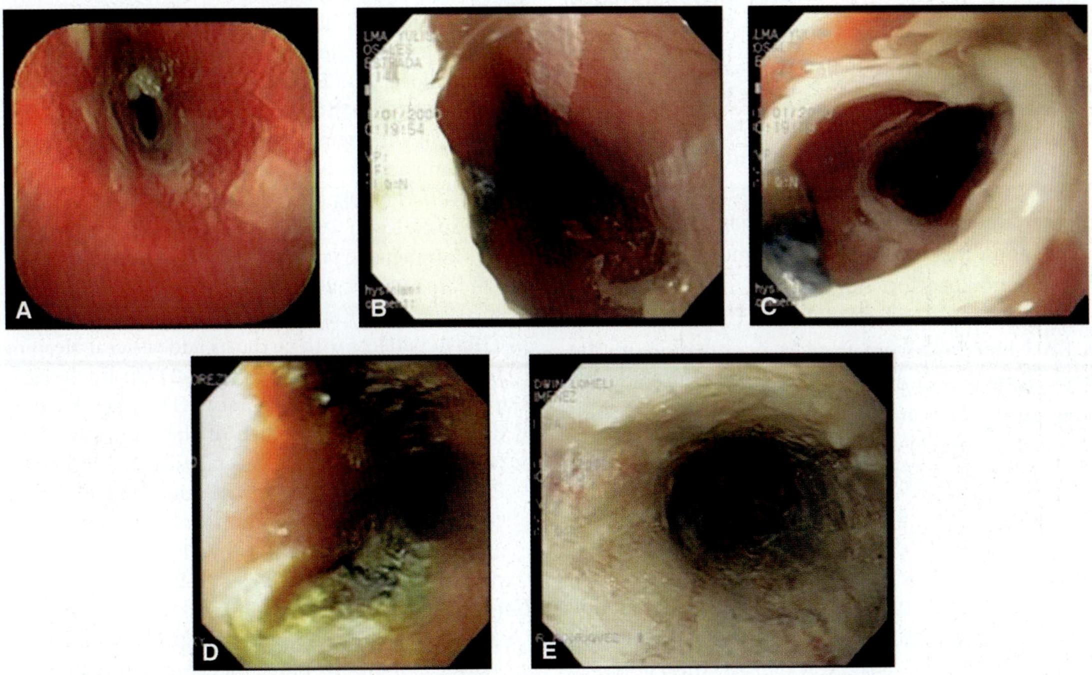

Figure 26.6 Modified Zargar endoscopic classification of mucosal injury caused by ingestion of caustic substances. **A.** Edema and erythema. **B.** Erosions and ulcers. **C.** Circumferential ulceration. **D.** Scattered areas of esophageal necrosis. **E.** Extensive esophageal necrosis. (Reprinted from Betalli P, Falchetti D, Giuliani S, Pane A, Dall'Oglio L, de Angelis GL, Caldore M, Romano C, Gamba P, Baldo V; Caustic Ingestion Italian Study Group. Caustic ingestion in children: is endoscopy always indicated? The results of an Italian multicenter observational study. *Gastrointest Endosc*. 2008 Sep;68(3):434-9, with permission from Elsevier.)

should be placed. Based on anatomic locations, the tenets of operative approach to the esophagus should be used. If necrosis is not addressed, patients are at high risk of progression to perforation, sepsis, and death. Further, if a patient fails to improve after initial operative management, reoperation is indicated to assess for missed transmural necrosis. If there is transmural necrosis of both the esophagus and stomach, a stripping esophagectomy and gastrectomy via a cervical and abdominal approach is indicated. It is imperative that esophageal reconstruction is delayed as the proximal and distal stricture formation rate with immediate reconstruction is too high. The management of necrosis isolated to the esophagus is controversial and many recommend attempts at nonoperative management over esophagectomy with gastric preservation. Additional extended resection of necrosis in adjacent organs may be required depending on the extent of injuries. In addition, adjunctive workups are always required in this setting including bronchoscopy for extension of necrosis, which may in itself require operative intervention. In a situation of pan-necrosis of the bowel, aggressive resections are not recommended due to unacceptably high morbidity and mortality.

SUMMARY

Esophageal perforation is a life-threatening condition with a variety of etiologies and presentations. A high index of suspicion must be maintained to ensure timely diagnosis and management. Treatment modalities vary greatly depending on patient factors and location but include medical, endoscopic, and surgical modalities. Upper gastrointestinal bleeding from varices is common in the cirrhotic population. Control of bleeding includes medical therapy, endoscopic and IR intervention, and rarely surgery. Management of foreign body ingestion depends on the patient age, symptoms, and objects ingested. First-line therapy remains endoscopy. Caustic ingestion is a life-altering event. Ingestion in children tends to be accidental with lower volumes, as opposed to the deliberate efforts in adults. CT has replaced endoscopy as the initial test for staging caustic injury. Therapy depends upon degree and location of caustic injury.

SUGGESTED READINGS

Aiolfi A, Ferrari D, Riva CG, et al. Esophageal foreign bodies in adults: systematic review of the literature. *Scand J Gastroenterol.* 2018;53(10–11):1171-1178.

Ali J, Rice R, David E, et al. Perforated esophageal intervention focus (PERF) study: a multi-center examination of contemporary treatment. *Dis Esophagus.* 2017;30(11):1-8.

Benjamin ER, Inaba K. Cervical esophagus. In: Demetriades D, Inaba K, Velmahos G, eds. *Atlas of Surgical Techniques in Trauma.* 2nd ed. Cambridge university Press; 2020:89-93.

Biffl W, Moore E, Feliciano DV, et al. Western Trauma Association critical decisions in trauma: diagnosis and management of esophageal injuries. *J Trauma Acute Care Surg.* 2015;79(6):1089-1095.

Chirica M, Bonavina L, Kelly MD, et al. Caustic ingestion. *Lancet.* 2017;389(10083):2041-2052.

Chirica M, Kelly MD, Siboni S, et al. Esophageal emergencies: WSES guidelines. *World J Emerg Surg.* 2019;14:26. doi:10.1186/s13017-019-0245-2

Chirica M, Resche-Rigon M, Bongrand NM, et al. Surgery for caustic injuries of the upper gastrointestinal tract. *Ann Surg.* 2012;256(6):994-1001.

Chirica M, Resche-Rigon M, Zagdanski AM, et al. Computed tomography evaluation of esophagogastric necrosis after caustic ingestion. *Ann Surg.* 2016;264(1):107-113.

Contini S, Scarpignato C. Caustic injury of the upper gastrointestinal tract: a comprehensive review. *World J Gastroenterol.* 2013;19:3918-3930.

Cowan T, Foster R, Isbister GK. Acute esophageal injury and strictures following corrosive ingestions in a 27 year cohort. *Am J Emerg Med.* 2017;35(3):488-492.

Ferrari D, Aiolfi A, Bonitta G, et al. Flexible versus rigid endoscopy in the management of esophageal foreign body impaction: systematic review and meta-analysis. *World J Emerg Surg.* 2018;13:42.

Fidelman N, Kwan SW, LaBerge JM, et al. The transjugular intrahepatic portosystemic shunt: an update. *AJR Am J Roentgenol.* 2012;199:746-755.

Garcia-Pagan JC, Caca K, Bureau C, et al. Early use of TIPS in patients with cirrhosis and variceal bleeding. *N Engl J Med.* 2010;326(25):2370-2379.

Garcia-Tsao G, Sanyal AJ, Grace ND, Carey W; Practice Guidelines Committee of the American Association for the Study of Liver Diseases, the Practice Parameters Committee of the American College of Gastroenterology. Prevention and management of gastroesophageal varices and variceal hemorrhage in cirrhosis. *Hepatology.* 2007;46(3):922-938.

Geevarghese SK, Hiatt JR, Busuttil RW. Management of portal hypertensive hemorrhage in the era of liver transplantation. In: Busuttil RW, Klintmalm GB, eds. *Transplantation of the Liver.* 2nd ed. Saunders; 2005:507-511.

Geng C, Li X, Luo R, et al. Endoscopic management of foreign bodies in the upper gastrointestinal tract: a retrospective study of 1294 cases. *Scand J Gastroenterol.* 2017;52(11):1286-1291.

Kim AW, Park C. Thoracic esophagus. In: Demetriades D, Inaba K, Velmahos G, eds. *Atlas of Surgical*

Techniques in Trauma. 2nd ed. Cambridge university Press; 2020:142-149.

Lampridis S, Mitsos S, Hayward M, et al. The insidious presentation and challenging management of esophageal perforation following diagnostic and therapeutic interventions. *J Thorac Dis*. 2020;12(5): 2724-2734.

Methasate A, Lohsiriwat V. Role of endoscopy in caustic injury of the esophagus. *World J Gastrointest Endosc*. 2018;10:277.

Ngan JH, Fok PJ, Lai EC, et al. A prospective study on fish bone ingestion. Experience of 358 patients. *Ann Surg*. 1990;211(4):459-462.

Richardson JD. Management of esophageal perforations: the value of aggressive surgical treatment. *Am J Surg*. 2005;190:161-165.

Ryu HH, Jeung KW, Lee BK, et al. Caustic injury: can CT grading systems enable prediction of esophageal stricture? *Clin Toxicol*. 2010;48:137-142.

Salam AA. Distal splenorenal shunts: hemodynamics of total versus selective shunting. In: Baker RJ, Fischer JE, eds. *Mastery of Surgery*. 4th ed. Lippincott Williams & Wilkins; 2001:1357-1366.

Sancheti MS, Fernandez FG. Surgical management of esophageal perforation. *Operat Tech Thorac Cardiovasc Surg*. 2015;20(3):234-250.

Temiz A, Oguzkurt P, Ezer SS, et al. Predictability of outcome of caustic ingestion by esophagogastroduodenoscopy in children. *World J Gastroenterol*. 2012;18(10):1098-1103.

Watkins J, Farivar A. Endoluminal therapies for esophageal perforations and leaks. *Thorac Surg Clin*. 2018;28(4):541-554.

CHAPTER

27 Surgical Complications and Surgical Rescue

Oscar D. Guillamondegui, Salina M. Wydo, and Nicole A. Stassen

INTRODUCTION

More than 1 million patient discharges in the United States are a result of surgical and medical complications. Acute Care Surgeons are often called upon to help manage patients with procedural and surgical complications. The incidence of surgical complications is associated principally with patient characteristics and may not be fully preventable. Further deterioration and death are often avertible if promptly identified and handled. The difference in morbidity and mortality from a complication stems primarily from the capacity to expeditiously and appropriately "rescue" patients from the complication. Each additional complication suffered by a patient increases the risk of failure to rescue. The "failure to rescue" is defined as "death after an adverse occurrence." Failures occur at each of three main time points including identification of a change in patient status, prompt communication of the change to senior staff, and implementation of treatment. The spectrum of "surgical rescue" techniques required in the care of these patients potentially includes operation, surgeon-guided resuscitation, critical care, interventional procedures, endoscopic procedures, and bedside procedures. This chapter will review the evaluation and management of the most common surgical rescue scenarios encountered by the Acute Care Surgeon including uncontrolled sepsis (surgical site infection, anastomotic leak, and enteric injury) and complications of endoscopy.

UNCONTROLLED SEPSIS

Surgical Site Infection

CASE PRESENTATION

A 37-year-old female is postoperative day 5 after undergoing a laparoscopic converted to open appendectomy for perforated appendicitis. She has noticed increased pain and swelling at her incisions with some drainage. Her past medical history includes endometriosis. Her past surgical history includes a laparoscopic cholecystectomy. She is febrile to 38.9 °C and tachycardic with an HR of 105 beats/min and a blood pressure of 103/49 mm Hg. On examination, she is ill appearing and has rapidly spreading cellulitis around her incision with purulent drainage. Labs are notable for a white blood cell count of 17 300/mm^3, lactate of 3.7 mmol/L, creatinine of 1.3 mg/dL, hemoglobin of 9.5 g/dL, and an INR of 1.1. Resuscitation with isotonic fluid is started through two large bore peripheral intravenous lines.

Question: *What is the most likely diagnosis?*

Answer: *Surgical site infection*

Etiology

Surgical site infections (SSI) remain one of the most common adverse events affecting hospitalized surgical patients. Data from the National Nosocomial Infection Surveillance System (NNIS) show an average incidence of SSI of 2.6%, accounting for 38% of nosocomial infections in surgical patients. SSI is a major contributor to patient morbidity and mortality in hospital settings with an annual cost in the United States estimated at 3.5-10 billion dollars. SSI negatively impacts not only the patient's physical health but also their mental health.

SSI is a complex problem influenced by numerous factors, only some of which are under the surgeon's control. These risk factors can be broadly separated into intrinsic (patient) factors that are modifiable or nonmodifiable, as well as extrinsic (eg, procedure, facility, preoperative, and operative) factors (**Table 27.1**). There can be a substantial increase in SSI risk, in urgent or emergent situations where there may not be an opportunity to optimize fully a patient's comorbid status. In the majority of SSIs, pathogens are introduced at the time of the operative procedure. The risk of wound

TABLE 27.1 ■ Risk Factors for SSI

Intrinsic Factors	Age Nutritional status Diabetes Smoking Obesity Coexistent infections at a remote body site Colonization with microorganisms Altered immune response Length of preoperative stay

Extrinsic Factors	Skin antisepsis
	Preoperative shaving
	Preoperative skin preparation
	Duration of operation
	Antimicrobial prophylaxis
	Operating room ventilation
	Inadequate sterilization of instruments
	Foreign material in the surgical site
	Surgical drains
	Surgical technique
	  Poor hemostasis
	  Failure to obliterate dead space
	  Tissue trauma

contamination and subsequent SSI also depends on location, the nature of the surgical wound/incision, and the procedure performed. The SSI rate increases with worsening of the Centers for Disease Control and Prevention (CDC) wound class (clean, clean-contaminated, contaminated, and dirty), with clean and low-risk operations having the lowest incidence and contaminated and high-risk operations having higher infection rates. The rate of SSI is also higher for an emergency surgery, as opposed to elective cases independent of solely clinical comorbidities. Even with multimodal strategies/guidelines to decrease SSIs that occur across a range of settings under the supervision of numerous providers, SSIs still occur.

Evaluation and Management

SSIs are classified into three categories determined by depth and tissue spaces involved. Superficial incisional SSI is confined to the skin and subcutaneous tissues. Deep incisional SSI involves the deep soft tissue, such as the fascial and muscular layers. Organ/space SSI extends further beyond these anatomic boundaries. The diagnosis of SSI starts with clinical evaluation. SSI symptoms include localized erythema, induration, warmth, and pain at the incision site. Purulent wound drainage and separation of the wound may occur. In morbidly obese patients or in those with deep, multilayer wounds such as after thoracotomy, external signs of SSI may be delayed. Some patients will have systemic evidence of their infection such as fever and leukocytosis. The presence of these systemic features in the absence of local signs of wound infection should raise suspicion for organ/space SSI, or for an infection arising from an alternate site. SSIs rarely occur during the first 48 hours after surgery, with fever during that period usually stemming from noninfectious or unknown causes. SSIs that do occur in this time frame are generally due to *Streptococcus pyogenes* or *Clostridium* species.

The key principle of SSI therapy remains identification and control of the source of infection. For superficial incisional SSI, the most important therapy is to open the incision, evacuate the infected material, and continue dressing changes until the wound heals by secondary intention. A variety of local wound care options are available, with the simplest being saline-soaked cotton gauze dressings. For uncomplicated superficial incisional SSI, no antibiotic therapy is required after opening the incision. Deep incisional SSI requires in addition to opening the incision and evacuating/debriding the infected material, antibiotic therapy in patients with systemic features, or widening erythema (>5 cm in diameter). Continued clinical monitoring follows to ensure an appropriate clinical response, with consideration of alternative diagnoses if atypical features appear (**Figure 27.1**).

Diagnosis of an organ/space SSI often requires diagnostic testing in addition to clinical evaluation to localize the site of infection. Computed tomography (CT) is the diagnostic standard as it allows cross-sectional visualization of the entire surgical area with excellent spatial resolution and delineation of the adjacent anatomic structures. CT is also not impaired in the setting of ileus, wound dressings, stomas, or the open abdomen. The use of intravenous contrast helps increase the diagnostic accuracy. The images often demonstrate a hypodense collection (between 0 and 30 Hounsfield units) associated with peripheral intensification. Ultrasound (US) is a useful adjunct. US is inexpensive, distinguishes between fluid and solid tissue without ionizing radiation, and can be performed at the bedside. However, some areas can be difficult to visualize because of body habitus, bowel gas, postoperative air, or postsurgical changes. An abscess on ultrasound generally appears as a multilocular complex mass with debris, septations, and irregular thick walls. Treatment of organ/

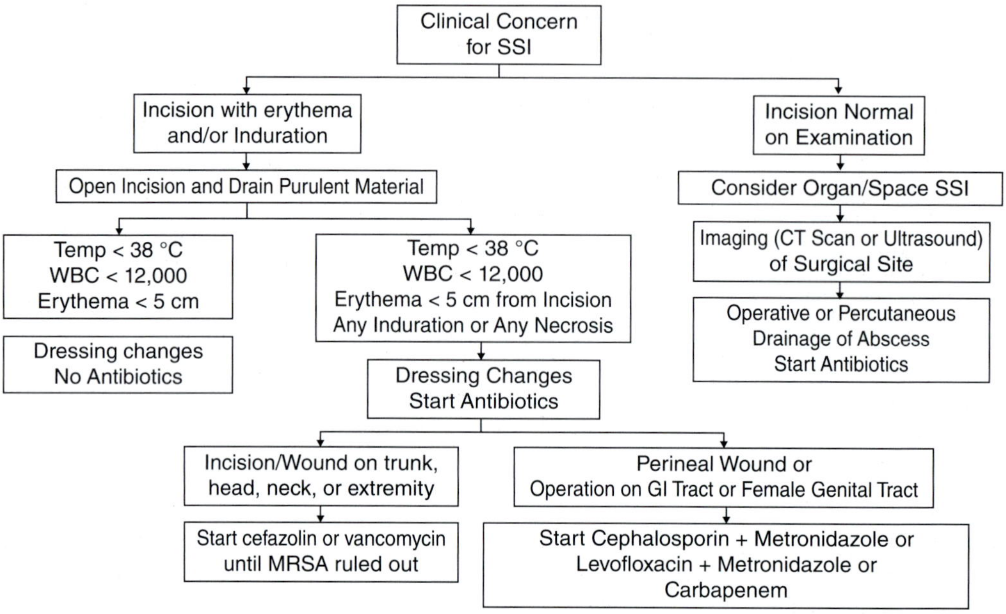

Figure 27.1 SSI evaluation algorithm. (Adapted from Stevens DL, Bisno AL, Chambers HF, et al. Practice guidelines for the diagnosis and management of skin and soft tissue infections: 2014 update by the Infectious Diseases Society of America. *Clin Infect Dis*. 2014;59:e10-e52.)

space SSI includes source control and initiation of appropriate antimicrobial therapy influenced by the local microbiological epidemiology. The least invasive, nonsurgical therapy is always the first approach for treatment of intra-abdominal collections, whenever feasible. Continued clinical examination follows to ensure an appropriate response to treatment. The principal cause for failure of percutaneous drainage is misdiagnosis of the magnitude, extent, complexity, or location of the abscess. In these rare cases of ineffective/nonfeasible minimal invasive interventional treatment of abscesses, operative drainage should be performed when possible.

Initiation of antibiotic therapy is appropriate in patients with more complicated infections and who are demonstrating signs of systemic shock. The principle of source control remains essential, with the appropriate selection of antibiotics based on the type of surgical procedure performed, and the expected microbial causes for the infection. From a general perspective, the microbes responsible for infection of surgical wounds originate from either the surrounding skin or associated structures that are contiguous with the regions of the surgical procedure. The most frequently identified pathogens are *Staphylococcus aureus*, *coagulase-negative Staphylococci*, *Escherichia coli*, *Enterococcus faecalis*, and *Pseudomonas aeruginosa*. Individual institutions may have variations in the proportions of specific species, due to differences in the volumes of various surgical specialties. There is a substantial growth in multidrug resistant (MDR) organisms including methicillin-resistant *S aureus* (MRSA), making obtaining microbial data paramount. If a culture is procured, an aspirate of pus in a syringe or a tissue specimen provides the most meaningful information vs swabs of wound drainage. Appropriate antibiotic stewardship, which generally favors a short course, narrower rather than broader coverage when possible, should be included in antimicrobial decision-making (see **Figure 27.1**).

Postoperative necrotizing soft-tissue infections are a rare but serious subset of surgical site infections. Clostridial myonecrosis is most frequently caused by *Clostridium perfringens* although other species of *Clostridium* have also been implicated. Clostridial myonecrosis can occur within a few hours of surgery and is characterized by high fevers and severe pain that extends beyond the original wound. The surrounding tissue and muscle become necrotic, resulting in skin discoloration and the formation of hemorrhagic bullae. Purulent drainage is often absent and a thin, serous discharge is more common. Necrotizing fasciitis caused by group A Streptococcus has also been reported in the postoperative period and may be associated with hypotension, renal failure, and respiratory failure. Both etiologies are

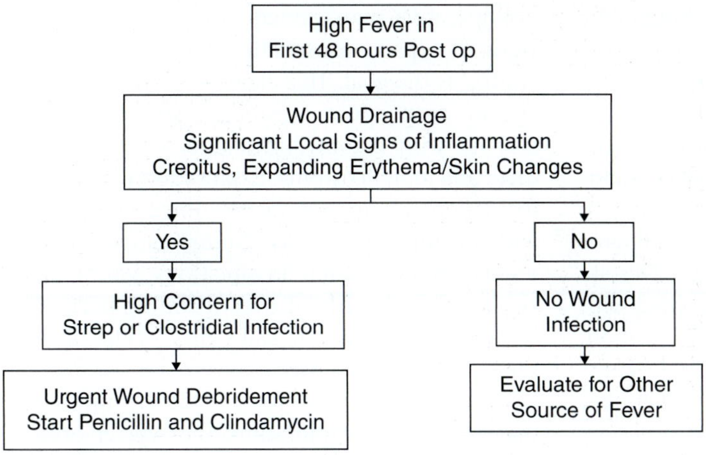

Figure 27.2 Algorithm for potential necrotizing SSI. (Adapted from Stevens DL, Bisno AL, Chambers HF, et al. Practice guidelines for the diagnosis and management of skin and soft tissue infections: 2014 update by the Infectious Diseases Society of America. *Clin Infect Dis.* 2014;59:e10-e52.)

emergencies and rapid surgical intervention is necessary to debride necrotic tissue. Antibiotics are secondary in importance to surgical resection; penicillins and clindamycin are considered the treatment of choice in concert with serial debridement (**Figure 27.2**).

Anastomotic Leak

CASE PRESENTATION

A 77-year-old female is postoperative day 8 after undergoing a right hemicolectomy for a near obstructing colon cancer. She had been tolerating a diet, but now her abdomen is distended and tympanic. Her past medical history includes hypothyroidism and hypertension. Her past surgical history includes a partial thyroidectomy, classic cesarean section, and laparoscopic cholecystectomy. She has a low-grade fever and mild tachycardia with an HR of 100 beats/min and a blood pressure of 123/49 mm Hg. On examination, she is toxic appearing, is distended, and has lower abdominal tenderness. Labs are notable for a white blood cell count of 16 300/mm^3, lactate of 2.9 mmol/L, creatinine of 2.1 mg/dL, hemoglobin of 9.5 g/dL, and an INR of 1.1. Intravenous access is obtained with two large bore peripheral intravenous lines and resuscitation is initiated with isotonic fluid is started.

Question: *What is the likely diagnosis?*

Answer: *Anastomotic leak*

Etiology

Anastomotic leak, both small and large bowel, are a major complication of bowel surgery. Leaks occur with the added detriment of increasing overall morbidities, length of stay, and mortality. The risk of leak varies depending on the type of surgery and the location of the anastomosis. The data suggest that leaks occur following 2%-20% of gastrointestinal anastomoses, depending on the population studied. Small bowel anastomoses leak approximately half as frequently as colonic anastomoses with both numbers more than doubling in the emergent setting. Although several factors may affect the outcome of surgical resection, the type of anastomosis, whether hand-sewn, single-layered/double-layered, or stapled, does not change the rate of leakage.

Many factors do play a role in the health of the anastomosis and the ultimate formation of a leak. The most common risk factor is an associated comorbidity, such as chronic liver disease, malnutrition, and cardiac disease, with the highest risk being multiple comorbidities. This risk may increase the incidence of leak up to five times that seen in an elective procedure. The site of anastomosis is also a factor in the development of a leak. Colonic anastomoses are twice as likely to develop a leak as small intestinal anastomoses. Although age has not been proven as a risk factor, the anastomosis in a male patient is over twice as likely to leak. Sepsis and blood transfusions also increase the risk of leak by over two times. Finally, neither surgeon experience level nor drain placement appears to have any effect on anastomotic outcomes. However, operative time >3 hours may increase the risk by over 50%. A diverting ileostomy performed with colonic anastomoses has a protective effect of nearly 50%.

Finally, the formation of a leak exposes the patient to an increased risk of secondary complications. These range from increased incidence of pneumonia, renal insufficiency, sepsis, ventilator dependence, wound dehiscence, and death. Despite efforts to decrease the risk factors associated with anastomotic leaks prior to operative intervention, these leaks are considered an unavoidable complication. Strategies to identify and treat them are necessary to decreasing further sequelae.

Evaluation and Management

The issue with the term "anastomotic leak" is that experts do not agree on what constitutes a leak. Nevertheless, the evaluation of a leak begins with the suspicion of loss of integrity of the anastomosis and the physiologic sequelae. The most common symptoms include prolonged ileus followed by fever, tachycardia, and leukocytosis. These findings are typically followed by local or frank peritonitis. Suspect a leak if the patient is not following a normal postoperative trajectory. Findings may be subtle, such as nausea or persistent ileus, general feeling of unwellness or intolerance to oral intake or tube feedings. If a drain is in place, enteral contents may be identified within the output and, if not present, progression to succus or stool noted in the wound bed may be the first sign. If there is suspicion of a leak without the identification of enteral fluids (from the wound or drain), computed tomography (CT scan) with oral contrast may help define the actual site of loss of integrity of the anastomosis or the associated fluid collection or abscess. The contention of some surgeons is that an identified abscess does not always constitute an actual leak at the anastomosis site and may be a deep space infection. If enteral content is drained from the fluid collection, then it should be assumed to be an anastomotic leak.

Once a leak is discovered, the management should focus on the situation that mitigated the pathology and the associated pathophysiology of the patient. The first decision point is operative or nonoperative management. Initially, if there are signs of sepsis, resuscitation followed by source control is the goal. This algorithm includes drainage of deep space infection, exploratory laparotomy with ostomy formation, or repair with diverting loop ileostomy. Exploration with ostomy formation occurs up to two-thirds of patients with postoperative leaks. Nonoperative management may be possible in situations with a small, contained leak without overwhelming peritonitis or sepsis. Anastomotic leaks may occur up to 1 month postanastomosis.

If the leak is discovered outside the time frame that allows safe exploration, the typical presentation is as an enterocutaneous fistula. The fistula may present as enteric content in the midline wound, manifesting from a drain site or as an intraperitoneal fluid collection. In the first two circumstances, getting control of the output is essential. In the third case, draining and forming an enterocutaneous tract diverted off the midline is preferred. Fistulae are described as low, moderate, or high output depending on the volume of content expressing from the site. Low output fistulae average <200 mL in any 24 hours with high output at >500 mL per 24 hours and moderate between 200 and 500 per day. Management of the late presentation anastomotic leak as an enterocutaneous fistula consists of first deciding on the likelihood of closure without operative intervention and, if not possible, management strategy toward surgical intervention. When possible, maintaining oral intake is the best route of supplementation to provide nutritional and fluid balance support. If increased oral intake raises the output of the fistula, the next step is total parental nutrition while halting per os intake. Whichever route allows appropriate intake, nutritional status should be continued for 3-6 months with reassessment for surgical intervention intermittently. Although the multitude of outcomes of an enterocutaneous fistula is beyond the scope of this chapter, ultimately, the goal is operative repair of the anastomotic leak with resection and continuity restoration of the pathologic segment of small or large bowel.

Enteric Injury

CASE PRESENTATION

A 56-year-old female presents to the emergency department with fevers, abdominal pain, and drainage from her incisions from her robotic hysterectomy. Her past medical history includes diabetes, obstructive sleep apnea, and hypertension. Her past surgical history includes the recent robotic hysterectomy (she is postoperative day 5 today), an open right hemicolectomy, and three caesarian sections. She is febrile with a temperature of 38.9 °C, heart rate of 110 beats/min, and a blood pressure of 90/45 mm Hg. On examination, her incisions are noted to have bilious drainage emanating from them (**Figure 27.3**) and she has frank peritonitis. Laboratory results are notable for a white blood cell count of 18 300/mm^3, lactate of 3.6 mmol/L, creatinine of 2.4 mg/dL, hemoglobin of 9.5 g/dL, and an INR of 2.1. Intravenous access is obtained with two large bore peripheral intravenous lines and resuscitation is initiated with isotonic fluid.

Question: *What is the likely diagnosis?*

Answer: *Enteric injury*

Etiology

With the ever-increasing popularity of robotic-assisted and laparoscopic surgery over the past decades, the literature reporting complications involving the use of this technology has also grown. Fortunately, the overall rate of serious complication with minimally invasive surgery remains low. Most complications occur during abdominal entry in minimally invasive surgery. Complications can be minor, including insufflation of the subcutaneous tissue leading to subcutaneous emphysema and extraperitoneal insufflation and postoperative infection. However, they can also be major and life threatening, including injury to major blood vessels or viscera. Safe peritoneal access necessitates an understanding of and comfort with multiple entry techniques; there is no foolproof technique for the creation of pneumoperitoneum. The patient's surgical history and risk of adhesive disease, particularly when considering abdominal entry for laparoscopic trocars, should be carefully considered. Familiarity with a variety of peritoneal access techniques facilitates selecting the safest and most effective abdominal entry approach for an individual patient. However, no significant differences in overall complication rates have been found for closed compared with open techniques for primary abdominal insufflation when performed by experienced surgeons. The risk of injury with Veress needle insertion increases significantly with additional number of placement attempts and reaches 44%-74% for three and 85%-100% for four or more attempts. It is therefore recommended that an alternate entry technique be used after three failed attempts with the Veress. Secondary trocar/ports should always be placed under direct laparoscopic vision with the abdomen insufflated. This portion of the chapter will focus on enteric injury during laparoscopy.

Enteric injury is the third leading cause of death, after anesthesia and major vascular injury, following a laparoscopic procedure. Injury to the gastrointestinal tract occurs in 0.03%-0.18% of patients undergoing laparoscopic surgery, with small bowel injuries being most common. Approximately one-third of bowel injuries occur during abdominal access, and the remaining two-thirds result from dissection, electrocoagulation/thermal conduction, or tissue grasping. Many of these injuries occur out of the surgeon's primary viewing field and are not recognized during the index operation. Delayed diagnosis of a gastrointestinal injury is a significant cause of morbidity and mortality and a major reason for legal action in the United States.

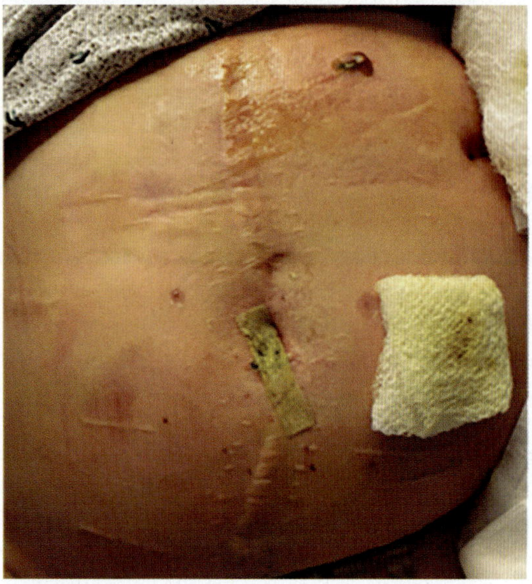

Figure 27.3 Appearance of patient's abdominal wall postoperative day 5 after robotic hysterectomy.

Evaluation and Management

Many bowel injuries (near 50%) are unrecognized intraoperatively. Symptoms related to gastrointestinal injury usually manifest within 12-36 hours postoperatively, but presentation can be delayed for up to 5 or 7 days. Clinical signs of a bowel injury range from frank peritonitis with enteric drainage from the port sites as in the case above to subtler clinical findings including intolerance to PO intake, abdominal distension, and increased abdominal pain. In general, if a patient does not gradually improve following laparoscopic surgery and continues to have abdominal pain, especially if associated with tachycardia or fever, bowel injury should be suspected and evaluation undertaken. Patients with peritoneal findings should undergo re-operation, open or laparoscopic, depending on the patient's clinical status. If the diagnosis is less clear, the most useful imaging modality is contrast-enhanced CT. Although demonstration of free intra-abdominal gas on CT is a sign of perforation, ~40% of patients will have more than 2 cm of free gas at 24 hours postlaparoscopy, despite the lack of any clinical evidence of bowel perforation. However, because laparoscopy utilizes carbon dioxide to insufflate the abdomen, any residual gas in the peritoneum should be absorbed quickly. The presence of free intra-abdominal air or free fluid in amounts greater than expected for the postoperative time frame suggests ruptured viscus until proven otherwise.

Initial management of the patient with suspected gastrointestinal perforation includes intravenous (IV) fluid therapy, cessation of oral intake, and broad-spectrum antibiotics along with source control. Emergent surgical intervention (open or laparoscopic) should be undertaken when perforation is confirmed or strongly suspected.

Iatrogenic stomach, duodenum, small bowel, colon, and rectal iatrogenic injuries are managed based upon their AAST injury grade (**Table 27.2**). Lower-grade injuries (grade I, II, or III) of the stomach, small bowel, colon, or rectum can usually be debrided and repaired primarily. On the other hand, higher-grade injuries (grade IV and V), which are less common, are generally not amenable to primary repair. High-grade injuries (IV, V) require resection and anastomosis as appropriate. Grade IV and V injuries to the stomach or duodenum often require complex repair or reconstruction depending upon the location and extent of injury as well as the patient's overall clinical status. Intestinal anastomoses can be performed using a one-layer or two-layer handsewn or stapled technique. The choice of technique depends upon the location of the injury, the patient's clinical status, and surgeon's experience and preference.

For patients with a delayed presentation or multiple injuries, consider a staged damage-control approach. The affected segments of bowel are resected using a gastrointestinal stapler and delaying restoration of gastrointestinal continuity and fascial closure until the patient has stabilized.

Endoscopy Complications

CASE PRESENTATION

A 50-year-old female presents to the emergency department with syncope and abdominal pain after undergoing a screening colonoscopy the day prior. Her past medical history includes hypertension. Her past surgical history includes a laparoscopic appendectomy. She is afebrile with a heart rate of 120 beats/min and a blood pressure of 93/48 mm Hg. On examination, she has abdominal pain. Labs are notable for a white blood cell count of 5300/mm^3, lactate of 3.6 mmol/L, creatinine of 2.4 mg/dL, hemoglobin of 8.5 g/dL, and an INR of 1.1. Intravenous access is obtained with two large bore peripheral intravenous lines and resuscitation with isotonic fluid is started.

Question: *What is the likely diagnosis?*

Answer: *Splenic injury postcolonoscopy*

Upper and lower gastrointestinal (GI) endoscopies are ubiquitous procedures, but major complications of concern to the acute care surgeon fortunately remain relatively infrequent. The most common complications of both upper and lower endoscopies are cardiopulmonary (eg, hypotension or hypoxia; 5%-10%), but the most common complications of relevance to the acute care surgeon are hemorrhage and perforation. The next sections will outline risks for, causes of, and management of common endoscopic complications. In some instances, the surgeon may be the endoscopist, and in others, the surgeon may be consulted for his or her knowledge and expertise, in the absence of the patient needing operative intervention. As such, the treatments outlined in the section will focus primarily on surgical rescue, but mention will be made of endoscopic management techniques where appropriate. A general rule is that the extent of morbidity and mortality of postendoscopic hemorrhage and perforation is largely dependent on time to diagnosis and treatment. Iatrogenic complications should be high on the list of differential diagnoses and care expedited until ruled out.

TABLE 27.2 ■ AAST Enteric Injury Grading Scales

Organ	Injury Grade	Description of Injury
Stomach	I	Contusion/hematoma Partial-thickness laceration
	II	Laceration <2 cm in GE junction or pylorus <5 cm in proximal 1/3 stomach <10 cm in distal 2/3 stomach
	III	Laceration >2 cm in GE junction or pylorus >5 cm in proximal 1/3 stomach >10 cm in distal 2/3 stomach
	IV	Tissue loss or revascularization of <2/3 of stomach
	V	Tissue loss or revascularization of >2/3 of stomach
Duodenum	I	Hematoma involving single portion of duodenum Partial-thickness laceration with no perforation
	II	Hematoma involving more than one portion Laceration with disruption of <50% of circumference
	III	Laceration with disruption of 50%-75% of circumference of D2 Laceration with disruption of 50%-100% of circumference of D1, D3, D4
	IV	Laceration with disruption of >75% of circumference of D2 Involving ampulla or distal common bile duct
	V	Laceration with massive disruption of duodenopancreatic complex Devascularization of duodenum
Small bowel	I	Contusion or hematoma without devascularization Partial-thickness laceration without perforation
	II	Laceration <50% of circumference
	III	Laceration ≥50% of circumference without transection
	IV	Transection of the small bowel
	V	Transection of the small bowel with segmental tissue loss Devascularized segment of small bowel
Colon	I	Contusion or hematoma without devascularization Partial-thickness laceration without perforation
	II	Laceration <50% of circumference
	III	Laceration ≥50% of circumference without transection
	IV	Transection of the colon
	V	Transection of the colon with segmental tissue loss Devascularized segment of colon
Rectum	I	Contusion or hematoma without devascularization Partial-thickness laceration without perforation
	II	Laceration <50% of circumference
	III	Laceration ≥50% of circumference
	IV	Full-thickness laceration with extension into the perineum
	V	Devascularized segment of rectum

Adapted from Moore EE, Cogbill TH, Malangoni MA, et al. Organ injury scaling, II: pancreas, duodenum, small bowel, colon, and rectum. *J Trauma*. 1990;30:1427-1429.

Hemorrhage

Etiology. Hemorrhage is unusual but warrants involvement of the acute care surgeon. Bleeding can be divided into two categories: local bleeding (ie, after polypectomy or therapeutic maneuver) or injury to surrounding structures (ie, splenic injury).

Local bleeding occurs in 0.1%-0.6% of therapeutic colonoscopy. Risk factors for bleeding include increasing size of polyp, sessile or thick-stalked polyps, patient antithrombotic or anticoagulant use (may increase incidence to 0.87%), and poor endoscopic technique. In the event of immediate bleeding, the cause is direct trauma and is more common when cut electrocautery is used. Delayed presentation is more common in cases in which coagulation electrocautery was used—as days' pass, the burned tissue sloughs and exposes raw mucosa, which then bleeds.

Damage to other organs (eg, the spleen) may result in intraperitoneal bleeding. The incidence of injury to the spleen is reported to be 0.004% but is likely underreported. It is thought to occur either while scoping a difficult-to-navigate sigmoid colon or at the splenic flexure itself; excessive force on the endoscope or insufflation causing the splenocolic ligament to avulse the splenic capsule results in hemorrhage. Patients with prior operations (particularly females with a history of gynecologic surgery) or a history of intra-abdominal infection or pancreatitis appear to be at higher risk, possibly due to adhesive disease.

Evaluation and management. Local bleeding can be recognized immediately at the time of endoscopy or delayed (1-14 days postprocedure), can present with hematochezia or melena, and may be accompanied by hemodynamic changes. Diagnosis is made by direct visualization (if immediate) or by history/examination. Obtain a CTA to localize bleeding and facilitate treatment. Initial interventions should focus on resuscitation and hemorrhage control. Discontinue all anticoagulation and consider reversal, based on risk-benefit analysis in the context of individual patient factors (severity of bleeding and likelihood of thrombosis). The majority of local bleeds after colonoscopy resolve with conservative management.

Occasionally, a patient will present with abdominal pain and hypotension/tachycardia. Immediate treatment should be started with IV fluids and blood product as indicated. A bedside ultrasound may help to rapidly identify intra-abdominal free fluid. While ultrasound is not specific for splenic injury, it may support the diagnosis in the appropriate clinical context. Labs and imaging should be obtained.

Given the rarity of this complication, data on optimal nonoperative management strategies are limited. Generally, these injuries are approached similarly to the management of blunt abdominal trauma and are graded using the AAST solid organ injury scale (**Table 27.3**). The grade may help guide management and stratify risk of nonoperative

TABLE 27.3 ■ AAST Splenic Organ Injury Grading Scale

Organ	Injury Grade	Description of Injury
Spleen	I	Subcapsular hematoma <10% surface area Parenchymal laceration <1 cm in depth Capsular tear
	II	Subcapsular hematoma 10%-50% surface area Intraparenchymal hematoma <5 cm Parenchymal laceration 1-3 cm
	III	Subcapsular hematoma >50% surface area Ruptured subcapsular or intraparenchymal hematoma ≥5 cm Parenchymal laceration >3 cm in depth
	IV	Any injury in the presence of a splenic vascular injury or active bleeding confined within the splenic capsule Parenchymal laceration involving segmental or hilar vessels producing >25% devascularization
	V	Any injury in the presence of splenic vascular injury with active bleeding extending beyond the spleen into the peritoneum Shattered spleen

Adapted from Kozar R, Crandall M, Shanmuganathan K, et al. Organ injury scaling 2018 update: spleen, liver and kidney. *J Trauma Acute Care Surg*. 2018;85(6):1119-1122.

treatment. Patients with hemodynamic instability or evidence of bleeding refractory to nonoperative management should be treated operatively with splenectomy, and blood product administration tailored to hemodynamic status rather than laboratory values. Damage control surgery may be indicated in cases of patient physiologic exhaustion to allow correction of coagulopathy. Patients who are hemodynamically normal/stable may be considered for nonoperative management. Consider angioembolization in cases with contrast extravasation or pseudoaneurysm on imaging. Monitor the patient for worsening abdominal exam, drop in hemoglobin, or hemodynamic changes. Any of these should prompt re-imaging and consideration of operative intervention. There are no data on the treatment of iatrogenic spleen injuries in the setting of splenic pathology (eg, tumor).

Upper GI Perforation

Etiology. Upper GI endoscopy has an overall 0.13% adverse event rate, which is increased in therapeutic (PEG, FB removal, dilatation, treatment of varices, stenting, and ablation) when compared to diagnostic procedures. The overall incidence of iatrogenic esophageal perforation may be 0.09%-2.2% for dilation of simple conditions, but higher for complex lesions (longer length, multiple areas, and strictures due to radiation). The rate may also be up to 3% for endoscopic mucosal resection (EMR) for Barret or endoscopic submucosal dissection (ESD) for squamous cell cancer. Additional risks include Zenker diverticulum, esophageal stricture, cervical osteophytes, and history of recurrent foreign body ingestion. Rarely are esophageal perforations due to biopsy.

Esophageal perforations are most commonly iatrogenic (60%) and carry high morbidity and mortality (10%-20%), increasing substantially as the time from injury to treatment widens. The perforation causes contamination of the surrounding spaces or body cavity with oral secretions and digestive fluids, which results in inflammation, severe sepsis, and possibly death. The most important factor in patient outcome is time to treatment.

Perforations of the stomach and duodenum are most commonly related to therapeutic instrumentation such as dilation of gastrointestinal anastomosis or with instrumentation during ERCP.

Evaluation and management. Given the morbidity of delayed diagnosis, iatrogenic perforation should be high on the differential diagnosis of patients with postendoscopy issues and evaluation with imaging should be performed in a timely fashion. Perforation of the different sections of the foregut has different presenting signs and symptoms.

Perforation of the esophagus may present as dysphonia, hoarse voice, dysphagia, subcutaneous air, respiratory compromise, pneumothorax, or pleural effusion. Perforations of the distal esophagus, stomach, and duodenum may be associated with abdominal pain and signs of sepsis/peritonitis. If plain films (chest and abdomen) are obtained, findings concerning for perforation include pneumoperitoneum, pneumomediastinum, subcutaneous air, or pleural effusion. A contrast-enhanced CT scan is useful to confirm suspicion (sensitivity 92%-100%) and identify extravasation of contrast, masses, abscesses, and fluid collections that may require additional therapy.

Treatment of esophageal perforation is dependent on which part of the esophagus is injured, as well as time to presentation and underlying pathology. Treatment modalities include nonoperative, endoscopic, or surgical repair. Criteria for nonoperative management are outlined in **Table 27.4.** Success rates are greater in noninflamed/nonpathologic tissue.

All patients with iatrogenic perforations should receive broad-spectrum IV antibiotics, NPO status, and proton pump inhibitor therapy (PPI). Early nutritional support (enteral route favored) is essential for healing. Endoscopic placement of NG decompression is recommended. Fluid collections (abscess and pleural effusion), if identified on imaging, should be drained via percutaneous techniques.

Primary endoscopic management is the preferred method of treatment for perforations that are recognized during the index procedure and selected patients with delayed presentation (poor surgical candidates and underlying pathology not amenable to surgical therapy). These endoscopic therapies include through-the-scope (TTS) or over-the-scope (OTS) clips, stenting, and endoscopic vacuum therapy. Clips are first line for small (<2 cm) injuries. Due to their relatively shorted arm length, TTS clips are typically reserved for smaller perforations, in benign (noninflamed) tissue. OTS clips may be successful in larger perforations, as the clips have longer arms with which to grasp tissue, and greater closing force.

Full- or partially covered self-expandable metal stents or self-expandable plastic stents are

TABLE 27.4 ■ Criteria for Nonoperative Management of Esophageal Perforation Postendoscopy

Delay in management	Early: <24 h
Clinical presentation	Absence of symptoms and signs of sepsis
Radiological criteria	Cervical or thoracic location of the esophageal perforation Contained perforation of surrounding tissues • Intramural • Minimal periesophageal extravasation of contrast material with intraesophageal drainage • Absence of massive pleural contamination
Esophageal characteristics	No preexistent esophageal disease
Other	Possibility of close surveillance by expert esophageal team Availability of round the clock surgical and radiological skills

Adapted from Chirica M, Kelly M, Siboni S, et al. Esophageal emergencies: WSES guidelines. *World J Emerg Surg*. 2019;31(14); epub.

particularly useful for larger perforations or perforations through malignant tissues. Careful stent selection is necessary to maximize therapeutic benefit while minimizing the risk of stent migration (8%-40% incidence) or crossing the UES or LES. Stents should remain for 2-4 weeks post-placement to ensure sealing of the perforation. Compared with open repair and diversion, stent placement for esophageal perforation is associated with decreased morbidity, length of stay, time to oral intake, and cost (88% success, 7.5% mortality for stent placement).

Endoluminal vacuum therapy is another advanced endoscopic technique, mainly reserved for poor surgical candidates, or those who have failed other treatment options. Analogous to other forms of negative pressure wound therapy (NPWT), endoluminal vacuum therapy is performed by the endoscopic placement of sponge/vacuum-tipped nasal tube into the defect/cavity. The tube is connected to negative pressure and allowed to granulate.

After endoscopic treatment, the patient should be observed and kept NPO until a contrast study can be obtained to confirm adequate sealing of the defect.

If patients are not candidates for NOM or endoscopic therapy fails, consider surgery. The outcomes for surgical treatment of esophageal perforation are 83% treatment success and 17% in-hospital mortality. There are reports of successful laparoscopic repair of esophageal perforation, but this approach should be performed at the discretion of the acute care surgeon. Regardless of approach, surgical management requires adequate exposure, debridement of nonviable tissue, closure of injury, use of adjacent tissue to buttress repair, and adequate drainage.

Perforation of the cervical esophagus is most likely to respond to nonoperative management due to containment of the local fascial planes. If surgery is required, attempt direct repair of the defect. The injury is approached from an incision along the anterior border of the left sternocleidomastoid muscle. A collar incision may be used if access to the contralateral side is necessary. The esophagus should be circumferentially mobilized, debrided to viable tissue, the defect repaired with single- or double-layer tension-free suture, and buttressed with local healthy tissue (eg, sternocleidomastoid muscle). Establish enteral access for feeding (either endoscopically placed NG tube or surgical jejunostomy tube) at the time of surgery. If the injury or extent of tissue damage is too large to be successfully repaired (>50% of the esophageal circumference), perform esophageal diversion and drainage.

Approach to injuries to the thoracic esophagus will be individualized based on the individual patient circumstances. Depending on the level, the best access may be achieved via either the left (distal esophagus) or the right (midthoracic esophagus) side. Imaging findings help guide selection of approach. Note that the mucosal defect is often longer than the externally visible muscular tear; a proximal and distal myotomy helps identify the true extent of injury. Once the defect has been exposed and nonviable tissue debrided, the defect is closed in two layers: the first being the mucosal layer, and second being the outer muscular layer. The repair should be free of tension and buttressed by local tissue (eg, pericardium, pleura, or intercostal muscle). Drainage of fluid collections, the mediastinum, and pleural cavity should be performed. Obtain nutritional access. If the defect is too extensive to be amenable to surgical repair, perform drainage and resection/diversion/

exclusion. Resection is preferred when there is underlying esophageal pathology, as the tissue is unlikely to heal.

Abdominal esophageal perforations are relatively uncommon and occur most frequently as a complication of an antireflux procedure. The general principles follow that of cervical and thoracic perforations: exposure, debridement to healthy tissue, tension-free repair, and local tissue buttressing. A gastric fundal wrap may be used to buttress the repair. Enteral access for nutritional support should be obtained, and the space drained.

Colonoscopic Perforation, Abdominal Compartment Syndrome

Etiology. The incidence of clinically demonstrable perforation ranges from 0.016% to 0.8% with diagnostic colonoscopy to 0.02%-8% with therapeutic colonoscopy. Risk factors for iatrogenic perforation include low BMI, advanced age, female gender, prior pelvic surgery, diverticulosis, colon obstruction, inflammatory bowel disease, and the use of advanced endoscopic therapies (eg, such as pneumatic stricture dilation, stenting, endoscopic mucosal resection [EMR], or endoscopic submucosal dissection [ESD]). Depending on the time to presentation/treatment, as well as the patient's comorbid factors, mortality may be as high as 5%-25%.

The rate of perforation also varies by colonic location: the rectosigmoid is the most common, representing 50%-60% of perforations, followed by cecum (15%-25%), hepatic flexure (10%-17%), transverse colon (7%-9%), and splenic flexure (5%-8%). Perforation may occur due to one of three mechanisms: shear or stretch pressure against the bowel wall, overinsufflation/barotrauma, or therapeutic instrumentation (eg, thermal injury, or full-thickness tissue resection). Shear/stretch injuries are more common in the rectosigmoid due to its sharp angles as well as the predilection for pelvic adhesions from prior surgeries or past episodes of diverticular disease. The cecum is most vulnerable to barotrauma due to its thin wall; the increased pressure causes linear tears along the relatively thin cecal wall, evolving into full-thickness defects. Therapeutic instrumentation injuries are more common in the transverse colon, although may occur along its entire length. Thermal injury is related to the intensity and duration of current applied, and risk may be reduced by utilizing the technique of saline injection to lift the mucosa away from the bowel wall. Thermal injury may not be full thickness and may not become apparent for several days as the injury transitions to full thickness.

Abdominal compartment syndrome is a rare, but an emergent complication of colonoscopic perforation. The insufflated air crosses into the peritoneal cavity, where intra-abdominal pressure builds. Once intra-abdominal pressure reaches a certain threshold, respiration becomes limited, and preload to the heart decreases, causing hypotension and tachycardia. (See also Chapter 10.)

Evaluation and management. The presentation, diagnosis, and treatment of colonic perforation depend on the time to recognition, patient condition, and degree of contamination. Methods of evaluation and treatment generally depend on the setting in which the perforation is recognized (intraprocedure or postprocedure), time to presentation (early/within 24 hours or delayed), and acuity of the patient. Conservative, endoscopic, and surgical therapies have all been described with some success. In general, patients who present in septic shock, with signs of peritonitis, or who exhibit gross spillage of luminal content on contrast studies require surgical treatment. Treatment is NPO, IVF hydration, and antibiotics. Parenteral nutrition should be considered in patients with signs of malnutrition or in patients who will be NPO for >7 days.

Diagnosis may be immediate (up to 68%) or delayed (23% on day 1 or 2; the remainder identified >2 days). Immediate diagnosis may be made by visualizing intraperitoneal structures, loss of insufflation, sudden pain, abdominal distention, or hemodynamic changes (in the case of increased abdominal pressures or abdominal compartment syndrome). In the event of hemodynamic collapse (hypotension and tachycardia) in the setting of immediate recognition of perforation, consideration should be given to emergent abdominal decompression.

The majority of perforations are recognized postprocedure. These typically present with worsening or unrelieved abdominal pain, inability to pass flatus, signs of sepsis (eg, tachycardia and fever), or signs of peritonitis. Diagnosis is made by imaging. Plain films may demonstrate free air under the diaphragm but are not particularly sensitive. CT is the imaging modality of choice. Sensitivity may be improved with IV and enteral contrast. Some patients will present with clinical peritonitis, but who otherwise lack imaging signs of perforation. Postpolypectomy syndrome (incidence 0.003%-0.1%) occurs due to a transmural burn to the bowel wall with localized peritonitis; there will be no radiographic evidence of perforation. Conversely, CT scan may demonstrate "false positives"—for example, up to 63% of ESD procedures may have pneumomediastinum or pneumoperitoneum on scan in the absence of true perforation. Such cases should be managed conservatively, with monitoring of the patient's examination and status.

Data are limited regarding the optimal method (endoscopic, laparoscopic, or open) of treatment of iatrogenic colon perforation. In 2018, the World Society of Emergency Surgery published a review of the data with summary recommendations (**Figure 27.4**). In general, goals of treatment are resuscitation, control of contamination, and restoration of function (either anatomic or extra-anatomic). If the perforation recognized during the endoscopic procedure is small (ie, <2 cm) and the patient remains hemodynamically appropriate, endoscopic clipping may be attempted, either by through-the-scope (TTS) clips or over-the-scope (OTS) clips. This technique is limited by the ability of the clips to grip deeper layers of colon wall and achieve adequate seal. Over-the-scope clips are available with longer clip arms than TTS clips and may have better success.

If the patient presents postprocedure, treatment is determined by the patient's clinical status and the degree of injury/contamination identified on imaging. Patients who are hemodynamically normal and free of overt signs of peritonitis or sepsis with no/minimal contrast spillage on contrast-enhanced CT scan may be monitored, kept NPO, treated with broad-spectrum antibiotics, and serially examined. Any deterioration of clinical status should prompt surgical treatment. Patients with sepsis, peritonitis, or gross extravasation of contrast on imaging should be evaluated for surgery.

Evidence is limited to support a standard method of surgical intervention. Laparotomy is the traditional approach, but iatrogenic injuries have been successfully treated via laparoscopy. Regardless of the approach, priorities of

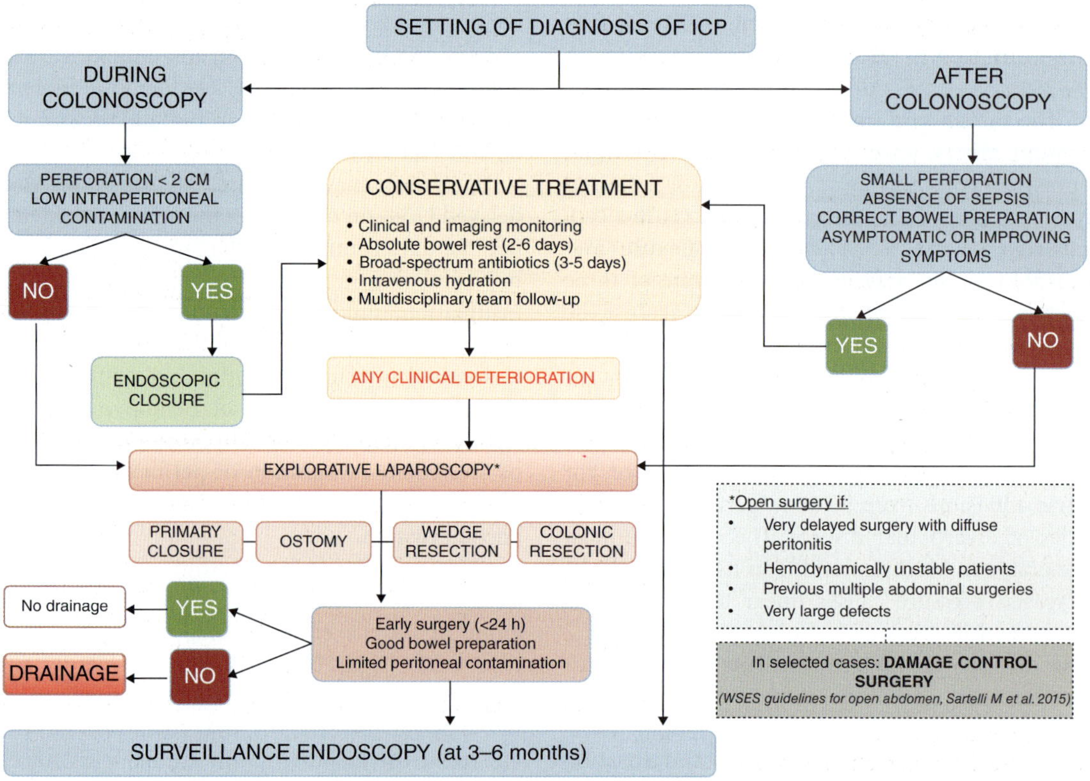

Figure 27.4 World Society of Emergency Surgery recommendations for the treatment of iatrogenic colonic perforation (ICP). (Adapted from de'Angelis N, Di Saverio S, Chiara O, et al. 2017 WSES guidelines for the management of iatrogenic colonoscopy perforation. *World J Emerg Surg*. 2018;13:5.)

operative management are control of contamination, debridement or resection of nonviable tissue, and restoration of function (either primary repair or resection, with or without proximal diversion). Simply a colotomy may be primarily repaired if small (<25% circumference), with a short time to presentation, in a hemodynamically normal patient. If the defect is too large to be successfully repaired without concern for stenosis, the area should be resected. Choice of an anatomic resection or wedge resection should be made with consideration of the patient's underlying colorectal pathology. After resection, perform a primary anastomosis in patients with appropriate tissue, comorbidities, and who are hemodynamically normal. In the setting of significant contamination, significant underlying colorectal pathology that would impair healing, or in the unstable patient, perform diversion. Damage control surgery may be appropriate in physiologically exhausted patients.

SUMMARY

In summary, acute care surgeons will continue to be called upon to manage complications as a result of operative and other invasive procedures. It is the failure to follow a normal postoperative or postprocedural course that should raise an alert that a complication may be present. The spectrum of techniques potentially required to care for these patients includes operation, surgeon-guided resuscitation, critical care, interventional procedures, endoscopic procedures, and bedside procedures. Early recognition and expeditious treatment of complications help decrease their morbidity and mortality and the "rescue" of these patients.

SUGGESTED READINGS

Ahmad G, Gent D, Henderson D, et al. Laparoscopic entry techniques. *Cochrane Database Syst Rev.* 2015;8:CD006583.

Anderson ML, Pasha TM, Leighton JA. Endoscopic perforation of the colon: lessons from a 10-year study. *Am J Gastroenterol.* 2000;95:3418-3422.

Andrade EG, Olufajo OA, Drew EL, et al. Blunt splenic injury during colonoscopy: is it as rare as we think? *Am J Surg.* 2018;215(6):1042-1045.

Badia JM, Casey AL, Petrosillo N, Hudson PM, Mitchell SA, Crosby C. Impact of surgical site infection on healthcare costs and patient outcomes: a systematic review in six European countries. *J Hosp Infect.* 2017;96:1-15.

Bakker IS, Grossmann I, Henneman D, Havnega K, Wiggers T. Risk factors for anastomotic leakage and leak-related mortality after colonic cancer surgery in a nationwide audit. *Br J Surg.* 2014;101:424-432.

Ban KA, Minei JP, Laronga C, et al. American College of Surgeons and Surgical Infection Society: surgical site infection guidelines, 2016 update. *J Am Coll Surg.* 2017;224:59-74.

Bassette M. Eckmann C, Giacobbe DR, Sartelli M, Montravers P. Post-operative abdominal infections: epidemiology, operational definitions and outcomes. *Intensive Care Med.* 2020;46:163–172.

Briggs A, Peitzman AB. Surgical rescue in medical patients—the role of acute care surgeons as the surgical rapid response team. *Crit Care Clin.* 2018;34:209-219.

Burch JM, Franciose RJ, Moore EE, et al. Single-layer continuous versus two-layer interrupted intestinal anastomosis: a prospective randomized trial. *Ann Surg.* 2000;231:832.

Chew C, Yeung J, Faragher I. Treatment of colonoscopic perforation: outcomes from a major single tertiary institution. *ANZ J Surg.* 2019;89(5):546-551.

Chirica M, Kelly M, Siboni S, et al. Esophageal emergencies: WSES guidelines. *World J Emerg Surg.* 2019;14:26.

Cirocchi R, Kelly M, Griffiths E, et al. A systematic review of the management and outcome of ERCP related duodenal perforations using a standardized classification system. *Surgeon.* 2017;15(6):379-387.

de'Angelis N, Di Saverio S, Chiara O, et al. 2017 WSES guidelines for the management of iatrogenic colonoscopy perforation. *World J Emerg Surg.* 2018;13:5.

Eisner IS, Wadhwa RK, Downing KT, Singhal PK. Prevention and management of bowel injury during gynecologic laparoscopy: an update. *Curr Opin Obstet Gynecol.* 2019;31:245-250.

Fuller J, Ashar BS, Carey-Corrado J. Trocar-associated injuries and fatalities: an analysis of 1399 reports to the FDA. *J Minim Invasive Gynecol.* 2005;12:302.

Global Guidelines for the Prevention of Surgical Site Infection. 2nd ed. World Health Organization; 2018.

Han ES, Advincula AP. Safety in minimally invasive surgery. *Obstet Gynecol Clin North Am.* 2019;46:389-398.

Härkki-Sirén P, Kurki T. A nationwide analysis of laparoscopic complications. *Obstet Gynecol.* 1997;89:108.

Hatchimonji JS, Kaufman EJ, Sharoky CE, Ma L, Garcia Whitlock AE, Holena DN. Failure to rescue in surgical patients: a review for acute care surgeons. *J Trauma Acute Care Surg.* 2019;87:699-706.

Horan TC, Gaynes RP, Martone WJ, et al. CDC definitions of nosocomial surgical site infections, 1992: a modification of CDC definitions of surgical wound infections. *Infect Control Hosp Epidemiol.* 1992;13:606-608.

Iwashita T, Lee JG, Nakai Y, et al. Successful management of perforation during cystogastrostomy with an esophageal fully covered metallic stent placement. *Gastrointest Endosc.* 2012;76:214-215.

Johnston MJ, Arora S, King D, et al. A systematic review to identify the factors that affect failure to rescue and escalation of care in surgery. *Surgery.* 2015;157:752-763.

Kang D, Ryu D, Choi C, et al. Clinical outcomes of iatrogenic upper gastrointestinal endoscopic perforation: a 10-year study. *BMC Gastroenterol.* 2019; 19(1):218.

Kelly M, Bhangu A, Singh P, Fitzgerald JEF, Tekkis PP. Systematic review and meta-analysis of trainee- versus expert surgeon-performed colorectal resection. *Br J Surg.* 2014;101:750-759.

Kirkpatrick AW, Baxter KA, Simons RK, et al. Intra-abdominal complications after surgical repair of small bowel injuries: an international review. *J Trauma.* 2003;55:399.

Ko CW, Dominitz JA. Complication of colonoscopy: magnitude and management. *Gastrointest Endosc Clin N Am* 2010;20:659-671.

Kowalczyk L, Forsmark CE, Ben-David K, et al. Algorithm for the management of endoscopic perforations: a quality improvement project. *Am J Gastroenterol.* 2011;106:1022-1027.

Kozar R, Crandall M, Shanmuganathan K, et al. Organ injury scaling 2018 update: spleen, liver and kidney. *J Trauma Acute Care Surg.* 2018;85(6):1119-1122.

Kuppusamy MK, Hubka M, Felisky CD, et al. Evolving management strategies in esophageal perforation: surgeons using nonoperative techniques to improve outcomes. *J Am Coll Surg.* 2011;213:164-171.

Kutcher ME, Sperry JL, Rosengart MR, et al. Surgical rescue: the next pillar of acute care surgery. *J Trauma Acute Care Surg.* 2017;82:280-286.

Lahat E, Batumsky M, Shapiro R, et al. Diagnosis and management of splenic injury following colonoscopy: algorithm and case series. *Tech Coloproctol.* 2016;20(3):163-169.

Lee SG, Russ A. Predicting and preventing postoperative outcomes. *Clin Colon Rectal Surg.* 2019;32:149-156.

Levy I, Gralnek I. Complications of diagnostic colonoscopy, upper endoscopy, and enteroscopy. *Best Pract Clin Gastroenterol.* 2016;30(5):705-718.

Maeda Y, Hirasawa D, Fujita N, et al. Mediastinal emphysema after esophageal endoscopic submucosal dissection: its prevalence and clinical significance. *Dig Endosc.* 2011;23:221-226.

Magrina JF. Complications of laparoscopic surgery. *Clin Obstet Gynecol.* 2002;45:469.

Mangram AJ, Horan TC, Pearson ML, Silver LC, Jarvis WR. Guideline for prevention of surgical site infection, 1999. Hospital Infection Control Practices Advisory Committee. *Infect Control Hosp Epidemiol.* 1999;20:250-280.

Martin KE, Moore CM, Tucker R, Fuchshuber P, Robinson T. Quantifying inadvertent thermal bowel injury from the monopolar instrument. *Surg Endosc.* 2016;30:4776-4784.

Merchea A, Cullinane DC, Sawyer MD, et al. Esophagogastroduodenoscopy-associated gastrointestinal perforations: a single-center experience. *Surgery.* 2010;148:876-880.

Michetti CP, Smeltzer E, Fakhry SM. Splenic injury due to colonoscopy: analysis of the world literature, a new case report, and recommendations for management. *Am Surg.* 2010;76:1198-1204.

Moore EE, Cogbill TH, Malangoni MA, et al. Organ injury scaling, II: pancreas, duodenum, small bowel, colon, and rectum. *J Trauma.* 1990;30:1427-1429.

Nduka CC, Super PA, Monson JR, Darzi AW. Cause and prevention of electrosurgical injuries in laparoscopy. *J Am Coll Surg.* 1994;179:161-170.

Okabayashi K, Ashrafian H, Zacharakis E, et al. Adhesions after abdominal surgery: a systematic review of the incidence distribution and severity. *Surg Today.* 2014;l44:405-420.

Paspatis GA, Dumonceau JM, Barthet M, et al. Diagnosis and management of iatrogenic endoscopic perforations: European Society of Gastrointestinal Endoscopy (ESGE) position statement. *Endoscopy.* 2014;46(8):693-711.

Patil N, Solanki N, Mishra P, et al. ERCP-related perforation: an analysis of operative outcomes in a large series over 12 years. *Surg Endosc.* 2020;34(1):77-87.

Raju GS, Fritscher-Ravens A, Rothstein RI, et al. Endoscopic closure of colon perforation compared to surgery in a porcine model: a randomized controlled trial (with videos). *Gastrointest Endosc.* 2008;68:324-332.

Reumkens A, Rondagh E, Bakker C, et al. Post-colonoscopy complications: a systematic review, time trends, and meta-analysis of population-based studies. *Am J Gastroenterol.* 2016;111(8):1092-1101.

Saur NM, Paulson EC. Operative management of anastomotic leaks after colorectal surgery. *Clin Colon Rectal Surg.* 2019;32:190-195.

Silber JH, Williams SV, Krakauer H, et al. Hospital and patient characteristics associated with death after surgery. A study of adverse occurrence and failure to rescue. *Med Care.* 1992;30:615-629.

Stevens DL, Bisno AL, Chambers HF, et al. Practice guidelines for the diagnosis and management of skin and soft tissue infections: 2014 update by the Infectious Diseases Society of America. *Clin Infect Dis.* 2014;59:e10-e52.

Stulberg JJ, Delaney CP, Neuhauser DV, et al. Adherence to surgical care improvement project measures and the association with postoperative infections. *JAMA.* 2010;303:2479-2485.

The Italian ColoRectal anastomotic Leakage (iCral) study group. Colorectal surgery in Italy: a snapshot from the iCral study Group. *Updates Surg.* 2019;71:339-347.

The Italian ColoRectal Anastomotic Leakage (iCral) study group. Risk factors for adverse events after elective colorectal surgery: beware of blood transfusions. *Updates Surg.* 2020;72:811-819.

Ukleja A, Afonso BB, Pimentel R, et al. Outcome of endoscopic balloon dilation of strictures after laparoscopic gastric bypass. *Surg Endosc.* 2008;22:1746-1750.

Vicente A, Jiminez P, Lopez M, et al. Management of esophageal perforation: 28-year experience in a major referral center. *Am Surg.* 2018;84(5):684-689.

Watkins JR, Farivar AS. Endoluminal therapies for esophageal perforations and leaks. *Thorac Surg Clin.* 2018;28(4):541-554.

Young PY, Khadaroo RG. Surgical site infections. *Surg Clin North Am.* 2014;94:1245-1264.

CHAPTER

28 Complications of Bariatric Surgery

Gary Alan Bass, Jonathan Imran, Paul P. Healy, and Noel G. Williams

INTRODUCTION

Obesity, an abnormal or excessive fat accumulation that may impair health, is routinely defined as a body mass index (BMI) over 30 kg/m^2. However, this is not a direct measurement of adiposity, and the UK National Institute for Health and Care Excellence recommends using waist circumference in conjunction with BMI. Worldwide, an estimated 900 million over 20 years are overweight, and 500 million people over 20 years are obese. In the United Kingdom, the Department of Health suggests that 61.3% of UK adults are either overweight or obese, with 24% of males and 26% of females being obese. Irish figures from the National Task Force on Obesity estimate that 39% of Irish adults are overweight, and 18% are obese.

Obesity impacts physical, psychological, and social health, and it is a significant risk factor for death from ischemic heart disease, diabetes mellitus, and cancer. The economic burden is substantial, with an estimated 2%-4% of health budgets in the European Union spent on adult obesity. Obesity costs the UK National Health Service £5.1 billion in 2006/2007, and data from Ireland estimated a spend of €1.13 billion in 2009 on direct and indirect obesity-related costs. Obesity reportedly costs the U.S. economy over $100 billion annually.

Lifestyle modifications form the basis of obesity interventions with adjuvants such as pharmacotherapy and surgery being employed in selected individuals. Despite advances in health promotion initiatives and pharmacotherapy, surgery has proven superiority over nonsurgical interventions in reducing weight. Consequently, there has been a trend toward an increase in surgical interventions targeting obesity, and worldwide, over 340 000 bariatric procedures are performed annually. These procedures are increasingly performed in high-volume specialist centers, and there is a further group of patients who seek such interventions abroad where follow-up and aftercare can be limited or even nonexistent.

A morbidity rate of 2.4%-10% has been reported internationally depending on the type of procedure, and recently, The National Bariatric Surgery Registry (United Kingdom) reported an overall complication rate of 2.6%. Should complications arise, many individuals may present to local and nonspecialist centers. Therefore, to manage such patients safely, acute care surgeons should know the commonly performed procedures and their associated complications.

This chapter aims to look at the standard surgical procedures performed for obesity, focusing on the associated late complications that present to emergency general surgeons and their management.

CASE PRESENTATION 1: GASTRIC BAND SLIPPAGE

A 34-year-old woman presented to the emergency department (ED) with a 4-day history of nausea, regurgitation, and upper abdominal pain. Past surgical history was significant for the insertion of a laparoscopic adjustable gastric band 3 years previously, in another country. An abdominal x-ray performed on admission revealed a "slipped" (mispositioned) gastric band (**Figure 28.1A and B**).

Question: *What would you do next?*

Answer: *A Huber needle (**Figure 28.2**) was placed into the subcutaneous port and used to aspirate the band's saline content to completion. Almost immediate symptomatic relief accompanied the band deflation. The patient proceeded to laparoscopic band removal during the same hospitalization.*

CASE PRESENTATION 2: GASTRIC BAND EROSION

A 62-year-old man presented to the ED with a 2-day history of his gastric band port protruding through the skin of his abdomen (**Figure 28.3**). He had the band inserted 8 years prior in another country and had successfully lost 63 kg. He was systemically well on admission. A computed tomography (CT) scan was performed on admission, which revealed fractured tubing and a band that had eroded into the gastric lumen (**Figure 28.4**).

Question: *What would you do next?*

Answer: *As the tubing was fractured, the patient went on to have an upper gastrointestinal endoscopy with attempted removal of the band; however, this was unsuccessful.*

Question: *What would you do next?*

Answer: *The following day, the patient underwent laparoscopic removal of the band (**Figure 28.5**). His total length of stay was 3 days.*

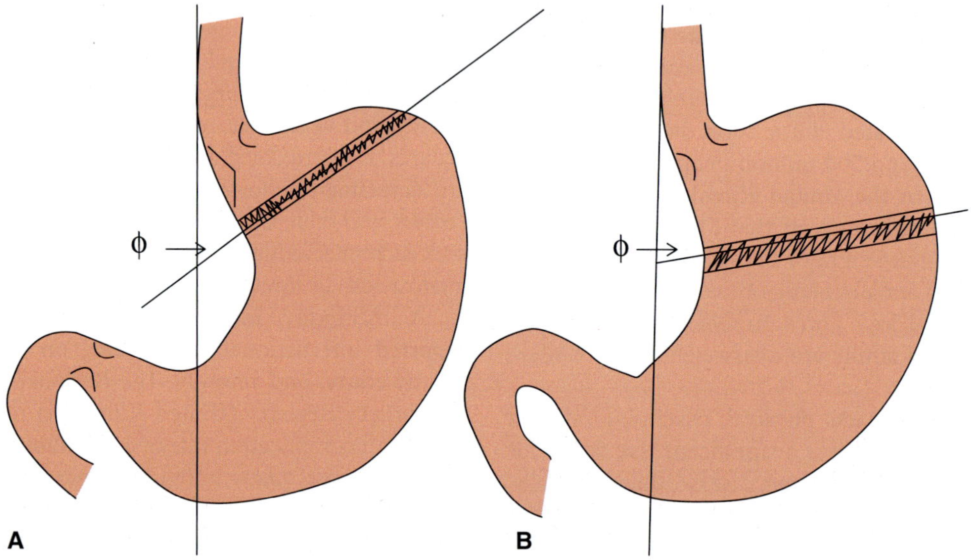

Figure 28.1 **A, B.** An abnormal Phi angle (see text) on a plain radiograph helps determine band slippage in the correct clinical context.

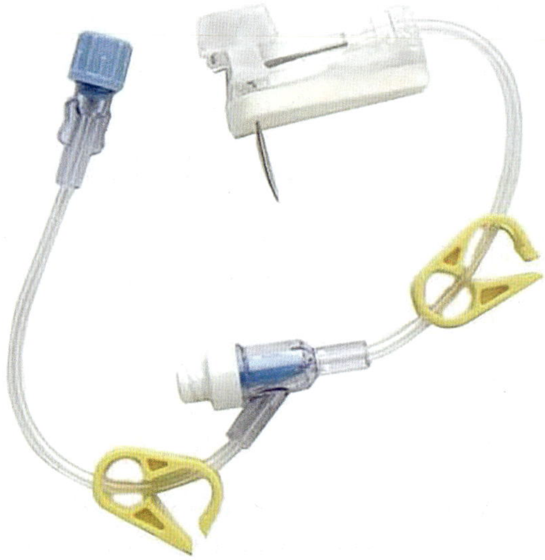

Figure 28.2 Huber needle used to access the subcutaneous port and deflate an indwelling band.

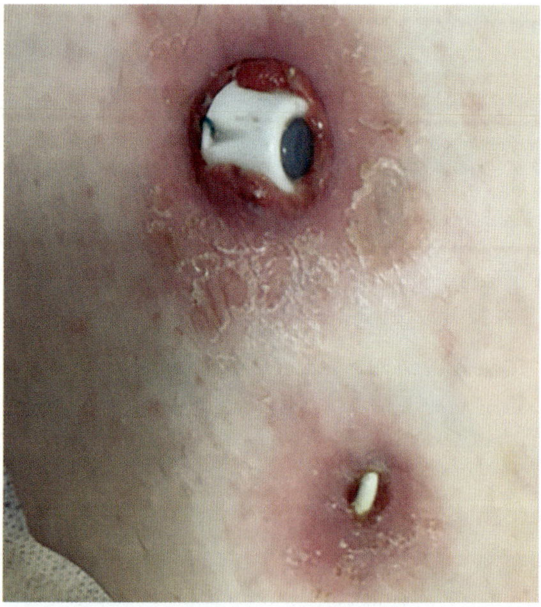

Figure 28.3 Cellulitis or skin ulceration overlying the port or tubing is often a sign of band erosion into the stomach.

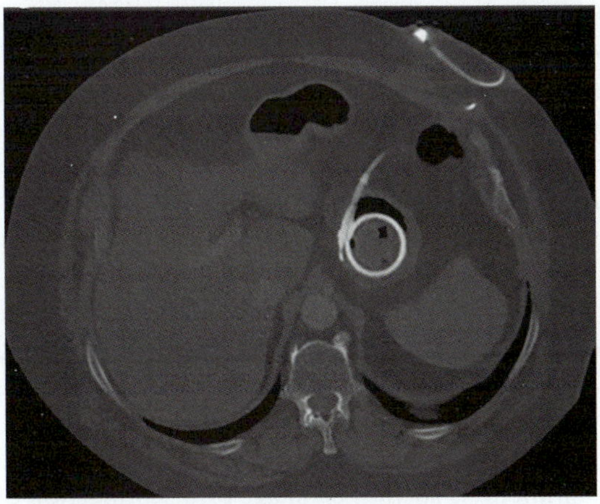

Figure 28.4 CT radiographic demonstration of band erosion in the same patient.

LAPAROSCOPIC ADJUSTABLE GASTRIC BANDING

Description

Laparoscopic adjustable gastric banding (LAGB) is a restrictive procedure where an adjustable silicone ring is placed below the gastroesophageal junction to create a pouch. It is connected to a port placed in the subcutaneous tissue and can be inflated or deflated to increase or decrease the degree of restriction. It is reversible and generally considered a safer procedure than other bariatric procedures as the GI tract is not entered, and there is no anastomosis. Nevertheless, late complications do arise, and a re-operation rate of 10%-20% has been reported. Band slippage, pouch enlargement, band erosion, and port site complications are the most common problems associated with LAGB. When evaluating patients with a history of LAGB, common presenting complaints are new-onset chest or epigastric pain, heartburn, dysphagia, or choking. Before proceeding with any interventions or further workup, it is prudent to deflate the gastric band. Most gastric bands have a balloon that is filled with 4-13 mL of fluid.

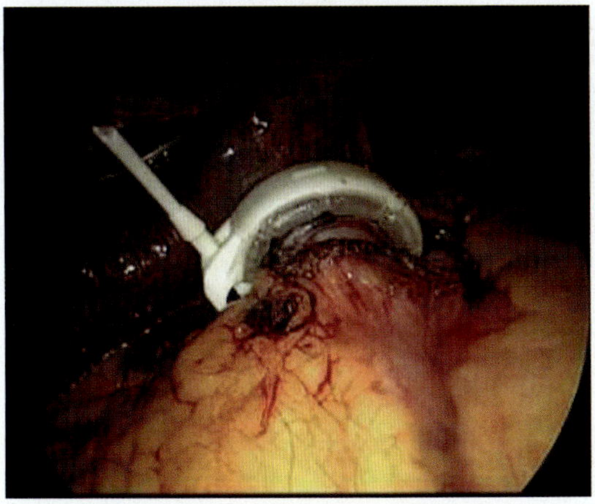

Figure 28.5 Eroded, malpositioned band on laparoscopy. Partially eroded bands may be removed laparoscopically or endoscopically. The patient should be counseled about the potential for gastric resection or gastrectomy.

Complications

Band slippage resulting in gastric prolapse occurs with cephalad prolapse of the body of the stomach or caudal movement of the band. Features suggestive of band slippage include acute dysphagia, vomiting, regurgitation, and pain (epigastric, left upper quadrant, and chest). If left untreated, the incarcerated stomach pouch may be at risk of ischemia. Investigations that can help in the diagnosis of band slippage include plain radiographs of the lower chest/upper abdomen, which show a shift in the band from a typically angled 2-8 o clock position (see **Figure 28.1A,B**) to a 4-10 o clock position. The angle formed between the spine's vertical axis and the band is the "phi angle" and should be no more than 58° (normal 4°-58°). The band's central ring may also be visible, and there will be dilation and prolapse of the gastric pouch. An upper gastrointestinal series or abdominal CT with water-soluble contrast can identify a dilated incarcerated gastric pouch.

The dilated portion of the GI tract proximal to the band with band slippage is differentiated from pouch dilation by this abnormally positioned band and acute symptoms. Urgent intervention is required to deflate the band (typically found in the left upper quadrant or over the sternum) using a Huber or spinal needle as complications can include gastric perforation and stomach necrosis. If access to the port is difficult, it can also be accessed via ultrasound guidance or fluoroscopy. If symptoms fail to improve with the band's full deflation or if the patient exhibits signs of sepsis and peritonitis, perform operative exploration via laparoscopy or exploratory laparotomy. When evaluating a band during exploration, we recommend beginning dissection of the band in the lesser sac to avoid mobilization or manipulation of the herniated stomach, especially if it appears ischemic. The band and surrounding capsule should be identified (see **Figure 28.5**), and the capsule divided. The buckle is identified and unbuckled, and the slippage is reduced. If the band cannot be released, it can be cut and removed from its tract. It is essential to identify and divide any remaining constricting capsules to prevent further problems. If the herniated stomach appears ischemic but not frankly necrotic, it may be useful to evaluate viability after re-perfusion. In this case, a second-look operation is indicated. In cases with frankly necrotic tissue, resection is the operation of choice. A sleeve gastrectomy or fundal resection may be accomplished with the aid of a bougie or endoscopic guidance.

Pouch enlargement is the dilation of the proximal gastric pouch with or without a change in the band angle and obstruction. The patient may present with a lack of satiety, heartburn, regurgitation, and occasional chest pain and is diagnosed with an upper GI contrast series. It occurs due to overinflation or overeating. Nonoperative management, which includes band deflation, a low-calorie diet, and reduced portion sizes, is successful in treating up to 77% of patients. If unsuccessful (ie, the pouch remains enlarged), surgical removal or replacement is needed.

As mentioned above, band slippage and pouch enlargement can be managed by the acute care surgeon with complete band deflation. Being familiar with the technique to deflate the balloon can remedy both clinical problems, particularly band slippage, and prevent complications such as necrosis or perforation.

Band erosion can occur both early or many years after surgery. A review of 15 775 patients reported an incidence of 1.46% and in other series the rate has been between 0.2% and 3.3%. Early erosion may occur due to gastric injury or a microperforation that initiates a chronic inflammatory process and eventual erosion. Late erosions are believed to result from chronic ischemia due to an excessively tight band. Band erosion may manifest with a loss of restriction, epigastric pain, gastrointestinal bleeding, or intra-abdominal abscess or port site infection. At endoscopy, the gastric band is visible within the gastric lumen on retroflection. If this is discovered, management involves band removal via laparoscopy or laparotomy and complete drainage. The repair of the site of erosion should not be attempted during initial exploration. It may be possible to remove the band at endoscopy. However, it is recommended that this be performed by a bariatric or endoscopic specialist.

Port site complications include infection and malfunctions such as breakage or disconnection of the tubing. Infection may manifest in the early postoperative period as localized erythema, swelling, and pain, which may be successfully treated with antibiotics. If unsuccessful, and infection is limited to the port, it can be removed and the tubing tied off with suture and reinserted once the infection resolves. Late port site infection may be due to band erosion, and loss of restriction may also be present in such a scenario. Port malfunction can occur as a result of disconnection of the tubing or when leakage occurs and may be suspected if weight regain occurs. Disconnection can be assessed by plain radiograph or fluoroscopic examination, and leakage will be evident by a discrepancy in the volume of saline injected and subsequently aspirated. It is also indicated if the injection of saline does not result in any restriction.

Both band erosion and port site complications can generally be safely referred back to bariatric surgeons or an upper gastrointestinal surgeon for further management. However, if the patient is unwell, the acute care surgeon may need to intervene sooner.

CASE PRESENTATION 3: SMALL BOWEL OBSTRUCTION

A 65-year-old woman was transferred from a peripheral hospital with severe central abdominal pain, distension, and vomiting for 24 hours. She had a background history of a gastric bypass 9 years previously. A CT in the peripheral hospital revealed small bowel obstruction secondary to an internal hernia with a 3-cm neck (**Figure 28.6A and B**).

Question: *What would you do next?*

Answer: *The patient underwent a laparotomy on the same day of transfer. Intraoperatively, the entire small bowel had herniated through the mesenteric defect from her previous surgery. It was decompressed via an enterotomy, the hernia was reduced, and the mesenteric defect closed.*

CASE PRESENTATION 4: ANASTOMOTIC/SUTURE LINE LEAK

A 37-year-old woman developed hypotension, tachycardia, and increasing abdominal pain on postoperative day 2 following a single-anastomosis laparoscopic gastric bypass. On physical examination, involuntary

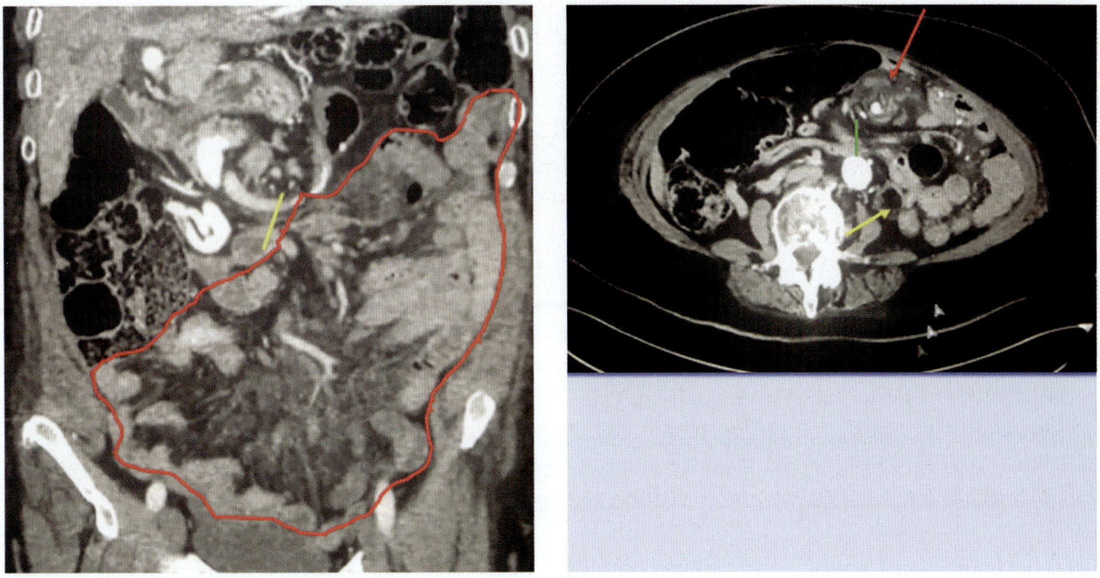

A B

Figure 28.6 Coronal **(A)** and axial **(B)** CT slices demonstrating internal herniation of small bowel through Peterson mesenteric defect following Roux-en-Y gastric bypass. Axial image shows the hernia neck (*green line*), "whorling" of the mesentery (*red arrow*), and the entire small bowel to the left of the large bowel (*yellow arrow*).

boardlike rigidity of the abdominal musculature was noted. Contrast-enhanced CT demonstrated extraluminal gas and the extravasation of water-soluble oral contrast at the esophagogastric angle of His.

Question: *What would you do next?*

Answer: *The patient was returned emergently to the operating room, where dehiscence of the suture line was oversewn.*

CASE PRESENTATION 5: SLEEVE GASTRECTOMY STAPLE LINE BLEED

A 28-year-old woman was found to be anxious, diaphoretic, and tachycardic and hypotensive in the surgical ward on the evening of postoperative day 1 following a laparoscopic sleeve gastrectomy. Abdominal distension and tenderness were noted on physical examination, as well as pallor of the conjunctiva. Complete blood count revealed a serum hemoglobin of 7.1. The patient was returned to the operating room for diagnostic laparoscopy where the clot was washed out and active ooze was noted at the resection staple line. Precise electrocautery was applied to the bleeding points, taking care not to cause a thermal gastrotomy.

Question: *What would you do next?*

Answer: *The patient was returned to the ward and was discharged well on postoperative day 3.*

ROUX-EN-Y GASTRIC BYPASS

Description

Roux-en-Y gastric bypass initially involves forming a gastric pouch of ~30 mL volume from the proximal stomach and the division of small bowel at a point 50-100 cm from the duodenojejunal flexure. The distal small bowel (Roux limb) is then anastomosed to the newly formed pouch to create a gastrojejunostomy. The bypassed segment of the stomach and proximal small bowel (biliopancreatic limb) is then anastomosed to the small bowel 100-150 cm from the newly formed gastrojejunostomy. Overall, the procedure produces weight loss by both restrictions of intake and malabsorption (**Figure 28.7**).

Complications

Surgical complications occur due to physiological changes and the alteration in anatomy and include obstruction (gastric remnant distention and anastomotic stenosis), hemorrhage, marginal

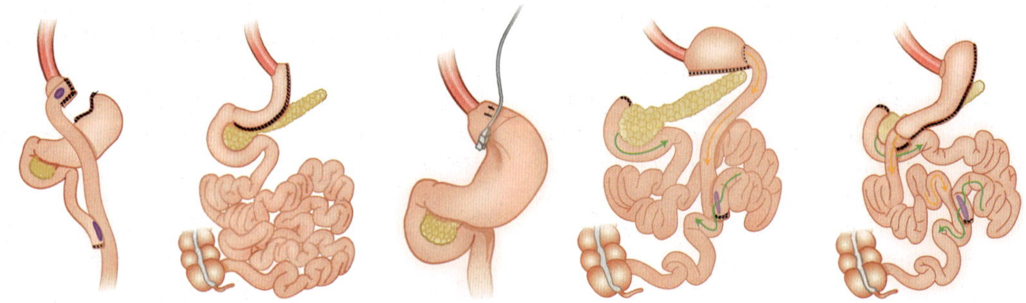

Figure 28.7 Current bariatric and metabolic operations. (Reprinted with permission, Cleveland Clinic Foundation ©2022. All Rights Reserved. In: Peitzman AB, Yealy DM, Fabian TC, et al. *The Trauma Manual: Trauma and Acute Care Surgery*. 5th ed. Wolters Kluwer; 2020. Figure 74.1.)

ulceration, and anastomotic leak. Other complications include short bowel syndrome, dumping syndrome, and nutritional deficiencies but may not present as primary surgical emergencies (**Table 28.1**).

Small bowel obstruction can occur at any point from the newly formed gastrojejunal anastomosis to the terminal ileum. In a review of 2395 patients, small bowel obstruction incidence has been reported at 3.9%. Potential causes include adhesions (48.4%), internal hernias (28%), and kinking of the jejunojejunal anastomosis (13%). Symptoms vary depending on the level of obstruction and include colicky abdominal pain, nausea and vomiting, abdominal distention, and constipation. Despite vomiting being a well-associated feature of small bowel obstruction, it may be absent if the obstruction is confined to the biliopancreatic limb. In a patient with a history of a gastric bypass procedure that presents with evidence of small bowel obstruction, assume it is due to an internal hernia until proven otherwise.

CT is useful in ruling out mechanical obstruction, but if an obstruction is identified it can highlight a transition point. Obstruction of any etiology distal to the jejunojejunal anastomosis can dilate the biliopancreatic limb, Roux limb, and gastric remnant. Bilious vomiting is a feature, and insertion of a nasogastric tube may decompress the proximal small bowel. Obstruction of the biliopancreatic limb results in a dilated biliopancreatic limb, duodenum, and gastric remnant and can give rise to abnormal liver function tests and an elevated serum amylase. An isolated dilation of the Roux limb occurs in obstruction proximal to the jejunojejunal anastomosis and bilious vomiting is unusual in this scenario. However, following gastric bypass, the sensitivity of CT in

TABLE 28.1 ■ Roux-en-Y Bypass (RYGB): Causes and Treatment of Small Bowel Obstruction

Cause	Time of Onset	Treatment
Jejunojejunal (JJ) obstruction	Early[a], Late[b]	Replace antiobstruction suture, revise JJ, lysis of adhesion(s)
Mesenteric window	Early	Reduce herniated Roux limb and resuture
Intraluminal hematoma	Early	Exploration and clot removal
Internal hernias	Early, late	Mesenteric defect/window, Petersen defect, biliopancreatic defect—operative reduction and repair for each
Jejunal intussusception	Late	Reduction or resection
Incisional/port site hernia	Early, late	Reduction and hernia repair

[a]Early <30 days postbariatric surgery.
[b]Late >30 days postbariatric surgery.
From Peitzman AB, Yealy DM, Fabian TC, et al. *The Trauma Manual: Trauma and Acute Care Surgery*. 5th ed. Wolters Kluwer; 2020.

identifying obstruction is reduced (51% vs 80%-90% in patients without gastric bypass).

Despite the well-documented benefits of laparoscopic surgery, its use in *Roux-en-Y* gastric bypass is associated with an increase in internal hernia formation. This is believed to be due to fewer adhesions that develop following a laparoscopic approach. Sites of potential herniation include the following:

A. The defect in the transverse mesocolon if the Roux limb is placed in a retrocolic position (mesocolic)
B. The space between the Roux limb mesentery and transverse mesocolon (Peterson hernia)
C. The mesenteric defect at the site of the jejunojejunostomy
D. The suture line between the Roux and biliopancreatic limbs (see Chapter 16, Figure 16.15)

These internal hernias can present acutely with evidence of strangulation or with recurrent episodes of colicky abdominal pain. Imaging may be nondiagnostic. The presence of mesenteric swirling on CT raises the suspicion of an internal hernia, but contrast reaching the colon does not exclude it from the differential diagnosis. Due to the risk of strangulation, have a low threshold for surgical exploration in an emergency setting. Operative management involves reducing the internal hernia, removing nonviable bowel, and closing any mesenteric defects.

Gastric remnant syndrome is a rare sequela of obstruction, but failure to recognize its occurrence can lead to perforation, peritonitis, and death. Features include epigastric pain, hiccups, a distended and tympanic upper abdomen, dyspnea, or tachycardia. A plain abdominal radiograph may show a gastric air bubble and diagnosis can be confirmed on CT imaging with oral contrast. A dilated gastric remnant with a collapsed duodenum can indicate an obstruction in the pyloric region, but this will not be amenable to standard interventions such as nasogastric tube decompression. Urgent decompression with a gastrostomy tube (operative or percutaneous) is warranted in such cases.

Stomal (anastomotic) stenosis has been documented in up to 6% and may present with symptoms of nausea, vomiting, gastroesophageal reflux, or dysphagia. Diagnosis can be established with an upper GI contrast series, although endoscopy is both diagnostic and therapeutic. Endoscopic dilatation is safe and effective, but some may require more than one dilation, and perforation can occur. It is appropriate that if anastomotic stenosis is identified and requires dilation, it should be referred back to the initial bariatric surgeon or upper gastrointestinal surgeon. It usually does not require emergency intervention.

Marginal ulcers usually occur on the jejunal aspect of the gastrojejunal anastomosis. An upper endoscopy is warranted in patients presenting with a history of Roux-en-Y gastric bypass and symptoms of a marginal ulcer (food intolerance, abdominal pain, dysphagia, nausea, or emesis). Most marginal ulcers will resolve with nonoperative management. This should include cessation of nonsteroidal anti-inflammatory drugs and aspirin use, as well as smoking cessation. A proton pump inhibitor should be started, and testing for Helicobacter pylori should be performed. If a perforated marginal ulcer is suspected, perform an upright chest x-ray or CT scan of the abdomen and pelvis. The patient should also be started on broad-spectrum antibiotics, resuscitated appropriately, and taken to the operating room for exploration. If a perforation is identified, contamination should be controlled, and when possible, an omental patch placed over the perforation, and adequate drainage should be accomplished.

Upper gastrointestinal hemorrhage is rare following Roux-en-Y gastric bypass and occurs more commonly in the early postoperative period due to marginal ulcers at the gastrojejunostomy. Suspected upper GI hemorrhage should be managed according to local and national guidelines and an upper gastrointestinal endoscopy performed. If the source of hemorrhage is not identified, further investigations include colonoscopy and angiography. In the context of ongoing hemorrhage without a definitive source, the gastric remnant and duodenum may need to be explored. However, rarely do these require surgical intervention for hemorrhage control.

LAPAROSCOPIC SLEEVE GASTRECTOMY

Description

Laparoscopic sleeve gastrectomy (LSG) results in a narrow tubular stomach formation by dividing and excising a significant portion of the stomach. Its effects as a weight loss procedure are mediated through both restriction and hormonal changes. These changes are believed to be related to reduced serum ghrelin levels, which generally stimulate hunger. The procedure maintains a functioning pylorus, avoids an anastomosis and insertion of a foreign body, and preserves normal intestinal absorption.

Complications

Long-term complications are related to strictures, which can occur at the gastroesophageal junction or incisura angularis and manifest with dysphagia and vomiting. As with stomal stenosis, these are usually investigated with an upper GI contrast study or endoscopy and can be treated with endoscopic dilation. However, if dilation is required, it should ideally be done by the bariatric or upper gastrointestinal surgeon.

Patients with a history of LSG are also at risk of leak and fistula formation. If re-operation for a gastric sleeve leak is required, the goal should be to drain the affected area widely. This is accomplished through laparoscopy, open exploration, or percutaneous drainage. It is also vital to evaluate for a distal stricture, as this is a risk factor for gastric sleeve leakage. Other repair options include sleeve resection with esophagojejunostomy, primary repair, or endoscopic stent placement. Placement of a T-tube through the anastomotic defect to create a controlled fistula while also inserting a feeding jejunostomy into the Roux limb has also been described. As with other GI-related complications, basic surgical principles of resuscitation, initiation of broad-spectrum antibiotics +/− antifungal agents, and bowel rest should be accomplished.

SUMMARY

The incidence of complications after bariatric surgery depends on the duration of follow-up, the type of complication, the specific bariatric procedure performed, and individual patient characteristics. Peritoneal signs are blunted and even absent in the severely obese patient. Patients who develop a small bowel obstruction after Roux-en-Y gastric bypass require prompt surgical, not conservative management, due to the likelihood of internal hernias and the high risk for bowel infarction. Anastomotic leaks occur early after RYGB, but staple line leaks can occur months later after LSG. The approach to choledocholithiasis in the RYGB patient requires alternate access to the common bile duct.

SUGGESTED READINGS

Copaescu C, Smeu B, Habibi M. Roux-en-Y feeding jejunostomy—the preferred surgical option for enteral nutrition in patients with leaks or fistula after gastric sleeve. *Chirurgia*. 2019;114:798-808.

El-Hayek K, Timratana P, Shimizu H, Chand B. Marginal ulcer after Roux-en-Y gastric bypass: what have we really learned? *Surg Endosc*. 2012;26(10):2789-2796.

Kawkabani Marchini A, Denys A, Paroz A, et al. The four different internal hernias occur after laparoscopic. Roux-en-Y gastric bypass performed for morbid obesity: is there any multidetector computed tomography (MDCT) features permitting their distinction? *Obes Surg*. 2011;21(4):506-516.

Lee YC, Wang HP, Yang CS, et al. Endoscopic hemostasis of a bleeding marginal ulcer: hemo-clipping or dual therapy with epinephrine injection, and heater probe thermocoagulation. *J Gastroenterol Hepatol*. 2002;17(11):1220-1225.

Leyba JL, Navarrete S, Navarrete Llopis S, Sanchez N, Gamboa A. Laparoscopic technique for hernia reduction and mesenteric defect closure in patients with internal hernia as a postoperative complication of laparoscopic Roux-en-Y gastric bypass. *Surg Laparosc Endosc Percutan Tech*. 2012;22(4):e182-e185.

Martin MJ. AAST Joint Panel. *Bariatric Emergencies and Damage Control for the Acute Care Surgeon, 2017 SAGES Annual Meeting in Houston, TX*. 2017.

Wendling MR, Linn JG, Keplinger KM, et al. Omental patch repair effectively treats perforated marginal ulcer following Roux-en-Y gastric bypass. *Surg Endosc*. 2013;27(2):384-389.

Wernick B, Jansen M, Noria S, Stawicki SP, El Charr M. Essential bariatric emergencies for the acute care surgeon. *Eur J Trauma Emerg Surg*. 2016;42:571-584.

CHAPTER

29 Complications of Wound Healing

David Silver, Rafael G. Ramos-Jimenez, and Matthew D. Neal

CASE PRESENTATION

A 75-year-old male with a past medical history of COPD and cirrhosis presents after a ground level fall and is diagnosed with a left hip fracture, with planned nonoperative management. His primary and secondary surveys are unremarkable, and further imaging reveals no other injuries but identifies multiple subsegmental pulmonary emboli. The patient is admitted for heparinization, pain control, and physical therapy evaluation. The patient passes no flatus and has no bowel movements during the first hospital day, and his abdominal examination revealed mild distension without tenderness or peritoneal signs. On the morning of hospital day 2, the patient is noted to be increasingly distended and exquisitely tender in the right upper and lower quadrants. Cross-sectional imaging reveals a colonic ileus with cecal pneumatosis and a cecal diameter of 10 cm.

The patient is taken to the OR for exploratory laparotomy. A dilated right colon and cecum are noted immediately upon entry to the abdomen, and a focal area of patchy necrosis is seen in the anterior aspect of the cecum without evidence of perforation or gross contamination. Given the distension of the remaining colon and the patient's ongoing anticoagulation, a right hemicolectomy and ileostomy are performed. The abdomen is closed and the subcutaneous tissues are loosely approximated.

Over the next 5 days, the patient tolerates limited oral intake. He develops serosanguinous drainage from his midline. There are no associated febrile episodes, skin erythema, or leukocytosis. On the night of postoperative day 6, the patient has a sudden increase in abdominal pain, tachycardia, and dehiscence of his laparotomy incision. The patient undergoes a laparotomy with fascial dehiscence repair, recovers uneventfully, and presents to the clinic 6 months later for ileostomy takedown and ventral hernia repair.

Questions: *What is the burden of surgical site infections (SSIs) in the EGS population? What are the evidence-based approaches for preventing and managing the complications of wound healing and SSIs in the EGS population? How can we reduce both the short- and long-term risk of wound complications in the EGS patient population?*

Answers: *Please see the sections that follow for question answers.*

INTRODUCTION

This chapter discusses the clinical aspects of wound healing, the added burden that wound complications impose on our patients, and the treatment of these complications. Wound healing is the process by which injured or infected tissue regains its integrity and function. Tissue can regain ~80% of its preinjury strength, architecture, and function. Physiologic stressors, such as those seen in emergency general surgery (EGS) patients, can compromise wound healing and lead to wound-related complications. We believe acute care surgeons can offer comprehensive risk reduction by bundling successful interventions in the preoperative, operative, and postoperative stages of the EGS patient.

In the United States, surgical site infections (SSIs) are the most common and costly hospital-acquired infections (HAIs). About 160 000-300 000 SSIs are documented every year, with an estimated annual cost of $3.5 billion to $10 billion. Patients with SSIs have a longer length of stay (LOS) and an increased risk of readmission. More importantly, they are twice as likely to die even when adjusted for age and comorbidity. It is estimated that 55% of all SSIs are "reasonably preventable" with adherence to existing wound care guidelines. However, despite evidence-based guidelines and quality improvement initiatives, provider compliance is still lacking.

PREOPERATIVE STRATEGIES

The optimization of chronic health issues and malnutrition is the foundation of successful wound healing (see **Table 29.1**). While these strategies are difficult to implement in the preoperative setting of emergency general surgery and trauma, careful consideration should be given to the risk benefit ratio of temporarily delaying an operation and

TABLE 29.1 ■ Chronic Illness and Wound Healing Complications

Disease	Risk Factor or Intervention	Effect	Level of Evidence (GRADE)
COPD	GOLD class 3 or 4	OR = 4.0	Low quality
Diabetes	$HbA_{1c} \geq 7\%$	OR = 2.13	Moderate quality
Chronic kidney disease	Stage 3 or stage 4 CKD is associated with a significant increase in wound infections	RR = 2.6	Moderate quality
Tobacco dependence	Heterogeneous but effect seen with at least 4 wk of preoperative smoking cessation	RR = 0.56	High quality
Alcohol dependence	Not an *independent* risk factor for surgical site infections	—	Moderate quality

Data from Britt LD, Peitzman AB, Jurkovich GJ, Barie PS, eds. *Acute Care Surgery*. Wolters Kluwer; 2018:92.

gaining the opportunity to correct acute physiologic derangements in an effort to maximize tissue perfusion, normothermia, normoxia, and glycemic control. Other nonmodifiable risk factors, at least in the emergent setting, such as smoking, contaminated wound, body mass index, and number of blood transfusions are important to recognize to properly risk stratify patients and plan future procedures. If an operation can be safely completed in an elective or semielective fashion, and the aforementioned variables can be optimized, wound complications are considerably reduced.

Evaluation of nutritional status assessment should be included in all preoperative assessments (see Chapter 7). Serum albumin is a predictor of perioperative morbidity and mortality. However, in the acute and critical care settings, traditional serum protein markers (albumin and prealbumin) are often a reflection of the acute physiologic response to inflammation. However, they do not reliably represent a patient's nutritional status. Other surrogate measurements such as muscle mass are still undergoing validity trials. In addition to targets for optimization, nutritional status evaluation can provide information for better patient counseling and shared decision-making. Nutrition Risk Screening Tool provides a granular assessment and was validated in patients undergoing abdominal surgery (**Table 29.2**). Ranging from 0 to 7, scoring >3 indicates significant nutritional risk. **Table 29.3** summarizes recommendations for preoperative nutritional optimization.

Early nutrition should be initiated within 24-48 hours in critically ill patients who are unable to maintain volitional intake. Enteral nutrition is preferred over peripheral nutrition if the gastrointestinal tract can tolerate feeds. In patients on stable or decreasing vasopressor requirements, initiating enteral nutrition is recommended.

Frailty describes a domain of risk that is *not* captured by malnutrition and comorbid illnesses. It can be conceptualized as a diminished ability to recover from physiological insults. Frailty is most commonly measured with 5 items: unintentional weight loss >10 lb in the past year, grip strength below the 20th percentile, self-reported exhaustion, low physical activity, and slow walking speed as measured by a 4-minute walking test. Intermediate frailty is a score of 2 or 3 and frail is a score of 4 or 5. A frailty score of 2 or 3 translates into a twofold increase in postoperative complications as defined by the National Surgical Quality Improvement Project (NSQIP); frailty has been linked to postoperative complications *independently* of age. Prehabilitation and nutritional counseling have been used to optimize frail patients with good results.

End-stage liver disease (ESLD) and cirrhosis are two medical comorbidities that deserve special attention. These disease processes are associated with poor surgical outcomes and wound healing complications. A multidisciplinary approach including hepatology is critical for appropriate preoperative and postoperative care. If unavailable, providers should consider transferring to a higher level of care. Coagulopathy, portal hypertension, ascites, and malnutrition are eventual sequelae of cirrhosis, requiring intensive evaluation and treatment to prevent catastrophic complications. Mayo, Meld, Childs-Pugh, and Vocal-Penn are validated risk stratification systems to help in informed decision-making for patients, families, and providers.

TABLE 29.2 ■ NRS-2002

Impaired Nutritional Status		Severity of Disease	
Absent (Score 0)	Normal nutritional status	Absent (Score 0)	Normal nutritional requirements
Mild (Score 1)	Weight loss >5% in 3 mo Food intake below 50%-75% of normal requirements in preceding week	Mild (Score 1)	Hip fracture Chronic patients, in particular with acute complications: cirrhosis, COPD Chronic hemodialysis, diabetes, oncology
Moderate (Score 2)	Weight loss >5% in 2 mo BMI 18.5-20.5 and impaired general condition Food intake 25%-60% of normal requirement in preceding week	Moderate (Score 2)	Major abdominal surgery Stroke Severe pneumonia Hematologic malignancy
Severe (Score 3)	Weight loss >5% in 1 mo (15% in 3 mo) BMI < 18.5 and impaired general condition or PO intake <25% of normal requirement in preceding week	Severe (Score 3)	Head injury Bone marrow transplantation Intensive care patients (APACHE > 10)
Age	If ≥70 years old add 1 to total score		

Data from Britt LD, Peitzman AB, Jurkovich GJ, Barie PS, eds. *Acute Care Surgery*. Wolters Kluwer; 2018:93.

Although most of the preoperative strategies discussed are not applicable in urgent or emergent scenarios, their use in the interventions that follow the index procedure will help minimize the risk of wound complications.

OPERATIVE STRATEGIES

To minimize wound complications, employ standard sterile and antiseptic technique for all surgical procedures as well as intraoperative management of oxygenation, volume and maintenance of normovolemia status, temperature, and tight glucose control (see **Table 29.4**).

After the operation, laparotomy closure can be completed with early primary (closure at the initial operation), early definitive (during initial hospitalization), or delayed primary closure (see Chapters 9 and 10). The consensus opinion

TABLE 29.3 ■ Preoperative Nutritional Interventions

Population Studied	Intervention	Effect	Level of Evidence (GRADE)
Patients undergoing abdominal surgery with an NRS ≥ 5	Minimum of 7 d of parenteral or enteral nutrition before surgery	Complication rate of 25.6% in those receiving nutritional support vs 50.6% in the control group	Moderate quality
Patients undergoing colorectal resection for cancer	Oral intake of arginine and n-3 fatty acids for 5 d before surgery	Infection rate of 12% in preoperative nutritional support group vs 32% in control	Moderate quality
Systematic review and meta-analysis of randomized trials involving surgical patients	Heterogeneous but mostly immunomodulatory nutrition (IN) vs standard oral nutrition supplements (ONS)	No significant difference between IN and ONS	High quality

Data from Britt LD, Peitzman AB, Jurkovich GJ, Barie PS, eds. *Acute Care Surgery*. Wolters Kluwer; 2018:93.

TABLE 29.4 ■ Standard Antiseptic Interventions and Intraoperative Management

Intervention	Description	Strength of Recommendation	Level of Evidence (GRADE)
Hand antisepsis	Use of waterless chlorhexidine scrub or traditional water-based scrubs prior to gowning and gloving is appropriate and equivalent.	Strong	Moderate
Surgical site preparation	Use of chlorhexidine preps is appropriate and superior to other preps.	Strong	Low-moderate
Antibiotic prophylaxis	Administer appropriate antibiotics within 1 h prior to procedure or 2 h for vancomycin or fluoroquinolones.	Strong	Moderate
Perioperative oxygenation	Use of 80% FiO_2 intraoperatively and postoperatively for 2-6 h.	Strong	Moderate
Normothermia	Avoidance of hypothermia with the use of warming devices.	Conditional	Moderate
Normovolemia	Intraoperative goal-directed fluid therapy.	Conditional	Low
Glucose control	Intraoperative blood glucose control (110-150 mg/dL).	Conditional	Low

Data from Britt LD, Peitzman AB, Jurkovich GJ, Barie PS, eds. *Acute Care Surgery*. Wolters Kluwer; 2018:94.

of hernia societies and our practice is to close by approximating viable tissues in a tension-free fashion with a 1:4 wound to suture ratio with continuous, slowly absorbable suture (see **Table 29.5**). In the setting of trauma and significant contamination, delayed skin closure should be considered to reduce the risk of superficial SSI. Of note, 7 RCTs comparing saline irrigation with povidone-iodine irrigation have shown that povidone-iodine irrigation significantly reduced SSIs.

Often, physiologic derangements limit delayed primary closure. In this case, the clinical team should complete daily assessments of limiting factors and consider abdominal closure a priority. Each day with an open abdomen, the risk of wound contraction, ventral herniation, and fistula formation are higher. The primary closure rates have a bimodal distribution, with early closure determined by postoperative ICU care and delayed closure impacted by the temporary

TABLE 29.5 ■ Midline Laparotomy Closure

Intervention	Recommendation	Effect	Strength of Recommendation	Level of Evidence (GRADE)
Continuous vs interrupted suturing	Continuous	OR 0.59 for VH	Strong	High
Mass closure vs single layer closure	Single layer	—	Weak	Low
Suture length to wound length ratio	4:1	OR = 3.7 for VH	Weak	Moderate
Suture material	Slowly absorbable	OR = 0.6 for VH	Strong	High
"Small bites" vs large bites	"Small bites" (0.5-0.8 cm from the wound edge separated by 0.5-cm intervals)	OR = 2.1 for SSI when large bites OR = 3.7 for VH when large bites used	Weak	Moderate

Data from Britt LD, Peitzman AB, Jurkovich GJ, Barie PS, eds. *Acute Care Surgery*. Wolters Kluwer; 2018:94.

abdominal closure technique. Of note, although some authors report no difference in outcomes between early mesh repair and early component separation, this is highly controversial. Recent recommendations from the World Society of Emergency Surgery and the European Hernia Society do not advocate early component separation with the open abdomen. Available data suggest that the risk of development of a hernia decreases with mesh placement as reinforcement for the fascial closure. However, this is at the expense of a higher rate of wound infection, at times requiring extirpation of the mesh. There is increasing interest in prophylactic mesh at the time of abdominal closure to prevent the occurrence of incisional hernia.

Commonly implemented strategies with insufficient evidence specifically for emergency general surgery include routine use of iodine-impregnated drapes, wound protectors, and antibiotic irrigation. Some of these applications, however, have evidence of benefit in elective general surgery. As such, guidelines from agencies such as the World Society of Emergency General Surgery support multiple interventions for EGS based on data from elective general surgery. These measures include the use of wound protectors, antibacterial sutures, perioperative antibiotics, normothermia, and negative-pressure wound therapy.

POSTOPERATIVE CARE

Careful, regular examination of surgical wounds for dehiscence, seroma, hematoma, or infection is the most important strategy to minimize complications. Prompt detection of wound complications is critical to good outcomes. Seroma is a fluid collection that develops in dead space, can delay wound healing, and increase risk of infection. An abdominal ultrasound can be used to diagnose and assist with aspiration or decompression, although typically seromas are left to resolve on their own unless symptomatic or compromising wound integrity. Hematoma is a collection of blood from inadequate hemostasis or spontaneous bleeding. If bleeding is persistent, local wound exploration may be required to avoid life-threatening hemorrhage or skin necrosis.

WOUND HEALING COMPLICATIONS AND PROBLEMS

Surgical site infections (SSIs) are defined as the infection of the superficial tissues, organs, or spaces exposed during an operation (classified in **Figure 29.1** and summarized in **Table 29.6**). The

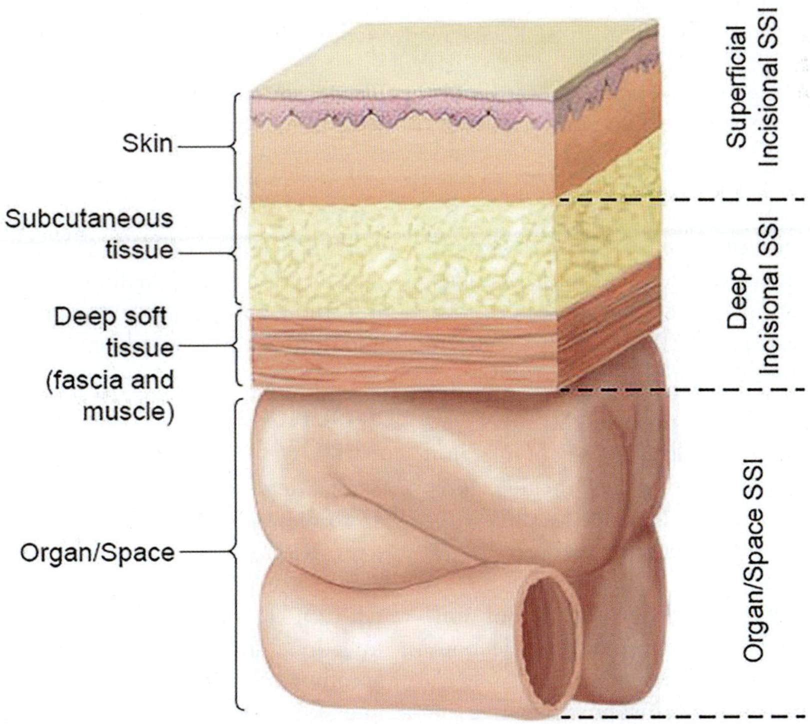

Figure 29.1 Cross section of the abdominal wall depicting U.S. Center for Disease Control and Prevention (CDC) classification for surgical site infection. (From Britt LD, Peitzman AB, Jurkovich GJ, Barie PS, eds. *Acute Care Surgery*. 1st ed. Wolters Kluwer; 2012:596. Figure 43.1.)

TABLE 29.6 ■ Criteria for Diagnosis of Incisional and Organ/Space Surgical Site Infections (SSIs) Within 30 days of All Procedures (1 Year if Prosthetic Material Implanted)

Incisional SSI
Superficial—infection involves skin or subcutaneous tissue of the incision *and* at least one of the following: 1. Purulent drainage from the superficial incision. 2. Organisms isolated from an aseptically obtained culture from the superficial incision. 3. One or more of the following: pain, localized swelling, erythema, or heat, and incision is opened deliberately by surgeon, unless incision is culture negative. 4. Diagnosis of superficial incisional SSI by a surgeon.
Deep—infection involves fascial or muscle layer of the incision *and* at least one of the following: 1. Purulent drainage from the deep incision, excluding organ/space.[a] 2. Incision that dehisces spontaneously or is opened deliberately by a surgeon in the presence of fever (>38 °C), or pain, unless site is culture negative. 3. Evidence of infection is found on direct examination, during repeat surgery, or by histopathologic or radiologic examination.[b] 4. Diagnosis of deep incisional SSI by a surgeon.
Organ/space SSI—infection of any part of the anatomy (eg, organs or surgically created spaces) opened or manipulated during an operation *and* at least one of the following: 1. Purulent drainage from a drain that is placed into the organ/space. 2. Organisms isolated from an aseptically obtained culture from the organ/space. 3. Evidence of infection is found on direct examination, during repeat surgery, or by histopathologic or radiologic examination.[b] 4. Diagnosis of an organ/space SSI by a surgeon.

For all classifications, infection is defined as occurring within 30 d after the operation if no implant is placed or within 1 y if an implant is in place and the infection is related to the incision.
[a]Report infection that involves both superficial and deep incision sites as a deep incisional SSI.
[b]Report an organ/space SSI that drains spontaneously through the incision as a deep incisional SSI.
From Britt LD, Peitzman AB, Jurkovich GJ, Barie PS, eds. *Acute Care Surgery*. 1st ed. Wolters Kluwer; 2012:598.
Adapted from Mangram AJ, Horan TC, Pearson MI, et al. Guideline for prevention of surgical site infection, 1999. Hospital Infection Control Practices Advisory Committee. *Infect Control Hosp Epidemiol*. 1999;20:250-278.

prevalence and severity of SSIs are related to operative factors, host factors, and the amount of microbial contamination preceding source control. Surgical procedures can be classified by the extent of microbial contamination into four classes:

1. Class I/Clean: no infection present, only exposure if colonized flora, 0%-2% risk of infection
2. Class II/Clean Contaminated: include entry into hollow viscus in a controlled setting without spillage or gross contamination, 2%-5% risk of infection
3. Class III/Contaminated: introduction of non-native bacteria into a normally sterile body cavity, 5%-10% risk of infection
4. Class IV/Dirty: wounds that present with a significant delay in which tissue necrosis or purulent material is present, 40% risk of infection

Management of wounds is dependent on the classification and likelihood of developing an infection, with treatment ranging from incision and drainage to reoperation.

WOUND DEHISCENCE (THE BURST ABDOMEN)

Fascial dehiscence results in 0.4%-3.5% of all laparotomies, usually in the first 7-10 postoperative days. Risk factors *independently* associated with dehiscence are emergency intervention, dementia, COPD, ascites, jaundice, anemia, deep space infection, and SSI. Fascial dehiscence may be accompanied by evisceration, which is an absolute indication for operative intervention in patients who can tolerate surgery. If a patient is not a surgical candidate, local wound care with nonadherent dressings should be promptly instituted to minimize the risk of peritonitis or enteric fistula. Although the routine uses of retention sutures to prevent fascial dehiscence is *not* recommended, Khorgami et al. demonstrate that high-risk patients, defined as those with >2 risk factors for dehiscence, experience reduced rates of fascial dehiscence and evisceration with retention sutures. Consider the risk of a second dehiscence (12%) or eventual hernia (up to 50%) in closure of the burst abdomen. No technique is strongly supported with data. Our recommended technique includes 3-cm bites of the fascia with steps of 5 mm (**Figure 29.2**). Running or interrupted sutures may be used.

VENTRAL HERNIA

As discussed in the operative strategies section, several strategies to manage ventral hernias (VH) have been shown to be equivalent; therefore, the management of VH should be guided by provider familiarity with the procedures and their complications. The preoperative recognition of the patient at high risk for postoperative ventral hernia is the first step in risk reduction. Independent risk factors include smoking, contaminated or dirty wound (class III and IV), body mass index (BMI) >25 kg/m^2, incisional SSI, blood transfusions, and thickness of the subcutaneous abdominal tissues. It is the opinion of the authors that elective incisional or ventral hernia repair in patients without obstructive symptoms should be deferred until *after* smoking cessation for a period of at least 4 weeks.

COMPLICATIONS OF ILEOSTOMIES AND COLOSTOMIES

The first question to ask: is a stoma really necessary? If a stoma is not created, the complication related to the stoma is avoided. As with many of the abovementioned complications, the best strategy to reduce the complications of stoma creation is prevention. In the preoperative setting, this consists of early consultation with enterostomal therapists and careful selection of stoma placement. This strategy should be considered in all patients who do not require emergent intervention. In the operating room, the decision to create a loop or end ileostomy vs a loop or end colostomy should take into account the patient's functional status, their preexisting medical comorbidities, risk of herniation, ease of future stoma takedown, and cosmesis. Medical comorbidities of particular relevance for surgeons considering stoma creation are renal disease, inflammatory bowel disease (IBD), morbid obesity, coronary artery disease (CAD), and chronic heart failure (CHF).

Once the decision on placement and type of stoma has been made, turn your attention to the

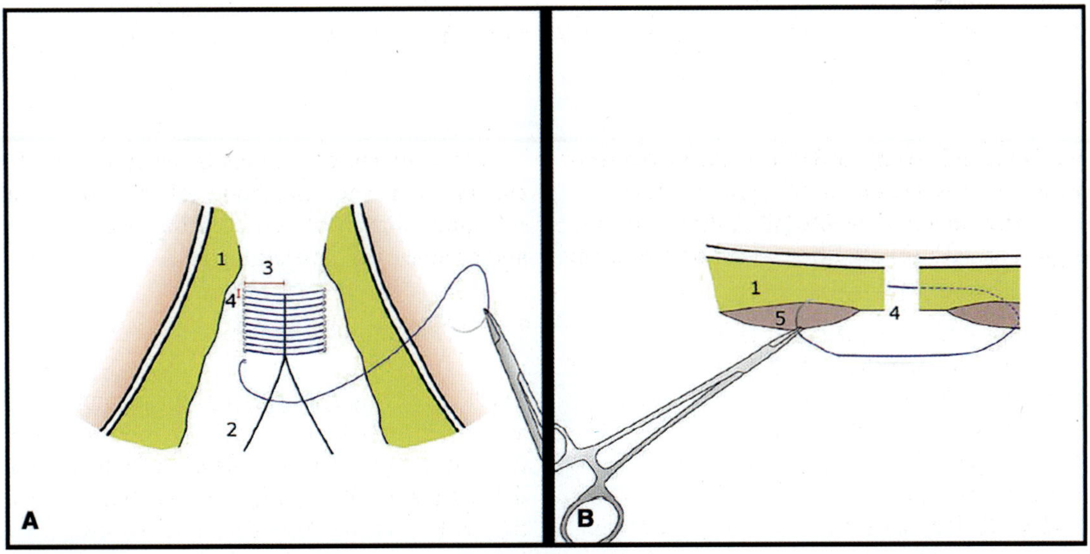

Figure 29.2 Mass closure technique with big bites and small steps. **A.** SQ fat (*1*), rectus muscle fascia (*2*), big bites of 3 cm (*3*), small steps of 5 mm (*4*). **B.** The stitch shown in cross-sectional view showing the relation to rectus muscle (*5*). (Reprinted by permission from Springer: Springer Nature. Jensen TK, Gogenur I, Tolstrup MB. High rate of incisional hernia observed after mass closure of burst abdomen. *Hernia.* 2021. https://doi.org/10.1007/s10029-021-02523-4)

technical aspects that reduce stoma complications such as confirming minimal tension is placed on the bowel, maintaining hemostasis of the stoma and abdominal wall, and everting ileostomies to minimize skin irritation. Immediately postoperatively, the fluid and electrolyte balance of patients with medical comorbidities and newly created stomas should be closely monitored. This will reduce the risk of hypovolemia and acute kidney injury (AKI), as well as provide an early intervention point for antimotility therapy or bulking agents such as fiber.

The morbidity of a stoma depends upon ileostomy or colostomy, end-stoma or loop, indication for the stoma, elective vs emergency operation, body habitus, and prior operations (**Figure 29.3**). Stoma complications may be early (with 30 days of stoma creation) or late. Early stoma complications include ischemia/necrosis, parastomal abscess, retraction, or mucocutaneous separation. Late stoma complications include parastomal hernia, retraction, prolapse, and, rarely, varices.

A parastomal hernia is more common with colostomy than ileostomy. Although most patients with parastomal hernias are symptomatic, they generally do not require operation. Absolute indications for repair of a parastomal hernia are obstruction or incarceration with strangulation. Relative indications for operation include prolapse, stenosis, difficulty with appliance fit, large hernia size, pain, incarceration, or intractable dermatitis. Several authors have advocated mesh reinforcement at the time of the stoma formation.

Operative repair of a parastomal hernia remains a challenge, with high recurrence rates. If possible, eliminate the stoma with restoration of GI continuity. Local, direct suture repair of the parastomal hernia fails in 75%. Stoma relocation is a second option, generally requiring laparotomy. Consider that three sites of potential hernia are then created. Mesh repair of the parastomal hernia as an onlay or keyhole recurs in over 20%. Sublay mesh (retrorectus) repair or a Sugarbaker technique recurs in ~10%.

Stoma prolapse occurs more frequently with loop colostomy than end colostomy, generally the distal limb. Uncommonly, prolapse may lead to strangulation or obstruction. Acute stomal prolapse is treated at the bedside with the application of ice and sugar. Stoma prolapse can be

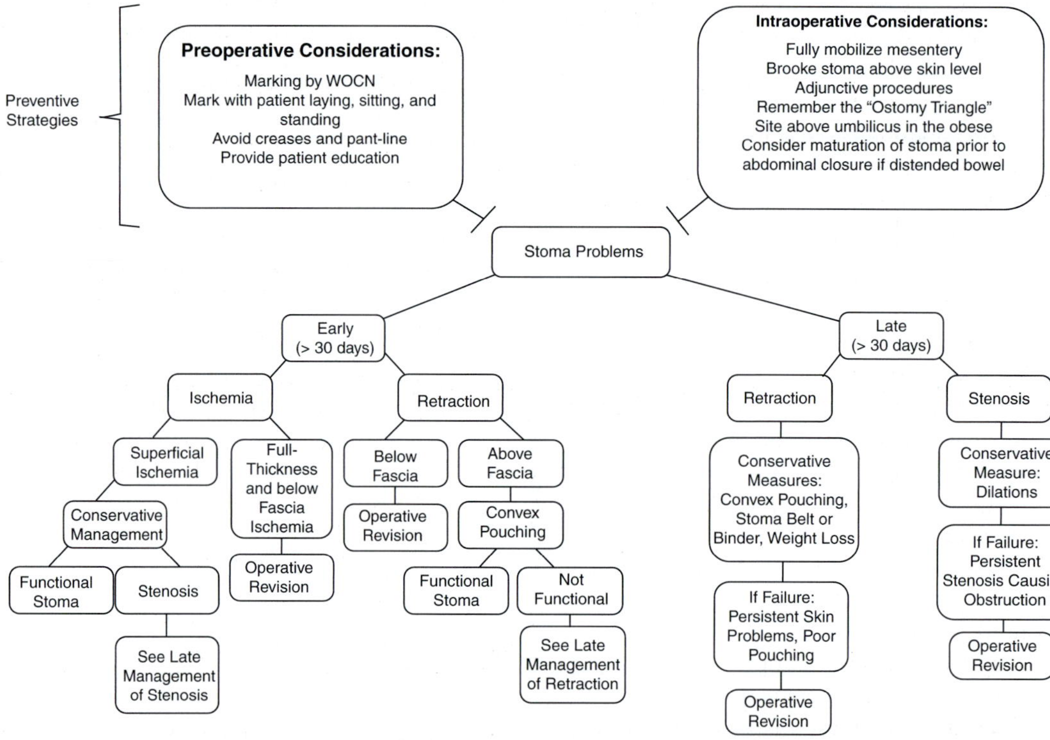

Figure 29.3 Management and avoidance of stoma problems. (From Suwanabol PA, Hardiman KM. Prevention and management of colostomy complication: retraction and stenosis. *Dis Colon Rectum* 2018;61:1344-1349.)

operatively treated with revision, resection, or relocation.

Stomal necrosis can be a surgical emergency. A dusky stoma postoperatively may represent venous congestion or arterial insufficiency. The venous congestion often resolves as edema lessens and venous outflow improves. Necrosis of the stoma is usually from devascularization of the conduit. Management of the ischemic stoma depends on the extent of the ischemia. If simply superficial, reoperation is not mandated. However, realize that retraction or stenosis ultimately will result. If the ischemia extends more proximally in the stoma (visualized with a glass tube and light), early revision may be required. Reoperation is mandated when the necrosis is deep to or near the level of the fascia.

To minimize stomal necrosis or later stricture, when you create the stoma, ensure good blood supply, mobilize the bowel sufficiently to avoid tension, create an opening in the fascia that is not too tight, and brook the stoma ensuring that it protrudes well above the fascia. The aperture in the skin should be just large enough that the mucocutaneous junction apposes. If the skin aperture is made too large, attempts to have the mucosa reach and adhere to the cutaneous junction will retract and fail. This can result in parastomal infection, stoma retraction or stricture, or difficulty with the appliance.

After the index hospitalization, stoma reversal and restoration of intestinal continuity should be performed as soon as patients can be medically and nutritionally optimized utilizing the strategies discussed in this chapter.

SUMMARY

- The majority of SSIs and their downstream effects are preventable.
- Understanding the comorbidities, nutritional status, and indication for surgery in our patients allows us to optimize them and reduce their risk of a wound complication.
- Incorporating evidence-based recommendations into our care in both the acute and chronic setting will decrease the overall risk of wound complications.
- Systematic diagnostic approaches and evidence-based management strategies of SSIs and wound complications can improve outcomes for our high-risk patient population.
- Acute care surgeons can provide global risk reduction by bundling successful interventions in the preoperative, operative, and postoperative stages.

SUGGESTED READINGS

Allegranzi B, Bischoff P, de Jonge S, et al. New WHO recommendations on intraoperative and postoperative measures for surgical site infection prevention: an evidence-based global perspective. *Lancet Infect Dis*. 2016;16:e288-e303.

Allegranzi B, Zayed B, Bischoff P, et al. New WHO recommendations on preoperative measures for surgical site infection prevention: an evidence-based global perspective. *Lancet Infect Dis*. 2016;16:e276-e287.

Anderson DJ, Podgorny K, Berríos-Torres S, et al. Strategies to prevent surgical site infections in acute care hospitals: 2014 update. *Infect Control Hosp Epidemiol*. 2014;35:605-627.

Ban KA, Minei J, Laronga C, et al. American College of Surgeons and Surgical Infection Society: surgical site infection guidelines, 2016 update. *J Am Coll Surg*. 2017;224:59-74.

De Simone B, Sartelli M, Coccolini F, et al. Intraoperative surgical site infection control and prevention: a position paper and future addendum to WSES intra-abdominal infections guidelines. *World J Emerg Surg*. 2020;15(1):10.

Itatsu K, Yokoyama Y, Sugawra G, et al. Incidence of and risk factors for incisional hernia after abdominal surgery. *Br J Surg*. 2014;101:1439-1447.

Jensen TK, Gögenur I, Tolstrup MB. High rate of incisional hernia observed after mass closure of burst abdomen. *Hernia*. 2021. Oct 21. doi: 10.1007/s10029-021-02523-4. Epub ahead of print. PMID: 34674087.

Justianiano CF, Temple LK, Swanger AA, et al. Readmissions with dehydration after ileostomy creation: rethinking risk factors. *Dis Colon Rectum*. 2018;61:1297-1305.

Khorgami Z, Shoar S, Laghaie B, et al. Prophylactic retention sutures in midline laparotomy in high-risk patients for wound dehiscence: a randomized controlled trial. *J Surg Res*. 2013;180(2):238-243. doi:10.1016/j.jss.2012.05.012.

Krishnamurty DM, Blatnik J, Mutch M. Stoma complications. *Clin Colon Rectal Surg*. 2017;30:193-200.

Lopez-Cano M, Garcia-Alamino JM, Antoniou SA, et al. EHS clinical guidelines on the management of the abdominal wall in the context of the open or burst abdomen. *Hernia*. 2018;22:921-939.

Magill SS, Edwards J, Bamberg W, et al. Multistate point-prevalence survey of health care–associated infections. *N Engl J Med*. 2014;370:1198-1208.

Makary MA, Segev D, Pronovost P, et al. Frailty as a predictor of surgical outcomes in older patients. *J Am Coll Surg*. 2010;210:901-908.

Mehdorn M, Groos L, Kassahun W, et al. Interrupted sutures prevent recurrent abdominal fascial dehiscence: a comparative retrospective single center cohort analysis of risk factors of burst abdomen and its recurrence as well as surgical repair techniques. *BMC Surg.* 2021;21:208. https://doi.org/10.1186/s12893-021-01219-x

Muysoms FE, Antoniou SA, Bury K, et al. European Hernia Society guidelines on the closure of abdominal wall incisions. *Hernia.* 2015;19(1):1-24.

Sørensen LT, Hemmingsen UB, Kirkeby LT, et al. Smoking is a risk factor for incisional hernia. *Arch Surg.* 2005;140:119-123.

Sørensen LT, Malaki A, Wille-Jørgensen P, et al. Risk factors for mortality and postoperative complications after gastrointestinal surgery. *J Gastrointest Surg.* 2007;11:903-910.

Suwanabol PA, Hardiman KM. Prevention and management of colostomy complication: retraction and stenosis. *Dis Colon Rectum.* 2018;61:1344-1349.

Tolstrup MB, Watt SK, Gögenur I. Reduced rate of dehiscence after implementation of a standardized fascial closure technique in patients undergoing emergency laparotomy. *Ann Surg.* 2017;265:821-826.

Umscheid CA, Mitchell M, Doshi J, et al. Estimating the proportion of healthcare-associated infections that are reasonably preventable and the related mortality and costs. *Infect Control Hosp Epidemiol.* 2011;32:101-114.

World Health Organization (WHO). *Report on the Burden of Endemic Health Care-Associated Infection Worldwide. WHO Library Cataloguing-in-Publication Data.* 2011. http://whqlibdoc.who.int/publications/2011/9789241501507_eng.pdf

CHAPTER

30 Spontaneous Hemoperitoneum

Angela M. Ingraham, Vanessa P. Ho, and Marie Crandall

CASE PRESENTATION

A 32-year-old woman presents to the emergency department with a 2-day history of abdominal discomfort and distension. She notes that she has felt slightly dizzy, short of breath, and light-headed, which started today. She states that she has had some right upper quadrant pain that became severe yesterday, but the pain has since improved. She is otherwise healthy and takes only oral contraceptives, which she has taken for 10 years. Initially, she does not recall any history of trauma but then noted that a few days prior to admission, her 6-year-old nephew accidentally kicked her in the abdomen while playing.

Vital signs are significant for a blood pressure of 86/64 mm Hg and a heart rate of 115/min. She is normothermic, and oxygenation is normal. Laboratory results are significant for a hemoglobin of 6.6 g/dL and a creatinine of 1.1 mg/dL; the remainder of the basic metabolic panel is normal. Lactate is 3.4 mmol/L. Pregnancy test and tumor markers are negative. A contrast-enhanced CT scan of the abdomen is obtained that showed a large volume of hemoperitoneum throughout the abdominal cavity and a well-circumscribed 8-cm liver mass, which appears suspicious for rupture due to evidence of active contrast extravasation. The hemoperitoneum appears to be heterogeneous in appearance throughout the abdominal cavity, suggestive of areas of clot.

Question: *What are the appropriate next steps in the management of this patient?*

Answer: *The patient is actively bleeding from her liver tumor, which is likely a hepatocellular adenoma. Initial management should focus on bleeding control and treatment, including consultation with interventional radiology, establishment of large bore intravenous access, maintaining normothermia, and resuscitation with blood products, as appropriate.*

INTRODUCTION

Spontaneous hemoperitoneum is defined as blood within the peritoneal cavity that is nontraumatic in origin. Spontaneous hemoperitoneum is not a singular diagnosis but is the result of an uncommon cause of acute abdominal pain, which can be life-threatening. Spontaneous hemoperitoneum may originate from vascular structures, visceral solid organs, gynecologic organs, or coagulopathy-related disorders. While rare, spontaneous hemoperitoneum has become more common, with 1434 discharges in the United States in 1993 (0.6/100 000 discharges) increasing to 4155 (1.3/100 000 discharges) in 2010. Spontaneous retroperitoneal or rectus sheath hemorrhage can be related to vascular structures or coagulopathy. In some cases of intraperitoneal or retroperitoneal hemorrhage, no direct source can be identified.

This chapter will outline the clinical presentation of spontaneous hemoperitoneum, as well as rectus sheath and retroperitoneal hemorrhage, describe possible sources of bleeding, outline principles of the diagnostic workup, and describe potential treatment options.

CLINICAL PRESENTATION

Patients with spontaneous hemoperitoneum typically present with nonspecific abdominal symptoms and sequelae of blood loss. Patients can have acute abdominal pain, abdominal distension, tachycardia, hypotension, or even abdominal compartment syndrome in extreme cases where arterial bleeding is the cause. Rectus sheath hemorrhage usually presents with acute abdominal pain with a palpable abdominal mass anteriorly because spread is limited to the rectus sheath space and therefore typically does not cross the midline. However, very large hematomas can dissect along the transversalis fascia or inferiorly toward the prevesical space anterior to the bladder. Spontaneous retroperitoneal hemorrhage presents similarly, with signs of hemorrhage or nonspecific pain, usually in the back or the abdomen, and possibly new sensations of fullness or bulging, depending on the location of the hemorrhage. Retroperitoneal bleeding can also lead to compression of vessels or nerves of the lower extremities and present with pulselessness, extremity numbness, or weakness. In this rare circumstance, emergent operative decompression of the retroperitoneal hematoma may be required. Patients may note abdominal or flank ecchymosis or discoloration, or an abdominal mass.

Hemorrhage can lead to nonspecific symptoms, such as syncope, altered mental status, light-headedness, dizziness, chest pain, dyspnea, or weakness. Depending on the extent and chronicity of the bleeding, laboratory and vital sign findings may show signs of hemorrhage or hemorrhagic shock such as tachycardia, orthostatic hypotension, persistent hypotension, acute anemia or chronic anemia with iron deficiency, elevated creatinine or other signs of acute renal insufficiency, acidosis, or elevated lactate. Early and rapid imaging is key to elucidate a diagnosis of spontaneous hemoperitoneum and to pinpoint a possible point of origin. A remote or mild history of trauma may be present, although typically the traumatic event is not the chief complaint.

Any organ or structure in the abdomen, retroperitoneum, or abdominal wall that has blood vessels can theoretically be the source of peritoneal, retroperitoneal, or abdominal wall bleeding. Spontaneous bleeding has been reported from the liver, spleen, kidneys, blood vessels of the abdomen including visceral and mesenteric vessels that develop arteriovenous malformations (AVM) or aneurysms, omental vessels, Meckel diverticulum, or gynecologic structures, such as ovarian cysts. Spontaneous hemoperitoneum also occurs in pregnancy.

Initial management of the patient with spontaneous hemoperitoneum is based primarily on the hemodynamic status of the patient. The basic principles of resuscitation and the management of hemorrhage should not be neglected when treating spontaneous hemoperitoneum or bleeding from the rectus sheath or retroperitoneum. The patient should be kept warm, which may necessitate increasing the temperature of the interventional radiology (IR) or operating room (OR) suite as well as transporting blood and fluid warmers to the location where the patient is being treated. Large bore intravenous access should be established and maintained. Balanced transfusions should be provided, and coagulopathy corrected.

The hemodynamically unstable patient may require emergent laparotomy to control exsanguinating bleeding. In the hemodynamically stable patient, the first line of management is computed tomography (CT), often followed by angiography and embolization. If IR techniques are unable to control the bleeding or the patient is persistently hypotensive, surgery may be necessary. Surgical options for bleeding control vary depending on the etiology of the hemorrhage but include ligation, repair (with native tissues or prosthetics), resection (complete or partial depending on the organ causing the bleeding), and other hemostatic techniques (eg, electro- and argon beam-coagulation, tissue sealants, and hemostatic agents [eg, Surgicel ® products]). Depending on the etiology, particularly in instances of a bleeding cancer, after hemorrhage is controlled, subsequent definitive treatment will need to be considered.

IMAGING

A variety of imaging methods can be utilized in the setting of suspected spontaneous hemoperitoneum as well as rectus sheath and retroperitoneal bleeding. However, the limitations and appropriateness of each methodology should be acknowledged and considered based upon the patient's clinical condition. Obtaining imaging is critical in cases of spontaneous hemoperitoneum. Imaging allows the clinician to establish the most likely etiology of the bleeding, identify if the bleeding is ongoing, and thus direct treatment accordingly. The choice of imaging should be dictated by the patient's hemodynamic status and the most likely suspected cause.

CT is the most commonly utilized method in patients presenting with acute abdominal pain that is suspected to be due to spontaneous hemoperitoneum. Magnetic resonance imaging (MRI) is rarely the first modality utilized to identify hemoperitoneum. However, ultrasound may be considered if the source is likely to be gynecologic in nature. Additionally, if the patient is hemodynamically unstable, ultrasound may be utilized to confirm hemoperitoneum, as unstable patients should not be transported to the CT or MRI suite. In the next several paragraphs, the benefits, drawbacks, and common uses of sonography, CT, and MRI will be reviewed.

Sonography can identify intraperitoneal blood in the pelvis and around the liver and the spleen. With sonography, blood appears as simple hypoechoic fluid. Hemoperitoneum is distinguished from simple ascites by the presence of foci of increased echogenicity. These foci represent clot formation. As the clot matures and becomes increasingly organized, the fluid becomes uniformly echogenic. Sonography is the imaging modality of choice for identifying gynecologic pathology that may be responsible for spontaneous hemoperitoneum. Sonography, however, has limitations in its use for diagnosing and directing treatment for spontaneous hemorrhage. Sonography cannot determine whether active extravasation of blood is present and has limited abilities to determine the source of the hemoperitoneum.

If available and the patient is hemodynamically stable, CT is an excellent imaging modality for hemoperitoneum, as it provides detailed information regarding the bleeding. Blood appears as high-attenuation fluid within the peritoneal cavity. The appearance of blood on CT imaging, however, is variable and dependent on the time interval between hemorrhage and imaging as well as the rate and volume of the hemorrhage. Once the diagnosis of hemoperitoneum has been made, the next steps are to identify a cause, to assess for the presence of active extravasation, and to determine the approximate duration of bleeding. Clots typically form first adjacent to the site of bleeding, which is referred to as the sentinel clot sign. CT can potentially identify a lesion in either the liver or the spleen or a vascular abnormality that may have resulted in the spontaneous hemoperitoneum. The identification of the lesion can, at times, be limited by the volume of hemorrhage. In these instances, if the patient is managed nonoperatively, interval repeat imaging should be performed after several weeks to elicit a treatable cause. At other times, when the etiology is not initially clear from the CT images, it can sometimes become apparent during angiography. For example, hepatic hemangiomas are characterized by early opacification or irregular areas with persistence of contrast after arterial emptying while a hemangioma may appear as a C-shaped lesion with an avascular center.

While a contrast-enhanced CT scan is the ideal, the patient's overall medical status and comorbidities must be taken into account, as hemoperitoneum can be identified if contrast is contraindicated. Intraperitoneal blood can be detected by CT imaging both with and without the use of intravenous contrast medium. On a noncontrast CT scan, hemoperitoneum is identified as high-attenuation fluid around the solid organs and bowel. However, it is difficult to assess for active extravasation with a noncontrast CT. The benefits of a contrast-enhanced CT scan include not only its ability to identify potential active extravasation but also to better identify a possible underlying cause. Delayed imaging (repeating a noncontrasted CT scan after a contrasted or noncontrasted CT scan has just been performed) aids further in the detection of active extravasation or characterization of an identified cause. Active extravasation on delayed imaging may result in a larger focus of high-attenuation extravasated blood and/or contrast medium compared with the initial noncontrast CT image. The advent of multidetector CT, particularly 16- and 64-row scanners, has also made the identification of active extravasation easier. On contrasted scans, active extravasation is identified when there is a high-attenuation area that is the same density as an adjacent vessel. The identification of active extravasation is important because it usually mandates acute intervention, either surgical or endovascular embolization.

Additionally, CT can provide clinicians with information about the duration of bleeding, as fresh as compared to clotted as compared to lysed blood will have different Hounsfield units (HU), also known as the "hematocrit effect." Acutely, hemoperitoneum has an attenuation value close to that of intravascular blood. On noncontrast imaging, blood from acute hemorrhage has an attenuation of 30-45 HU because of its high protein content. Within the first several hours, clotted blood appears hyperdense (HU > 60) due to an increase in the concentration of hemoglobin. Areas of high attenuation, which represent clot, may be surrounded by areas of lower attenuation, which is made up of serum. Additionally, if new bleeding is present in addition to older, clotted blood, a mixed-attenuation pattern will be present. As blood hemolyzes over 3-4 weeks, the attenuation value becomes closer to that of water. As with sonography, a fluid-fluid level may be identified on CT if the blood has had a chance to settle; denser cellular elements will pool in the dependent portions and have a higher attenuation value than the less-dense superficial fluid. A fluid-fluid layer is diagnostic of intraperitoneal hemorrhage.

MRI can identify both hemoperitoneum and the underlying cause of spontaneous hemoperitoneum but is not useful in identifying active extravasation. In particular, MRIs are useful to determine if the hemoperitoneum is due to an underlying hepatic or splenic mass that may have ruptured. MRIs are also often used to further characterize a hepatic mass identified on an initial CT scan. Acute intraperitoneal blood (<1 day old) on MRI is of intermediate signal intensity on T1-weighted imaging and low signal intensity on T2-weighted imaging. Over the next several days, blood will become high signal intensity on both T1- and T2-weighted imaging. After many days, the signal intensity of blood decreases on both T1- and T2- weighted imaging. Intraperitoneal hematoma may demonstrate heterogeneous signal on both T1- and T2-weighted imaging. Old hematoma will demonstrate a low signal peripheral rim with central high or mixed signal intensity on both T1- and T2-weighted imaging.

LABORATORY STUDIES

In addition to imaging, laboratory evaluations should be conducted based upon the likely etiology of the bleeding. For example, if the bleeding is of hepatic origin, measures of liver function as well as the presence of cirrhosis and the potential impacts of liver dysfunction on coagulation should be pursued. Additionally, tumor markers (eg, carcinoembryonic antigen, CA 19–9, and alpha-fetoprotein) should be drawn.

Additional laboratory tests should especially considered if the source is thought to be of an adrenal origin. Because operating on a patient with an occult pheochromocytoma could be catastrophic, if an adrenal mass is suspected and if time allows, a biochemical workup, including glucocorticoid and catecholamine excess, may be able to be performed to rule out a hormonally active tumor. While physiologic stress can increase cortisol and catecholamine levels, catecholamine levels in patients with pheochromocytoma are often more than four times the upper limit of normal. Adrenocorticotropic hormone (ACTH) levels can help differentiate elevated cortisol due to physiologic stress (elevated ACTH) or due to a functional adrenal tumor (suppressed ACTH). Should the patient be amenable to nonoperative management, consider repeat biochemical evaluation after the acute stress is over. If emergent surgical intervention is needed and prohibits a biochemical workup, the possibility of pheochromocytoma or Cushing syndrome should be communicated to the anesthesiologist, and the use of beta-blockade without alpha-blockade should be avoided. The development of adrenal insufficiency requiring stress doses of glucocorticoids postoperatively should be anticipated.

ETIOLOGIES OF SPONTANEOUS HEMOPERITONEUM

Solid Organs

Hepatic Bleeding

The most frequently reported cause of spontaneous hemoperitoneum is spontaneous rupture of a liver lesion (see also Chapter 23: Complex Liver Masses). Often, the liver lesion is previously undiagnosed. Precipitating or related factors can include recent minor trauma or hormonal changes. Liver lesions can be benign (adenoma, hemangiomata, and focal nodular hyperplasia [FNH]) or malignant (hepatocellular carcinoma [HCC] or metastatic liver lesions) (**Table 30.1**). Rupture of a hepatic lesion is typically characterized by right upper quadrant pain or fullness and can be punctuated by sudden and severe pain with hypotension; changes in liver function enzymes or hyperbilirubinemia may also be present.

Hepatocellular adenoma. The most common benign lesion that can rupture is a hepatocellular adenoma, also known as hepatic adenoma. Hepatic adenomas are typically solid lesions that occur in otherwise normal hepatic tissue. They are more common among females and often associated with oral contraceptive use, pregnancy, or anabolic androgen steroids. Estrogen use is thought to be related to adenoma development in a dose-dependent fashion, and oral contraceptive use is thought to be associated with an ~30- to 40-fold increase in adenoma incidence compared to nonusers. Obesity and metabolic syndrome are associated with the development of adenomas in men. Hepatic adenomas over 5 cm are at risk for both bleeding as well as malignant transformation. In addition, in male patients, the presence of a hepatic adenoma should always prompt intervention due to the higher incidence of beta-catenin subtypes, which have a much higher malignant potential (see Chapter 23: Complex Liver Masses for details). Single bleeding adenomas are often amenable to selective angioembolization. Patients who are diagnosed with hepatic angiomas should be referred for follow-up by a hepatic specialist.

Hepatic hemangiomas. Hepatic hemangiomas are the most common primary liver tumors, present in 0.4%-20% of the population. These lesions are typically diagnosed incidentally for nonspecific abdominal complaints. The majority of new cases occur in patients between the age of 30 and 50, with female incidence three times higher than in men. Hepatic hemangiomas may increase in size with estrogen therapy or during pregnancy. Hemangiomas of >10 cm in size are considered to be giant hemangiomas; symptomatic or giant hemangiomas should also be followed by a specialist in case treatment is needed after the bleeding episode has resolved. For bleeding related to a hepatic hemangioma, potential surgical treatments include anatomic/nonanatomic resection or enucleation, selective portal vein embolization, and liver transplantation. Giant hemangiomas, particularly superficial lesions, are preferentially treated with enucleation to preserve hepatic parenchyma and minimize bleeding.

TABLE 30.1 ■ Spontaneous Hemoperitoneum: Solid Organ Sources and Considerations

Liver	

Sources:
• Neoplasms
  • Adenoma
  • Focal nodular hyperplasia
  • Hepatocellular cancer
    • Hemangioma
    • Metastases
    • Angiosarcoma
• HELLP syndrome
• Amyloidosis
	Additional considerations:
	• Malignancy workup
	• Potential for embolization
	• Liver function
	• Tumor function
	• Potential for transplant

Spleen	

Sources:
• Infectious
  • Malaria
  • Infectious mononucleosis (EBV)
  • CMV
  • HIV
• Malignancy
  • Lymphoma
  • Leukemia
  • Angiosarcoma
• Amyloidosis
	Additional considerations:
	• Pathologic splenomegaly workup
	• History of trauma
	• Potential for embolization
	• Postsplenectomy vaccination

Kidney	
Sources: • Renal cell cancer • Angiolipoma	Additional considerations: • Malignancy workup • Potential for embolization • Posttreatment renal function
Adrenal Gland	
Sources: • Metastases • Pheochromocytoma • Adenocarcinoma	Additional considerations: • Malignancy workup • Tumor markers (CEA, CA19-9, AFP) • Assessment for tumor function • Adrenal insufficiency

Focal nodular hyperplasia. Focal nodular hyperplasia (FNH) is the second most frequent benign tumor of the liver. While CT studies have shown incidental FNH to be present in 0.3%-3%, clinical studies suggest a clinically relevant prevalence that is even lower. Ninety percent of patients with FNH are female. FNH can occur at any age, although the most common age at presentation is 35-50 years of age. Despite the increased rate in females, hormones such as oral contraceptives are not thought to be associated with increased risk for the development of FNH. FNH tends to be incidentally diagnosed as a solitary solid liver lesion that is described as having a central stellate scar on imaging studies, usually being <5 cm in size, and typically not changing in size over time. FNH can be associated with other lesions that have the potential to have malignant conversion, but isolated typical FNH lesions do not usually need to be followed over time.

Hepatocellular cacinoma. Hepatocellular carcinoma (HCC) can present with tumor rupture leading to hemoperitoneum (see also Chapter 23: Complex Liver Masses). Tumor rupture, similar to the rupture of other lesions, can present with sudden abdominal pain, distension, an acute drop in hemoglobin, and hypotension. HCC patients may present with a history compatible with other signs and symptoms of cancer, such as with vague upper abdominal pain, weight loss, early satiety, or a palpable mass in the right upper quadrant. HCC is also associated with paraneoplastic syndromes that lead to hypoglycemia, hypercalcemia, and electrolyte disturbances. Serum tumor markers may be present in HCC, the most common of which is alpha-fetoprotein. Contrast-enhanced CT imaging can diagnose the tumor as well as the hemoperitoneum, and emergent angiogram with embolization is the treatment of choice for acute life-threatening hemorrhage.

For bleeding related to a spontaneous hepatic hemorrhage, particularly that related to HCC, several factors should be considered. First, many patients have concomitant diagnoses of cirrhosis or fibrosis, which make them unfavorable operative candidates. Depending on the patient's specific health status, goals of care discussions and potential pursuit of palliative care may be considered. For all patients with bleeding from HCC, conservative management is successful in almost half of patients. In those who fail conservative management, most (80%) bleeding can be controlled with embolization. In the 20% of patients for whom embolization is not possible, challenges encountered include but are not limited to thrombosis of the main portal vein and arteriovenous shunting. However, rebleeding after embolization is substantial (up to 22% in some series), which carries a high mortality rate (up to 52%). Embolization should be carried out using gel foam as opposed to coils to allow for future chemoembolization; embolization should also follow a selective or subselective approach to maximize postembolization hepatic function.

For patients who either fail or are not candidates for embolization, surgical management of spontaneous hepatic hemorrhage may be necessary. Surgical management options include plication and packing, ligation of the feeding hepatic artery or its branches, and resection. Attempts should be made to avoid resection of the HCC at the initial operation as out-comes are better when the resection is performed in a delayed manner.

Nontraumatic Splenic Hemorrhage

The spleen is the most commonly injured solid organ in the abdomen due to trauma. However, nontraumatic splenic rupture is relatively rare. Often, patients present with a history of very minor trauma, and their hemorrhagic shock is inconsistent with the seemingly minor trauma. Atraumatic splenic bleeding, because it is uncommon, is often difficult to diagnose and can lead to a delay in diagnosis. Nontraumatic splenic rupture rarely occurs in the normal spleen but usually occurs as a consequence of pathologic splenomegaly. Causes of pathologic splenomegaly include infection, malignancy, or disorders of metabolic, hematologic, or vascular origin. Hematologic or metabolic disorders, such as hemophilia, polycythemia, or amyloidosis, may be previously diagnosed but this is not always the case. Primary malignant tumors of the spleen are extremely rare; the most common tumor is angiosarcoma, which has a very poor prognosis. Depending on the severity of bleeding and rupture, nonoperative management, angioembolization, and splenectomy are possible treatment options.

Kidney

The most common causes of perirenal bleeding are neoplasms, with 50% being malignant. Renal angiolipomas may also present with acute bleeding. Preferred treatment of a renal angiolipoma is angioembolization. If found incidentally, most angiolipomas can be observed. Whether those >4 cm require intervention is currently debated.

Vascular Lesions

Vascular aneurysms within the abdomen are another rare cause of hemoperitoneum. Management of ruptured abdominal aortic or iliac aneurysms is covered in Chapter 20: Vascular Emergencies. Systemic vascular connective tissue diseases, such as Ehlers-Danlos syndrome, can also lead to vascular fragility with rupture (**Table 30.2**). Pancreatitis with associated vascular involvement, such as splenic artery aneurysm rupture, can lead to retroperitoneal or intraperitoneal hemorrhage. Symptomatic visceral aneurysms are at high risk for rupture and should be treated. A herald bleed may precede uncontained rupture. In general, asymptomatic visceral artery aneurysms should be treated when >2-3 cm, when identified during pregnancy, in the liver transplant patient, or when multiple aneurysms are present. Eighty percent of ruptured visceral artery aneurysms are pseudoaneurysms, which highly correlate with rupture. Although relatively uncommon, pancreaticoduodenal artery (PDA) and hepatic artery aneurysms are at high risk of rupture, as they are generally pseudoaneurysms. The average size of ruptured PDA pseudoaneurysms is only 12.7 mm. The risk of rupture thus depends primarily on the presence of a pseudoaneurysm and the high risk locations.

TABLE 30.2 ■ Spontaneous Hemoperitoneum: Vascular Causes

Arterial	

Sources:
• Ruptured abdominal aortic aneurysm
• Ruptured iliac aneurysm
• Ruptured visceral artery aneurysm
• Ruptured mycotic aneurysm
• Ruptured pseudoaneurysm
	Other considerations:
	• Rapid enlargement of aneurysm size (>0.5 cm over 6 months)
	• High-risk anatomic locations
	  • Pancreaticoduodenal arcade
	  • Gastroduodenal arcade
	  • Intraparenchymal hepatic artery
	• Workup for connective tissue disease
	• Open or endovascular approach
	• Potential for embolization
	• Monitoring for thrombosis or embolism
	• Long-term monitoring

Venous	
Sources: • Omentum • Abdominal varices • Pelvic veins	

AVMs may also lead to spontaneous nontraumatic hemoperitoneum. AVMs from the gastrointestinal tract and from the uterus have been reported to cause hemoperitoneum but are rare.

For bleeding related to ruptured visceral artery aneurysms, endovascular intervention has been documented to be superior to open repair. Endovascular repair is associated with a 30-day mortality rate of 7.4% and a complication rate of 8.9% compared to the 28.6% rate of major complication and mortality in the open group. However, patient selection in the endovascular treatment of aneurysms is critical as treatment of large saccular aneurysms by coil embolization may lead to poor long-term results. Technical failure of obliterating large aneurysmal sacs can be due to turbulence of the blood flow within the aneurysm, which promotes coil displacement, as well as difficulty completely packing a large aneurysm with coils, which causes persistent expansion of the residual sac. In these cases, open surgical treatment may be preferred.

When feasible, endovascular treatment is usually performed through transcatheter embolization or stent grafting. Interventional procedures can normally be performed under local anesthesia, with high technical success rates and shorter hospital stays. Patients should be monitored for the following complications after the procedure: arterial thrombosis or embolism resulting in organ infarctions or abscesses, coil migration, aneurysm recurrence, and a hematoma or a pseudoaneurysm at the arterial puncture site.

Gynecologic/Obstetrical Causes

In women of childbearing age, the most common source of spontaneous hemoperitoneum is the reproductive organs (**Table 30.3**). The patient with a ruptured ectopic pregnancy can present in profound hemorrhagic shock; this diagnosis must be considered and excluded early in the management of the female with spontaneous hemoperitoneum (see also Chapter 24: OB/GYN). Other sources include rupture of an ovarian cyst, such as a corpus luteum cyst or a follicular cyst. Vascular lesions of gynecologic organs can also be culprits. Patients with hemoperitoneum from rupture of a uterine lesion or endometriosis may also present in shock.

The HELLP syndrome presents in the pregnant patient with hemolytic anemia, elevations in transaminases, and thrombocytopenia (hemolysis, elevated liver enzymes, and low platelets). It is thought

TABLE 30.3 ■ Obstetrical/Gynecological Sources for Hemoperitoneum

Obstetric/Gynecologic	
Sources: • Ruptured ectopic pregnancy • Ruptured uterus • Ruptured uterine vessel • HELLP syndrome • Ruptured ovarian cyst • Ruptured endometrioma • Endometriosis	Other considerations: • Specialist availability • Potential for embolization • Treatment of primary pathology

to share a similar etiology to eclampsia/preeclampsia. Spontaneous hepatic hemorrhage can occur in HELLP resulting in a subcapsular hepatic hematoma that may breach the liver capsule, resulting in hemoperitoneum. This complication carries significant risk of mortality. HELLP usually presents between 28 and 36 weeks of gestation, most commonly (75%) involving the right hepatic lobe. CT angiogram may be diagnostic. At times, these patients require emergent delivery of the placenta and fetus to reverse the syndrome. Angiography/embolization may be effective for hemostasis. On occasion, the patient will be hemodynamically unstable requiring emergent operative intervention.

Retroperitoneal and Rectus Sheath Bleeding

Prior to widespread use of therapeutic anticoagulation, retroperitoneal and rectus sheath hematomas were very rare. These complications of anticoagulation have increased and are reported to occur with an incidence between 0.1% and 0.6% of anticoagulated patients. There is limited consensus on the treatment of these hematomas, although single-institution observational studies have provided some insight into current management principles.

The retroperitoneum is a vascular space, and retroperitoneal bleeding can be a result of hemorrhage from any retroperitoneal organ or blood vessel, which includes the aorta, the kidneys or adrenal glands, the pancreas and associated vasculature, the duodenum and associated vasculature, and the muscles that line the retroperitoneal cavity. Gynecologic conditions can also rupture into the retroperitoneum rather than the peritoneal cavity. Coagulopathy, including intentional and iatrogenic coagulopathy, or minor trauma can also contribute to development of retroperitoneal hemorrhage. Options for treatment include medical management and reversal of coagulopathy, angiography, or surgical intervention and evacuation of the hematoma. Retroperitoneal hemorrhage can also occur after percutaneous intervention utilizing femoral access, as a posterior vascular puncture can lead to hemorrhage into the retroperitoneal space.

Unlike the peritoneal cavity or the retroperitoneum, the rectus sheath has limited contents. Typically bleeding within the rectus sheath occurs as a result of rupture of the epigastric artery or a muscular tear. Rectus sheath hematomas usually occur in the setting of coagulopathy and systemic anticoagulation and may be precipitated by coughing, pregnancy, or minimal abdominal trauma. Iatrogenic causes of rectus sheath hematomas include recent needlesticks, such as subcutaneous injections of insulin or heparin as well as femoral vascular access.

Rectus sheath and retroperitoneal bleeding will often cease with conservative management as the bleed is related to microangiopathy. Anticoagulation discontinuation and reversal with transfusions as needed often are sufficient. Surgical management has a limited role, as the ability to identify the source of bleeding once the hematoma is opened is low and opening the hematoma releases the established tamponade and can provoke additional bleeding. Active bleeding, as indicated by a blush on contrast-enhanced CT imaging, predicts potential failure of conservative treatment and often prompts evaluation by IR colleagues. As novel anticoagulants often do not have reliable antidotes, angioembolization can prove to be a useful adjunct in the cases of rectus sheath and retroperitoneal bleeding. The hemodynamic stability of the patient and the degree of blood loss generally drive the decision to pursue embolization. In patients who are unstable due to bleeding from a rectus sheath hematoma, empiric embolization of the ipsilateral inferior epigastric artery should be considered.

Given that spontaneous retroperitoneal and rectus sheath hematomas are relatively rare, there are no large studies on this topic. Several small studies (Warren et al., Baekgaard et al.) have suggested that the patient population is high risk, often with serious chronic comorbidities and are on therapeutic anticoagulation for medical causes. As a result, bleeding can result in hemorrhagic shock requiring transfusion. However, <20% of patients undergo a therapeutic intervention for hemorrhage as most bleeding episodes are self-limited and resolve as the coagulopathy is reversed. Unfortunately, in-hospital mortality has been reported to be as high as 25%, often for reasons other than the acute hematoma. These studies suggest that spontaneous retroperitoneal hemorrhage is a relatively rare condition that is associated with severe medical comorbidities and high mortality. Palliative care and symptom management are also appropriate in these circumstances for patients with serious underlying illness.

SUMMARY

In summary, spontaneous peritoneal hemorrhage is an acute and life-threatening problem that requires a high index of suspicion. Contrast-enhanced (if possible) imaging is the most important diagnostic tool to localize the source of the bleeding, which then can prompt the clinician to pursue treatment that is appropriate for the causative entity. Bleeding can originate from solid organs, abdominal vasculature, or the soft tissues of the retroperitoneum or rectus sheath. Also, key for the treatment of these diseases is the reversal of coagulopathy and, for patients with severe comorbidities, the treatment of any underlying conditions and/or the application of palliative care principles when appropriate.

SUGGESTED READINGS

Agency for Healthcare Research and Quality Healthcare Cost and Utilization Project. *Free Health Care Statistics*. Accessed September 2, 2020. https://hcupnet.ahrq.gov/#setup

Aubrey-Bassler FK, Sowers N. 613 cases of splenic rupture without risk factors or previously diagnosed disease: a systematic review. *BMC Emerg Med*. 2012;12:11. http://www.biomedcentral.com/1471-227X/12/11

Baekgaard JS, Eskesen TG, Lee JM, et al. Spontaneous retroperitoneal and rectus sheath hemorrhage—management, risk factors and outcomes. *World J Surg*. 2019;43(8):1890-1897.

Chaer RA, Abularrage CJ, Coleman DM, et al. The Society for Vascular Surgery clinical practice guidelines for management of visceral aneurysms. *J Vasc Surg*. 2020;72:3S-39S.

European Association for the Study of the Liver (EASL). EASL Clinical Practice Guidelines on the management of benign liver tumours. *J Hepatol*. 2016;65(2):386-398.

Furlan A, Fakhran S, Federle MP. Spontaneous abdominal hemorrhage: causes, CT findings, and clinical implications. *AJR Am J Roentgenol*. 2009;193(4):1077-1087.

Ibrahim F, Dunn J, Rundback J, et al. Visceral artery aneurysms: diagnosis, surveillance and treatment. *Curr Treat Options Cardiovasc Med*. 2018;20:97. doi:10.1007/s11936-018-0696-x

Kasotakis G. Spontaneous hemoperitoneum. *Surg Clin North Am*. 2014;94(1):65-69.

Lai ECH, Lau WY. Spontaneous rupture of hepatocellular carcinoma. *Arch Surg*. 2006;141:191-198.

Lubner M, Menias C, Rucker C, et al. Blood in the belly: CT findings of hemoperitoneum. *Radiographics*. 2007;27(1):109-125. doi:10.1148/rg.271065042

Lucey BC, Varghese JC, Soto JA. Spontaneous hemoperitoneum: causes and significance. *Curr Probl Diagn Radiol*. 2005;34(5):182-195.

Marti JL, Millet J, Sosa JA, et al. Spontaneous adrenal hemorrhage with associated masses: etiology and management in 6 cases and a review of 133 reported cases. *World J Surg*. 2012;36:75-82.

Shukla AJ, Eid R, Fish L, et al. Contemporary outcomes of ruptured visceral artery aneurysms. *J Vasc Surg*. 2015;61:1442-1448.

Tataria M, Dicker RA, Melcher M, Spain DA, Brundage SI. Spontaneous splenic rupture: the masquerade of minor trauma. *J Trauma*. 2005;59(5):1228-1230.

Warren MH, Bhattacharya B, Maung AA, Davis KA. Contemporary management of spontaneous retroperitoneal and rectus sheath hematomas. *Am J Surg*. 2020;219(4):707-710.

Index

Note: Page numbers followed by *f* indicate figures; those followed by *t* indicate tables.

D

Q

R

T

U